Community Supports
for Aging Adults with Lifelong Disabilities

Community Supports
for Aging Adults with Lifelong Disabilities

edited by

Matthew P. Janicki, Ph.D.
University of Illinois at Chicago

and

Edward F. Ansello, Ph.D.
Virginia Commonwealth University
Richmond

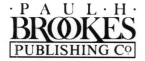

·P A U L·H·
BROOKES
PUBLISHING CO

Baltimore • London • Toronto • Sydney

Paul H. Brookes Publishing Co.
Post Office Box 10624
Baltimore, Maryland 21285-0624

www.brookespublishing.com

Typeset by Pro-Image Corp., Techna-Type Division, York, Pennsylvania.
Manufactured in the United States of America by
Hamilton Printing Company, Rensselaer, New York.

Some of the case studies and personal stories in this book represent actual people and actual circumstances. In most instances, the names and other identifying information of individuals have
been changed to protect their identities. Some case studies and personal stories are composite
accounts that are based on several different actual people and various circumstances; these case
studies do not represent the lives or experiences of specific individuals, and no implications
should be inferred. Case studies that are based on real people or circumstances are presented
herein with the written consent of the individuals or their legal guardians.

Library of Congress Cataloging-in-Publication Data
Community supports for aging adults with lifelong disabilities / edited by Matthew P.
Janicki and Edward F. Ansello.
    p. cm.
  Includes bibliographical references and index.
  ISBN 1-55766-462-5
  1. Developmentally disabled aged—Services for. 2. Community health services.
3. Handicapped—Services for. 4. Developmentally disabled aged—Care. I. Janicki,
Matthew P., 1943–. II. Ansello, Edward F.

RA427 .C6185 2000
362.4'084'6—dc21

                                            00-021580

British Library Cataloguing in Publication data are available from the British Library.

Contents

VI   Assessing the Present, Designing the Future

About the Editors

Matthew P. Janicki, Ph.D., Research Associate Professor of Human Development, College of Associated Health Professions, University of Illinois at Chicago, 1640 West Roosevelt Road, Chicago, Illinois 60608

Dr. Janicki is a research associate professor of human development at the Institute of Disability and Human Development at the University of Illinois at Chicago and serves as Director for Technical Assistance at the Rehabilitation Research and Training Center on Aging with Mental Retardation at that university. He also is a research professor and co-director at the Centre on Intellectual Disabilities at the University at Albany (New York). Formerly, he was Director for Aging and Special Populations at the New York State Office of Mental Retardation and Developmental Disabilities. Dr. Janicki was a Joseph P. Kennedy, Jr. Foundation public policy leadership fellow, spending a sabbatical year at the National Institute on Aging and the U.S. Senate. He was responsible for founding several aging and intellectual disabilities interest groups within American and international intellectual and gerontological professional societies. He is the author of numerous books and articles in the areas of aging, dementia, public policy, and rehabilitation with regard to people with intellectual and developmental disabilities and has lectured and provided training in aging and intellectual disabilities around the world. Dr. Janicki is a fellow of the American Psychological Association, the Gerontological Society of America, and the International Association for the Scientific Study of Intellectual Disabilities.

Edward F. Ansello, Ph.D., Director, Virginia Center on Aging; Professor of Gerontology, Virginia Commonwealth University, 520 North 12th Street, Box 980229, Richmond, Virginia 23298

Dr. Ansello is Director of the Virginia Center on Aging and is a professor in the Department of Gerontology, Medical College of Virginia Campus, Virginia Commonwealth University (VCU) in Richmond. He joined VCU after a 20-year career at the University of Maryland, where he was a co-founder of the Maryland Center on Aging and Coordinator of the Nursing Home Administrators 100-Hour Program. Much of his work seeks to bring the aging and disabilities systems into greater cooperation. He co-developed and co-hosted the 1987 Wingspread Conference on Aging and Lifelong Disabilities and has written articles, book chapters, and books on aging and developmental disabilities for gerontological audiences. He has directed or co-directed several research and demonstration projects on aging with disabilities in the community, including Partners Project I in Maryland (1987–1990), Partners Project II in Virginia (1990–1992), and Partners Project III in Virginia and Maryland (1993–1996). These projects sought to determine public policy on aging and lifelong developmental disabilities, to establish mechanisms of collaboration between service systems, and to build the capacities of agency staff, older people, and family members with regard to coping with growing old with lifelong impairments. Dr. Ansello is a fellow of the Gerontological Society of America and a charter fellow of the Association for Gerontology in Higher Education.

About the Contributors

Rick Berkobien, M.S.W., Committee Administrator, Policy, Research, and Committee Services, Oregon State Legislature, 453 State Capitol, 900 Court Street NE, Salem, Oregon 97301. Prior to accepting his position with the Oregon state legislature and at the time he wrote his chapter in this book, Mr. Berkobien served as Assistant Director of the Department of Research and Program Services at The Arc of the United States. He assisted in directing The Arc's coalition-building effort directed at outreach for at-risk, two-generation elderly families and served as the Principal Investigator for a project examining guardianship and family trusts that could help older families prepare for the future. His areas of professional interest include aging and developmental disabilities, financial planning, and family supports.

Christine Bigby, Ph.D., M.S.W., Lecturer, Department of Social Work and Social Policy, La Trobe University, Bundoora, Victoria 3083, Australia. Dr. Bigby has practiced as a social worker in a range of organizational contexts, specializing in the field of intellectual disabilities since the mid-1980s. Her research has focused on the nature of policy, formal services, and informal supports for older people with intellectual disabilities. She was awarded the National Research Award of the Australian Society for the Study of Intellectual Disability in 1993. Dr. Bigby coordinates the first year of the La Trobe University social work program and teaches an elective on policy and practice for adults with intellectual disabilities. She maintains strong links with the field by providing regular case consultations with a regional disabilities services team and serving as the joint coordinator of the Australian network on aging and disability.

Patricia A. Bloom, Ph.D., Research Professor, Department of Psychiatry and Behavioral Sciences; Director of Education and Training, Center on Aging and Developmental Disabilities, University of Miami School of Medicine, Dominion Tower, Suite 601 (D-305), 1400 N.W. 10th Avenue, Miami, Florida 33136. Dr. Bloom has master's degrees in education and international relations and a doctoral degree in psychology with national certification in gerontology. She has published articles and a manual, *Portrait of Survival*, based on her research with older adults and has developed curricula and training programs for professionals working with older adults in a variety of areas, including crisis response and family and community interventions. She has administered a number of statewide initiatives and was the project coordinator for the FLAGs, or Florida's local action groups, during their 2 years of development and implementation.

Anne L. Botsford, Ph.D., ACSW, Associate Professor, Director of Fieldwork Education, Department of Social Work, School of Social and Behavioral Sciences, Marist College, Dyson Center 340, Poughkeepsie, New York 12601. Dr. Botsford has worked extensively with older families of adults with intellectual disabilities and has developed and evaluated the effectiveness of group intervention in assisting older families with planning for the future. She is the senior co-author of the community education manual *End-of-Life Care: A Guide for Supporting Older People with Intellectual Disabilities and Their Families,* published by NYSArc, Albany, New York.

Nancy Breitenbach, Chief Executive Officer, Inclusion International, 13D Chemin du Levant, F-01210 Ferney-Voltaire, France. Ms. Breitenbach is Chief Executive Officer of Inclusion International (formerly known as the International League of Societies for Persons with Mental Handicap), a worldwide federation of associations whose objective is to defend and support people with intellectual disabilities and their families. Previously, she served as head of programs for people with disabilities for the Fondation de France in Paris. She is the author of several French-language textbooks on aging and disability.

Roy I. Brown, Dip. Psych., Ph.D., Foundation Professor and Dean, School of Special Education and Disability Studies, Flinders University, Post Office Box 2100, Adelaide 5001, South Australia, Australia. Dr. Brown has developed a wide range of programs for people with disabilities and tertiary education for personnel, and he has published extensively based on research and practical demonstration projects in the field of intellectual disabilities, including individuals in the 20- to 70-year-old age bracket.

Timothy L. Bruckner, Director of Aging and Day Support Services, Lakeshore Community Services, 1352 West 26th Street, Erie, Pennsylvania 16508. Mr. Bruckner completed his education at St. Mary's Abbey, Seton Hall University, and the University of Pittsburgh and completed an internship at the University of Pittsburgh. A contributing member of the American Society on Aging and the Gerontological Society of America, he is a published author in the area of applied gerontology. Mr. Bruckner is one of only 25 master trainers worldwide who are authorized by the American Association on Mental Retardation to conduct training on "Definition, Classification and Systems of Support for People with Intellectual Disabilities."

Phillip G. Clark, Sc.D., Professor and Director, Program in Gerontology and the Rhode Island Geriatric Education Center, University of Rhode Island, White Hall G-15, Kingston, Rhode Island 02881. Dr. Clark previously was Director of the Rhode Island Family Futures Planning Project, funded by the Administration on Aging. He has published extensively on health and human services policy for older adults, ethical issues in geriatric health care policy, and interdisciplinary collaboration and teamwork. He has been Project Director/Principal Investigator for grants from the Administration on Aging, the Bureau of Health Professions, the National Institute on Aging, and the Rhode Island Foundation.

Constance L. Coogle, Ph.D., Assistant Director of Research, Assistant Professor of Gerontology and Psychology, Virginia Center on Aging, Virginia Commonwealth University, 520 North 12th Street, Room B-25, Richmond, Virginia 23298. Dr. Coogle has extensive experience in conducting evaluation research for a number of grant-funded projects supported by the Administration on Aging, the Andrus Foundation of the American Association of Retired Persons, and the National Institute of Mental Health. She served as Evaluation Director for the Partners II Project and as Associate Director for the Partners III Project. Dr. Coogle is the Director of Evaluation for a 3-year project on geriatric interdisciplinary team training conducted by the Virginia Geriatric Education Center with support from the Bureau of Health Professions, Health

Resources and Services Administration, U.S. Department of Health and Human Services.

Sally-Ann Cooper, M.D., M.R.C.Psych., Professor, Department of Psychological Medicine, University of Glasgow, Academic Centre, Gartnavel Royal Hospital, 1055 Great Western Road, Glasgow G12 0XH, Scotland, United Kingdom. Dr. Cooper is a professor of learning disabilities at the University of Glasgow and Honorary Consultant in Learning Disabilities Psychiatry at Greater Glasgow Primary Care National Health Service Trust. She has a particular interest in the mental health needs of adults and older people with intellectual disabilities and has published extensively on this topic.

Arthur J. Dalton, Ph.D., Research Scientist, New York State Institute for Basic Research in Developmental Disabilities, 1050 Forest Hill Road, Staten Island, New York 10314. Dr. Dalton is Deputy Director for the Center on Aging Studies at the institute. He has 25 years of research experience in the field of intellectual disabilities and developmental disabilities, and he served as an associate professor in the Department of Physiology in the Faculty of Medicine at the University of Toronto, Canada. He has more than 10 years of voluntary experience in working directly with families, health care professionals, and individuals with Alzheimer's disease. He was one of the founders and for 3 years was President of the Alzheimer Society of Canada, the world's first self-help, nonprofit national organization devoted to family support, public education, and advocacy for individuals affected by Alzheimer's disease. Dr. Dalton is a member of the Board of Directors of the National Down Syndrome Congress.

Philip W. Davidson, Ph.D., Professor of Pediatrics and Psychiatry; Director, Strong Center for Developmental Disabilities, School of Medicine and Dentistry, University of Rochester, Box 671 URMC, 601 Elmwood Avenue, Rochester, New York 14642. Dr. Davidson has been Director of the Strong Center for Developmental Disabilities, an Administration on Developmental Disabilities–funded university affiliated program, since 1975. Dr. Davidson's research interests include psychiatric and behavior disorders of children and older adults with intellectual disabilities. Since 1991, he has been a senior investigator in the Seychelles Child Development Study, examining the developmental neurotoxicity of methylmercury. He has published extensively on a range of topics related to intellectual disabilities, has served on numerous editorial boards of professional journals, and has been elected to leadership offices within the American Association on Mental Retardation, the American Psychological Association, the Society of Pediatric Psychology, and the American Association of University Affiliated Programs.

DiAnn L. Davies, M.A.R., Director of Development, Research Foundation for Mental Hygiene, Housing Office, 44 Holland Avenue, 4th Floor, Albany, New York 12229. Ms. Davies directs the grants and development program for the New York State Research Foundation for Mental Hygiene's Innovative Models for Housing Independence Partnerships (IMHIP) program. She has been working with individuals with disabilities since the mid-1970s in the fields of education, housing, vocational rehabilitation, service coordination, recreation, ministry, and art in the United States, England, and Australia. She has conducted workshops and presented at conferences, nationally and internationally, on finding alternative funding sources, coalition and collaboration building, program development, and negotiation and influence.

Robert J. Davies, M.P.A., Assistant Director, New York State Office of Mental Retardation and Developmental Disabilities, 44 Holland Avenue, Albany, New York 12229. Mr. Davies is Assistant Director of Housing and Family Care for the New York State Office of Mental Retardation and Developmental Disabilities. He has worked in the field of developmental disabilities since the 1970s, starting in direct care and sheltered workshops. He has worked in vocational rehabilitation, service coordination, and recreation but primarily in program development. He is a leader in the development of person-controlled housing for people with disabilities and serves as a master trainer on housing options.

Sharon Davis, Ph.D., Director of Research and Program Services, The Arc of the United States, 1010 Wayne Avenue, Suite 650, Silver Spring, Maryland 20910. Dr. Davis is Director of the Department of Research and Program Services at The Arc of the United States in Silver Spring, Maryland. She oversees The Arc's coalition-building endeavors and provides guidance for the implementation of a variety of projects focusing on inclusion and choice for people with developmental disabilities and their families. Dr. Davis also oversees The Arc's position statement development and publications program.

Sharon M. Desmond, Ph.D., Associate Professor, Department of Health Education, University of Maryland, 2376 Health and Human Performance Building, College Park, Maryland 20742. Dr. Desmond is an associate professor in health education at the University of Maryland at College Park (UMCP) and is Co-Director of the Minority Health Research Laboratory in that department. She has worked at UMCP since 1989, with an emphasis on community health, health behavior, and survey research. Her current research focus is on implementing programs to decrease health disparities among underserved populations.

Ezra D. Ehrenkrantz, FAIA, Sponsored Chair and Executive Director, Center for Architecture and Building Science Research, New Jersey Institute of Technology, 323 Dr. Martin Luther King Boulevard, Campbell Hall Room 335, University Heights, Newark, New Jersey 07102. Mr. Ehrenkrantz holds the Sponsored Chair for the Center for Architecture and Building Science Research at New Jersey Institute of Technology. In addition, he is a founder and principal of Ehrenkrantz, Eckstut, and Kuhn, a New York City–based architecture and planning firm. As a researcher, architect, and teacher, he has pioneered developments in many areas of housing and construction and is a fellow of the American Institute of Architects.

Alan R. Factor, Ph.D., Associate Director, Rehabilitation Research and Training Center on Aging with Mental Retardation, Department of Disability and Human Development, University of Illinois at Chicago, 1640 West Roosevelt Road, Chicago, Illinois 60608. Dr. Factor is Associate Director for Training and Dissemination at the Rehabilitation Research and Training Center on Aging with Mental Retardation and is a senior research specialist at the Institute on Disability and Human Development, University of Illinois at Chicago. Dr. Factor has conducted national studies of innovative services and community supports for older adults with developmental disabilities. He has directed projects funded by the Administration on Aging and the Administration on Developmental Disabilities to promote later-life planning by adults with developmental disabilities and their families. Dr. Factor is on the Leadership Council of the Aging, Disability, and Rehabilitation Network of the American Society on Aging, is a disciplinary director of the Illinois Geriatric Education Center, and chairs the Developmental Disabilities Special Interest Group of the Gerontological Society of America. He has been a consultant on aging and developmental disabilities to various organizations. Dr. Factor has lectured widely, has co-authored several articles on aging and developmental disabilities, and was a co-editor and contributor to *Older Adults with Developmental Disabilities: Optimizing Choice and Change* (Paul H. Brookes Publishing Co., 1993).

Lucinda Grant-Griffin, Ph.D., Policy Analyst, New York State Office of Mental Retardation and Developmental Disabilities, 44 Holland Avenue, Albany, New York 12229. Dr. Grant-Griffin has more than 30 years of experience in education and human services. She is employed as a policy development specialist at the New York State Office of Mental Retardation and Developmental Disabilities (OMRDD), where she coordinates federal and state activities within the Bureau of Policy Analysis. Prior to taking her current position, she directed OMRDD's Office of Minority Services, Multicultural Professional Development Institute (MPDI). Dr. Grant-Griffin has been employed as a research assistant and policy consultant with the New York State School Boards Association, an instructor at Clark-Atlanta University (formerly Clark College), and a teacher in the elementary and middle school systems of South Carolina and New York.

Katharine S. Hacker, Ph.D., M.S.W., Consultant/Senior Planner, Niagara County Office for the Aging, 100 Davison Road, Lockport, New York 14094. Dr. Hacker managed one of the demonstration sites on which the New York State Caregiver Outreach Program was based and later served as a consultant to the project.

Stanley L. Handelman, D.M.D., Professor Emeritus, Eastman Dental Center, University of Rochester, 625 Elmwood Avenue, Rochester, New York 14620. Dr. Handelman is the former Chair of the Department of General Dentistry at Eastman Dental Center. He has extensive experience in dental education and has numerous publications, including publications in the field of developmental disabilities.

Jane E. Harlan-Simmons, M.A., Research Associate, Indiana Institute on Disability and Community, 2853 East 10th Street, Bloomington, Indiana 47408. Ms. Harlan-Simmons has been a research associate at the Institute for the Study of Developmental Disabilities, the University Affiliated Program of Indiana, since 1988. Ms. Harlan-Simmons's work within the Institute's Center for Aging Persons with Developmental Disabilities includes the provision of training and consultation as well as the production of educational publications and videotapes. She has participated in several demonstration components of the federally funded projects awarded to the center, including working as a community builder for the Community Membership Project.

Tamar Heller, Ph.D., Professor, Director of Rehabilitation Research and Training Center on Aging with Mental Retardation, Department of Disability and Human Development, University of Illinois at Chicago, 1640 West Roosevelt Road, Chicago, Illinois 60608. Dr. Heller is also Associate Head for Academic Affairs and Director of Graduate Studies of the Department of Disability and Human Development (DHD), University of Illinois at Chicago. She also directs the Rehabilitation Research and Training Center (RRTC) on Aging with Mental Retardation and several projects on transition issues and support interventions for individuals with developmental disabilities and their families. The RRTC is a national center in the United States that brings together researchers and advocacy organizations to study disabilities and aging and to promote progressive public policies. Dr. Heller has written extensively and has presented papers at major conferences on the topics of aging and developmental disabilities, family adjustment over the life course, and family support interventions for people with disabilities.

C. Michael Henderson, M.D., Assistant Professor, Departments of Internal Medicine, Pediatrics, and Psychiatry, University of Rochester School of Medicine and Dentistry, 601 Elmwood Avenue, Rochester, New York 14642. Dr. Henderson is a geriatrician and a specialist in developmental disabilities at Strong Memorial Hospital in the Department of Medicine and Psychiatry in Rochester, New York, and is an associate at the Strong Center on Aging and Developmental Disabilities at the University of Rochester. Dr. Henderson has many years of experience in clinical settings assessing older adults with a variety of developmental disabilities.

David B. Henry, Ph.D., Assistant Professor of Psychology, Institute for Juvenile Research (MC 747), Department of Psychiatry, University of Illinois at Chicago, 907 South Wolcott Avenue, Chicago, Illinois 60612. Dr. Henry's research focuses on the ways in which people with disabilities are perceived and evaluated by others. He is one of the developers of the Community Living Attitudes Scales (CLAS) (*Mental Retardation,* 1996), an instrument used to assess attitudes and values with respect to people with disabilities. In addition, Dr. Henry is a co-investigator on several federally funded projects aimed at the prevention of antisocial behavior.

B. Lynn Hutchings, M.Arch, Research Architect, Center for Architecture and Building Science Research, New Jersey Institute of Technology, 323 Dr. Martin Luther King Boulevard, Campbell Hall Room 335, University Heights, Newark, New Jersey 07102. Since 1990, Ms. Hutchings has conducted a number of research projects and analyzed the social and environmental needs of people with developmental disabilities, physical disabilities, and people who are aging with dementia. She is a trainer in home modifications.

Elizabeth A. Kennedy, Ph.D., Assistant Professor of Social Science, Community and Technical College, University of Akron, Associate Studies, Polsky 133H, Akron, Ohio 44325. Dr. Kennedy serves as Curriculum Coordinator for the "Death and Dying" course in the Community and Technical College at the University of Akron. She is a fellow of the Institute for Life-Span Development and Gerontology at the University of Akron and is the Project Coordinator/Consultant for the Person-Centered Planning for Later Life: A Curriculum for Older Adults with Mental Retardation training program for that agency. Dr. Kennedy also is a bereavement services provider for Hospice of Medina County in Medina, Ohio. Her research interests include aging and older adulthood, with a special emphasis on issues related to death and dying.

Christopher B. Keys, Ph.D., Professor, Department of Disability and Human Development, University of Illinois at Chicago, 1640 West Roosevelt Road, Chicago, Illinois 60608. Dr. Keys is a professor of psychology and of disability and human development. He is the Chair of the Division of Community and Prevention Research in the Department of Psychology. A fellow of the American Psychological Association, Dr. Keys has served as President of the Society for Community Research and Action and as Chair of the Council of Community Psychology Program Directors. He has worked with and studied disability service providers and advocacy organizations since 1980 in order to improve organizational functioning and empower people with disabilities and their family members. His current work focuses on promoting awareness of disability rights and the success of high school students with disabilities in communities of color.

Phyllis Kultgen, Ph.D., Director, Center on Aging and Community, Indiana Institute on Disability and Community, Indiana University, 2853 East 10th Street, Bloomington, Indiana 47408. Prior to her retirement in May 2000, Dr. Kultgen was the Director of the Center for Aging Persons with Developmental Disabilities at the Institute for the Study of Developmental Disabilities, the University Affiliated Program of Indiana. She has been involved in the field of aging and developmental disabilities since the mid-1980s, writing and directing numerous grants, teaching, and providing training and consultation in an array of topics related to aging with disabilities. Dr. Kultgen has been active in promoting community connections for elders since 1983.

Jennifer B. Mactavish, Ph.D., Assistant Professor and Graduate Program Coordinator, Health, Leisure, and Human Performance Research Institute, University of Manitoba, 102 Frank Kennedy Centre, Winnipeg, Manitoba R3T 2N2, Canada. Dr. Mactavish is an assistant professor and researcher who is interested in the social-psychological effects of recreation and leisure in the lives of individuals with intellectual disabilities. In particular, her work has focused on enhancing understanding of the relationship between recreation and leisure and quality of life (e.g., social integration, independence, interdependence) from the perspectives of these individuals and their families. Dr. Mactavish is the author of numerous publications in this area, an active volunteer in a variety of community service agencies, and a frequent presenter at national and international conferences.

Michael J. Mahon, Ph.D., Dean of the Faculty of Physical Education and Recreation, University of Alberta, P-421 Universiade Pavilion, Edmonton, Alberta T6G 2H9, Canada. Dr. Mahon received his graduate education at the University of North Carolina at Chapel Hill. He has been actively involved as both a practitioner and an academic in the fields of therapeutic recreation, disability, and aging since the mid-1970s. His present research is concerned with later-life planning for older adults with mental disabilities. He is the co-author of the text *Introduction to Recreation Services for People with Disabilities: A Person-Centred Approach* (Sagamore Publishing, 1997). Dr. Mahon was previously associated with the University of Manitoba. He is the author of numerous publications and has presented at both national and international conferences.

Kevin J. Mahoney, Ph.D., Associate Professor, Graduate School of Social Work, Boston College, McGuinn Hall 306, Chestnut Hill, Massachusetts 02167. Dr. Mahoney is the National Program Director for the Cash and Counseling Demonstration and Evaluation funded by the Robert Wood Johnson Foundation and the U.S. Department of Health and Human Services. Dr. Mahoney has served in a number of policy-making and administrative positions in state governments. From 1978 to 1987, he was Chief of Research and Program Development at the Connecticut Department on Aging, where he was responsible for that state's home care programs for the frail elderly. From 1987 to 1995, Dr. Mahoney developed and implemented innovative partnerships between private insurance and Medicaid to finance long-term care, first in Connecticut and then in California. He speaks and writes extensively on consumer direction, the roles of the public and private sectors in financing long-term care, long-term care insurance, and care management.

Hans Malmström, D.D.S., Associate Professor, Eastman Dental Center, University of Rochester, 623 Elmwood Avenue, Rochester, New York 14620. Dr. Malmström is Program Director for the Advanced Education in General Dentistry program at the University of Rochester and the Clinical Chief for General Dentistry Clinic at Eastman Dental Center. He received his doctor of dentistry degree from the University of Gothenburg, Sweden, and completed a general practice residency program at the University of Connecticut. He has had experience in dental education, including the dental care of adults with developmental disabilities.

Philip McCallion, Ph.D., Associate Professor, School of Social Welfare, University at Albany, 135 Western Avenue, Albany, New York 12222. Dr. McCallion is a faculty research associate at the Ringel Institute of Gerontology and Co-director of the Centre on Intellectual Disabilities. He was formerly the Executive Director of the Training School at Vineland (New Jersey). His research is focused on caregiving issues, particularly the interaction of informal care with formal services, and the experiences of multicultural families. Most recently, his research has included evaluation of the effectiveness of select interventions, including work on improving interactions between aging and developmental disabilities service providers, the development of exemplary outreach strategies to families that are not connected to service systems, and demonstrating the effectiveness of community-based interventions for grandparents who are caregivers. Dr. McCallion has published on interventions for caregivers of older people who are in frail health, those caring for people with Alzheimer's disease, and those caring for adults with developmental disabilities. He is the co-author of *Maintaining Communication with Persons with Dementia: An Educational Program for Nursing Home Staff and Family Members* (Springer Publishing Co., 1998).

Mark E. Moss, D.D.S., Ph.D., Assistant Professor, Eastman Department of Dentistry, University of Rochester, 625 Elmwood Avenue, Rochester, New York 14620. Dr. Moss's research interests relate broadly to oral disease epidemiology and oral health services research. He received his doctor of dentistry degree from Marquette University, a master's degree in preventive medicine from the University of Wisconsin–Madison, and a doctoral degree in epidemiology from the School of Public Health at the University of North Carolina at Chapel Hill.

Dawna Torres Mughal, Ph.D., RD, FADA, Director, Dietetics Program, Associate Professor, College of Sciences, Engineering, and Health Sciences, Gannon University, 109 University Square, Erie, Pennsylvania 16541. Dr. Mughal is Director of the Coordinated Dietetics and Medical Technology Programs and the Consortium Program in Dietetics at Gannon University. She teaches clinical dietetics, which includes nutrition throughout the life cycle, rehabilitation, and behavioral health. She has developed and conducted continuing education programs on many nutrition topics for various groups and has served as an adjunct faculty member at Lake Erie College of Osteopathic Medicine in Erie. She is a registered dietitian and certified as a charter fellow of the American Dietetic Association.

Richard V. Olsen, Ph.D., Director of Health Care and Aging Environments Research, Health and Aging Division, Center for Architecture and Building Science Research, New Jersey Institute of Technology, 323 Dr. Martin Luther King Boulevard, Campbell Hall Room 335, University Heights, Newark, New Jersey 07102. Dr. Olsen is an environmental psychologist specializing in design research and evaluation of facilities for people with physical, cognitive, and emotional disabilities.

Rosemeire R. Santos-Teachout, D.D.S., M.S., Assistant Professor, Developmentally Disabled Dental Clinic Coordinator, Eastman Department of Dentistry, University of Rochester, 625 Elmwood Avenue, Rochester, New York 14620. Dr. Santos-Teachout is the Program Coordinator of the Dental Clinic for the Developmentally Disabled at the University of Rochester. She received her doctor of dentistry degree from the Universidade Federal de Minas Gerais in Brazil and her master's degree from Ohio State University. She has extensive clinical experience and several publications regarding adults with developmental disabilities.

Christine N. Sears, Director of Development and Public Relations, Madison County Arc, 639 Lenox Avenue, Oneida, New York 13421. Ms. Sears has served as Director of Planning and Public Relations for the Office for the Aging in Madison County, New York, one of the few private, not-for-profit area agencies on aging in New York State (most are agencies of county governments). Ms. Sears is the recipient of the 1998 Madison County Mental Health and Community Services Board Award for her work countywide on aging and developmental disability issues.

Chad M. Sed, M.A., Research Associate, Institute for Life-Span Development and Gerontology, University of Akron, Akron, Ohio 44325. Mr. Sed is a doctoral candidate in the University of Akron's industrial organizational psychology program with a specialization in gerontology. His research involvement has included Person-Centered Planning for Later Life: A Curriculum for Older Adults with Mental Retardation, the Death and Dying module for that curriculum, the employability of adults with intellectual disabilities, the training of workers who are ages 40 years and older, personality and aging, and the work and retirement of older people. His research has been presented at international conferences. His research interests include the employability of adults with intellectual disabilities and adult postretirement work.

Peter Sheridan, Senior Housing Specialist, Research Foundation for Mental Hygiene, 44 Holland Avenue, Albany, New York 12229. Mr. Sheridan is a senior housing specialist for the New York State Research Foundation for Mental Hygiene's Innovative Models for Housing Independence Partnership Program. He is a member of the National Affordable Housing Task Force, the New York State Consolidated Plan Partnership Advisory Committee, and the New York State Accessibility Committee (which oversees revisions to the New York State Building Code to meet requirements of the Americans with Disabilities Act [ADA] of 1990 [PL 101-336]). He is a graduate of the Pratt Institute Community Economic Development internship program.

Jean M. Sherman, Ed.D., RN, Director of Education and Training, Center on Aging and Developmental Disabilities, University of Miami School of Medicine, Dominion Tower Suite 601 (D-305), 1400 N.W. 10th Avenue, Miami, Florida 33136. Dr. Sherman received her doctoral degree in adult education and also is a registered nurse. Before working in the disability field, she spent more than 10 years in leadership positions in the aging network. In these positions, she worked with several community coalitions. Dr. Sherman was the primary author of the manual that resulted from the project described in her chapter. She also has written a comprehensive training program for families of adults with developmental disabilities as well as other professional publications. Dr.

Sherman has conducted conference workshops locally and nationally, including cross-training workshops for professionals in the fields of aging and disabilities.

Dawn M. Shoop, Ph.D., Faculty Research Associate, Center on Aging, University of Maryland, 2367 Health and Human Performance Building, 255 Valley Drive, College Park, Maryland 20742. Dr. Shoop is a developmental psychologist who works in health education/research. Her research areas have included identity development, risk taking, and human immunodeficiency virus (HIV) prevention and education. She is a member of the research faculty of the University of Maryland Center on Aging, where she conducts research on aging, disability, and health policy.

Lori Simon-Rusinowitz, M.P.H., Ph.D., Deputy Project Director, Cash and Counseling Demonstration and Evaluation, Center on Aging and Department of Health Education, University of Maryland, Health and Human Performance Building, 255 Valley Drive, College Park, Maryland 20742. Dr. Simon-Rusinowitz is a faculty member in the Department of Health Education. She has been interested in aging and disability issues since 1987. As part of the Cash and Counseling Project, she has overseen a study of consumers' preferences for consumer-directed personal care. Dr. Simon-Rusinowitz earned her doctoral degree in health policy at the University of Illinois at Chicago and her master of public health degree from the University of Michigan.

Jo-Ann Sowers, Ph.D., Adjunct Associate Professor, Department of Public Health and Preventive Medicine, School of Medicine, Oregon Health Sciences University, 3608 S.E. Powell Boulevard, Portland, Oregon 97202. Dr. Sowers is a principal investigator at the Center on Self-Determination, a program of the Oregon Institute on Disability and Development at the Oregon Health Sciences University. Dr. Sowers's work has focused on the demonstration of self-determination models and strategies for youth and adults with developmental disabilities. Her areas of professional interest also include employment, community integration, and natural supports for individuals with developmental disabilities.

Marie R. Squillace, M.A., Faculty Research Associate, Center on Aging, University of Maryland, 2367 Health and Human Performance Building, College Park, Maryland 20742. Ms. Squillace is a faculty research associate at the University of Maryland's Center on Aging. As part of the Cash and Counseling Project, she has coordinated the operations of the Interdisciplinary Health Research Laboratory in a study of consumers' preferences for consumer-directed personal care. She is a doctoral candidate in the Department of Health Education at the University of Maryland.

Harvey L. Sterns, Ph.D., Professor of Psychology, Director of the Institute for Life-Span Development and Gerontology, University of Akron; Research Professor of Gerontology, College of Medicine, Northeastern Ohio Universities, Polsky 326, Akron, Ohio 44325. Dr. Sterns is a professor of psychology and Director of the Institute for Life-Span Development and Gerontology at the University of Akron. Dr. Sterns has been involved in gerontology since the 1960s and is considered a leading expert in his field. Dr. Sterns serves in leadership roles on numerous national committees related to aging and disability issues, and his credits include numerous publications and presentations. He is a fellow of the Gerontological Society of America and a charter fellow of the Association for Gerontology in Higher Education.

James A. Stone, M.F.A., FAAMR, Executive Director, Third Age, Inc., 1548 Deer Lake Drive, Lexington, Kentucky 40515. Mr. Stone is an assistant professor in the College of Social Work at the University of Kentucky. Mr. Stone has more than 20 years of experience in gerontology and developmental disabilities, including 6 years as a coordinator on a national project examining small-family housing and reverse equity mortgage options for older adults. He served as the Project Coordinator for the Aging with Developmental Disabilities Project of the Texas Department on Aging during the project's inception and implementation. He has been involved in developing and implementing community programs based on person-centered individualized plans of support for older adults with developmental disabilities in rural areas that offer few services. He is the author of research reports, book chapters, monographs, and training manuals on a variety of issues concerning older families and individuals with developmental disabilities.

Connie B. Susa, M.Ed., Mentorship Coordinator, Rhode Island Parent Information Network, 175 Main Street, Pawtucket, Rhode Island 02860. Ms. Susa was the Coordinator of the Family Futures Planning Project, Program in Gerontology, at the University of Rhode Island in Kingston. She has consulted widely throughout New England on issues related to people with disabilities and has worked for the Rhode Island Developmental Disabilities Council and the Rhode Island Department of Education. She is a consultant on community inclusion for agencies serving the needs of adults with developmental disabilities and their families.

Janene N. Suttie, Ph.D., Coordinator of Disability Studies, School of Human Services, Griffith University, Brisbane, Queensland 4111, Australia. Dr. Suttie served as the Coordinator for the demonstration project described in her chapter while she was an assistant professor at the University Affiliated Program at the University of Hawaii at Manoa from 1992 through 1996. She is State President and National Councilor of the Australian Society for the Study of Intellectual Disabilities and sits on the Intellectually Disabled Citizens Council of Queensland.

Jennie Todd, Field-Based Coordinator, Indiana Institute on Disability and Community, Indiana University, 2853 East 10th Street, Bloomington, Indiana 47408. Ms. Todd has worked with people with disabilities and their families since 1980. She was instrumental in facilitating the transition from traditional facility-based services to nontraditional community supports focusing on typical community roles at Community Incentives, Inc., in Martinsville, Indiana. Ms. Todd leads the community building team at the center.

Kuo-yu Wang, Ph.D., Associate Professor, Department of Social Welfare, National Chung-Cheng University, 160, San-hing, Ming-Hsiung, Chia-yi, Taiwan, Republic of China. Dr. Wang teaches courses on social policy analysis, welfare and rights, and disability policy. She is a leading researcher in the area of aging and intellectual disabilities in Taiwan. Her research has included studies on estimating life expectancy for adults with intellectual disabilities who live in residential programs in Taiwan. Her work has been in rural communities, where she has collected information on families that include an adult with an intellectual disability living at home. She has a grant from the National Science Council of Taiwan to collect data on dementia among institutional residents older than 35 years of age. Dr. Wang is a leading advocate for disability rights in Taiwan and is active in Pacific Basin disability organization activities.

Jean B. Zink, M.S., Faculty Research Assistant (Retired), University of Maryland Center on Aging, College Park, Maryland 20742. Before her retirement, Ms. Zink was Project Manager for the Partners Project on aging and developmental disabilities. She also served as a consultant to the Partners II Project. Ms. Zink taught "Aging and Disabilities" at the University of Maryland, University College, Institute for Gerontological Practice, and has given numerous workshops on "Aging with a Lifelong Disability" and "Communicating with Your Physician." Ms. Zink had polio in 1951 and has had post-polio syndrome since 1995.

Foreword

I am pleased to introduce to you this most valuable book, *Community Supports for Aging Adults with Lifelong Disabilities*, edited by my distinguished friends Drs. Matthew P. Janicki and Edward F. Ansello. It addresses a matter of vital concern: We must ensure that our fellow citizens with lifelong developmental disabilities are able to grow old among us in the communities that we call home. Through my 30 years in the Special Olympics movement and as the Executive Vice President of the Joseph P. Kennedy, Jr. Foundation, I have had the privileged opportunity to meet literally thousands of people with mental retardation and their families. I have witnessed the extraordinary progress we have made as a society in overcoming the health and medical problems they have faced, as well as the social stigma that sometimes accompanies them. As a result, people with mental retardation and others with lifelong disabilities are living longer and fuller lives. Growing old is no longer the privilege of the few.

The World Health Organization (WHO) has recognized both the opportunities and the challenges that people who are aging with lifelong disabilities present. WHO's (2000) report, *Healthy Aging: Adults with Intellectual Disabilities*, notes the right of people with developmental disabilities to live a full, healthy life and, at the same time, notes that their needs will put demands on both developed and developing countries to create new types of living arrangements and community supports as they age with these disabilities. The WHO estimates that there are currently 500 million people around the world who have some disability requiring special health and social supports. As these individuals age, their needs change, as do their disabilities.

As more and more of our fellow citizens with lifelong disabilities age, we learn more about the various challenges that these individuals and their families and other caregivers encounter. Many of these needs may be remarkably similar to what all of us hope for in our later years—a safe home, a secure financial situation, physical well-being, and independence. We also know how important it is in later life to stay connected to family and to the lives of others. Aging adults with lifelong disabilities must be part of the social fabric of our communities and our families, with their contributions celebrated and cherished.

Yet, as this book illustrates so well, aging adults with developmental disabilities face unique challenges. For example, we know that many of these adults "age in place" in their families, with their caregiving parents. Adults with disabilities often outlive their parents. In the United States alone, we estimate that 500,000 people with developmental disabilities have reached the age of 60, and their most common living arrangement is with their families in the communities. They now, or will soon, require an array of supports to remain meaningfully in their communities. With appropriate recognition and support, they can experience lives that are interwoven with the lives of their families, neighbors, and friends.

There is much that all of us—parents, family members, advocates, and human ser-vices and health care professionals—must learn in order to help people with mental retardation and other developmental disabilities age with dignity and experience a rich and rewarding fullness of years.

Community Supports for Aging Adults with Lifelong Disabilities answers the needs of these caregivers. It offers rich, practical information drawn from successful experiences in meeting both the opportunities and the demands of aging with lifelong disabilities. It recognizes the central role of family caregivers and the talents of older people with developmental disabilities, as well as the importance of community services. This book offers sound and innovative ideas and strategies. Drs. Janicki and Ansello have assem-bled contributing authors from around the world who are leaders in the field of aging. The contributors are researchers, consumers, planners, advocates, and others who have lived with individuals with lifelong disabilities, in their professional work and in their personal lives. Collectively, they offer insights and lessons learned on the critical mat-ters that enable community living for this population.

I believe that this book will be an enormous benefit to consumers, family care-givers, and professionals. For individuals with lifelong disabilities, as for all of us, growing old must be a gift to enjoy.

Eunice Kennedy Shriver
Executive Vice President
Joseph P. Kennedy, Jr. Foundation

Preface

The attainment of late life by large numbers of people with lifelong developmental disabilities was one of the significant achievements of the late 20th century. It embodies two of the era's demographic evolutions: the aging of nations and the longevity of people with serious disabilities. In addition, it brings together the formerly parallel fields of gerontology and disabilities. We compiled this book to examine how these fields have become more inclusive and interwoven.

Disabilities are a fact of later life for many people. Although the percentage of older people with disabilities appears to be declining, their absolute numbers are increasing substantially. The prospect of an extended, full life for a person with a lifelong developmental disability is both real and present. The same is true for the prospect of survival after a serious late-onset disability such as stroke or dementia. The prospects for meaningful lives in either situation are far less certain. Careful study of the intersection of aging and lifelong disabilities, then, potentially has beneficial implications for all three fields of concern: aging, developmental disabilities, and late-onset disabilities.

We launched *Community Supports for Aging Adults with Lifelong Disabilities* with the understanding that most people wish to grow old and to live their lives in their own communities, with neighbors and neighborhoods, with services and opportunities of a typical life. We asked, "What enables someone with a lifelong disability to realize this common wish?" Growing numbers of older adults with lifelong disabilities are in need of a variety of residential, activity, and other day-to-day supports. Many of these older adults live on their own or with their families; others reside in a variety of housing provided or supported by private agencies or government authorities. We decided that this book would focus on these adults, their families, and the various human services delivery systems with which they come into contact as the three key elements that enable them to remain meaningfully in their communities. Accordingly, the core of this book addresses, respectively, the pertinent issues that older people face as they age, models of aiding families, and designs for making the human services infrastructure responsive to their needs. We intend this book for applied use. It should offer practical content for managers, practitioners, planners, educators, advocates, families, and others who are concerned about the meaningful continuation of community living for aging adults with lifelong impairments.

This book's content reflects the progress made during the last quarter of the 20th century at the intersection of aging and lifelong disabilities. Early work focused on primary issues of demography and adaptation to later-life stages, especially the unprecedented emergence of larger numbers of older adults with lifelong disabilities and the implications for systems without a history of meaningful interaction. In retrospect, we can see that the early work progressed somewhat unevenly through overlapping stages that might be referred to as *demographic, exploratory, model building and testing,* and *implementation.* Initially, representatives from the fields of aging and disabilities worked to understand the magnitude of aging with lifelong disabilities and the principal contributing factors in its emergence as an issue in need of attention. Next they examined each other's system to comprehend better its complexities of priorities, funding streams, practices, and values. Cross-training translated these understandings. With awareness of this growing special population, communities, states, and nations then supported the building and testing of models to partner the fields of aging and lifelong disabilities more effectively in order to benefit older people with disabilities. This building and testing stage continues even while the processes of implementation multiply.

The latest initiatives go beyond the previously defined primary areas of study and substantiate the realities that community living has become a fixture in the lives of individuals with lifelong disabilities and that aging affects all facets of their lives. Thus, we have structured this book to reflect what might be called the *new primary areas*, such as changing service philosophies and their effect on older people with lifelong disabilities, emerging research and service models for supporting families and individuals in community living, rising knowledge and research in health and wellness, and practical applications of models that further community development. We hope that compilation of these "new primaries" sets off the next wave of exploration and the development of even newer primaries.

We have adopted the term *intellectual disabilities* instead of *mental retardation* fairly consistently. *Intellectual disability* represents a more respectful, inclusive, effective, and recognizable representation of the disability under discussion, providing a more natural parallel to other descriptors used to characterize life's conditions, such as physical or sensory disabilities. In like manner, we use the terms *lifelong disabilities* as well as *developmental disabilities* because of the former's immediate comprehendability.

We are impressed by the forward-thinking editors at Paul H. Brookes Publishing Co., who saw this book as the vehicle for chronicling the new areas of development in our fields of study and practice. We also are pleased with the responses that we received from our contributing authors. In every instance, they gave thoughtful consideration to what they had done in their work and how it complemented the thinking about the new primaries. They contributed energetically, thereby enhancing the breadth and depth of ideas presented. We purposely sought contributors from North America, Europe, Australia, and Asia, engaging and cajoling them into sharing their most important experiences and insights, realizing that the broadest dialogue would stimulate the most progress. As a result, the book's sections are based on the best and most productive ideas and experiences in the field represented.

We asked Mrs. Eunice Kennedy Shriver to write the foreword to this book in recognition of her life's work as an advocate for people with lifelong disabilities. Her three decades of commitment have helped to produce the older adults who are the focus of this book. We honor Mrs. Shriver's life, and we are honored in turn by her foreword.

Each of us has been involved in projects related to aging and lifelong disabilities since the 1980s. Edward F. Ansello was instrumental in assembling the first joint meeting of state administrators of aging and of disability services in the United States that followed. The meeting also resulted in the report *Aging and Lifelong Disabilities: Partnership for the 21st Century* (University of Maryland/Elvirita Lewis Foundation, 1989), which Edward F. Ansello co-authored with Thomas Rose, that set the tone for similar efforts in the years that followed. Matthew P. Janicki co-edited with Henryk M. Wisniewski the first comprehensive textbook on aging and developmental disabilities,

Aging and Developmental Disabilities: Issues and Approaches (Paul H. Brookes Publishing Co., 1985), which explores the extant primaries and stands as a primer for its time. Subsequently, both of us worked within our respective domains to further the cross-fertilization of our fields and to encourage applications of community supports that would promote the most inclusive societies. With *Community Supports for Aging Adults with Lifelong Disabilities,* we have drawn from our separate and collective experiences to develop a book that we hope will serve as a primer for the new century. We trust that it will be as useful and reflective as the books that have preceded it.

1

The Aging of Nations

Impact on the Community, the Family, and the Individual

Edward F. Ansello and Matthew P. Janicki

Growing old with lifelong developmental disabilities is, at once, a recently acquired privilege for many individuals, an unexpected event for families who have raised them, and a challenge to policy makers who guide, and practitioners who deliver, the various support services these individuals need to remain in their communities. Reaching later life with lifelong disabilities reflects the triumph of the individual, the family, and the community over history that consigned people with lifelong developmental disabilities to truncated lives. Helping them to enjoy their newly acquired longevity and to live lives more fully and typically than before requires purposeful interactions among the individuals with disabilities, their families, and their communities.

In this chapter, we focus on the individual, the family, and the community as three interrelated elements necessary to help ensure continued meaningful living for aging adults who want to grow old in their communities. We also review in reverse order how all three have been affected by the aging of nations. Beginning with a macroscopic perspective, we examine the concept of community in a larger sense, demonstrating that the aging of nations has come about largely through developments that are neither gerontological nor geriatric, and that have added little to aging-related expertise. We then examine the concept of community in a more local sense, noting the growth in numbers of aging adults and of those who grow old with disabilities, whether lifelong or late onset, as well as the creation of attendant "systems" to serve these populations. With regard to these systems, we use the United States as a point of reference.

Next, we examine the reformulation of the family engendered by the aging evolution. Longer life expectancies have produced multigenerational families and have introduced new concerns into daily life, such as balancing work and family, but have not diminished the family's commitment to providing chronic care to dependent relatives. Finally, this chapter considers the individual newly arrived on the stage of later life, the aging person with lifelong developmental disabilities. The wide broadcast of the "gift of time" (Ansello & Eustis, 1992) has benefited him or her, creating the potential for continued community living for an extended life course; however, ensuring that this potential is realized requires recognition of needs, capacities, and contexts. We acknowledge qualitative differences in orientation to community living between older people (e.g., those 50 years old or older) who have grown up without legislated services and younger people who have grown older with them. With this in mind, we review the supports needed to help the aging adult with lifelong disabilities to achieve "assisted autonomy" while living in the community.

UNPRECEDENTED CHANGES: THE COMMUNITY

There have been two great demographic evolutions within developed nations in the 20th century: the explosion in numbers of older people and the survival to later life of people with formerly life-shortening disabilities. These evolutions share a common denominator, surviving early life. Throughout the centuries, childhood and the bearing of children have been fraught with dangers. These have included exposures to diseases, infections, bacteria, and viruses that caused high infant and maternal mortality. A relatively abbreviated life expectancy legitimated, and even required, a focus on what we now consider early life in most aspects of civilized living: social relations and marriage, education, health care, government, and the workplace. The 20th century changed all of this. Improved hygiene, rising levels of education, and medical breakthroughs, especially the discovery of antibiotics to combat bacterial infections and vaccines to counteract viruses, combined to affect a fundamental, and as yet incomplete, alteration in not only how life is lived, but also in how social institutions such as government, education, and services in the community respond to this extended life span.

In 1900, with high infant mortality and vulnerability of women to death during or near childbirth, the average life expectancy at birth in the United States and in other developed nations hovered near or less than 50 years. Today, because of the aforementioned improvements, life expectancy at birth in the developed nations approaches 80 years, being about 78 years in Western Europe, 76 years in North America, and 69 years in Latin America and the Caribbean (U.S. Bureau of the Census, 1998).

The aging of nations can be seen in Table 1, which projects changes in demographics for representative nations between 1998 and 2010. Breitenbach (Essay I) notes correctly that "problems" of aging and of aging with developmental disabilities are the privileged concerns of the developed nations. Developing nations do not have the luxury of these problems. Generally, lower infant mortality rates, pronounced aging of the population, and the stage of development of the nation are correlated, with more developed nations having lower infant mortality rates and larger older populations (Peterson, 1999). Conversely, high infant mortality rates tend to occur because of high fertility rates, which, in turn, are associated with an overall younger population in a developing nation (Murray & Lopez, 1996). Sub-Saharan Africa illustrates these relationships. Most of the nations in this part of the world continue to cope with relatively high infant mortality rates, and there is projected to be little change in the percent of

I

AGING ADULTS AND
THEIR LIFE SITUATIONS

No contemporary text on aging and lifelong disabilities can disregard the impact of the aging-related demographics and social change that the developed world will continue to experience during the next several decades. The high birth rate after the second world war produced what was earlier designated as the "baby boom" generation and what is slowly becoming the "senior boom" generation. Given this, in Chapter 1, we explore the aging of developed nations and discuss implications for nations, communities, families, and aging adults with lifelong disabilities. We assess the readiness of health care and supportive service providers to respond meaningfully to increased numbers of older adults with lifelong disabilities, and we introduce the concept of *assisted autonomy.*

Closely related to these demographic and ethnographic phenomena are issues of quality of life. This phrase has assumed diverse meanings, and Brown, an eminent social scientist, in Chapter 2 undertakes the considerable task of exploring this concept as it applies to older adults with lifelong disabilities. We were particularly keen to diverge from traditional theses on this subject and delve into what the dimensions, principles, and practices associated with the quality-of-life models mean for us in the area of gerontology. The applications of such models will enable us to look at disability in fresh ways, affecting how people with disabilities take control of their own lives, how we develop and manage supports and services to assist them, how we apply assessment and intervention strategies, and how we provide both professional education and service evaluation.

In Chapter 3, we take the philosophical underpinnings of human services applications one step further. Mahon and Mactavish, two Canadian social researchers, observe how social integration, as a critical component of quality of life for individuals with dis-

1

abilities, needs to be considered from the experiential perspective of older adults. There has been little effort to determine whether older adults consider social integration to be an important facet of their lives. Mahon and Mactavish share the results of a 3-year interdisciplinary study undertaken in Canada that contrasts perspectives of older adults with those of service providers and social supports. They present a model for understanding social integration and quality of life, noting the implications of this model for the provision of services for older adults with lifelong disabilities.

In this same vein, Bigby, in Chapter 4, provides an overview of the research literature on informal support networks at two stages in the life course of adults with lifelong disabilities. Drawing on both her research inquiries and a major study undertaken in Australia, she concludes that the type of support that parents, siblings, more distant family members, and friends provide early on to middle-age adults who live with aging parents is in contrast to what will be available when these same adults are older and in the postparental care stage. As a keen observer of family dynamics, she explains that adults in the postparental care phase often retain a key network member who takes responsibility for advocacy and oversight of their well-being. Among older adults in their 50s and 60s, siblings (sometimes more distant relatives or family friends) tend to replace parents in fulfilling such roles. However, as adults age, that central parental role is not replaced and often older adults have to become more reliant on formal services.

Breitenbach's essay closes Section I. An observer of the world scene, she grounds many of these foundational issues in an international perspective, noting that issues of aging with lifelong disabilities are currently the privileged concern of the developed nations.

Table 1. Infant deaths, life expectancies, and percentage of older adults in select countries

	Infant deaths per 1,000 live births		Life expectancy at birth (in years)		Percentage of population ages 60 years and older	
	1998	2010	1998	2010	1998	2010
Asia						
Cambodia	107	82	48.0	52.8	4.6	4.5
India	63	39	62.9	68.4	6.9	8.3
Japan	4	4	80.0	81.1	22.1	29.1
Malaysia	22	15	70.4	73.7	6.3	7.9
People's Republic of China	45	25	69.6	73.2	9.9	12.4
Republic of China (Taiwan)	6	5	76.8	80.5	11.6	14.5
Europe						
Germany	5	5	77.0	78.9	22.1	26.1
Italy	6	5	78.4	79.8	23.4	27.4
The Netherlands	5	5	78.0	79.5	18.0	22.5
Norway	5	4	78.2	79.7	19.6	22.1
Poland	13	9	72.8	75.9	16.3	18.5
United Kingdom	6	5	77.2	79.0	20.4	22.8
North America						
Canada	6	5	79.2	80.7	16.4	20.0
Mexico	26	15	71.6	75.5	6.3	8.1
United States	6	5	76.1	77.4	16.5	18.7
South America						
Argentina	19	14	74.5	76.8	13.9	14.8
Brazil	37	22	64.4	67.7	7.6	10.2
Chile	10	7	75.2	77.9	10.1	13.4
Ecuador	32	19	71.8	75.5	6.4	8.1
Paraguay	37	26	72.2	74.6	6.7	7.4
Venezuela	28	18	72.7	75.7	6.6	8.6
Sub-Saharan Africa						
Angola	132	95	47.9	54.5	4.7	4.7
Cameroon	77	64	51.4	49.8	5.2	5.1
Ghana	78	62	56.8	60.6	5.0	5.1
Kenya	59	54	47.6	43.7	4.1	4.9
Malawi	134	113	36.6	34.8	4.3	4.5
Uganda	93	69	42.6	47.6	3.5	3.0

Adapted from U.S. Bureau of the Census (1998, December).

older people. Although acknowledging that even the best estimates are estimates and that demographic projections are based on data whose sources are sometimes less than reliable or are subject to nationalistic exaggerations, it seems evident that surviving childhood and maternity help to produce the aging of nations.

The demographic evolutions in the developed nations have produced millions of older people without necessarily producing the aging-related expertise to go along with them. Because late life has been achieved by preventing or controlling the causes of death in the early years, late life remains relatively unexplored territory in health care, public policy, education, the work place, and other social arenas. Witness the near-constant retooling of government-funded pension schemes such as Social Security. Most were enacted in the first half of the 20th century by legislators socialized to a reality of a shorter life expectancy, one where attaining 60 or 65 years was the privilege of the few. Witness, too, the slow growth in the number of geriatricians in some developed nations, especially in the United States, where only 6,800 physicians of the nearly 700,000 who are licensed had earned added qualifications in geriatric medicine by 1996 (Alliance for Aging Research, 1996).

The aging of nations has increased the numbers of mainstream older people and older people with disabilities, whether lifelong or late onset. As noted elsewhere (Ansello & Eustis, 1992), the total number of older Americans with lifelong disabilities can be debated. First, being primarily community dwellers rather than institutional residents and, in many instances, not being known to formal services or programs, many are not figured in agency "counts." Second, number estimates are complicated by disagreements over what is a lifelong disability and which people to include under the lifelong disabilities umbrella, which historically has been dominated by people with intellectual disabilities. Third, there has been too little history of interaction among the various constituencies that can make up a population of people with lifelong disabilities and an insufficient sharing of data. Finally, the perceptions by formal service providers of their capacities to meet current and future demands of the population they serve may influence census attempts. Therefore, earlier estimates by developmental disabilities professionals of about 4 or 5 of every 1,000 people older than the age of 60 having a developmental disability (Jacobson, Sutton, & Janicki, 1985) might reasonably be conservative. Quite possibly, a higher estimate of about 1 in 100 elders is more realistic when we take the above factors into account (Ansello & Eustis, 1992; Ansello & Rose, 1989).

Moreover, the number of people who need assistance is expected to increase substantially in the next 15 years, as more community-dwelling older adults with lifelong disabilities are discovered in two-generation elderly families. This is likely to happen in families in which the parent or other caregiver has died or become frail and the situation is called to the attention of the aging network or another service system. The numbers of aging adults with intellectual and developmental disabilities being revealed also includes those who were inappropriately labeled in their childhoods. Labels such as "mentally retarded" were more frequently applied before the 1970s for reasons unacceptable or unlikely today, such as poor education, behavior considered unruly or asocial, coincident physical deformities or impairments, or because of inadequate screening for such conditions as hearing loss or other physical causes of "abnormal" behavior. As a result, people labeled "mentally retarded" some 40 or 50 years ago, or "developmentally disabled" up until recently, who have survived to late life today include large numbers of relatively quite capable, minimally impaired older adults. They also include those people whose mislabeling may have meant institutionalization, socialization to a "retardation provider" system, and separation from the mainstream of education, work, and community life. In addition, there are increasing numbers of adults surviving to middle age and older who have physical limitations because of early life conditions, such as cerebral palsy or polio (and who are now experiencing deconditioning or postpolio syndrome), or from traumatic damage resulting in spinal cord and closed head injuries (leading to unexpected additional later-life impairments).

One must note, as well, that late-onset impairments are increasingly a factor in late life. Although not the issue at hand, the greater prevalence of older adults with late-onset disabilities has helped to create a broadened societal sensitivity to matters of aging and disability. In the United States, for instance, there are approximately 6.5 million people older than the age of 65 with chronic vision impairments or blindness; the majority of all blind and visually impaired Americans are adults who lost their vision after becoming elderly (Crews & Whittington, 2000). Some 11 million people older than the age of 65 have hearing impairments or deafness. In addition, approximately 6 million older adults have communication impairments (Ansello & Eustis, 1992). The estimates of older people with Alzheimer's disease or other forms of dementia keep increasing. There are unknown millions of older people with multiple impairments, and survival to later life now brings greater numbers of older adults experiencing late-onset impairments on top of lifelong impairments, such as Alzheimer's disease among older adults with Down syndrome (Janicki & Dalton, 1999).

The aging of nations has commonly outpaced developed nations' social-institutional responses to that aging (United Nations, 1998). In the United States, for example, the Social Security System of the 1930s seems not to have known a period of stability since its inception. The Older Americans Act of 1965 (PL 89-73), which addresses services for people ages 60 and older, has undergone amendments in its mandates that seemingly personify the progressive aging of America. Consider the functions of the area agencies on aging. Since 1965, their priorities and programs have evolved in focus from providing congregate meal sites to sustain the nutritional requirements of the large numbers of older adults living at the poverty level, to serving those most "at risk," the frail and the dependent, while meeting the social-recreational and self-developmental needs of older adults who may not be fully able to sustain themselves in their own homes.

Coinciding with these shifts in focus to more frail and elderly Americans have been economic considerations, especially the fiscal conservatism dictated by recession and political ideology. These generated or reinforced imperatives to serve those most in need, reshaping Older Americans Act services toward vulnerability (e.g., adult day care, ombudsman, home care services). Even the limited funds for discretionary programs that remain in the Older Americans Act have been targeted to support Medicare watchdog projects to protect vulnerable older people. The aging network, composed of the federal Administration on Aging, state units on aging, and local area agencies on aging, has become more oriented toward disabilities in later life, but this has come about essentially by medicalizing the network's existing program-centered infrastructure, which is sometimes criticized as being rather controlling or paternalistic. These matters raise the possibility of conflict with the person-centered, person-directed values that the disabilities system espouses.

The system of policy makers and practitioners in the field of developmental disabilities has itself only recently begun focusing on the aging of people with lifelong disabilities (Ansello & Rose, 1989; Janicki & Wisniewski, 1985; Seltzer, 1988). Just as the aging network has, for several reasons, become more disabilities oriented recently, so has the disabilities system become more aware of the aging of its population. The disabilities system has operationalized the belief that a focus on the early years, especially early intervention, and all the professional training, staff development, and resources that go along with it, can improve the person's life for the life course. Insightful leaders in the field (e.g., Dybwad, 1962) began calling attention to this life-span approach many years ago and are continuing to do so (Dybwad, 1999a, 1999b).

Within our communities, the increased longevity of people with serious disabilities, especially those with lifelong developmental disabilities, is an evolution every bit as significant as the mainstream aging evolution, but it is one with fewer participants. Also, this evolution seems more a product of the late 20th century; therefore, it does not enjoy the benefit of decades of increments in public consciousness. As a result, efforts to improve the quality of life of people growing old with lifelong disabilities have been sporadic, uncoordinated, and, perhaps most important, recent (Coogle, Ansello, Wood, & Cotter, 1995). There has been little history to this concern. Practitioners at the intersection of aging and developmental disabilities have, nevertheless, energized their "wit to win" (LePore & Janicki, 1997) in addressing the demands of the evolution in longevity with developmental disabilities.

Research and model projects focused on community living have broadened understanding of the needs of aging adults with lifelong disabilities and have increased awareness of the system's abilities and inabilities to meet those needs (see Section IV). Pointedly, these first efforts have often brought the aging and disabilities service systems into contact with one another. A period of mutual exploration by the systems at this intersection has demonstrated that opportunities exist for joint initiatives, exchanges, and collaborations that benefit the aging adult with lifelong disabilities.

UNPRECEDENTED CHANGES: THE FAMILY

The aging of developed nations has affected families both qualitatively and quantitatively (Hagestad, 1986). Indeed, the effect is sometimes inextricably intermixed, as when added life has triggered the creation of life stages that did not exist in either popular nomenclature or scientific study before the 20th century. The stage of life known as "adolescence" emerged at the beginning of the 20th century, made possible, and even required, by business demands for a more educated labor force and the need to limit numbers in that body. The late 20th century saw "young adulthood" recognized as a stage distinct from and interposed between adolescence and full maturity. Similarly, a prolonged life expectancy has produced the phenomenon of the "third age" (Laslett, 1991), and has stimulated both examination of the complexities inherent in having numerous years remaining beyond the satisfaction of jobs and careers and reassessment of the insufficiencies of awkwardly labeling this period as consisting of the "young-old" and "old-old."

Families now contend with offspring being at home initially for a longer period than in the past, that is, young adults still living at home in their 20s; adult children with impairments living at home or elsewhere with assistance through their young adult and middle years; and aging parents and grandparents becoming less capable and more frail with advanced age. Caregiving has become, among the aging nations, not only bidirectional but also multidirectional.

Until the mid-20th century, families of four or more generations were rare. The popular notions of the "way it used to be," with extended families pulling together for mutual benefit, has achieved mythic dimensions. Even three-generation families were not commonplace. Butler (1975) observed that, in 1920, the chance of a 10-year-old having at least two grandparents was only two in five. The aging of developed nations has meant that half of today's families contain four generations (Brody, 1985) and that caregiving may be shared among various family members. This phenomenon is particularly striking in new-immigrant or "multicultural" families (McCallion, Janicki, & Grant-Griffin, 1997).

Four generations alive means the likelihood of two generations being old or nearly so; thus, the two-generation elderly family is becoming more of a reality in disability circles. Studies (e.g., Janicki, McCallion, Force, Bishop, & LePore, 1998; McCallion & Janicki, 1997) suggest bidirectionality of exchanges between these two older generations in the case of aging with disabilities. Family caregiving by the oldest generation to the next younger is typical when the latter has aged with lifelong impairments, and, recently, skipped-generation caregiving has received attention with grandparents assuming caregiving roles for relatives with disabilities (McCallion, Janicki, Grant-Griffin, & Kolomer, 2000). Family caregiving by the second-oldest generation to the oldest describes the overwhelming majority of chronic care provided to support elders with late-onset disabilities. Seltzer (1988, 1992) cited programs to train families to be case managers for older relatives with disabilities. Doty, Jackson, and Crown (1998), using data from the 1989 National Long-Term Care Survey and the Informal Caregivers Survey, reported that almost half of the primary caregivers of older people with disabilities are themselves age 65 or older.

One of the two more significant contributors to the aging of adults with lifelong developmental disabilities is improved health care. The other contributor is the lengthened survival of parents. Advances in health care are of signal importance because improvements in treating such conditions as cardiovascular disease, diabetes, hypertension, and obesity have meant that people with lifelong impairments are better able to survive what were formerly life-stunting diseases (Evenhuis, 1999). Pharmacotherapeutic agents, such as beta blockers, have made breakthroughs in treating hypertension, angina, and irregular heartbeat. The increased longevity of parents has relevance because the majority of all people with developmental disabilities live in the community with their families. For example, Seltzer, Begun, Seltzer, and Krauss (1991) noted that across all ages fewer than 20% of people with intellectual disabilities live in a licensed residential setting. Rose and Ansello (1987) estimated that 60% of older adults with intellectual and developmental disabilities are aging in their communities without the assistance of aging, developmental disabilities, or any other formal service systems.

Families and family caregiving are central to supporting aging adults with lifelong impairments in the community (Seltzer, Begun, Magan, & Luchterhand, 1993). Families are especially critical to the relatively older members among these adults, those who have aged in their communities without assistance from formal service systems, because families provide both the money and the time necessary to sustain them (Seltzer & Krauss, 1994). Family caregiving reflects the simultaneous realities of 1) community, not institutional, living being the norm; 2) chronic care occurring in "convoys" of family and friendship networks (e.g., through parental and sibling involvement; Seltzer et al., 1991); and 3) underrecognized reliance on, and insufficient assistance to, caregivers in the family (Ansello, Coogle, & Wood, 1997). Eustis and Fischer (1992), Racino and Heumann (1992), and other researchers, of course, have argued persuasively for further incorporation of the independent living movement's emphasis on autonomy and paid, client-directed personal assistance. These calls tend to resonate with the relatively younger and middle-age adults with developmental disabilities. For older adults, families have been the sustenance of their community living (Roberto, 1993).

Family Caregivers Need Recognition

With no major increase in funding for aging network and developmental disabilities services on the horizon, especially in the United States, it seems prudent and practical to work to strengthen the capacities of family caregivers to continue their care. For them to do so, they need, at the least, recognition of their central role in the lives of so many aging adults with lifelong disabilities. Family caregivers are the unrecognized core of the long-term care system, saving governments (local, state, federal) billions of dollars in chronic care costs, and saving aging and developmental disabilities service systems from becoming further overwhelmed. Recognition is the least tangible of the needs of family caregivers, but it sets in motion ways of meeting family caregivers' other needs of reinforcement and reliable resource.

Family Caregivers Need Reinforcement

Family caregivers need added skills and knowledge to continue doing what they want most, to be left alone. Family caregivers deserve to be associated mentally and practically as part of the service system, receiving training on matters related to aging with developmental disabilities, conditions and impairments, self-health, environmental press, community resources, advocacy, and so on. Often, family caregivers have postponed their own "midlife crises" and other recognitions of their own aging because of the unrelenting requirements of their caregiving. As a result, permanency planning ("futures planning") is not common (Chapter 5). It would be prudent to strengthen the abilities of family caregivers to continue their caregiving (see Chapter 7). For policy makers, potential avenues of strengthening family caregivers include appropriations for training families, caregiving stipends or grants, tax deductions, tax credits, and service credit banking.

Family Caregivers Need Reliable Resources

Family caregivers need information on various topics (e.g., health insurance, government programs, services) that is coordinated rather than scattered among various locations, and reliable, coming from a source that is likely to be there when needed. Aging and disabilities agencies tend to overestimate the likelihood that family caregivers desire and will accept direct services from them. Outreach projects, such as those carried out in Maryland and Virginia (Ansello et al., 1997; Coogle et al., 1995), have demonstrated that outreach initiatives are a two-way bridge, carrying information to caregivers and individuals with developmental disabilities and bringing data back to agencies on the status of the caregiver and individual. Pointedly, these initiatives reveal both the family's desire to remain independent of agency direct service and the frequent frustration of that desire, by the absence of a reliable resource for the family to call upon for diverse information needs.

Amidst the aging of nations and the varying degrees of change in societal norms thereby set in motion, the family stands firmly as a major contributor to the aging in the community of adults with lifelong disabilities. To continue their commitment, families need recognition, reinforcement, and a reliable resource of information. They need, as well, to be included in service agencies' initiatives.

UNPRECEDENTED CHANGES: THE INDIVIDUAL

The aging of developed nations has meant, of course, more aging individuals. But individual "aging" is notoriously difficult to define. Reasons are multiple, from the physiological to the political. Each of us grows less alike as we grow older. The dynamic of human development increases differentiation within a group as it ages. Individuals express their aging through a variety of physical, psychological, social, and other changes, and each happens at a different rate. Indeed, within the human body the various organs (e.g., heart, lungs, kidneys, liver) age at different rates. Faced with these variabilities, legislatures have artificially pegged aging to certain chronological points; for instance, in many countries at age 60 or 65 a person typically becomes eligible to receive benefits in his or her national pension scheme.

From public policy to direct service, the practice is to generalize to groups of people of a certain age, called cohorts, rather than to recognize individuals. So, one may refer to the cohort of 1930 and plan for the group's characteristics. At the same time, one must acknowledge that biomedical advances and health-promoting lifestyles may alter the expression of aging. What was "typical" of groups of people at 65 years of age a generation ago may be more relevant today at an older chronological age, say 70 or 75 years of age. The plans for services carefully developed after studying the characteristics of the cohort of 1930 may not apply to the cohort of 1940, and so on. In any event, because group members grow less alike with age, heterogeneity increases. With larger within-group variance, there will always be individuals who do not reflect the norm, no matter how diligently the cohort is studied. In essence, the gerontological imperative of individuation makes the person-centered approach particularly relevant with aging adults with lifelong disabilities.

Individuals with lifelong disabilities are enjoying more years of life than ever before. Their "gift of time" has enabled more years as members of families and, potentially, more years of community involvement, contributions to others, and participation in disabilities and aging day programs and center activities. Longer lives also mean that aging people with lifelong disabilities may survive beyond their caregiving parents, siblings, and family members and beyond the relevance of traditional skills development or job programs (Bigby, 1997). Longer lives also mean that retirement from these work experiences, or at least a change in them, becomes a more common expectation. Furthermore, not the least of the consequences of this "gift of time" for older people with lifelong disabilities is that they enter new territory, the uncharted area between the established expertise of those who work in the field of developmental disabilities and those who work in the field of aging.

Articulate adults with lifelong disabilities, such as Kailes (1992), who spoke of her aging with cerebral palsy, and Zink (1992; Essay IV), who examined her experiences with postpolio syndrome, illustrate the challenges of aging for people with lifelong disabilities. They are growing older amidst social institutions, especially health care, that not only are unprepared to meet their needs, but also are intransigent in maintaining erroneous beliefs and practices. Kailes (1992) described the fallacy of medical opinion that her cerebral palsy was static and would not progress. She reported experiencing the natural processes of aging being superimposed on her impairments, impairments that may have been worsened by her lifelong actions to overcome them. Similarly, Zink observed (1992) that the individual reaching later life with lifelong disabilities often has fundamentally different perspectives on self-image and acceptance of assistance from a person who experiences late-onset disabilities after a life without impairments.

What might an individual with lifelong disabilities expect while growing old? What are "reasonable" responses from social institutions such as government, health care, family, and community services? At the most basic, older adults with lifelong disabilities have the same rights to personal growth as do others without such disabilities (Nowak, 1999). They are entitled to an array of services generally available to the broader, older population, that is, to have access to and to participate in various community resources that maintain, encourage, and reward us as members of our communities. Beyond this, they are entitled to the privacy, demands, wants, and other trials and tribulations that other people typically experience as they age, including the expression through self-advocacy of what they will do with their own lives.

Integral to personal growth is the exercise of choice and self-determination (Dybwad, 1999a, 1999b; Levitz, 1999). Choice needs to be informed, so aging adults can define, when it is appropriate, what long-range planning can be most useful to them. This planning may emphasize skills acquisition, promote independent self-care, and introduce rewarding use of leisure time, as well as help sustain current skills. Individuals with lifelong disabilities may require lifelong assistance. However, such assistance does not need to subrogate the individual or eliminate the exercise of choice. Individuals with lifelong disabilities are entitled to "assisted autonomy" to help them remain as independent in their community as possible.

Moody (1992) maintained that the concept of autonomy has an uneasy application to the elderly. The concept has become distorted and misunderstood in contemporary culture, being evoked and chanted unthinkingly such that it has achieved sacred status, like human rights and justice, and is "acclaimed, publicly at least, as our supreme virtue" (Moody, 1992, p. 3). The theory of autonomy is translated in practice as individualism, self-control, and independence from others. Moody resisted extending this practice to older people because the concept fails to consider their deepest needs. Blindly upholding autonomy ignores the conditions into which their years and impairments may have placed them and contradicts their fundamental human needs for respect, meaning, care, and social connections.

> We are compelled, I believe, to widen our perspective and to shift our attention to another ideal, the ideal of human dignity. The conventional discourse of modern ethics, deriving from Kant and the Enlightenment, tends to make "dignity," "respect for persons," "individual rights," and "autonomy" all somehow equivalent to one another or at least bound together in essential ways. That conceptual equivalence is one I want to resist. Dignity does not completely coincide with the ideals of autonomy and individualism enshrined in our liberal culture and in the language of bioethics. Dignity is far more bound up with the interpersonal and social fabric than with isolated acts of rational deliberation or consent. (Moody, 1992, p. 4)

Moody (1992), discussing the ethics of long-term care, differentiated between "choice" autonomy (being able to select options) and "resolution" autonomy (being able to carry out those options). For aging individuals with impairments, exercising either form of autonomy, as well as settling a disconnection between choice and resolution, will likely require negotiation with and assistance by others. This process, being interpersonal and social, confirms the individual's human dignity rather than denying it. The process that we call *assisted autonomy* is relevant to aging with lifelong disabilities.

Consistent with assisted autonomy are initiatives on cash and counseling personal assistance models (see Chapter 13); modifying home environments (see Chapter 14); planning for later life and retirement (see Chapter 11); and health promotion and disease prevention (see Chapters 12 and 17), as well as several others that not only recognize the human needs of aging adults with lifelong disabilities, but also act to respond positively to them.

Successful aging is the goal modern gerontologists have espoused for aging adults. The definition of "successful," however, has eluded consensus over the years. Lengthy, multidisciplinary, multisite collaborations (e.g., Rowe & Kahn, 1998) supported by the MacArthur Foundation in the United States have culminated in definitions of and prescriptions for success that are receiving approbation from many in the scientific and gerontological communities. Rowe and Kahn maintained that aging has different dimensions. At its most basic, aging is either pathological or normal. Pathological aging occurs when adults are affected by diseases or age-related disabilities. Normal aging is further differentiated as either usual or successful. Usual aging is seen as nonpathologic; that is, it describes elders who are functioning well, yet are at substantial risk for disease and disability. The problem, Rowe and Kahn (1998) maintained, is that we accept decline as being normal with age. Many succumb to this categorization of aging. Successful aging is when there is a low risk for pathology and strong evidence of high function. Because successful aging is seen as the ideal and the model evolving from this concept has gained broad attention, it is worth exploring its applicability to older adults with lifelong disability (Janicki, 1999).

Successful aging, as defined by Rowe and Kahn (1998), includes three main components: avoiding disease or disease-related disability, maintaining high cognitive and physical function, and engaging with life. Behind this theory are the questions of how aging affects older adults and whether the adults are functioning adaptively as they age. A connecting factor is the extent to which older adults are actively engaged with life. Rowe and Kahn (1998) operationalized the three components as follows:

- Low probability of disease reflects the absence, presence, or severity of risk factors for disease.
- High functional level draws on a combination of physical and cognitive capacities for personal activity (i.e., what a person can or cannot do).
- Active engagement concerns productive activity and interpersonal relations (defined as contacts and transactions with others, exchange of information, emotional support, and direct assistance).

Successful aging, thus, draws on the confluence of demonstrated good health, capacity for and display of socialization and productivity, and faculty for self-discipline. It means having the ability to maintain one's physical and cognitive health, having control over life choices, and giving of oneself in a manner that is fulfilling and productive. There is ample support for this conceptualization. As Strawbridge, Cohen, Shema, and Kaplan (1996) noted, those adults considered to be aging successfully generally have greater involvement in their community, engage in more physical activity, and demonstrate better mental health. In addition, lifelong exercise of control may be a critical factor in successful aging (Schulz & Heckhausen, 1996), as may interaction with social structures (Riley, 1998).

What are this concept's implications for growing older with a lifelong disability? Can it be argued that successful aging does not apply to adults already compromised by disability? Rowe and Kahn (1998) are silent in this regard; yet inherent in their conceptualization is the equation that the presence of disability may be incompatible with successful aging. However, this may not be the case, particularly when applied to adults with lifelong disabilities whose physical status is not further compromised (see Schulz & Heckhausen, 1996). A lifelong disability may not be an impediment to healthy or successful aging if there are no significant medical aspects to the disability, if the individual has developed productive coping skills and compensatory mechanisms during adulthood, and if the individual has maintained lifelong autonomy or control over his or her life activities.

Because Rowe and Kahn (1998) viewed successful aging as the combination of avoiding debilitation, disease, and disability (as opposed to impairment); maintaining high physical and cognitive function; and sustaining engagement in social and productive activities, a range of support strategies must figure in addressing these aspects. Assisted autonomy may help individuals with lifelong disabilities realize successful aging. Through a process of negotiated assistance, supports can be designed to help maintain health and physical capacities, provide intellectually and physically stimulating environments, and ensure that meaningful social networks and community engagement reinforce the process of aging.

IMPLICATIONS FOR AN AGING NATION

The implications of the aging of nations are at once both simple and profound. On the large scale, nations and their communities need to adjust to the demographic imperative of aging, the widespread broadcast of the gift of time that is bringing longer lives to all members of the population. Families need recognition and reinforcement so that their vital roles in the well-being of aging adults with lifelong disabilities can be sustained. At the personal level, individuals themselves need encouragement to exercise choice and self-determination, and the correlated supports to make these happen. They need assisted autonomy to become an everyday reality in their lives.

Having said this, we note that implementing these simple needs presents profound challenges. There is no historical text to which we can refer. The aging of nations is an unprecedented phenomenon. Some fundamental responses to the implications are as follows.

For the Population

Indications are that the aging of populations in developed nations will increase, and that this imperative will progressively affect the developing nations as well over the next several decades (see Figure 1). Each nation will need to develop a more comprehensive accounting of the number of its aging citizens whose needs are driven by their lifelong physical or cognitive disabilities. This accounting will need to be the engine that drives a more inclusionary public policy at each level of governance. At the same time, nations

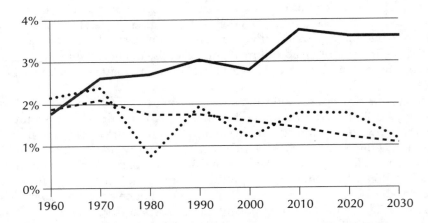

Figure 1. Average annual percentage growth in the segment of nations' populations ages 60 years and older, showing that elderly populations are growing fastest in developing countries because of their initially low numbers of older people. (*Key:* ▬▬ , less developed countries; ▪ ▪ ▪ , more developed countries; ••••, worldwide. Adapted from U.S. Department of Commerce, Economics and Statistics Administration, U.S. Bureau of the Census. [1999, December]. *Global aging into the 21st century* [Wallchart]. Washington, DC: Author.)

will have to recognize the principle of individuation within the growth of their older populations, that is, the fact that aging individuals are not a unitary phenomenon, that each age cohort differs from others, and that people and their needs are both different and diverse. The contemporary generations of aging adults tend to be relatively healthy and vigorous, expecting to be involved in their communities and to be less reliant upon social and health care structures. There is every reason to believe that these expectations will materialize among aging individuals with lifelong disabilities as well.

For Families

As the nature of disabilities included under the umbrella of lifelong intellectual and developmental disabilities expands, so must the recognition that families are the primary caregivers for many older adults with lifelong disabilities. As researchers conduct more investigations with a family-oriented focus, we are learning more about the dynamics of family caregiving, futures planning, and transitions. This expanded interest is of great value because it will provide the necessary information to design responsive services and supports. Families need recognition, reinforcement, and reliable resources in their communities. Actions to strengthen families can occur at national and various jurisdictional levels; these can include legislated initiatives such as tax credits and grants for family caregivers, community-based education and training on disabilities-related and self-care topics, simpler referral to existing resources, flexible employment schemes to sustain work and caregiving, and so on. Strengthening the family caregivers of aging individuals will also help younger parents to prepare for the future and enable individuals with lifelong disabilities to move toward greater independence without compromising their relationships with their parents or other family caregivers.

For the Individual

Aging adults with lifelong disabilities vary greatly in their life settings, orientations to formal and informal supports, aspirations, and the gamut of physical, behavioral, and psychosocial characteristics that mark each human as an individual. Broadly speaking, older cohorts of individuals with lifelong disabilities tend to have grown old in their communities with the help of family caregivers who may or may not have sought assistance from formal service systems. Their experiences of assisted autonomy are qualitatively different from those of younger cohorts who more often have benefited from legislated support services, coordinated formal service systems, and advocated for rights and self-care. The most basic implication is that, for aging individuals, one size does not fit all.

Individuals with lifelong disabilities should expect to grow older with the same rights to personal growth that others enjoy. Negotiated assistance should enable their participation in community activities, their taking opportunities for interpersonal relationships, and their living of lives that allow for privacy, success, and failure.

CONCLUSIONS

The risk of a huge evolution like the aging of nations is that the single case, the individual, is lost in a sea of consequences. The intention of this chapter's overview has been to keep sight of the individual, while fixing him or her in a larger perspective, whether it be a family context, a neighborhood or community, or a state or nation. The purpose of formalized service systems must be to sustain the individual's human dignity, regardless of the level of the individual's disabilities.

It is hoped that the community supports that we describe (and that the other contributors to this book amplify) put flesh to the skeleton of assisted autonomy. Collectively, the contributors speak from their experiences at the broader macrospective level. They relate their involvement with families and others who provide support. They share their acquired expertise on what helps to make everyday community living work for aging adults with lifelong disabilities.

REFERENCES

Alliance for Aging Research. (1996). *Will you still treat me when I'm 65?* Washington, DC: Author.

Ansello, E.F., Coogle, C.L., & Wood, J.B. (1997). *Partners: Building inter-system cooperation in aging with developmental disabilities.* Richmond: Virginia Center on Aging, Virginia Commonwealth University.

Ansello, E.F., & Eustis, N.N. (1992). A common stake? Investigating the emerging intersection of aging and disabilities. *Generations, 16,* 5–8.

Ansello, E.F., & Rose, T. (1989). *Aging and lifelong disabilities: Partnership for the twenty-first century.* Palm Springs, CA: Elvirita Lewis Foundation.

Bigby, C. (1997). Later life for adults with intellectual disability: A time of opportunity and vulnerability. *Journal of Intellectual and Developmental Disabilities, 22,* 97–108

Brody, E.M. (1985). Parent care as a normative family stress. *Gerontologist, 25*(1), 19–29.

Butler, R.N. (1975). *Why survive? Being old in America.* New York: Harper & Row.

Coogle, C.L., Ansello, E.F., Wood, J.B., & Cotter, J.J. (1995). Partners II—Serving older persons with developmental disabilities: Obstacles and inducements to collaboration among agencies. *Journal of Applied Gerontology, 14,* 275–288.

Crews, J.E., & Whittington, F.J. (Eds.). (2000). *Vision loss in an aging society: A multidisciplinary perspective.* New York: American Foundation for the Blind Press.

Doty, P., Jackson, M.E., & Crown, W. (1998). The impact of female caregivers' employment status on patterns of formal and informal eldercare. *Gerontologist, 38,* 331–341.

Dybwad, G. (1962). Administrative and legislative problems in the care of the adult and aged mentally retarded. *American Journal on Mental Deficiency, 66,* 716–722.

Dybwad, G. (1999a). Foreword. In S.S. Herr & G. Weber (Eds.), *Aging, rights, and quality of life: Prospects for older people with developmental disabilities* (pp. xv–xviii). Baltimore: Paul H. Brookes Publishing Co.

Dybwad, G. (1999b). Self-determination: Influencing public policy. In M.A. Allard, A.M. Howard, L.E. Vorderer, & A.I. Wells (Eds.), *Selected speeches of Gunnar Dybwad: Ahead of his time* (pp. 145–149). Washington, DC: American Association on Mental Retardation.

Eustis, N.N., & Fischer, L.R. (1992). Common needs, different solutions? Younger and older homecare clients. In E.F. Ansello & N.N. Eustis (Eds.), *Aging and disabilities: Seeking common ground* (pp. 25–37). Amityville, NY: Baywood Publishing Co.

Evenhuis, H. (1999). Associated medical aspects. In M.P. Janicki & A.J. Dalton (Eds.), *Dementia, aging, and intellectual disabilities: A handbook* (pp. 103–118). Philadelphia: Brunner/Mazel.

Hagestad, G.O. (1986). The aging society as a context for family life. *Daedalus, the Journal of the American Academy of Arts and Sciences, 115*(1), 119–139.

Jacobson, J.W, Sutton, M.S., & Janicki, M.P. (1985). Planning for an older developmentally disabled population. In M.P. Janicki & H.M. Wisniewski (Eds.), *Aging and developmental disabilities: Issues and approaches* (pp. 143–160). Baltimore: Paul H. Brookes Publishing Co.

Janicki, M.P. (1999). Public policy and service design. In S.S. Herr & G. Weber (Eds.), *Aging, rights, and quality of life: Prospects for older people with developmental disabilities* (pp. 289–310). Baltimore: Paul H. Brookes Publishing Co.

Janicki, M.P., & Dalton, A.J. (Eds.). (1999). *Dementia, aging, and intellectual disabilities: A handbook.* Philadelphia: Brunner/Mazel.

Janicki, M.P., McCallion, P., Force, L., Bishop, K., & LePore, P. (1998). Area agency on aging outreach and assistance for households with older carers of an adult with a developmental disability. *Journal of Aging and Social Policy, 10,* 13–36.

Janicki, M.P., & Wisniewski, H.M. (Eds.). (1985). *Aging and developmental disabilities: Issues and approaches*. Baltimore: Paul H. Brookes Publishing Co.

Kailes, J.I. (1992). Aging with a disability: Educating myself. In E.F. Ansello & N.N. Eustis (Eds.), *Aging and disabilities: Seeking common ground* (pp. 149–156). Amityville, NY: Baywood Publishing Co.

Laslett, P. (1991). *A fresh map of life: The emergence of the third age*. Cambridge, MA: Harvard University Press.

LePore, P., & Janicki, M.P. (1997). *The wit to win: How to integrate older persons with developmental disabilities into aging network programs*. Albany: New York State Office for the Aging.

Levitz, M. (1999). Self-advocacy for a good life in our older years. In S.S. Herr & G. Weber (Eds.), *Aging, rights, and quality of life: Prospects for older people with developmental disabilities* (pp. 279–287). Baltimore: Paul H. Brookes Publishing Co.

McCallion, P., & Janicki, M.P. (1997). Area agencies on aging: Meeting the needs of persons with developmental disabilities and their aging families. *Journal of Applied Gerontology, 16*, 270–284.

McCallion, P., Janicki, M.P., Grant-Griffin, L., & Kolomer, S.R. (2000). Grandparent caregivers II: Service needs and service provision issues. *Journal of Gerontological Social Work, 33*(3), 63–90.

McCallion, P., Janicki, M.P., & Grant-Griffin, L. (1997). Exploring the impact of culture and acculturation on older families caregiving for persons with developmental disabilities. *Family Relations, 46*, 347–357.

Moody, H.R. (1992). *Ethics in an aging society*. Baltimore: The Johns Hopkins University Press.

Murray, C.J.L., & Lopez, A.D. (1996). *The global burden of disease: A comprehensive assessment of mortality and disability from diseases, injuries, and risk factors in 1990 and projected to 2030 (Summary)*. Geneva: World Health Organization.

Nowak, M. (1999). International human rights standards: Aging and disabilities. In S.S. Herr & G. Weber (Eds.), *Aging, rights, and quality of life: Prospects for older people with developmental disabilities* (pp. 33–43). Baltimore: Paul H. Brookes Publishing Co.

Older Americans Act of 1965, PL 89-73, 42 U.S.C. §§ 3001 et seq.

Peterson, P.G. (1999). Gray dawn: The global aging crisis. *Foreign Affairs, 78*(1), 42–55.

Racino, J.A., & Heumann, J.E. (1992). Independent living and community life: Building coalitions among elders, people with disabilities, and our allies. In E.F. Ansello & N.N. Eustis (Eds.), *Aging and disabilities: Seeking common ground* (pp. 79–90). Amityville, NY: Baywood Publishing Co.

Riley, M.W. (1998). Response to "successful aging." *Gerontologist, 38*, 151.

Roberto, K.A. (1993). *The elderly caregiver: Caring for adults with developmental disabilities*. Thousand Oaks, CA: Sage Publications.

Rose, T., & Ansello, E.F. (1987). *Aging and developmental disabilities: Research and planning*. Final Report to the Maryland Planning Council on Developmental Disabilities. College Park: The University of Maryland Center on Aging.

Rowe, J.W., & Kahn, R.L. (1998). *Successful aging*. New York: Pantheon.

Schulz, R., & Heckhausen, J. (1996). A life span model of successful aging. *American Psychologist, 51*, 702–714.

Seltzer, G.B., Begun, A., Magan, R., & Luchterhand, C. (1993). Social supports and expectations of family involvement after out of home placement. In E. Sutton, T. Heller, A.R. Factor, B.A. Hawkins, & G.B. Seltzer (Eds.), *Older adults with developmental disabilities: Optimizing choice and change* (pp. 123–140). Baltimore: Paul H. Brookes Publishing Co.

Seltzer, G.B., Begun, A., Seltzer, M., & Krauss, M. (1991). Adults with mental retardation and their aging mothers: Impacts of siblings. *Family Relations, 40*, 310–317.

Seltzer, M.M. (1988). Structure and patterns of service utilization by elderly persons with mental retardation. *Mental Retardation, 26*, 181–186.

Seltzer, M.M. (1992). Family caregiving across the full lifespan. In L. Rowitz (Ed.), *Mental retardation in the year 2000* (pp. 85–100). New York: Springer-Verlag.

Seltzer, M.M., & Krauss, M.W. (1994). Aging parents with coresident adult children: The impact of lifelong caring. In M.M. Seltzer, M.W. Krauss, & M.P. Janicki (Eds.), *Life course perspectives on adulthood and old age* (pp. 3–18). Washington, DC: American Association on Mental Retardation.

Strawbridge, W.J., Cohen, R.D., Shema, S.J., & Kaplan, G.A. (1996). Successful aging: Predictors and associated activities. *American Journal of Epidemiology, 144*, 135–141.

U.S. Bureau of the Census. (1998, December). *International data base* [On-line]. Available http://www.census.gov/cgi-bin/ipc/idbsum.

U.S. Department of Commerce, Economics and Statistics Administration, U.S. Bureau of the Census. (1999, December). *Global aging into the 21st century* [Wallchart]. Washington, DC: Author.

United Nations. (1998). *International plan of action on ageing and United Nations principles for older persons*. New York: Author.

Zink, J.B. (1992). Adjusting to early- and late-onset disability: A personal perspective. In E.F. Ansello & N.N. Eustis (Eds.), *Aging and disabilities: Seeking common ground* (pp. 111–114). Amityville, NY: Baywood Publishing Co.

2

Learning from
Quality-of-Life Models

Roy I. Brown

Since the late 1970s, the concept of quality of life has been expanded considerably as it relates to developmental disabilities. Much of this change has occurred with adolescents and adults, but there are obvious implications for older adults. Raphael (1996) and Brown (1989) suggested that quality-of-life concepts and the research associated with them have the potential to help optimize the aging experience, and Ory and Cox (1994) noted that a change in attitudes toward elderly people has brought new emphasis to the relevance of quality-of-life concepts for this age group. With this in mind, this chapter draws on studies that are particularly concerned with adults and relate to middle- and older-age adults with intellectual disabilities (defined as individuals 45 years of age and older).

As a sensitizing process, the concept of quality of life has much to recommend because it enables us to view disability from a different and personal perspective (Taylor, 1994). Much of the early work in this area (e.g., Andrews & Withey, 1976) set the scene by recognizing the importance of personal perception in promoting behavior (i.e., subjective or perceptual and objective measures of behavior being recognized as determinants of well-being). Authors such as R.I. Brown (1997a, 1997b), Dossa (1989), Goode (1994), Renwick, Brown, and Nagler (1996), and Schalock (1998) contributed to conceptualizations of quality of life as it relates to the field of intellectual disabilities.

Edgerton, in his foreword to Goode, noted the importance of the person–environment interaction and believes, whatever the difficulties, that developments in intellectual disabilities focus "squarely on quality of life issues" (1994, p. ii). Many of the authors noted previously recognize that quality of life as a field of interest needs to focus on the perceptions of the individual with a disability, on that person's views of interactions with the environment, and on concerns relating to the construct of the environment by people with disabilities. In many ways, these issues have been developing over the years within the field of intellectual disability, and now have been incorporated into the quality-of-life framework, with the result that we now look at disability from a new standpoint. Assessment, service delivery, intervention, policy development, research, and evaluation for older adults with intellectual disabilities are all influenced by such thinking.

Edgerton (1994) and others recognized that it is only too easy to trivialize the concept of quality of life, for it is complex and not easily measured. It is diverse in character and its qualities are as individual as the number of people involved in defining it. Furthermore, there are those such as Wolfensberger (1994) who believe that defining such concepts as quality of life is dangerous. Wolfensberger's fears are centered on several issues related to definition and measurement. He proposed that the notion of quality of life, if reduced simplistically to quantitative units and assessment and based purely on tools designed to measure life quality from only a professional perspective, would lead to a travesty of science. Wolfensberger recognized that the concept and attributes of a quality-of-life model can be "hijacked" by different parties who have their own agendas for "purifying" society. But this is true of all sciences, and all discoveries can be used by any community for inappropriate means.

It is important at the outset to clarify that this chapter does not discuss some of the medical and economic applications by which quality of life is defined and calibrated in terms of scales based on professional and allied judgments, which result in such measures as quality-of-life years (QALYS). Cummins (1997), similar to Brown (1997c), believes that such methods are scientifically and socially unacceptable and serve to support Wolfensberger's (1994) argument regarding the potentially negative impacts of concepts such as quality of life. Such arguments are directed specifically to the needs of individuals with the accent on perceptions of life as recognized by these individuals. Thus the questions are, "How do individuals with an intellectual disability view their experiences?" and "What type of needs do they say they have and what form of experiences do they seek?" Despite the need to see quality of life from the individual's perspective, Andrews suggested that there are "broad similarities across people both in the structure of their perceptions of life components and in how they integrate those perceptions in evaluating well-being" (1974, p. 289).

A range of quality-of-life principles have now been established and are accepted by researchers and practitioners, such as I. Brown (1996), R.I. Brown (1997c), Cummins (1997), Goode (1994), Parmenter (1994), and Schalock (1997), who practice in the field of intellectual disability, and other researchers, such as Renwick and colleagues (1996), who have detailed this notion within the field of acquired immunodeficiency syndrome (AIDS), adolescent development, mental health, and allied areas. Raphael (1997) and Hatton (1998) discussed critically these conceptualizing principles. Because both improving and deteriorating quality of life, as phenomena, cannot be judged effectively by professionals separately from the individual experiencing these changes, a sociological and psychological conceptualization of quality of life has been established, which, although complex, relates clearly and specifically to personal perceptions and choices within the context described here. However, this conflicts with the health and economical rationalist views of quality of life, a topic that is discussed in some detail by Brown (2000).[1]

Thus, there appears to be a lack of unanimity as to how to approach these issues. Romney, Brown, and Fry (1994) itemized some of the controversies. Some of the concerns relate to the plethora of definitions, the varieties of taxonomies in terms of classification of the main features of quality of life, and the problems of viewing quality of life from the standpoint of specific professionals who are specializing in a specific disease disability (e.g., cardiac problems). Furthermore, there are issues raised around the development of theoretical foundations for quality-of-life models and the fact that the multidimensionality of the concept makes it difficult to understand the interaction of the multiplicity of variables in establishing an individual's quality of life. Added to this is the fact that quality of life can change over time and, because it may vary in relation to minor changes in personal or environmental factors, a host of scientific challenges must be addressed. Cultural factors complicate the issue further because different values may have diverse effects and therefore structure individual perceptions differently in various societies. Despite this, it is apparent, as Romney et al. (1994) stressed, that considerable gains have been made in theoretical construction and multimeasurement at both the quantitative and the qualitative levels. Gradually, in terms of application, an effort has been made to enhance individual well-being, and these concepts are being applied to the aging population with disabilities (Ory & Cox, 1994).

DEFINING QUALITY OF LIFE

Definitions of *quality of life* abound (see Table 1). They tend to be value-laden, differ between and within societies and different professional groups, and are influenced by the ephemeral nature of some of the components involved. If one accepts this, then the attributes of diversity, individuality, and change become important constructs in both the definition and application of quality of life. However, similar to Crick (1994) in trying to define *consciousness*, any attempt to bring exact precision to the definition would restrict the changing and growing understanding of the construct.

In this chapter, *quality of life* is defined as a multidimensional concept involving personal well-being across life domains within the context of an individual's met and unmet needs and desires (see Brown, Bayer, & MacFarlane, 1989; Felce & Perry, 1997). Felce and Perry (1997) noted that, although this form of conceptualization has developed in the field of intellectual disability, it also is relevant to the greater population. Brown (2000) noted that the construct is not necessarily disability based and, from psychological and sociological perspectives, enables us to view the individual and his or her needs rather than examine the label of disability. Brown, Bayer, and MacFarlane (1988) also suggested that *quality of life* can be defined as the extent to which an individual increasingly controls his or her environment, regardless of initial baseline.

---

[1]Brown (2000) believes that the development of the quality-of-life model is a direct challenge to economic rationalism in that it accents individual needs and perceptions, recognizes the importance of personal empowerment, and requires recognition of choice. It therefore precipitates arguments about the nature of government policy and service management, and the ways in which funds are deployed. It argues that personal control enhances self-image and, therefore, motivation and growth, thus conflicting with the prevailing attitudes toward congregate or group settings, education, and training within and beyond the disabilities field.

Table 1.   Definitions of quality of life

Author(s)	Quality of life is . . .
Cummins (1997)	Both objective and subjective, involving material well-being, health, productivity, intimacy, safety, community and emotional well-being
Felce and Perry (1997)	A multidimensional concept involving personal well-being; is concerned with intimate relationships, family life, friendships, standard of living, work, neighborhood, city or town of residence, the state of the nation, housing, education, health and self
Goode (1997)	An emphasis on promoting general feelings or perceptions of well-being, opportunities to fulfill potential and feelings of positive social involvement
Goode (1988)	Experienced when a person's basic needs are met and when he or she has the opportunity to pursue and achieve goals in major life settings
Brown, Bayer, and MacFarlane (1989)	The discrepancy between a person's unmet needs and desires, refers to the subjective or perceived as well as objective assessment, relates to all life domains, and recognizes interaction between individual and environment.
Renwick, Brown, and Nagler (1996)	The degree to which an individual enjoys important possibilities of his or her life

Schalock (1997) provided a simple and pragmatic definition involving a person's desired conditions of living, which relate primarily to home and community living, school or work, and health and wellness. Happiness also comes into some definitions. This gives rise to some conceptual problems because, as R.I. Brown (1996b) indicated, perceived quality of life can increase while happiness decreases as the individual gains control of choice and increases his or her range of perception in relation to needs. Renwick and Brown viewed quality of life as "the degree to which a person enjoys the important possibilities of his or her life" (1996, p. 80). They also provided a useful and practical conceptualization of the concept in terms of "being" (i.e., who the person is as an individual), "belonging" (i.e., how environments and others fit with the person), and "becoming" (i.e., what a person does to achieve hopes, goals, and aspirations).

PRINCIPLES OF QUALITY OF LIFE

At this juncture, it is useful to provide a brief account of the major principles recognized within the field of quality of life as they apply to aging and intellectual disabilities. The application of such ideas takes away from traditional labeling systems (e.g., intellectual disability and its subcategories) and moves toward a range of general principles that can apply regardless of classification. Although levels of well-being as perceived by people with disabilities may change over time, requiring adjustments to practice and intervention, the principles are fundamental and represent a reasonable consensus amongst those working in this field.

Well-Being

This notion represents an individual's range of experiences. Certain aspects may predominate at certain stages of the life span and differ in accent from individual to individual. A broad range of relevant areas can apply; however, Felce and Perry (1997) reduced these to five major categories: social well-being, emotional well-being, productive well-being, material well-being, and physical well-being. Under each of these constructs is a wide range of subcategories (see Figure 1). Schalock (1998) also included a dimension of individual rights that should not be overlooked. This last dimension, along with home and community issues, companionship, recreation, reminiscence, and fitness, is particularly important to defining well-being in the lives of aging adults. Ory and Cox (1994) noted the importance in conceptualizing health and behavior, as well as of the interaction between social and physical environments and health conditions and their influences on whether disabilities become handicaps.

Holism

This notion refers to the need to consider quality of life from the perspective of the whole individual, recognizing that different aspects of life as perceived from the inside have a different and frequently unintegrated meaning from the individual's perspective. The individual's perspective also is influenced by his or her experiences and personal hopes. Thus, each area of well-being is related to the other. To intervene or provide support to an individual in one domain requires examination, understanding, and frequently intervention in other domains. In other words, aspects of life cannot be separated at a practical level. Improvement in an area of well-being may require primary intervention in other aspects of well-being (e.g., improvement in leisure may influence well-being in health or accommodation). Likewise, deterioration in one aspect of well-being may result in a decline in another (e.g., loneliness may adversely influence physical health and activity levels). Furthermore, the introduction of physical and environmental adaptations can influence both health and behavior.

Life Span

The extension of life span among people with lifelong disabilities highlights the importance of optimizing experiences prior to old age. What occurs to individuals at any one developmental stage is determined to a considerable degree by what has previously occurred to them, including the attitudes and values of those people with whom they have been involved, such as members of their family and other primary caregivers. Each age stage, then, is not isolated from the previous or following experiences and must be recognized as forming part of the whole and, in part, determining future outcomes. The absence of a close partner or marriage is likely to reduce longevity and supports in later life. The quality of life in individuals' later years is, to some considerable degree, affected by their previous experiences.

Choice

Quality of life requires that we recognize the choices of people with disabilities and that we actively seek these while designing and developing programs, health systems, or social policies. It has been argued that responding to choice may be difficult when working with people with very limited intellectual abilities. However, as indicated by Brown

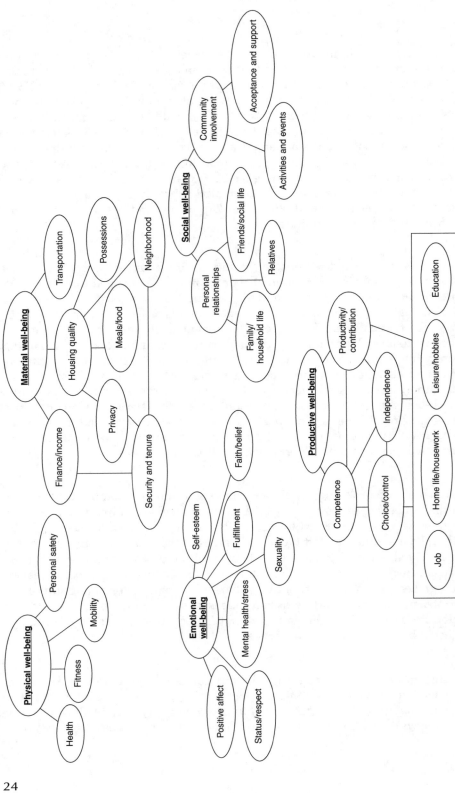

Figure 1. Domains relevant to quality of life for people with disabilities. (From Felce, D., & Perry, J. [1997]. Quality of life: The scope of the term and its breadth of measurement. In R.I. Brown [Ed.], *Quality of life for people with disabilities: Models, research and practice* [p. 57]. Cheltenham, UK: Stanley Thornes; reproduced with the permission of Nelson Thornes, copyright © 1997.)

24

et al. (1989), it is important that choices, however simple, should be explored despite the fact that the individuals may have minimal control of their environment for, without such attention, individuals will not be empowered and self-image and motivation are likely to decrease. In older individuals, particularly if they share accommodation with people other than life partners, choices over privacy, quiet times, or even where personal belongings are placed, are likely to be restricted (Brown, 1999). Different situations bring "trade-offs" in choices—but who decides the range of the "trade-offs"?

Personal Perception

One of the major aspects of the quality-of-life models is the critical role of personal perception. It is recognized, and perhaps best expressed by Andrews (1974), that people respond to what they perceive rather than objective reality. Perception is the way people view their experiences and environment, and is an interaction of sensations modified by previous experience and motivation. Perceptions of external events are much influenced by self-image. The way people perceive their environment is critical for their behavior and development, and has often been dismissed or minimized within habilitation or intervention practices, as well as within our support structures. In many quality-of-life studies, personal perceptions are regarded as subjective, and it is this subjective view that has brought about criticism (see Cummins, 1997). There is little doubt that complexities associated with personal perception give rise to problems and challenges in terms of measurement. However, most researchers agree that both subjective and objective measures are important. Studies suggest that such perceptions may be regarded as much more objective than has been previously recognized. Brown, Bayer, and Brown (1992), for example, suggested that the views of individuals can be recognized through verbal statement or action, and are frequently found to be repeatable and reliable, characteristics that are important for any objective scientific study. Changes in behavioral performance over time are more likely to relate to changing experiences and variation in the person's control of the environment than unreliable measurement. This, in itself, has major implications for the development of self-image, motivation, and empowerment, which are critical for effective development as well as control of one's environment. The perceptions that older adults with disabilities have of their care and support staff are likely to be a prime determinant of their cooperation, health, and longevity.

Empowerment

Quality-of-life models argue for empowering environments, that is, providing environments that encourage activity, decision making, and control by the individual. An individual's autonomy is enhanced through internal locus of control—in other words, the individual attempts to make his or her own decisions and carry out his or her intended actions without direction from others. The degree to which this can be done depends partly on the individual and requires flexible policy making and sensitive personnel. An agency that does not encourage individual autonomy can effectively reduce an individual's quality of life, not only in terms of satisfaction and well-being, but also in terms of experience and well-being in the longer term. Internal locus of control, even when support is required, ensures greater autonomy and, therefore, not only enhances activity but also often reduces the likelihood of abuse, which is physically and psychologically more likely to occur when the individual is totally dependent and under the control of others (see H. Brown, 1997).

Variability

Quality-of-life models accent the notion of within-group variability. Researchers have often been concerned with differences between groups. In quality-of-life research, however, there is interest in the differences that occur between individuals in the same group. This has often been regarded from a statistical point of view as error, but here it is considered to include aspects of individual responses, which are associated with personal variables. Indeed, this underscores the impact of quality-of-life models on research design by questioning the appropriateness of traditional control variables and recognizing that such variables as personal choice and self-image may play dominant roles in determining individual responsiveness to changes in the environment. Thus, it would be expected that such variability is increased through recognition of choice and that the older adult should be accepted in terms of his or her presenting needs, regardless of classification or label. Responses of professionals need to be at an individual level, and it is recognized that in responding this way, traditional group situations may be found to be unsuitable.

These features are critical to an understanding of quality of life in the field of aging and in people with lifelong disabilities. Evaluating these principles in the context of any aging individual with a lifelong disability will result in the development of fresh policies, more personally oriented planning, and sensitive professional involvement. The following section discusses these principles within the context of quality-of-life applications for such adults.

APPLICATION OF THE QUALITY-OF-LIFE MODEL

The previous discussion underscored the relevance of well-being across life domains, along with personal control and input into lifestyles at all stages of the life span. As Hogg and Moss (1990) indicated, the application of these concepts is critical for any lifespan practice for successful aging. Furthermore, they appear necessary as a foundation for service planning (Hogg & Lambe, 1997). Such concepts have implications for policy development, management, and service delivery for those who are aging and have lifelong disabilities (Brown, 1999).

Successful aging (i.e., aging associated with optimum health, psychological stability, and personal/social control; see Rowe & Kahn, 1998, for a fuller explanation) within this context implies the recognition of an individual's perceptions and the acceptance of these perceptions within models of intervention or support. This does not necessarily mean that anything an older individual says is accepted as objectively or externally valid. It assumes statements or behavior (when nonverbal) reflect interests or concerns of the older individual, and that overtly recognizing these affects both self-image and satisfaction. Other factors, such as the views of other parties and external objective data, also are relevant, even though quality-of-life research points out the dangers of accepting the opinions of relevant others as valid from the older individual's perspective. Even highly skilled caregivers can misunderstand what is desired or is desirable from the individual's perspective and, increasingly, quality-of-life research recognizes that such different views may arise from different perspectives and realities. Each may have validity in its own right but the individual's perception has a special relevancy because it directly reflects that individual's concerns.

Accenting Consumer Control

When individuals are older and have disabilities, there is a danger of services dehumanizing the individual by removing access and control. Quality-of-life models require policy makers, managers of organizations, practicing professionals, and family members to ensure that there is maximization of consumer control. The effects of changing environment and unfamiliarity are known to diminish responsiveness in older people with disabilities, and the loss of possessions and the rearrangement of lifestyles from individualized to congregate care facilities for the elderly can result in reduction of personal control and expression.

Accessibility and Control

In care provision there are concerns over the nature of and accessibility to the physical environment. Such concerns may cause environments to be redesigned; however, such adaptations may not meet the aspects of safety and access perceived as important by aging individuals (Ferguson, 1997). Frequently, their issues may relate to perceptions that, from a policy point of view, may seem inconsequential. Having ensured that the environment is physically safe, it may be regarded by authorities as a suitable environment for people who are elderly and who have disabilities. Yet the individuals themselves may not perceive safety within their environment and may have concerns that can cause anxiety and reduce responsiveness. Brown, Matthews, and Taylor (1997), for example, in carrying out quality-of-life assessments, found that aging individuals with intellectual disability who are said to be in a safe environment can have a wide range of fears and anxieties that relate to their lack of control over the events that take place. Furthermore, an aging person may have a sensory difficulty, such as poor dark adaptation, that leaves him or her less able to interpret the signs and signals within the environment, thus causing anxiety and frustration (I. Brown, 1994).

Sensory Skills Affect Quality of Life

Environmental stimuli must, as far as possible, be meaningful and interpretable by the older adult with a disability. Sensory impairments among older adults with intellectual disabilities are as high as or higher than in the general population (Janicki & Dalton, 1998), yet their ability to self-report any sensory losses or difficulties is less, thus putting quality of life at risk. For those who read, for example, there may be a requirement for larger print. For those who attend theaters, there may be a need for direct and easy access with appropriate lighting. This may mean enabling such individuals to attend events during daytime hours, which encourages people to feel safe on the streets, in corridors, and in meeting places (R.I. Brown, 1992). It means taking into account individuals' activity cycles, so they carry out social and other activities at their preferred time. This may challenge the routine procedures within care facilities and group homes as well as requiring changes to the community environment (R.I. Brown, 1992).

Perception and Assessment

Any individual's positive and negative perceptions are likely to have an effect on performance and well-being, and the links of these perceptions to external reality are likely to become more distorted through the intervention of aging processes and disability. It is because of this that assessment involving quality of life and well-being has been constructed. Such assessments frequently take into account both subjective (i.e., personal perceptions) and objective components, but researchers often assume that high intercorrelations need to occur if the measures are to be valid. This is not necessarily the case because perceptions from different individuals can have their own validities. If this is recognized, then different data can be seen to have therapeutic uses (see below). Furthermore, tests have often been employed to isolate dimensions or factors, and this frequently begs the question of test purpose. Intervention (i.e., changes to the environment to meet individuals' needs) is a critical and important consideration in looking at the validity of such assessment. In terms of reliability, test–retest coefficients are often quite high (0.6 or greater), whereas intercorrelations between subjects, spouses and family, and caregivers may be considerably lower. It seems important to measure the impressions and choices separately from those of personnel or caregivers. This does not mean that one view is more or less important than the other, but the views of individuals—consumer, parent, or caregiver—reflect different perceptions and entail different realities. All are important in coming to conclusions about an individual's lifestyle and well-being.

Within a quality-of-life model, R.I. Brown (1997c) argued that perceptual measures are not in error in relation to an objective assessment, but are recognized as different. For example, an individual who feels lack of safety in an environment is expressing a view that is important to address, even though the physical precautions have been taken and caregivers believe the individual is safe. We are aware of many staff who have "corrected" the views of older people with intellectual disabilities because they believe their statements are inaccurate. Within a model of quality of life, the views of older people are not seen as incorrect statements about external reality, but represent perceptual information that needs to be treated with respect, and are taken into account both in the design of environments and in the counseling processes that take place. Such discrepancies have been used as a basis for carrying out interviewing and counseling (Brown et al., 1992). A more effective view of individual needs can be obtained and more effective services devised by taking perceptions into account.

Assessment Instruments   Cummins (1995, 1997) listed 229 quality-of-life instruments and noted those most useful for people with some kind of cognitive impairment. Unfortunately, few such tests have been designed for older adults with intellectual disabilities. To be fully appropriate, questions need to be added to such scales that relate to reminiscence, adaptations to environment (within home and community), personal feelings of safety, loneliness and worries, and identification and maintenance of rights in the context of social and psychological well-being. In developing questionnaires, it must be recognized that the questions should only be used as a guide by the person who is presenting the information. The individual must be able to grasp the language spoken by the interviewer, and the interviewer should attempt to use the individual's terminology to elicit answers. The approach is largely a qualitative one with exploration through naturalistic inquiry. Examples of select instruments that might apply to older adults are shown in Table 2.

Empowerment, Aging, and Challenge   It is recognized that the purpose of seeking the older individual's perceptions and choices is to provide an environment that sets the scene for the individual's empowerment. As R.I. Brown (1996b) indicated, the development of such environments may lead to individuals being more assertive and thus challenging and making more demands on their environment. It is suggested that this is not a negative phenomenon, but rather an issue that needs to be handled with the greatest sensitivity by caregivers and professionals who may not always regard

Table 2.   Quality-of-life instruments relevant to older adults with intellectual disabilities

Scale/instruments	Description
Comprehensive Quality of Life Scale (Cummins, 1993)	Measures both objective and subjective areas across seven domains according to satisfaction and importance
Lifestyle Satisfaction Scale (Heal & Chadsey-Rusch, 1985)	Measures satisfaction of the individual with regard to life space, friends, and community participation opportunities
Resident Lifestyle Inventory (Bellamy, Newton, LeBaron, & Horner, 1990)	Used with people with severe intellectual disability and is completed by a caregiver only
Residential Satisfaction Inventory (Burnett, 1989)	Can be completed on a self-report basis
Rehabilitation Questionnaire: A Personal Guide to the Individual's Quality of Life (Brown, Bayer, & Brown, 1992)	Assesses individual responses and, separately, family responses to 11 categories, including Home Living, Things You Do, Family and Friends, and Self Image, completed by trained interviewers
30-Item Quality of Life Questionnaire (Schalock & Keith, 1993)	Uses a 3-point rating scale in the areas of environmental control, social integration, and community integration
Quality of Life Instrument Package (Brown, Raphael, & Renwick, 1997)	Involves input from the individual, family members, and professional caregivers within the contexts of "being, belonging, and becoming"; like the Brown and Bayer questionnaire, this package has been used with older people with intellectual disabilities
Quality of Life Interview Scale (QUOLIS) (Oullette-Kuntz & McCreary, 1996)	Covers dimensions such as support, access, participation, and contentment and is made up of 12 domains, including health, housing, safety, and case management; assessment is conducted by trained interviewers
Quality of Life Profile, Seniors Version (Raphael, 1996)	Self-report questionnaire that contains nine subdomains covering perceived importance of each item to the individual's personal satisfaction and individual control; long questionnaire (111 items), but use of a shortened version is recommended

such behavior as an asset. Unfortunately, it is easier for staff if consumers are nondemanding and quiescent.

In this regard, reminiscence can be a helpful and valuable process encouraging older individuals to retrieve and cope with long-term memories (Coleman, 1986; Gillies & James, 1994). They should be encouraged to do this if it is their own choice. However, it may be difficult for personnel to relate to the substance of the reminiscences because they may concern events that happened before the involvement of the caregiver. More important, it may be very difficult to appreciate the memories of people who have lived in institutions. Many people who have lived their early lives in institutions can give detailed, vivid, and exciting stories about their experiences, very often about escaping from them or about playing jokes among themselves or with staff (Brown et al., 1997). Others, having experienced a wide range of painful or unpleasant events, have cause to worry and may prefer not to discuss these matters. Whether one should pursue these memories is a delicate question and should be carried out only by gentle exploration and under very skilled counseling, within the volition of the older person.

Life-Span Planning One common ingredient of quality-of-life models is the importance of locus of control. If individuals have developed internal locus of control, they will be able to make decisions concerning their environments and select appropriate choices more easily. Internal locus of control is a developmental process—a lifelong process that needs to be supported at each stage of development—but choice and internal locus of control do not develop in a vacuum, and an ability to recognize the need for structure in their development is a professional skill resulting from training, experience, and the development of both personal and professional values (R.I. Brown, 1997b). Given the amazing changes in life expectancy in the field of disability, and very large life-span increases in particular subgroups (e.g., those people with Down syndrome [Stratford & Gunn, 1996] or Prader-Willi syndrome [James & Brown, 1992]), it becomes important that those who are involved during a person's early developmental years should have a clear notion that most individuals are likely to live much longer than previously expected. In many cases, individuals may be the first of their generation to outlive their parents.

Such individuals are much more likely to become dependent on others, rather than on their parents (see Chapter 5). In other words, unless personnel at every stage of development recognize the need for long-term planning and development, additional difficulties will arise during the final years of life. This change in life-span alters our expectations in terms of parental and professional images of the individual and his or her future. For example, the practitioners in neonatal care and new parents who have limited expectation of the child are likely to restrict the image the child has of him- or herself. This restricted self-image is likely to limit the development of internal locus of control and, therefore, increase dependencies in later life. This is one major reason why life-span planning is a necessary component of service and policy systems.

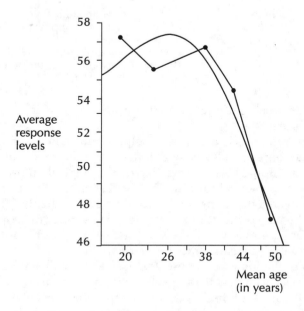

Figure 2.   Average responses of individuals (by age group) participating in leisure activities. (*Source:* Brown, R.I., & Bayer, M.B. [1992]. *Rehabilitation questionnaire and manual: A personal guide to the individual's quality of life* [pp. 21–23]. Toronto: Captus Press.)

Recreation and Leisure   The notions and practices of leisure and recreation among older people with intellectual disabilities are of interest. According to studies we have conducted, certain people (e.g., those with Down syndrome) seem to differ in activity level and decline at earlier ages than other people with intellectual disabilities. Figure 2 illustrates activity levels summarized across four domains of leisure (i.e., spectator, social, physical, and self-actualization; Nash, 1953). The results suggest that around the mid-20s, the leisure activities in people with intellectual disability are at their greatest and individuals show most interest in active leisure pursuits. They are most able to develop their own activities. Such abilities tend to decline fairly rapidly during the ensuing years, and self-actualization and choice ranges diminish. This may be a result of earlier, as well as current, experience. It also may be an expression of choice (i.e., individuals like to enjoy relaxing). Thus, choices need to be encouraged within the experience of developmental structure. Encouraging choice at any age may be desirable, but it is less likely to be effective if it has not been encouraged across the life span.

It also appears that activities flourish when they relate one to the other (i.e., in the context of a holistic approach). For example, people who have effective leisure skills are likely to be more effective in other domains and are more likely, at one extreme, to continue with vocational activities and, at another, are less likely to become dependent and devoid of initiative. The decline of leisure activity to the spectator level at earlier ages is of grave concern because this decline can have a marked effect on health and community integration. Lifestyle planning and active involvement in recreation across the life span are likely to be much more effective.

Forward Planning and Mental Imagery   One of the findings from intervention studies of quality of life is the notion of forward planning (R.I. Brown, 1996a). Many people with intellectual disabilities have difficulty in recognizing the effects of the present on later behaviors or the need to plan for subsequent events. Much of this appears to come about through the process of mental imaging, and stimulation of mental imagery may well be critical to continued well-being in old age. Poor mental imagery has been noted in people with brain injury since at least the 1950s, and Graham (1995) not only provided account of individuals with poor or no visual mental imagery, but she also underscored the stress in Western society of the verbal mode. In addition, Brown and Bullitis (1998) suggested that some older people with intellectual disability might have problems in retaining and/or using imagery. For example, one older individual noted that he experienced "pictures in his head" when he was younger, but no longer does. It seems to be taken for granted, as Brown and Bullitis (1998) noted, that people with intellectual disability have adequate mental imagery processes. As they found, many may not whereas others seem to experience some diminishing of these skills in later life. Yet, reminiscence in the elderly is recognized for many people as a resource and as a satisfying activity.

To help stimulate mental imagery, caregivers may want to gather a list of events that have taken place in the life of the older person. This information may come from the individual or from others. Photographs and newspaper pictures relating to events can enrich the material. Many caregivers are young and unfamiliar with such events and, therefore, have little in common with older people. Coleman (1986) stressed the importance of having personnel who are familiar with the major life events of older adults. The mental imagery thus stimulated can be a rich resource as the individual grows older and less active.

Control of Choices   Without intention, many family members and staff tend to exercise control over older people, including controlling the choices they make. This control over choice often involves very minor items—the types of drink or meals eaten, access to a local amenity or store, where one sits in a particular room, whether one can sit next to a person one likes, and when and with whom one seeks solace and/or privacy. There is some evidence to suggest that people with intellectual disabilities are particularly susceptible to control and that quite minor choices are not recognized or understood despite very willing staff and concerned parents (see Brown & Timmons, 1994; Brown et al., 1989).

Because choice takes place in a structured paradigm, this is a problematic issue for personnel. Experience suggests that most people do not make dangerous choices, and level of choice tends to be within an individual's grasp. That is not to say that inappropriate choices are not made, but the danger is that, if staff decide for any reason that choice is better not exercised, then well-being may be affected. This is unfortunate, as it is the making and enjoyment of choice that enhances lifestyle. Staff should discuss these issues in considerable detail and always keep the desires and needs of the individual in mind. This aspect should be a major part of personnel training. There are at least four components to bear in mind—choices over type, time, and place of activity and with whom one carries out the activity (Brown & Hughson, 1993). Staff need to have a clear understanding of the environment from which the individual has come and the ways in which he or she has behaved over time, including the types of choices he or she has made. Choice may mean that staff need to recognize the difference between what they would like for themselves and what the person wants. Sometimes these may be at variance, but the desires of the individual should be of primary concern.

Increasingly, we will find older individuals who have had a much wider range of choice and autonomy than previously because of the more open and flexible services being developed for younger age groups. If these individuals eventually move to a system that is insensitive or restrictive , the change is likely to jeopardize quality of life and may shorten life span. It is important that individual staff know much about their own value system and that they understand and help to build the value system of the services involved with as much participation as possible from the people served. Apart from diverse and collective knowledge about health and aging, the psychology and social aspects of aging suggest that staff will require training in the area of counseling, because the abilities to elicit information and to guide and help are important, particularly in relation to consumer and caregiver perceptions.

QUALITY OF LIFE: SOME CONCERNS

Drew, Logan, and Hardman (1986) noted that the standards of quality of life of people with intellectual disabilities who are older might be questionable. Increasingly, among older individuals, families are often absent. Because of greater longevity, individuals are outliving their parents, and siblings may not be a reliable source of care and support (see Chapter 5; Seltzer & Krauss, 1987). They, too, are often aging and want to have a less demanding lifestyle. Again, one is forced to the conclusion that preparation for aging must start early in the life cycle and that it must be a continuous process; every skill gained and every experience nurtured must be done with a view to enhancing and widening the person's environmental control. Although the nature of intellectual disability differs widely, it is important to recognize that, despite differences in level of control and ability to control, expansion of personal controls must be encouraged wherever possible.

Partnership

Issues of partnership become important. More people with intellectual disabilities are becoming partnered or married and, among those adults with conditions such as Down syndrome who tend to age earlier than others with intellectual disabilities, partnership also is becoming an important aspect of expectation and actuality. Partnership has many advantages that may extend longevity (R.I. Brown, 1996a). These include presence of a close friend and companion, increased motivation, greater emotional development, satisfaction and stability, sexual satisfaction, rewards of intimate affection, sharing tasks, using strengths and compensating for limitations, greater social contact with community, greater physical activity, improved physical fitness and health, improved skill levels, improved self-image, development of internal locus of control, more rewards, and someone to abreact to about concerns, worries, and anxieties. The challenge is to ensure that individuals who age and are partnered can remain together and can support one another, even when they move to elder care facilities (R.I. Brown, 1999).

Choice

It is suggested that most individuals with intellectual disabilities, young or old, frequently express contentment with their lives (Brown et al., 1989). Measures of satisfaction and happiness have been used in a variety of quality-of-life scales. Measures in these domains may not adequately reflect the improvements and changes based on the individual's choices. Frequently, if individuals discover that choices can be put into effect, they may become more dissatisfied with other aspects of their environment. Indeed, Brown et al. (1992) noted that as individuals gained increasing control they would start to expand control of other aspects of their lives. This is often challenging for staff or family who see requests and changes to requests as difficult or awkward. Perceptions are likely to change, and choices should be encouraged and, if possible, met. The art of good service is not to keep people quiet, but rather to enable individuals to express themselves and maximize their overall satisfaction levels. In this way, they can maintain or develop a self-image, enabling them to be as effective as possible in various aspects of living.

Brown, Matthews, and Taylor (1999) noted that older people value being able to move around their community despite having a disability. They also frequently appear to see themselves as ageless, except for age-related changes such as hair loss or changes in stamina. It appears that it is their life experiences that change and because they do not perceive change in themselves they often wonder why they have, for example, to move to a different residence, give up employment, or no longer attend a local occupational center. Cleanliness, choice of accommodation, privacy, having your own room, and being able to keep your own things tidy are all important. Furthermore, in a field that has stressed that activities are age-appropriate, the reemergence of choices associated with behaviors from younger days should not be overlooked or restricted. Playing simple games, uncomplicated model building, looking at personal collections (e.g., photographs), requesting to meet friends from the past, and other usual activities should be accommodated when possible. Many individuals want to play a role in carrying out a wide range of activities to support their own needs, particularly personal matters. Support may be needed from caregivers, but caregivers should not take over when this is not necessary, even though the individual may be slow and make minor mistakes. Individuals with mild or moderate impairments generally do not require regular and intensive care, although support for certain activities, such as buying clothes or referral to professionals for emergencies, particularly at the health level, may be necessary. When adults are more severely impaired, there is an even greater challenge to ensure that choice and stimulating but supportive environments remain present.

The use of perceptual measures in assessment has far-reaching consequences, because when an individual's perception differs from those of caregivers and other professionals, disagreement and frustration may occur. If counseling can be directed to differences between professional staff and the individual, then the development of a coherent and accepted perception can increase the sense of well-being and internal locus of control experienced by the individual. This should not be taken to mean that the individual is simply helped to understand the perception of professional or family members. However, it should mean that through discussion and demonstration all parties are helped to come to a common and practical understanding of the situation and the needs of the individual. It is at this point, at a clinical level, that changes in individual stability and awareness have been noted (Brown et al., 1992). This is, of course, a construct that is well recognized and practiced within the counseling domain (Robertson & Brown, 1992). The issue is not whether personal perception matches objective reality, but rather a recognition that what a person feels, interprets, and perceives become major markers in terms of how that individual responds and behaves. Indeed, the very fact that such views do not match with external reality may be extremely important and should not be ignored as incorrect. Table 3 illustrates select subjective or perceptual measures in this context that are illustrative to understanding aging and intellectual disability.

Table 3.   Personal perceptions contributing to quality of life

Acceptance by family, peers, employers, employees, and the local community

Access to the local community (e.g., shopping centers, theaters, churches)

Choices from the simple (e.g., what one drinks and when) to the complex (e.g., being alive)

Contribution to others (i.e., giving help)

Control over activities (e.g., employment, leisure, living at home)

Control over environment (e.g., house, bedroom, noise level)

Control over funds and where one lives

Control over home activities (e.g., meal selection [time, content, who prepares])

Control over personal effects (e.g., clothing, furnishings, photographs, magazines)

Control over privacy

Satisfaction

Emotional needs (e.g., companionship, relatedness, social and sexual needs, anxiety, worries, plans for the future)

Friendship network

Intimacy needs

Needs and control over change

Recognition of rights

Safety

Spiritual needs

Status (i.e., adulthood)

Employment and Activity

The desire and right to work after normal or early retirement are now accepted in the general population. It also must be taken into account among people with intellectual disabilities. Some individuals may want to retire and want to be involved in leisure pursuits. Yet, as described in this chapter, quality of life recognizes that work and leisure may be very important pursuits in providing individuals with an active and satisfactory lifestyle. Not only should such variation be taken into account in service development, but also in liaison between different services. It means that the rules of age determination have to be removed and criteria of choice, well-being, and personal need substituted. This is not to argue that all structures disappear, but rather that need and choice become important determinants within policy and management planning.

It is often accepted that later life involves a period when vocational independence or vocational reliance on occupational centers may no longer be viewed as appropriate. Yet the need to address personal issues from the individual's perspective still remains, because it is important to take into full account the choices of the people concerned. From a planning and management perspective, this requires taking into account both the specific and the indicated needs of a person and assessing to what extent these needs can be met through generic services or specialized services and the degree to which the individual remains or wants to become entirely centered in his or her home environment. Choice and well-being may mean that individuals retire at different ages and under differing conditions.

Depression

It is recognized that elderly people are prone to depression, and it appears that many of the problems of memory are associated with this (see Fry, 1986). Other work in the intellectual disability field has suggested that both depression and associated poor self-image are high contenders for low behavioral output and diagnosis of intellectual disability (R.I. Brown, 1992). Image issues, self-awareness, locus of control, and depression are matters over which staff need to be particularly knowledgeable. In this context, an understanding of personal, physical, and psychological space seems to be critical, and this is underlined in the quality-of-life literature (see Schalock, 1997). These issues also are clearly recognized in the goals and future concerns raised by Drew et al. (1986).

GENERIC VERSUS SPECIALIZED SERVICES

Quality-of-life models imply that no one approach to service delivery is preferred. It is not a matter of whether services should be generic or specialized, but rather what is most effective for a particular individual. This is likely to vary from person to person and service to service. It implies looking at the needs of the individual as he or she expresses them and observing the extent to which a particular individual's needs are best fulfilled. It also relates to selecting services that can ensure that abilities are maintained. Thus, the suitability of a service depends on whether it recognizes and practices specific principles. For example, would the service concerned allow the adult choice over contact staff? Is there a policy that ensures that personnel seek out and are sensitive to choices, whether expressed verbally or nonverbally? Do they recognize and accommodate privacy and familiar personal belongings and accept the individual's input and activities within this area? Does the service have a positive record in readily and effectively dealing with issues of access? Are policies and practices regarding discrimination and abuse appropriate? Will the person with intellectual disability be accepted as an individual in his or her own right? Does the service agency provide or select staff who have skills consistent with the constructs described earlier (e.g., the importance of consumer perception)? But the issue goes further than this. For example, is lifestyle regarded as successful and appropriate if the elderly individual lives in the community but is lonely and unable to access local resources despite being supported by generic services? In other words, placement and services have to be viewed within the context of physical, social, and personal actualization.

Quality of life, as Schalock (1997) pointed out, also must include the issue of rights—the right to grieve, the right to die with dignity, the right to continue to assert one's sexual preferences and sexual behaviors, and the right not to be abused. Individuals have the right to participate in the communities of their choice. Individuals should not merely be moved from the community because it is difficult to make arrangements for them or because they are believed to be physically frail. Psychological and social needs, although often seen as less important than health, must be given appropriate recognition. Individuals need to be observed and consulted, and, if they are largely nonverbal, their reactions to different situations need to be noted and their nonverbal behavior taken into account. These issues stress the importance of observational skills and understanding personal attitudes and values, so that there is less chance of limiting the choices of consumers.

Inclusion in generic services may be attractive from a policy perspective, but it is of little value to the person concerned if it cannot accommodate his or her personal issues. Policy and professional practice need to go hand in hand. Services need to demonstrate that they can effectively accommodate individuals with intellectual disabilities. In many countries, generic accommodation services are not able to do this and, when it comes to issues of intellectual disability, staff may be untrained, making a specialized service more attractive if personnel are experienced and individuals can be with friends they have known for many years. However, even here, monitoring and evaluation are required in an ongoing fashion with appropriate consumer, advocate, and independent appraisal. In the long run, the requirements noted here could be a stimulus to the effective development of all services and, therefore, need to be examined by all services. In short, applications of quality of life do not argue for or against generic or specialized services. They provide a basis against which services can be considered for and by any individual. Policy makers, managers, and personnel need to address this issue because the services that do this best are most likely to have positive responses from people with intellectual disabilities.

CONCLUSIONS

This chapter examines the development of quality-of-life models and considers their relevance to older people with lifelong disabilities. The main issue centers on maximizing independence and choices in the context of well-being and appropriate support. In the short term, policy and management systems need to adjust to these requirements. Furthermore, the training and practice of professionals working with older adults need to explore and make use of the practical implications arising from quality-of-life principles. An understanding and recognition of concepts such as empowerment, choice, and self-perception is likely to influence the behavior of such individuals. We now recognize that the life span of people with disabilities dating from the early years has expanded beyond expectations, creating new views and needs amongst elderly people with lifelong disabilities. The application of quality-of-life concepts is likely to change such views further because elderly individuals whose control of their environment is enhanced are likely to show increments in behavior and learning. In other words, the period that we regard as one for reminiscence and leisure also can be a time for regaining or even attaining new skills (Lifshitz & Rand, 1999).

In the longer term, the application of quality-of-life concepts across the full life span is likely to result in individuals with lifelong intellectual or developmental disabilities functioning at higher levels, thus requiring everchanging policies, management, and professional skills for serving those who are elderly and have a disability. This means that we need to have not only highly skilled personnel at the technical level, but also individuals who are able to understand conceptual changes and their implications for the aging people who they support and encourage. In the end, the issues addressed in this chapter are processes that should form part of service evaluation. Evaluations, as Schalock (1995) pointed out, should employ consumer input and description. Perceptions and qualitative data form a part of the evaluation process, once again empowering consumers, heightening their self-image, and giving them a critical role wherever possible in the services they experience.

REFERENCES

Andrews, F.M. (1974). Social indicators of perceived life quality. *Social Indicators Research, 1*, 279–299.

Andrews, F.M., & Withey, S.B. (1976). *Social indicators of well-being: Americans' perceptions of life quality.* New York: Plenum Publishing Corp.

Bellamy, G.T., Newton, J.S., Lebaron, N.M., & Horner, R.H. (1990). Quality of life and lifestyle outcomes: A challenge for residential programmes. In R.L. Schalock (Ed.), *Quality of life: Perspectives and issues* (pp. 127–137). Washington, DC: American Association on Mental Retardation.

Brown, H. (1997). Sexual rights and sexual wrongs in the lives of people with intellectual disabilities. In R.I. Brown (Ed.), *Quality of life for people with disabilities: Models, research and practice* (pp. 228–250). Cheltenham, UK: Stanley Thornes.

Brown, I. (1994). Promoting quality within service delivery systems. *Journal on Developmental Disabilities, 3*(2), i–iv.

Brown, I. (1996). The quality of life of marginal citizens: Homelessness. In R. Renwick, I. Brown, & M. Nagler (Eds.), *Quality of life in health promotion and rehabilitation: Conceptual approaches, issues, and applications* (pp. 204–216). Thousand Oaks, CA: Sage Publications.

Brown, I., Renwick, R., & Raphael, D. (1997). *Quality of life instrument package for adults with developmental disabilities.* Toronto: University of Toronto, Centre for Health Promotion.

Brown, R.I. (1989). Aging, disability and quality of life: A challenge for society. *Canadian Psychology/Psychologie Canadienne, 30*, 551–559.

Brown, R.I. (1992). Aging and the arts and disability: A community issue, arts: The soul of the community. In R.I. Brown, H. Coward, & J. Dugan (Eds.), *Arts: The soul of the community* (Community Seminar Series #2, pp. 21–46). Calgary, Alberta, Canada: University of Calgary, Calgary Institute for the Humanities..

Brown, R.I. (1996a). Growing older with Down syndrome. In B. Stratford & P. Gunn (Eds.), *New approaches to Down syndrome* (pp. 436–450). London: Cassell.

Brown, R.I. (1996b). People with developmental disabilities: Applying quality of life to assessment and intervention. In R. Renwick, I. Brown, & M. Nagler (Eds.), *Quality of life in health promotion and rehabilitation: Conceptual approaches, issues and applications* (pp. 253–267). Thousand Oaks, CA: Sage Publications.

Brown, R.I. (Ed.). (1997a). *Quality of life for people with disabilities: Models, research and practice.* Cheltenham, UK: Stanley Thornes.

Brown, R.I. (1997b). Quality of life and professional education. In R.I. Brown (Ed.), *Quality of life for people with disabilities: Models, research and practice* (pp. 310–326). Cheltenham, UK: Stanley Thornes.

Brown, R.I. (1997c). Quality of life: The development of an idea. In R.I. Brown (Ed.), *Quality of life for people with disabilities: Models, research and practice* (pp. 1–11). Cheltenham, UK: Stanley Thornes.

Brown, R.I. (1999, June). *Quality of life for older adults in communities and institutions.* Paper presented at the 6th International Conference on Aging and Disability, Rapid City, SD.

Brown, R.I. (2000). Quality of life: Challenges and confrontation. In K.D. Keith & R. Schalock (Eds.), *Cross-cultural perspectives on quality of life.* Washington, DC: American Association on Mental Retardation.

Brown, R.I., & Bayer, M.B. (1992). *Rehabilitation questionnaire and manual: A personal guide to the individual's quality of life.* Toronto: Captus Press.

Brown, R.I., Bayer, M.B., & Brown, P.M. (1992). *Empowerment and developmental handicaps: choices and quality of life.* London: Chapman & Hall.

Brown, R.I., Bayer, M.B., & MacFarlane, C. (1988). Quality of life amongst handicapped adults. In R.I. Brown (Ed.), *Quality of life for handicapped people* (pp. 111–140). London: Croom Helm.

Brown, R.I., Bayer, M.B., & MacFarlane, C. (1989). *Rehabilitation programmes: Performance and quality of life of adults with developmental handicaps.* Toronto: Lugas.

Brown, R.I., & Bullitis, E. (1998). *Images of consciousness and Down syndrome: Proceedings of the 1st Biennial Scientific Conference on Down Syndrome: Down Syndrome in the 21st Century.* Vancouver, British Columbia, Canada: Down Syndrom Research Foundation.

Brown, R.I., & Hughson, E.A. (1993). *Behavioural and social rehabilitation and training.* Toronto: Captus Press.

Brown, R.I., Matthews, B., & Taylor, J. (1997, August). *Quality of life: Ageing and Down syndrome.* Paper given at the 16th Congress of the International Association of Gerontology, Adelaide, South Australia, Australia.

Brown, R.I., Matthews, B., & Taylor, J. (1999). Quality of life: Ageing and Down syndrome. *Down Syndrome Research and Practice, 6*(3), 111–118.

Brown, R.I., & Timmons, V. (1994). Quality of life: Adults and adolescents with disabilities. *Exceptionality Education Canada, 4,* 1–11.

Burnett, P.C. (1989). Assessing satisfaction in people with an intellectual disability: Living in community-based residential facilities. *Australian Disability Review, 1,* 14–19.

Coleman, P.G. (1986). *Ageing and reminiscence process: Social and clinical implications.* Chichester, UK: John Wiley & Sons.

Crick, F. (1994). *The astonishing hypothesis: The scientific search for the soul.* New York: Scribner.

Cummins, R.A. (1993). *The Comprehensive Quality of Life Scale–Adult* (4th ed.; ComQol–A4). Melbourne, Australia: Deakin University, School of Psychology.

Cummins, R.A. (1995). On the trail of the gold standard for subjective well-being. *Social Indicators Research, 35,* 179–200.

Cummins, R.A. (1997). Assessing quality of life. In R.I. Brown (Ed.), *Quality of life for people with disabilities: Models, research and practice* (pp. 116–150). Cheltenham, UK: Stanley Thornes.

Dossa, P.A. (1989). Quality of life: Individualism or holism? A critical review of the literature. *International Journal of Rehabilitation Research, 12,* 121–136.

Drew, C.J., Logan, D.R., & Hardman, M.L. (1986). *Mental retardation: A life cycle approach.* Upper Saddle River, NJ: Merrill.

Edgerton, R.B. (1994). Foreword. In D. Goode (Ed.), *Quality of life for persons with disabilities: International perspectives and issues* (pp. i–ii). Cambridge, MA: Brookline Books.

Felce, D., & Perry, J. (1997). Quality of life: The scope of the term and its breadth of measurement. In R.I. Brown (Ed.), *Quality of life for people with disabilities: Models, research and practice* (pp. 56–71). Cheltenham, UK: Stanley Thornes.

Ferguson, R.V. (1997). Environmental design and quality of life. In R.I. Brown (Ed.), *Quality of life for people with disabilities: Models, research and practice* (pp. 251–269). Cheltenham, UK: Stanley Thornes.

Fry, P.S. (1986). *Depression, stress, and adaptations in the elderly: Psychological assessment and intervention.* Gaithersburg, MD: Aspen Publishers.

Gillies, C., & James, A. (1994). *Reminiscence work with old people.* London: Chapman & Hall.

Goode, D.A. (1997). Assessing the quality of life of adults with profound disabilities. In R.I. Brown (Ed.), *Quality of life for people with disabilities: Models, research, and practice* (pp. 72–90). Cheltenham, UK: Stanley Thornes.

Goode, D.A. (1988). *Quality of life for persons with disabilities: A review & synthesis of the literature.* Valhalla, NY: Mental Retardation Institute.

Goode, D.A. (Ed.). (1994). *Quality of life for persons with disabilities: International perspectives and issues.* Cambridge, MA: Brookline Books.

Graham, H. (1995). *Mental imagery in health care: An introduction to therapeutic practice.* London: Chapman & Hall.

Hatton, C. (1998). Whose quality of life is it anyway? Some problems with the emerging quality of life consensus. *Mental Retardation, 36,* 104–115.

Heal, L.W., & Chadsey-Rusch, J. (1985). The Lifestyle Satisfaction Scale (LSS): Assessing individuals' satisfaction with residence, community setting, and associated services. *Applied Research in Mental Retardation, 6,* 475–490.

Hogg, J., & Lambe, L. (1997). An ecological perspective on the quality of life of people with intellectual disabilities as they age. In R.I. Brown (Ed.), *Quality of life for people with disabilities: Models, research and practice* (pp. 201–227). Cheltenham, UK: Stanley Thornes.

Hogg, J., & Moss, S. (1990). Social and community integration. In M.P. Janicki & M.M. Seltzer (Eds.), *Aging and developmental disabilities: Challenges for the 1990s. Proceedings of the Boston roundtable on research issues and applications in aging and developmental disabilities* (pp. 25–51). Washington, DC: American Association on Mental Retardation.

James, T., & Brown, R.I. (Eds.). (1992). *Prader-Willi syndrome: Home, school and community.* London: Chapman & Hall.

Janicki, M.P., & Dalton, A.J. (1998). Sensory impairments among older adults with intellectual disability. *Journal of Intellectual and Developmental Disability, 23(1),* 3–11.

Lifshitz, H., & Rand, Y. (1999). Cognitive modifications in adult and older people with mental retardation. *Mental Retardation, 37,* 125–138.

MacFarlane, C., Brown, R.I., & Bayer, M.B. (1989). Rehabilitation Programmes Study: Quality of life. In R.I. Brown, M.B. Bayer, & C. MacFarlane, *Rehabilitation programmes: Performance and quality of life of adults with developmental handicaps* (pp. 56–67). Toronto: Lugus.

Nash, J.B. (1953). *Philosophy of recreation and leisure.* Dubuque, IA: Wm. C. Brown Communications.

Ory, M.G., & Cox, D.M. (1994). Forging ahead: linking health and behaviour to improve quality of life in older people. *Social Indicators Research, 33(1–3),* 89–120.

Ouellette-Kuntz, H., & McCreary, B. (1996). Quality of life assessment for persons with severe development disabilities. In R. Renwick, I. Brown, & M. Nagler (Eds.), *Quality of life in health promotion and rehabilitation: Conceptual approaches, issues, and applications* (pp. 268–278). Thousand Oaks, CA: Sage Publications.

Parmenter, T.R. (1994). Quality of life as a concept and measurable entity. *Social Indicators Research, 33,* 9–46.

Raphael, D. (1996). Quality of life of older adults: Toward the optimization of the aging process. In R. Renwick, I. Brown, & M. Nagler (Eds.), *Quality of life in health promotion and rehabilitation: Conceptual approaches, issues and applications* (pp. 290–306). Thousand Oaks, CA: Sage Publications.

Raphael, D. (1997). Quality of life of persons with developmental disabilities: Five issues concerning its nature and measurement. *Journal of Developmental Disabilities, 5(2),* 44–66.

Renwick, R., & Brown, I. (1996). The Centre for Health Promotion's conceptual approach to quality of life. In R. Renwick, I. Brown, & M. Nagler, *Quality of life in health promotion and rehabilitation: Conceptual approaches, issues, and applications* (pp. 75–88). Thousand Oaks, CA: Sage Publications.

Renwick, R., Brown, I., & Nagler, M. (1996). *Quality of life in health promotion and rehabilitation: Conceptual approaches, issues, and applications.* Thousand Oaks, CA: Sage Publications.

Robertson, S.E., & Brown, R.I. (Eds.). (1992). *Rehabilitation counselling: Approaches in field of disability* (Vol. 5). London: Chapman & Hall.

Romney, D.M., Brown, R.I., & Fry, P.S. (1994). Improving the quality of life: Prescriptions for change. In D.R. Romney, R.I. Brown, & P.S. Fry (Eds.), *Improving the quality of life: Recommendations for people with and without disabilities* (pp. 237–272). Dordrecht, The Netherlands: Kluwer.

Rowe, J.W., & Kahn, R.L. (1998). *Successful aging.* New York: Pantheon.

Schalock, R. (1997). The concept of quality of life in the twenty-first century disability programmes. In R.I. Brown (Ed.), *Quality of life for people with disabilities: Models, research and practice* (pp. 327–340). Cheltenham, U.K.: Stanley Thornes.

Schalock, R.L. (1998). Three decades of quality of life. In M. Wehmeyer & J.R. Patton (Eds.), *Mental retardation in the 21st century* (pp. 335–354). Austin, TX: PRO-ED.

Schalock, R.L. (1995). *Outcome-based evaluation.* New York: Plenum Publishing Corp.

Schalock, R.L., & Keith, K.D. (1993). *Quality of Life Questionnaire.* Worthington: OH: IDS.

Seltzer, M.M., & Krauss, M.W. (1987). *Aging and mental retardation: Extending the continuum.* Washington, DC: American Association on Mental Retardation.

Stratford, B., & Gunn, P. (1996). *New approaches to Down syndrome.* London: Cassell.

Taylor, S.J. (1994). In support of research on quality of life, but against QOL. In D. Goode (Ed.), *Quality of life for persons with disabilities: International perspectives and issues* (pp. 260–265). Cambridge, MA: Brookline Books.

Wolfensberger, W. (1994). Let's hang up "quality of life" as a hopeless term. In D. Goode (Ed.), *Quality of life for persons with disabilities: International perspectives and issues* (pp. 285–321). Cambridge, MA: Brookline Books.

3

A Sense of Belonging

Older Adults' Perspectives on Social Integration

Michael J. Mahon and Jennifer B. Mactavish

Physically and socially including people with a developmental disability as members of our communities has been a central goal of the disability movement since the mid-1960s. *Integration,* the term coined to describe this aim, was defined by Nirje (1976) as referring to those relationships between individuals that are based on recognition of each other's integrity and shared basic values and rights. Furthermore, the notion of social integration was seen as the interpersonal or impersonal social relationships in neighborhoods, schools, work situations, and the community at large. Within this general notion, manners, attitudes, respect, and esteem are mutually involved, and the interface is affected by public attitudes of the media and by the public images of people with disabilities (Nirje, 1976). These definitional concepts reflect a shift in societal attitudes that slowly came to life in the 1960s and that continue as we begin the 21st century. Since the mid-1960s, we appear to have accepted the notion that people with developmental disabilities have a right to live in the community. Or have we? Although it is true that fewer of these individuals reside within the walls of institutions, it also is true, as Lord and Pedlar stated, that being "*in* the community does not mean [being] *of* the community" (1991, p. 217; emphasis added). As Lord and Pedlar's words imply, integration is not achieved by a person's physical presence alone, but is contingent on establishing meaningful social connections with other members of the community.

Recognizing how critical the social component is in integration, a considerable body of literature focuses exclusively on social integration (Blatt & Kaplan; 1966; Hutchison & Lord, 1979; Nirje, 1969; Wolfensberger, 1972). Much of this work chronicles the ongoing struggles of people with developmental disabilities to become full members of their communities (Anderson, Lakin, Hill, & Chen, 1992; Burchard, Hasazi, Gordon, & Yoe, 1991; Lord & Pedlar, 1991; Pedlar, 1990; Ralph & Usher, 1995). It also is within this body of literature that the relationship between social integration and other key concepts in the field of developmental disabilities becomes evident. For example, Wolfensberger and Thomas (1983) argued that social integration provides the path whereby individuals with disabilities assume valued social roles, which further supports the development of relationships with other members of their communities, particularly those who are not devalued. Similarly, social integration is frequently presented as a means for enhancing the quality of life of individuals with disabilities. In fact, social integration is recognized as one of the dimensions that defines quality of life (Haring, 1991; Schalock, 1996; Wehmeyer & Schwartz, 1998). Beyond this conceptual link, social integration and quality of life also are acknowledged as highly complex, personally variable, socially constructed notions that defy precise definition (Storey, 1997; Taylor & Bogdan, 1990).

Our understanding of these socially constructed concepts, however, is rooted in the knowledge and opinions of researchers, service professionals, and other individuals who work to support people with developmental disabilities (Goode, 1988; Rosen, Simon, & McKinsey, 1995; Schalock, 1996). Consequently, a number of researchers have criticized this body of knowledge because of its failure to include the perspectives of individuals with developmental disabilities (Biklen & Moseley, 1988; Schalock, 1996; Taylor & Bogdan, 1990, 1996). Characterizing these criticisms, Biklen and Moseley argued that researchers are "outsiders" who "cannot take for granted the views or positions of insiders (people with a developmental disability) . . . but must formulate enhanced understanding by directly studying the perspectives of 'insiders'" (1988, p. 155).

Going beyond being concerned about whose definition and understanding of social integration we use in attempting to understand this phenomenon, we have to consider the notion of lifespan. Most of what has been written about social integration has not taken into consideration how social integration and the factors that influence it may vary across the lifespan of people with developmental disabilities. Do the factors that facilitate or constrain social integration change as people grow older? Does the meaning of social integration and its importance vary with advancing age? These types of questions have not received much attention from researchers. One exception to this was a study by Mahon and Goatcher (1999), which revealed that many older adults with developmental disabilities fear losing important social contacts at work and, as a result, are often reluctant to retire. Erickson, Krauss, and Seltzer (1989) came to similar conclusions in a study that also focused on the perspectives of older adults with developmental disabilities.

These two areas—personal perspectives of people with developmental disabilities and lifespan issues—served as the basis of a 3-year qualitative research project carried out in Canada. Drawing on the results of this study, this chapter concentrates on social integration and the factors that facilitate and constrain these experiences from the perspectives of older adults with developmental disabilities. In addition, we compare these individuals' understanding of social integration with the viewpoints of service providers and family members and others who serve as social supports.

COLLECTING PERSONAL PERSPECTIVES ON SOCIAL INTEGRATION

It is important to include the personal perspectives of people with developmental disabilities in research that aims to enhance understanding of notions such as social integration. Questions about effectively including these individuals in the research process and concerns about their ability to provide credible information, however, continue to be a challenge. Some researchers have attempted to address these questions by presuming the reliability and inherent value of all perspectives, collecting data intensively over a long period of time, building rapport with research participants, and using concrete processes to elicit data. Building on these approaches, we used three strategies, grounded in a qualitative research tradition, to collect information (Morgan, 1997). These strategies included individual interviews, focus groups, and follow-up meetings to confirm and/or disconfirm the emerging findings (Mactavish, Lutfiyya, & Mahon, 1998). The individual interviews were conducted first and provided an opportunity for the participants to get to know us and learn about the focus group process. This was followed by the focus groups, which served as a forum for the participants to share their personal perspectives on the meaning of social integration and the factors that facilitated and constrained their experiences of social integration. Of the eight focus groups that were held, each included at least four participants and two moderators. A structured questioning guide and verbal prompting were the principal techniques used by the moderators to stimulate discussion (Krueger & Casey, 2000). Finally, follow-up meetings were conducted with a cross-section of the original focus group participants to determine whether we had accurately captured their perspectives on social integration. In these meetings, a hierarchy of questions, verbal and visual prompting, and visual cues were used to present the findings in a way that was structured yet flexible enough for the participants to express their opinions.

Defining Social Integration

It is clear from reviewing the transcripts of the focus groups with older adults that the participants' understanding of social integration was rooted in the sense of belonging that came from sharing time, activities, and experiences with families and friends. Illustrating the nature of these discussions, an older woman—Sylvia—started the discussion by stating:

> Social integration . . . means feeling like I'm a part of things. I don't work, but I go to the Salvation Army and a woman's travel group . . . when I take part in things with my friends it makes me feel good—like I'm part of it. When I don't [take part], I feel left out.

Other participants then added to Sylvia's points by declaring:

> Being with my family!
> Going to my girlfriend's house.
> Going out—to the bar, dancing—with my friends.
> Not being bored. Belonging.

On the surface, this understanding appears to be consistent with discussions of social integration in the literature. That is, being involved in meaningful social relationships within a variety of contexts (e.g., recreation, family) is often presented as a key outcome of social integration, which, in turn, influences perceptions of community membership, belonging, and quality of life (Hutchison & McGill, 1992; Keith, 1990). A closer examination of the literature, however, suggests that "true" social integration is contingent upon interactions and relationships between individuals with and without developmental disabilities (Wolfensberger & Thomas, 1983). The participants in this study made no such distinction. The participants' thoughts suggest a meaning of social integration in which a sense of belonging is derived from friendships with people—independent of whether these people have disabilities.

Without delving into the debate about the meaning of *friendship*, it seems that social integration is not an outcome exclusive to interactions between people with and without disabilities, but is equally, and perhaps more frequently, the result of relationships that include peers with disabilities. Although this is an intuitively logical suggestion, it is not one that has received a great deal of attention in the literature, possibly because the perspectives of individuals with disabilities have been inadequately represented in previous discussions about social integration.

Factors that Can Help or Hinder Social Integration

Although the information from each focus group was analyzed individually, four themes consistently emerged as factors that affected social integration. These themes (context, structured recreation and leisure activities, friendships, and family) served both as facilitators and constraints. Namely, when a particular factor (e.g., structured recreation and leisure activities) was present, it enhanced social integration and, when it was absent, social integration was inhibited. Although the themes were consistent across the lifespan, the meaning and relative importance that older adults attached to the themes did vary, to some degree, from the perspectives of the other participants in our focus groups.

Context   When people with developmental disabilities spoke about social integration, they tended to zero in on the context or setting within which social integration took place. The contexts for social integration that were most prevalent for adolescents and adults were school and work. Those older adults who were still working also viewed work as a key context for social interaction. In contrast to some of the adolescents and adults who participated in the study who had varied work experiences (from supported employment to occupational centers), all the older adults were employed in occupational centers. For these individuals, the opportunities for social integration involved interaction with coworkers and staff members. That is, the occupational center provided a frequent and reliable meeting place where people could foster and maintain personally meaningful social connections with other people with disabilities and staff without disabilities. Illustrating this point are the thoughts of three participants—Mike, Sarah, and Jessica:

> Every day at work we do the same things. Every day! I don't like doing the same thing every day. But I've got lots of friends at work, and that's the good thing about it. You get to meet your friends and different people. My job (at the workshop) is the most important thing in my life . . . all my friends are at work as is my boyfriend, Shawn. I sometimes go out with Leslie and Wanda, but mostly I see them at work [at the workshop]. That's the place where I get to be with my friends. Being with my friends makes going to work fun.

Also emerging from the theme of contexts for social integration were two subthemes: valued social roles and day program/living situations.

Valued Social Roles   Independent of age, school attendance, or work setting, the act of fulfilling social roles that the participants valued enhanced their perceptions of being socially integrated. Although the participants identified themselves as fulfilling a number of valued roles (e.g., friends, aunt, uncle, student, artist), securing a job and being a paid employee were the symbols of community membership—of belonging—that were most consistently discussed. The following collection of quotes clearly articulates the importance of this subtheme:

> Jobs are hard to come by, but basically you have to work. Get a job and pay your own bills. That's the only way to go . . . be like everybody else . . . paying your own way. Having a job and making money are the most important . . . if you don't work and make money you're not like everyone else and you don't have money for doing the stuff you like—friends, movies. I'm interested in my job. I love getting paid—I love money a lot and love spending it more! Going out with my friends. I feel more important.

Tying this subtheme—valued social roles—back to the contexts in which people had consistent social contacts (i.e., school and work), it seems that these contacts in tandem with fulfilling socially appropriate and valued roles (as students, aspiring employees, and workers) acted together to enhance feelings of belonging and community membership. Put another way, the study participant's perceptions of social integration were not simply based on the presence or absence of social exchanges with other people, but were influenced by the roles they saw themselves fulfilling within society.

Day Placement/Living Situation   The second subtheme presents an alternative to school and work as contexts in which opportunities for social integration occur. Some of the older adults in our study no longer attended school and no longer worked. Two of these individuals lived in independent units within a personal care home, which afforded readily accessible and frequent opportunities for social interaction with other residents of the center. Two of the urban participants resided in independent apartments where they supported younger roommates who also have disabilities. These older adults seldom had visitors and, because of declining health and safety concerns, rarely ventured out to meet with friends or to take part in activities. Jean and Margaret's words characterize the contrasting experiences of these two distinct groups of older adults:

> I live in an apartment in the unit (personal care home). I've got a little kitchen, a bedroom, my own TV and stuff. I have neighbors on all sides. I go to the dining room to have my meals every day. Always eat with my friends Ben and Erica—they eat slow too. During the day I sometimes watch TV and do puzzles. I go to the common room and visit with the ladies a lot. Every day there is something going on. Some days, if I want to, I take part. Other times I just do what I want. I live in my own apartment, with Michelle. I look after her—do the cleaning and the cooking. Michelle goes to work. I don't. I hardly ever go out much anymore. My leg's not so good and it's just not safe—especially at night. So I stay home by myself. Watch TV and sleep. Sometimes I'm lonely, but I like being my own person. Doing my own thing.

Jean and Margaret's descriptions clearly reflect different experiences of social integration. In most cases, however, the older adults did not equate the quality of their daily lives with day programs and living situations that facilitated opportunities for social interaction. Apparently of greater importance to these individuals were a personal living space—a home to call their own—and the freedom to do as they pleased.

Structured Recreation and Leisure Activities   Outside people's regularly scheduled daily activities (e.g., school, work), recreation and leisure emerged as another important factor in facilitating social integration. Participants of all ages spoke at length about the many activities they most frequently enjoyed:

> I watch TV . . . do my puzzles in the morning, read. Sometimes I bake cookies. But mostly I just relax and watch TV by myself. (Stacy, a 39-year-old woman)

I ride my bike around if it's nice. . . . Once I had an accident on my bike, so now I only go out if it is nice. . . . If it's not nice I stay home. Watch TV. (Sam, a 50-year-old man)

As is evident in these comments, the most common activities were home based and, although not always clear from the participants' words, most of these activities were done with little if any social interaction. It was not clear from the data to what extent involvement in isolated forms of recreation contributed to social integration. It was clear, however, as the following statement shows that the participants typically did not recreate with other people unless it was within structured recreation settings:

Living on your own makes doing things with other people hard. Your friends cannot always come over, aye. And where are you going to find other people? I get to see other people at my travel meetings—if I can get there. The rest of the time it's easier just to do my puzzles and reading. I mostly do activities on my own. Watch TV, listen to music, just do nothing. If I do things with other people—my friends—I'm usually bowling or at the Legion.

It was not surprising, therefore, that structured recreation, as opposed to isolated home-based recreation, was identified by the participants as a central factor that contributed to their social integration. Establishing the basis for this theme, Tom described the importance of structured recreation in fostering his feelings of membership and belonging:

I answered an advert in the paper for a team who needed a dart player. I joined up. Now I'm part of the league, part of a team. We're regulars on Wednesday and Tuesday nights at the Inn.

Generally, however, older adults have fewer family- and community-based opportunities for structured recreation and, as such, most engage in higher frequencies of isolated and home-based activities than younger adults. This may reflect older adults' gradual withdrawal from more socially oriented recreation and leisure activities in the community and limited contact with their families. The reminiscence of two older women (ages 72 and 79) captures this gradual process of withdrawal:

I used to be a lot more active. Out all the time. Doing things. Bowling, going to 55-Plus meetings. Now there just seems to be less going on—or I don't know about it. So I spend more time at home, alone, doing my own thing . . . watching TV, fancy work. I would plan activities with other people more, like I used to. But they all seem too far away from where I am. At my age and health, I don't like to go to far from home. Especially at night. So I do crafts at home, if I'm not too tired.

Implicit in these comments is that the opportunities for some older adults to engage in structured recreation were constrained by a number of factors—perceived lack of opportunities close to home, lack of people with whom to do activities, and concerns about health and personal safety. These constraints were not exclusive to the experiences of older adults; however, declining participation was most pronounced within this group. Consequently, although structured recreation had served as a vehicle for social integration in the past, gaining access to these opportunities became increasingly difficult as the participants reached older age.

Friendships   Engaging in meaningful social relationships—having friends—is generally identified by people with developmental disabilities as one of the key ingredients to social integration across the lifespan. Defining the meaning of friends and friendships continues to be a topic of considerable debate within the disability literature (Green & Schleien, 1991). Much of this debate stems from apparent differences in the ways that people with developmental disabilities understand these terms and the perspectives of academics and service providers. Without getting into the details of this debate, our experience has revealed that friendship could be defined in a variety of ways. For older adults with developmental disabilities, their understanding typically assumed one of two perspectives: friendships as relationships that are based on mutuality and reciprocity, and friendships as relationships that simply involve shared interactions with "nice" people. Although interesting, these contrasting views on the meaning of friendship had little, if any, affect on the participants' perspectives on the importance of friends in promoting social integration. Supporting this contention, four people who subscribe to different views of friendship noted the following:

> Friends to me are people who like each other. Doing things with friends makes me feel part of things. Not left out. Isabelle and I have been friends for years. Too many years! We do all sorts of things together—things we both like . . . puzzles, movies. That's what makes us both happy. We belong together. Lisa [a service provider] is my friend. She's nice. She helps me do things that are hard to do on my own. Without my friend, Lisa, I'd have no friends. I'd be really lonely. Tom [also a service provider] helps me make sure I do the things I have to do so I can live on my own. Grocery shopping, going to the bank. Goes with me to get my bus pass. Tom's a really good friend. That's what friends are for . . . to help you out with things. So you're not alone.

From a social integration perspective, the definition of friendship seemed less relevant to the participants than whether they shared personally meaningful interactions with individuals whom they regarded as friends. Although being able to stand alone is a theme that facilitates social integration, friendship also was linked to the contexts in which the participants were active on a regular basis (i.e., contexts' theme—day placement). Specifically, as illustrated in the following quote, most friendships can be confined to the contexts in which they were initiated and seldom include interactions in other settings:

> When I go to work, I'm with my work friends. My friends at work are important to me. It's like being part of a team . . . we work together making lawn chairs, we work fast together. We get along. After work, I go home. My work friends go to where they live. So after work, I do things with Lana and Alexa—they're the two friends I live with.

In summary, although important in fostering social integration, the compartmentalized nature of friendships resulted in "islands of social integration" that varied with people's activities and experiences.

Family   Family, another theme identified by older adults with developmental disabilities, contributed to perceptions of social integration in a number of different ways. For those adults younger than the age of 35, families were most consistently described as playing a key role in promoting social integration both at home and in the community. Articulating the views of these individuals, two participants stated the following:

> I live with my parents. They're great! We do lots of things as a family. We're really close. I also depend on them for transportation. So I can get from home to work and from home to "Special O" [the Special Olympics]. My parents are always there for me and help to keep me involved. I live on my own, but I see my family a lot. Play golf and go fishing with my brothers. I have my grandpa, too. He's 88. I call him every day. He's always asking me about how things are going. He's really interested in whatever interests me—just like the rest of my family—they're all like that.

However, with advancing age, the nature and frequency of family contact changed. These changes were attributed to a number of factors including the death of parents and the more mobile nature of our society that often resulted in family members living great distances from one another:

> When my parents died, I used to go and visit my sister in British Columbia. That's when I was younger. Now not so much . . . I'm getting older and traveling is tiring. My family lives everywhere. My parents are in heaven. My sister is in Edmonton and my brother is in Toronto. I don't see them very often anymore.

The changing nature and frequency of family contact can lead to families playing a less direct role in fostering the social integration of older adults. Specifically, for these participants, assuming valued social roles (e.g., as sons, daughters, brothers, sisters, aunts, and uncles) facilitated enhanced feelings of belonging and connection within their families. Capturing the spirit of this perspective, two older adults noted the following:

> I used to have brothers, but they're all gone. They all died. I still got sisters-in-law, and I've got a whole bunch of nephews, and a bunch of cousins. I still visit with them so I still feel like part of a family. I'm an auntie eight, no, six times over. Four nephews—Ryan, Sean, Jason, and Christopher. Two nieces—Rachel and Pasadena. They're great! It's like being part of another family all over again.

Overall, the participants' views suggest that the role of families in facilitating social integration changes over the lifespan. For older adults, these changes are reflected in less contact with their families and less direct support for fostering social integration within the community. Nevertheless, fulfilling socially valued roles within their families continued to enhance the older adults' perceptions of belonging and social membership.

CONTRASTING PERSPECTIVES AMONG OLDER ADULTS, SERVICE PROVIDERS, AND FAMILY MEMBERS

The beginning of this chapter discusses the importance of collecting multiple perspectives on the meaning of socially constructed notions such as social integration. Traditionally, service providers, families, and other social supports have defined these concepts with little, if any, consideration of the perspectives of individuals with developmental disabilities. As such, chronicling the views of these individuals has been our primary focus to this point. Within our research, however, we also conducted focus groups with family members and others who serve as social supports and completed in-depth interviews with service providers. With the findings in Table 1 as the basis for discussion, the remainder of this chapter concentrates on how the perspectives of these two groups compare with those of individuals with developmental disabilities.

Service Providers

The service providers' column in Table 1 highlights eight themes that were derived from interviews with this group. Of these themes, four relate to the perspectives shared by older adults (i.e., personal environment, community, friends, families). Service providers indicated that people's personal environments affected social integration. By this, they were specifically referring to the person's residential setting (e.g., group home, living at home), as well as the type of community in which the person resided. Service providers also believed that rural communities were more conducive to social integration than urban centers. In comparison, the older adults identified their places of

Table 1. Contrasting perspectives on social integration: Themes from older adults with developmental disabilities, family members/social supports, and service providers

Service providers	Older adults with developmental disabilities	Families and other social supports
Community	Context	Valued social roles
The person	Structural recreation and	The person
Friends	leisure	Friends
Families/social supports	Friends	Care/advocacy
Organizational issues	Families	Vulnerability
Empowerment		Range of services
Process versus product		
Personal environment		

work and, to a lesser extent, their residential settings as the most common contexts for social integration.

Recreation was a theme common to older adults and service providers alike. Identified by service providers as a community subtheme, recreation was viewed as a medium for fostering social integration. As one person noted,

> What's really important, too, is to find that leisure or recreation activity that you're really interested in, so that when you're going to that place, you have something in common to talk about with the individuals there and that's how we often start our relationships.

Although service providers and older adults both shared the belief that recreation plays a role in social integration, their perspectives diverged on an important point. Service providers talked generally about recreation as a facilitator of social integration, whereas the older adults clearly focused on structured recreation as the key. For the older adults, this distinction probably lays in the fact that most of their self-initiated recreation included solitary activities at home, whereas their recreation within the community tended to be structured in a way that encouraged social contacts with other individuals.

Service providers, similar to older adults, described friends as an important cornerstone of social integration. Service providers believed that friendship was, in essence, the defining element of social integration. One noted,

> If friendships occur, then the social integration, I mean, it's there, it's just a normal thing and friendships, those are the difficult things to get established because friends sort of grow through being together and sharing experiences.

In further discussing the role of friendship, a critical point of contrast emerged between service providers' and older adults' perspectives on these relationships and their contributions to social integration. As noted earlier, older adults defined friendship in different ways, but these differences did not influence their opinions about the importance of these relationships in fostering feelings of belonging. Consequently, for some older adults, their friendships with paid staff members were central to their social integration. In contrast, service providers emphasized that relationships with paid staff members were not "true" friendships and, therefore, did not enhance social integration.

As with older adults, many service providers identify families as playing a crucial role in fostering social integration. Having said that, older adults tend to concentrate on families as providers of opportunities to fulfill valued social roles, whereas service providers focus on families as active promoters of social integration by including older adults in family events and encouraging participation in community activities. In addition, we observed that service providers often introduce the possibility that concerns about safety and vulnerability could result in family-imposed constraints to social integration. Although not discussing this issue directly, the older adults' views on declines in family contact also imply that families may contribute, positively and/or negatively, to social integration.

Beyond the four themes that overlapped with those identified by older adults, our interviews with service providers revealed four unique themes. Among the most notable of these were personal characteristics of the individual with a disability and community attitudes and education. The first of these themes captures service providers' perspectives on individual attributes (e.g., personal hygiene, physical appearance, personality, social and communication skills, degree of disability) that may help or hinder social integration. The second theme, community attitudes and education, reflects service providers' beliefs that community attitudes and knowledge of disability issues have strong influences on social integration. Taken together, these two themes highlight discrimination as one of the most pervasive barriers people with disabilities encounter in attempting to become socially integrated.

Service providers tend to view organizational issues (e.g., agency philosophy on social integration, staff training and turnover) and inadequate funding for individualized programming as major challenges to social integration. Overall, this theme can be quite negative in terms of its implications for social integration. Service providers seem to believe that staff should play an important role in the process of social integration, but are unable to do so because of various organizational constraints, including a lack of staff training and staff turnover. On a more positive note, service providers hold the opinion that when an organization's philosophy supports social integration, many of the staffing and funding concerns can be overcome.

Empowerment was another theme unique to the service providers' perspectives on factors that relate to social integration. This is not surprising because the literature is replete with assertions of the importance of empowerment and self-determination for people with developmental disabilities (Mahon, 1994; Sands & Wehmeyer, 1996; Ward & Kohler, 1996). Interviewees were in almost unanimous agreement that older adults with developmental disabilities have few opportunities to make decisions for themselves and that this lack of opportunity directly affects their social integration. Summing up the connection between decision making and integration, one service provider noted, "They should be able to make just as many decisions as anybody else. If they're not allowed to, then they're not being integrated."

In addition to decision making, service providers also identified interdependence as a key to promoting social integration. According to many of those interviewed, the aims of social integration are advanced when older adults have opportunities to engage in mutually reliant relationships in the community and have access to valued social roles. Clearly, this assertion is consistent with Wolfensberger's (1983) notion of social role valorization.

The final theme that emerged from the service provider interviews is what we call "process versus product." During the course of the interviews, numerous comments were made about the changing nature of social integration. In some cases, these comments related to the life spans of individuals, whereas in others, they were more focused on the evolution of social integration as a reality within our communities. In all cases, these comments stressed the importance of recognizing social integration as a process versus a product.

Families and Others Providing Social Supports

Focus groups that included family members and others who provide social supports yielded two themes that were consistent with ones identified by the older adults—friends and valued social roles. From both viewpoints, the presence of friends and the opportunity to fulfill valued social roles were recognized as important ingredients in social integration. It is interesting to note that on the issue of friendship, family members and others who provide social supports talked at length about the challenges that older adults face in initiating and sustaining these relationships and the need for families to support these efforts. Older adults, in contrast, did not describe their families as facilitators of friendship but as contexts for assuming valued social roles.

Family members and people providing social supports also mentioned work and living situations as influences on social integration. Unlike the older adults who talked about these contexts as presenting opportunities for social interactions, family members and people providing social supports concentrated on the constraining effects of constantly having to "fight" for services, lack of information about appropriate options, and more generally, about the shortage of available service options. Extending these concerns about availability and access to services, family members and social supports identified two additional themes—care/advocacy and vulnerability—as constraints or challenges to socially integrating older adults.

The personal characteristics of the individual with a developmental disability was the final theme that arose from focus groups with family members and social supports. Consistent with service providers' opinions, personal hygiene, physical appearance, behavior, social and communication skills, degree of disability, and health status were all viewed as factors that affect, usually by limiting, social integration.

CONCLUSIONS

Much of what we know about social integration is based on the perspectives of people without disabilities. While acknowledging that it is important to listen to the views of families and service providers, we also must listen to the voices of people with developmental disabilities. Supporting this contention, our research showed that service providers, family members, and social supports viewed social integration in ways that were not always consistent with the perspectives of older adults with developmental disabilities.

For example, the older adults did not distinguish between people with and without disabilities when they talked about friendships and how these contributed to social integration. This is in stark contrast to the perspectives of other informants, and a good deal of the literature that defines "true" friendship and social integration as outcomes of relationships among people without disabilities (Crapps & Stoneman, 1989; Green & Schleien, 1991). The older adults also identified structured recreation as providing very important opportunities for social integration. Service providers suggested that recreation, in general, is important, whereas family members and people providing social supports did not. Furthermore, the themes that were not identified by the older adults, but were consistent across the other informant groups (e.g., service providers, families, people who provide social supports), also are important because they point to the overarching theme of our study. Specifically, service providers, families, and people providing social supports tended to concentrate on constraints to social integration (e.g., personal characteristics, organizational issues, negative societal attitudes, lack of communication about available services). Conversely, older adults focused on factors that did not always capitalize on their full potential but did enhance their social integration.

What does this discrepancy in perspectives mean? Obviously, a number of interpretations are possible, depending on one's point of view. From our perspective, it seems that although well intentioned, service providers, families, and social supports may be preoccupied with what they see as the challenges of social integration. As a result, not enough attention is paid to supporting opportunities for social integration that are valued by older individuals with developmental disabilities. The significance of this possibility becomes apparent when recalling our earlier discussion about the link between social integration and quality of life. That is, social integration is recognized as one of the defining elements of quality of life, and both are regarded as complex ideas that mean different things to different people (Schalock, 1996). Including the perspectives of individuals with developmental disabilities, therefore, is imperative if our understanding of socially constructed concepts is to be enhanced. Furthermore, by increasing our knowledge, we will be in a better position to provide programs, services, and supports that assist people in becoming socially integrated and, in turn, achieving their own visions of what it means to lead meaningful and fulfilling lives.

REFERENCES

Anderson, D.J., Lakin, K.C., Hill, B.K., & Chen, T.H. (1992). Social integration of older persons with mental retardation in residential facilities. *American Journal on Mental Retardation, 96,* 488–501.

Biklen, S.K., & Moseley, C.R. (1988). "Are you retarded?" "No, I'm Catholic": Qualitative methods in the study of people with severe handicaps. *Journal of The Association for Persons with Severe Handicaps, 13,* 155–162.

Blatt, B., & Kaplan, F. (1966). *Christmas in purgatory: A photographic essay of mental retardation.* Needham Heights, MA: Allyn & Bacon.

Burchard, S.N., Hasazi, J.S., Gordon, L.R., & Yoe, J. (1991). An examination of lifestyle and adjustment in three community residential alternatives. *Research in Developmental Disabilities, 12,* 127–142.

Crapps, J.M., & Stoneman, Z. (1989). Friendship patterns and community integration of family care residents. *Research in Developmental Disabilities, 10,* 153–169.

Erickson, M., Krauss, M.W., & Seltzer, M.M. (1989). Perceptions of old age among a sample of aging mentally retarded persons. *Journal of Applied Gerontology, 8,* 251–260.

Goode, D. (1988). *Discussing quality of life: The process and findings of the work group on quality of life for persons with disabilities.* Valhalla, NY: Westchester County Medical Center, Mental Retardation Institute.

Green, F.P., & Schleien, S.J. (1991). Understanding friendship and recreation: A theoretical sampling. *Therapeutic Recreation Journal, 25*(4), 29–40.

Haring, T.G. (1991). Social relationships. In L.H. Meyer, C.A. Peck, & L. Brown (Eds.), *Critical issues in the lives of people with severe disabilities* (pp. 195–217). Baltimore: Paul H. Brookes Publishing Co.

Hutchison, P., & Lord, J. (1979). *Recreation integration: Issues and alternatives in leisure services and community involvement.* Ottawa, Ontario, Canada: Leisurability Publications.

Hutchison, P., & McGill, J. (1992). *Leisure, integration, and community.* Concord, Ontario, Canada: Leisurability Publications.

Keith, K.D. (1990). Quality of life: Issues in community integration. In R.L. Schalock & M.J. Begab (Eds.), *Quality of life: Perspectives and issues* (pp. 93–100). Washington, DC: American Association on Mental Retardation.

Krueger, R.A., & Casey, M.A. (2000). *Focus groups: A practical guide for applied research* (3rd ed.). Thousand Oaks, CA: Sage Publications.

Lord, J., & Pedlar, A. (1991). Life in the community: Four years after the closure of an institution. *Mental Retardation, 29,* 213–221.

Mactavish, J., Lutfiyya, Z., & Mahon, M.J. (1998). *"I can speak for myself": Involving individuals with a mental disability as research participants. Abstracts from the 1998 Symposium on Leisure Research.* Arlington, VA: National Recreation and Park Association.

Mahon, M.J. (1994). The use of self-control techniques to facilitate self-determination skills during leisure in adolescents with mild and moderate mental retardation. *Therapeutic Recreation Journal, 28*(2), 58–72.

Mahon, M.J., & Goatcher, S. (1999). Later life planning for older adults with mental disabilities: A field experiment. *Mental Retardation, 37,* 371–382.

Morgan, D.L. (1997). *Focus groups as qualitative research* (2nd ed.). Thousand Oaks, CA: Sage Publications.

Nirje, B. (1969). A Scandinavian visitor looks at U.S. institutions. In R. Kugel & W. Wolfensberger (Eds.), *Changing patterns of residential services for the mentally retarded* (pp. 51–57). Washington, DC: President's Committee on Mental Retardation.

Nirje, B. (1976). The normalization principle and its human management implications. In M. Rosen, C.R. Clark, & M.S. Kivitz (Eds.), *The history of mental retardation: Collected papers* (Vol. 2, pp. 363–376). Baltimore: University Park Press.

Pedlar, A. (1990). Normalization and integration: A look at the Swedish experience. *Mental Retardation, 28,* 275–282.

Ralph, A., & Usher, E. (1995). Social interactions of persons with developmental disabilities living independently in the community. *Research in Developmental Disabilities, 16,* 149–163.

Rosen, M., Simon, E.W., & McKinsey, L. (1995). Subjective measure of quality of life. *Mental Retardation, 33,* 31–34.

Sands, D.J., & Wehmeyer, M.L. (Eds.). (1996). *Self-determination across the life span: Independence and choice for people with disabilities.* Baltimore: Paul H. Brookes Publishing Co.

Schalock, R.L. (1996). Reconsidering the conceptualization and measurement of quality of life. In R.L. Schalock (Ed.), *Quality of life: Vol. I. Conceptualization and measurement* (pp. 123–139). Washington, DC: American Association on Mental Retardation.

Storey, K. (1997). Quality of life issues in social skills assessment of persons with disabilities. *Education and Training in Mental Retardation and Developmental Disabilities, 32,* 197–200.

Taylor, S.J., & Bogdan, R. (1990). Quality of life and the individual's perspective. In R.L. Schalock & M.J. Begab (Eds.), *Quality of life: Perspectives and issues* (pp. 27–40). Washington, DC: American Association on Mental Retardation.

Taylor, S.J., & Bogdan, R. (1996). Quality of life and the individual's perspective. In R.L. Schalock (Ed.), *Quality of life: Vol. I. Conceptualization and measurement* (pp. 11–22). Washington, DC: American Association on Mental Retardation.

Ward, M.J., & Kohler, P.D. (1996). Promoting self-determination for individuals with disabilities: Content and process. In L.E. Powers, G.H.S. Singer, & J. Sowers (Eds.), *On the road to autonomy: Promoting self-competence in children and youth with disabilities* (pp. 275–290). Baltimore: Paul H. Brookes Publishing Co.

Wehmeyer, M., & Schwartz, M. (1998). The relationship between self-determination and quality of life for adults with mental retardation. *Education and Training in Mental Retardation and Developmental Disabilities, 33*(1), 3–12.

Wolfensberger, W. (1972). *The principle of normalization in human services.* Toronto: National Institute on Mental Retardation.

Wolfensberger, W. (1983). Social role valorization: A proposed new term for the principle of normalization. *Mental Retardation, 21,* 234–239.

Wolfensberger, W., & Thomas, S. (1983). *PASSING (Program Analysis of Service Systems' Implementation of Normalization Goals): Normalization criteria and ratings manual* (2nd ed.). Toronto: National Institute on Mental Retardation.

4

Informal Support Networks
of Older Adults

Christine Bigby

This chapter examines the nature of informal support available to adults with intellectual disabilities at two distinct periods along the aging continuum: first, when adults are middle-age and still living at home with an elderly parent and, second, when they are older and have entered the postparental care phase of their lives. Both periods are of interest for research and yet remain largely unexplored. As Seltzer and Krauss noted, "Little is known about the course of intrafamilial change and development across the full life course for families with a child with mental retardation" (1994, p. 3). Informal support is a multidimensional concept, broader than just the provision of direct assistance or supervision with personal care and the tasks of everyday living. It can fulfill a broad spectrum of functions from tangible direct care tasks, emotional support, and companionship to indirect tasks such as care management, advocacy, and intangible roles such as caring about and oversight of well-being. Although the roles fulfilled may vary, informal sources can be equally significant in providing support to people who live independently, reside in residential services, or continue to live with their family.

Informal supports can be defined as those assistance arrangements made by families that are unpaid or not reimbursed and not provided by a "formal" organization. Thus, they are characterized by exchanges that are not formalized but provided by family, friends, neighbors, and acquaintances, *pro bono*, or by reciprocity. The nature and extent of an individual's informal support network changes through his or her life course, determined by the interaction of a multiplicity of factors, including individual characteristics and situational factors, mediated, in particular, by gender and family ties (Antonucci & Akiyama, 1987; Kahn & Antonucci, 1980). Adults who remain at home with parents have smaller, less diverse informal networks in which parents fulfill a more central role compared with those who have left parental care (Krauss & Erickson, 1988). As they age, they are likely to become part of a two-generation aging household, cared for by elderly parents. Their own aging, coupled with that of their parents and life course changes of other family members, will inevitably bring associated changes to family relationships and informal support. However, remaining at home and receiving lifelong parental care may no longer be a permanent option as increased life expectancy means that adults with intellectual disabilities have a greater chance of surviving into mid- and late adulthood and outliving their parents. Parental death or incapacity will cause a major life transition, precipitate a shift to nonparental care, and mark a major upheaval and rearrangement of their informal support networks. An understanding of the roles that informal supports can fulfill and acknowledgment of the type of informal supports available to an individual can provide important indicators of the nature of formal services they may require.

INFORMAL SUPPORTS FOR ADULTS LIVING WITH AGING CAREGIVERS

Estimates of numbers vary both within and between nations but it is clear that, through choice, commitment, or simply a lack of alternative options, many adults with intellectual disabilities live in families where parents are central to their support network (Beange & Taplin, 1996; Seltzer & Krauss, 1994; Walmsley, 1996). As parents age, their support networks shrink, lone parental caregivers increase, and the use and availability of formal services are reduced (McGrath & Grant, 1993; Smith, Fullmer, & Tobin, 1994). Grant (1993) suggested that networks of adults with intellectual disabilities living at home are typically family embedded and community insulated. Prosser and Moss (1996) drew similar conclusions, characterizing support networks of adults older than 40 years of age who live at home as operating on a hierarchical basis with defined parameters within which parents provide the bulk of care with little practical assistance from either other family members or the wider community of friends and neighbors. Although parents (predominantly mothers) appear to provide the bulk of instrumental support, other family members do play supportive roles to both the adult with an intellectual disability and aging caregivers. Their roles, however, tend to be affective, such as providing companionship or emotional support, rather than being instrumental and assisting with direct care tasks (Grant, 1986, 1987, 1988; Krauss & Erickson, 1988; Krauss, Seltzer, & Goodman, 1992; Prosser & Moss, 1996; Seltzer, Krauss, & Heller, 1991).

Studies show remarkable similarities in the size, composition, and dominance of family members in networks of adults living at home with aging caregivers. For example, Grant (1987) found that networks comprised 77% family members, 17% friends, and 6% professionals. Krauss and her colleagues (1992) found that approximately three quarters of networks were made up of family members, including parents (33%), siblings (25%), and other relatives (16%). Networks tend to be small, with the average size varying from five to seven people (Grant, 1987; Krauss & Erickson, 1988; Krauss et al., 1992). They are characterized by frequent contact, long-term relationships, and members who are predominantly older than the adult with intellectual disability (Krauss et al., 1992). Friends and neighbors are often connected to the adult with intellectual disability through their parents, which results in a larger than expected overlap between the parents' network and that of their adult child (Grant, 1986; Krauss et al., 1992). In the study by Krauss et al. (1992), 50% of the members of adults' networks also were members of parental networks. The vast majority of shared network members were close relatives (83%). However, it was notable that 40% of the friends of adults with intellectual disabilities also were included in their mothers' network.

Friends appear to play only a minimal role; for example, an estimated 40% to 50% of adults with intellectual disabilities living at home do not have friends (Grant, 1986; Krauss et al., 1992). These figures may, however, be misleading because studies have relied on caregiver perceptions rather than self-reports. Where friends are identified, they tend to be older and either shared with parents or others with intellectual disability met through specialist day centers or social clubs (Grant, 1986).

Relationships with Siblings

Seltzer and Krauss suggested the following:

> The perceived availability, quality and functions of sibling relationships for adults with retardation are important, although poorly understood. The potential of these relationships to provide a foundation for long-term care planning and for contributing to the emotional well-being of the adult with retardation is simply unknown. (1993, p. 113)

Studies (Begun, 1989; Lobato, 1983; Simeonsson & Bailey, 1986) of the sibling relationships where one sibling has intellectual disability are concentrated on childhood and adolescence. These studies point to the negative effects that having a sibling with intellectual disability has on children. These effects stem from disproportionate parental attention to siblings with disabilities, family isolation, imitation of the child with a disability, and anxiety or guilt about the reasons and nature of their sibling's disability (Begun, 1989; Lobato, 1983; Simeonsson & Bailey, 1986). An "affect neutral" model suggests that children are more involved in caregiving, training, and treatment activities with their sibling with intellectual disability and progressively less involved in normative types of affectively charged interactions. Consequently, it is suggested that affective disengagement occurs and relationships are less competitive, less intimate, and less intense than those with siblings without disabilities (Brody & Stoneman, 1986).

When a person has more than one sibling, the relationship with each sibling differs and usually the tie to one sibling will be stronger than the tie to the others (Begun, 1989; Seltzer, Begun, Seltzer, & Krauss, 1991; Zetlin, 1986). Similar to other relationships, those between siblings alter as participants develop and change throughout their lives. Zetlin (1986) suggested that middle-age siblings with an established, stable lifestyle can provide closer and more reliable support to an adult with intellectual disability than can younger siblings with less stable lives.

Zetlin (1986) identified five relationship types between young adults with intellectual disabilities and their siblings. The most common type of relationship (27 pairs) was characterized by warm feelings, minimal contact, and minimal involvement. Siblings did not have regular contact or regular responsibilities with their brother or sister with intellectual disability. Twenty sibling pairs had a relationship characterized by resentful feelings, minimal contact, and minimal involvement, whereas 12 sibling pairs were typified by warm feelings, regular contact, and moderate involvement. These siblings assisted elderly parents as caregivers and also were social companions for the adult with intellectual disability. Eight sibling pairs were characterized by warm feelings, frequent contact, and extensive involvement. In 4 of these pairs, a sibling had assumed the role of surrogate parent following the death or frailty of parents. Hostile feelings and no contact or involvement between siblings were rare. Only 7 sibling pairs had such a relationship, and only one person with intellectual disability had this type of relationship with all siblings.

Begun (1989) found that relationships between a broad age range of people with intellectual disabilities (12–69 years) and their sisters were generally positive. These relationships, however, were less competitive and intimate, with different patterns of nurturance, admiration, and domination than the relationships between the sister and her sibling without disabilities. Although relationships between people with intellectual disabilities and their sisters appeared to be affectively neutral, descriptions of these relationships were characterized by similar levels of affection and companionship as the relationships described with siblings without disabilities. Begun (1989) suggested that interpretations of relationships should be functionally based as they are less intimate, more dominant, and involve more caregiving because of the functional realities and competencies of the person with an intellectual disability.

Findings from a longitudinal study (Seltzer et al., 1991) of adults with intellectual disabilities living with an aging caregiver highlighted the significance of sibling roles. They concluded the following:

> As adults siblings have sustained contact with and rather extensive knowledge about the contemporary needs of their brother or sister with mental retardation and have engaged in a variety of familial experiences that signal continuing and meaningful roles in adulthood. (Krauss, Seltzer, Gordon, & Friedman, 1996, p. 90)

The involvement of siblings with a brother or sister with intellectual disability living with their parents appears to be both similar to (characterized by a low level of instrumental assistance) and different from (the salience of their involvement with respect to their mothers' well-being) patterns reported among typical adult siblings (Seltzer & Krauss, 1993). Siblings most commonly provide affective support to a brother or sister with intellectual disability. Affective support from at least one sibling was received by 80% of adults and, on average, 66% of all the siblings in a family provided such support (Seltzer et al., 1991). Similarly, Prosser and Moss (1996) found that support provided by siblings was more likely to be of an affective or recreational nature rather than help with day-to-day tasks. However, similar to Zetlin (1986), they found tremendous variation in the involvement of siblings with their brother or sister with intellectual disability, which ranged from extensive engagement and contact several times a week to visits once or twice per year.

Many factors affecting the relationship between an adult with an intellectual disability and their siblings are similar to those identified in the literature about siblings in general (Cicirelli, 1985; Connidis, 1994). For example, siblings who live together have more intense relationships than those who live apart, and co-residence increases the likelihood of a sibling providing instrumental support, although this may not extend to personal care tasks (Begun, 1989; Grant, 1987; Seltzer et al., 1991). Siblings who are substantially older than the person with intellectual disability are more satisfied and attribute more importance to the relationship than do siblings who are substantially younger. Sisters are more likely to be primary caregivers than brothers, although gender does not seem important when a person has only one sibling; in these situations, brothers are as involved as sisters (Begun, 1989). Families with higher levels of cohesion and expressiveness and who are more oriented toward achievement and independence have a higher level of sibling involvement than families without these traits (Seltzer et al., 1991).

FACTORS AFFECTING NETWORKS

The size of support networks declines as caregivers age. This may be due to loss such as death or life cycle moves, for example, a sibling leaving home (Grant, 1986, 1988; Heller & Factor, 1991; Suelze & Keenan, 1981). Nevertheless, family members are more stable than friends. Grant (1988) found that 49% of adults in his study had either a net loss or gain of friends over a 2-year period, whereas only 10% had a change of primary caregiver. Individual characteristics and the family's socioeconomic background affect the size of networks and the balance between family and friends. People with more severe disabilities have smaller networks with fewer younger members and, for them, friends are more likely to be shared with their caregiver (Krauss et al., 1992). Working-class families provided greater support, whereas adults from middle-class families are more likely to have friends in their network (Grant, 1987).

Relationships with Support Network Members

Krauss et al. (1992) suggested that relationships between adults with intellectual disabilities and members of their support networks are generally not reciprocal. In their study, on average, the adult received 3.7 types of support and returned 1.9. However, other researchers (Grant, 1987; Heller & Factor, 1988; Prosser, 1989; Todd, Shearn, Beyer, & Felce, 1993; Walmsley, 1996) point to evidence of reciprocal relationships between adults with intellectual disabilities and their primary caregivers. Strong bonds of mutual aid and a sense of interdependence may develop between an elderly caregiver and the adult with intellectual disability. Adults with intellectual disabilities who are living at home undertake domestic chores and, in addition, the financial viability of the household may depend on their pension. Their presence also may ensure that their elderly parent(s) can continue to live in their own home (Grant, 1986; Walmsley, 1996).

Predictors of Support Networks in Later Life

The nature of support networks while parents are alive and parental centrality as primary caregivers and as a pivotal link to other family and friends presage the occurrence of a significant upheaval when parents die or become incapacitated. As most people with intellectual disabilities will not have married or had children (Ashman, Suttie, & Bramley, 1993), in later life they will lack a spouse and children who typically provide the bulk of care to older people. Their closest relatives in the postparental care phase will be siblings, aunts, uncles, or cousins. Mainstream gerontological studies suggest that relatives such as these are much more likely to provide affective support and do not normally play significant instrumental or caregiving roles (Cicirelli, 1992; Johnson & Catalano, 1981; Wenger, 1987). Also, the nature of support from these relatives, particularly siblings, while parents are alive suggests that informal support may be limited and that replacement of parental roles, particularly in the realm of direct caregiving, may be problematic.

Litwak's (1985) theory of differential primary groups suggests that, because of their different group structures, members of an informal support network cannot easily substitute for one another. Thus, it is unlikely that other kin will replace the day-to-day personal care and supervisory tasks that a parent has fulfilled because they will not have the required characteristics (e.g., commitment, proximity, frequent contact, available resources). Replacement is only likely to occur where a network member with atypical characteristics exists, such as an unmarried sibling who lives in close proximity (Litwak, 1985). However, other close family members are likely to continue in their existing roles and may substitute for those tasks, previously fulfilled by a now absent network member, that match their characteristics. An example of this may be a task such as financial management, which requires long-term commitment but not proximity. However, Litwak (1985) suggested that, siblings, because they also may be elderly and have their own family commitments, may have a limited capacity to provide support and may not have the necessary resources to substitute for missing network members.

There appear to be no clear rules of family obligation that determine which kin will provide what support. Finch and Mason suggested that kin responsibilities to each other develop and change over time, built on and reflecting the history and nature of relationships between individuals, and that "specific responsibilities emerge as part of a long standing relationship between the parties which have a past as well as a present and anticipate a future" (1993, p. 28). Sets of commitments by particular family members will develop over time through a process of implicit or explicit negotiations that appear to follow certain patterns. Thus, people in similar kin positions may negotiate very different responsibilities. The structural position of people in respect to gender and genealogy will influence the commitments they negotiate, but the influence will be relative to each individual biography without any logically predictable pattern. This model suggests the difficulty of predicting from kin relationships alone what kind of support will be provided. People who lack close family members may have other more distant kin with strong commitments to them. This suggests the importance of understanding relationships among family members and informal agreements when considering the nature of informal support that may be available.

Finch and Mason's (1993) model underlines the importance that individual family dynamics play in determining the later-life support networks and perhaps also the salience of parental plans and expectations. Parents often have high expectations about the role siblings will play in future care but, as they are reluctant to make plans, such expectations often remain informal or implicit (Bigby, 1996; Heller & Factor, 1991; Kaufman, Adams, & Campbell, 1991). Most commonly, siblings are expected to take over a supervisory/management role for their brother or sister with intellectual disability rather than to provide direct care (Grant, 1989; Krauss, 1990; Richardson & Ritchie, 1989; Seltzer, Begun, Magan, & Luchterhand, 1993). Seltzer and her colleagues (1996) suggested that the current involvement of a sibling is an important predictor of his or her expected and intended future role in provision of support to his or her brother or sister with intellectual disability.

The norms of caring developed by parents over many years often include a fierce sense of independence, reluctance to seek help, and the protection of their adult child against a hostile community. Parents may have controlled many aspects of their adult's child's life, including mediating their contact with the community (Engelhardt, Brubaker, & Lutzer, 1988; Engelhardt, Lutzer, & Brubaker, 1987; Grant, 1987, 1988; Grant & McGrath, 1990; Prosser, 1989). Consequently, adults with intellectual disabilities may have been insulated from the community and have had few opportunities to make their own choices or extend and build their social networks. The protected lives that many adults experience makes predicting their future network characteristics and support needs difficult as their potential for building relationships and coping in a less protective environment will not have been tested and may be largely unknown.

Summary

Individual, family, and social contextual factors all affect the nature of an individual's support network. However, adults living with aging parents generally live in a social world dominated by family, with few friends of their own. Although the provision of hands-on care is primarily a mother's responsibility, siblings and other relatives provide support and companionship to both parents and the adult with intellectual disability. Predicting the size and scope of an adult's support network in later life when his or her parents are dead is difficult, though various theoretical propositions suggest that networks may lack those members who generally provide the bulk of direct care and support to the elderly. However, it is suggested that family history, negotiated commitments, and planning could be fundamental to the form of later-life social networks.

INFORMAL SUPPORT NETWORKS OF OLDER ADULTS IN THE POSTPARENTAL CARE PHASE

Beginning when a person is in his or her 50s, an age span of 30 years or more defines being an "older" person with intellectual disability. Because this is a period characterized by transitions, residential changes, and shifting support networks, generalizations about this group's characteristics are problematic (Bigby, 1997a). In addition, older people with intellectual disabilities are often treated as one homogenous group, thereby obscuring intragroup differences. For example, differential life experiences, care background, and current living situation all affect the nature of informal support networks. Much of the data about informal support networks of older people with intellectual disabilities are derived from large surveys, where frequency of contact is reported rather than the nature, quality, and content of interactions.

Several distinct threads are identified in the literature concerning informal support networks of older people with intellectual disabilities. The most dominant thread refers to the limited nature of networks and characterizes this group as "the family-less elderly" (Hogg, Moss, & Cooke, 1988). These older people with intellectual disabilities, unlike their "normal" peers, may have had no significant others in their lives since middle age because they did not marry, were not employed, or did not live in the community to develop friendships with neighbors and because their caregivers (often parents) have already died (Gibson, Rabkin, & Munson, 1992). It is suggested that friends and professionals will be more important than family in support networks and that the few family members involved will be mainly siblings, nieces, and nephews (Krauss & Erickson, 1988; Seltzer, 1985). Due to their network characteristics and their perceived difficulty in replenishing any losses to their support networks, older people with intellectual disabilities are believed to be particularly vulnerable to social isolation (Kropf, 1994; Seltzer & Seltzer, 1985). Some studies suggest that older people with intellectual disabilities have a high need for formal services. For example, Walz, Harper, and Wilson noted that "Late adult 'placement' in a care facility or nursing home is the probable alternative for a disabled person who has lost his or her parents" (1986, p. 626), and Lakin, Anderson, Hill, Bruininks, and Wright wrote that "Parents who have maintained their adult children at home are reaching ages where they must place their middle-aged children into residential settings" (1991, p. 66). Although supported accommodation is the most commonly identified service necessary in later life, other areas such as advocacy and care management also have been suggested as being important (Gibson et al., 1992). It is striking that when the loss of parents is anticipated, the continuing or additional roles that remaining informal network members may play are often ignored.

A different, more positive thread, but one for which there is little evidence, points to the intergenerational transmission of caregiving, suggesting that informal support, particularly that provided by siblings, will be important in the provision of care to older people with intellectual disabilities. For example, Janicki and Seltzer suggested the following:

> The public sector would not be able to absorb the wave of new clientele if, upon death of the parent, all adults with developmental disabilities who remained at home up to that point needed publicly supported residences. Rather, it is the extended family, primarily the siblings, who step in as primary caregivers when the parents are no longer able to fulfill this function. (1991, p. 103)

Furthermore, Roberto stated, "for aging persons with developmental disabilities, parents then siblings take on the primary responsibility of providing care. In both situations women (i.e., wives, mothers, daughters) tend to be responsible for providing day to day care for the recipient" (1993, p. 16). Much of the focus is on the replacement of the primary caregiver and, as a result, the other more intangible roles that informal sources may fulfill are largely neglected.

Network Characteristics

A common characteristic of the informal support networks of older people with intellectual disabilities is the absence of an informal primary caregiver. An indicator of this is that consistently less than one fifth of older people are reported to live in private homes (Ashman et al., 1993; Bigby, 1994, 2000; Community Services Victoria, 1992; Hand & Reid, 1989; Hogg & Moss, 1993; Prosser & Moss, 1996; Seltzer, 1985). A study that tracked the life changes of a group of older people after they left parental care in middle age demonstrated that people were less likely to have an informal primary caregiver as they aged. Until the age of 40 years, the entire study population had a parental primary caregiver. In the initial postparental care phase, when the average age of the sample was 52.5 years, just more than half still had an informal primary caregiver; however, this proportion had dropped significantly to less than one fifth when the average age of the group increased to 65 years (Bigby, 2000). In sharp contrast, Edgerton's (1988) longitudinal study of ex-institutionalized older people found that all the study cohort lived in private homes in the community (most were without a primary caregiver). This serves as a reminder that not all people with intellectual disabilities require such a caregiver.

Several qualitative studies give an indication of who, if anyone, replaces parents as informal primary caregivers (it should be noted that some studies have used broad age groupings and include younger adults as well). In the absence of parents, informal primary care is provided predominantly by siblings and occasionally by more distant relatives or family friends (Bigby, 1997b; Grant, McGrath, & Ramcharan, 1995; Heller & Factor, 1991; Moss, Hogg, & Horne, 1989; Prosser & Moss, 1996). For example, Moss et al. (1989) reported that 17 out of 121 people older than 50 years of age lived with a relative: 7 people with a parent, 6 people with sisters, 1 person with a cousin, 1 with a niece, 1 with a nephew, and 1 with a son. Characteristics associated with replacement primary caregivers are living with or being close to the parent and the person with intellectual disability before transition, caring for the parent in later life, a close long-term relationship with the older person, being single, being female, and being a sibling (Bigby, 1997b). The limited evidence available suggests that primary caregivers who replace parents do so only on a short-term basis and that a period of informal non-parental primary care is often followed by a move to supported accommodation (Bigby, 1997b; Grant, 1988; Prosser, 1989).

Bigby (1997b) found that, apart from the absence of parents, the networks of older adults in the postparental phase were quite similar to those of adults living with aging caregivers: small (with an average of six members), dominated by family, dense, and comprising chiefly people from a similar or older generation. People who were in contact with the older person at least twice per year were included as network members. Family comprised more than half the network for more than two thirds of the sample, less than one fifth had no family, and more than one third had no friends. Affective was the most common type of support provided, which, with varying intensity, was provided by all network members. More than three quarters of the sample also received one or more types of instrumental support; however, this usually came from one source only, most often a family member.

A difference between pre- and postparental care networks is that siblings, more distant relatives, or friends are more likely to fulfill instrumental roles in the postparental phase than previously. Some aspects of parental roles may be taken over by other network members who became more involved in the life of the older person after parents died or became incapacitated. For example, in Bigby's study (1997b, 2000), she found that tasks involving "caring about" the person were more likely to be taken over by a network member than those involving more direct "caring for." Despite the absence of spouses and children, a striking feature of most networks was a "key person" who proactively oversaw the well-being of the older person by managing their affairs and negotiating service provision. They took a strong advocacy role and combined three or more instrumental tasks with frequent contact, strong attachment, and a high level of commitment. Contact with key people generally provided opportunities for shared social activities, and most had a long-standing strong emotional bond with the older person. Key people were primarily siblings, but also included more distant relatives and friends/church connections. A close long-term relationship with the older person and the foreshadowing of their role by parents were the basis of key person relationships rather than genealogical relationship alone. Just as parents had done, key network members often nominated their own successor. For example, a sister may negotiate with one of her children to assume the role of key person in the future (Bigby, 1997b, 2000). However, despite such planning, the proportion of older people without a key network member increases with age.

The significance of long-term family care to the nature of later-life networks is suggested by the contrast between Bigby's findings and those from Edgerton's (1988) study of a group of older people with an institutional rather than a family care background. Edgerton (1988) found that roles played by family members in support networks of members of his study cohort were largely inconsequential and that reliance on a main benefactor diminished as they aged. However, despite the absence of a "key person," a very positive picture of their social networks emerged. Edgerton suggested that older individuals were "embedded in worlds of meaningful and reciprocal relationships with other people" (1988, p. 333).

INFLUENCE OF FAMILY RELATIONSHIPS

Survey data show that, with some exceptions, older people with intellectual disabilities are childless and unmarried (Ashman et al., 1993; Hand, 1994; Moss et al., 1989). Thus, for the majority, a sibling will be their closest relative, but for the estimated 30% without siblings it will be aunts, uncles, cousins, nieces, or nephews (Ashman et al., 1993). In spite of these atypical family constellations, Hogg and Moss (1993) suggested that family remain the chief providers of informal support as people with intellectual disabilities grow older. Blacher (1993) suggested that family members may be the only people with a long-term relationship to the older person and a perspective broad enough to encompass all of a person's service needs.

The proportion of older people with intellectual disabilities to have at least occasional contact with relatives varies considerably. For example, Bigby (1997b) found that 92% were in contact; Hand (1994) found that 71% were in contact; and Kearney, Krishnan, and Londhe (1993) found that 45% were in contact. Seltzer (1985) concluded that probably no more than one third of aging people with intellectual disabilities had contact with their siblings. A study of older residents in British long-stay hospitals found that just more than half had no contact with family members, which is similar to findings from an Australian national survey (Ashman et al., 1993; Kearney et al., 1993). Similarly, a U.S. study of older people in some type of residence found that half had no living family or were never visited by them, and of the other half, 6% saw a relative weekly, 8% monthly, and 35% less than monthly (Anderson, Lakin, Hill, & Chen, 1992).

Ties with siblings are their most significant relationships, as well as the closest, for most older people with intellectual disabilities. Seventy-nine percent of the older people in Bigby's (1997b) study had a sibling. Ninety-six percent of those with a sibling saw one of them at least twice per year, and 82% of all the subject's' siblings had contact with their brother or sister with intellectual disability at least twice per year, with most seeing them more frequently (Bigby, 1997b). Fulfilling the role of a key network member was the most common type of relationship between an older person with intellectual disability and their sole or closest sibling. Relationships with other siblings fell into two broad types: siblings as social contacts and alienated sibling. At most, siblings who were social contacts fulfilled only one instrumental role and were not substantially involved in the supervision of the older person's affairs. Typically, these siblings were named as next of kin or provided backup to other support network members. They had warm friendly relationships with the older person that provided opportunities for social interaction and companionship. Alienated sibling relationships were rare and characterized by little or no contact with the older person and a history of a poor relationship (Bigby, 1997b).

The nature of family relationships, need, and parental expectations are associated with sibling roles. Indicators suggest that siblings may fulfill or exceed the expectations of their parents regarding their involvement in the life of their brother or sister with intellectual disability (Bigby, 2000; Griffith & Unger, 1994). Relationships with more distant family members reflect family traditions or are associated with negotiated commitments between individuals and parents. Bigby (1997b) found that one third of older people had contact with extended family, although much of this contact was incidental and occurred at family functions.

The contrast between findings of two Australian studies suggests the significance of care background to family contact in later life. Ashman et al.'s survey (1993), which included people from all care backgrounds, found that about half (47%) of the older people in the study sample had at least yearly contact with relatives, which consisted primarily of visits on special occasions. Bigby's (1997b) study, which focused on people who had lived with parents until midlife, found a much higher level of family contact (92%). Studies of older people who are or previously have been institutionalized also indicate the salience of care background. For example, Skeie (1989) found that, when institutional residents had spent much of their lives at home, siblings were more likely to replace parents as regular visitors than they were for residents who had been institutionalized for most of their lives. Similarly, Edgerton (1988) suggested that family members were unimportant in the support networks of his ex-institutional cohorts.

Hogg and Moss (1993) suggested that the age, functional level, or type of residence of the person with intellectual disability does not affect contact with relatives. However, their study and several others (Ashman et al., 1993; Hand, 1994) tend to indicate that place of residence may be a factor. People in institutions have the least contact with relatives, whereas those living with family tend to have the most (Hogg & Moss, 1993). This variability may, however, be due more to their residential and family history than simply a function of their current place of residence. Ashman, Hulme, and Suttie (1990) suggested that locations also may be factors in that people in rural areas are more involved with their relatives than people who live in more urban areas.

INFLUENCE OF FRIENDS AND ACQUAINTANCES

Studies indicate that most friendships of older people with intellectual disabilities are tied to a specific context, and only about half of those with friends have contact with them outside their place of residence or day activity (Anderson et al., 1992; Ashman et al., 1993; Bigby, 1997b; Hogg & Moss, 1993). For example, Ashman et al. (1993) indicated that, while 70% to 90% of people had social contact with friends or staff at work or in their place of residence, only 40% had contact with them outside these settings. Context-specific friendships pose the challenge of ensuring the maintenance of friendships as people age and retire from day centers or move from house to house. It appears, however, that maintenance of friendship ties across contexts rarely occurs and that severed long-term ties with friends who have disabilities are not replaced by new friendships with peers who do not have disabilities (Bigby, 2000; Grant et al., 1995).

With the exception of Edgerton's (1988) sample, it has been generally observed that approximately one third of older people with intellectual disabilities are believed to be without friends (Bigby, 1997b; Grant et al., 1995). However, accounts and perceptions of friendships differ among respondents. Bigby (1997b) found that family and service providers were often unaware of friendships or discounted them thinking that, because of their poor social skills, older people had no friends.

Grant and his colleagues (1995) found that most older people with intellectual disabilities claimed to have access to a network of social acquaintances and friends in their community. However, they suggest that subtle differences exist between these two types of social relationships and, although everyone had acquaintances, friendships involving intimacy and reciprocity were rarer (Grant et al., 1995). A similar differentiation between friends and acquaintances was made in Bigby's (2000) study, in which many informants referred to unnamed groups of people as friends. For example, one person stated, "the people in Coles canteen all know me"; however, such groups were classified as acquaintances (Bigby, 2000). Both studies highlight the significance of acquaintances in social networks and suggest that older people are more likely to lack friends than acquaintances. Acquaintances can provide a sense of identity or belonging to the community, while also placing few expectations on people. Despite the existence of acquaintances in the community, older people do not appear to have strong relationships with their communities. For example, Grant et al. concluded that individuals "experienced degrees of physical, functional and organizational integration in their social lives but lacked personal, social and societal integration in a variety of ways" (1995, p. 42). Anderson et al. (1992) found that only 45% of older people, surveyed from a variety of residential situations, had met a neighbor.

The residential mobility experienced by people with intellectual disabilities, especially those who have lived with parents, disrupts longstanding relationships and connections with local communities (Bigby, 1997b; Grant et al., 1995). For example, Bigby (2000) found that people who remained in the locality of their family home regarded one or more neighbors as friends. Such people were an important source of affective and, sometimes, instrumental support. In contrast, most people who changed location did not retain contact with previous neighbors and, although people who moved to supported accommodation found acquaintances or friends among co-residents, they rarely had any interaction with people in their new neighborhood (Bigby, 2000). Furthermore, it seems that individual characteristics affect friendships more than family relationships, such that more competent people are likely to have more contact with friends (Moss et al., 1989).

Environmental factors also have a significant influence on friendship patterns. Nahemow (1988) suggested that older people are particularly affected by the environment in which they live. Older people with intellectual disabilities who live independently in the community or in group homes have consistently been shown to have more contact with friends than those living in institutions or with family (Anderson et al., 1992; Ashman et al., 1993; Hogg & Moss, 1993). An extensive review of friendships and social behavior of people of all ages with intellectual disabilities shows that opportunity, aspects of the social group, and the environment are more powerful determinants of an individual's social behavior and relationships than are personal traits (Landesman-Dwyer & Berkson, 1984). The strong tendency for older people with intellectual disabilities to live in restrictive residential settings that present a poor fit between level of functional competence and environmental opportunities provides some explanation for the vulnerability and limited nature of their friendship ties (Baker, Seltzer, & Seltzer, 1977; Bigby, 2000; Seltzer, Finlay, & Howell, 1988; Seltzer, Seltzer, & Sherwood, 1982).

CONCLUSIONS

The growing body of research suggests that in the postparental care phase the informal support networks of older adults with intellectual disabilities are more robust than some researchers have speculated. Most are not without family ties, and normative family roles such as "protector" and "facilitator" are fulfilled informally despite the absence of spouses or children (Sussman, 1985). For many, siblings assume a key pivotal role in their network, replacing some parental functions, mostly those involving "caring about" rather than "caring for." The caring about role, which includes advocacy, monitoring, and negotiation with agencies, is crucial to ensure the overall well-being of older people with intellectual disabilities and indispensable for this group of people who are highly reliant on formal services to replace the direct primary care previously provided by parents.

Family history, the quality of previous relationships, and negotiated commitment are fundamental to ensuring that siblings and others maintain and increase their involvement in the life of the older person after parental death. Supportive later-life networks evolve from relationships formed throughout the life course. This reinforces the critical importance of agencies, serving people with intellectual disabilities of any age, focusing attention and devoting resources to network building, and the recognition, nurturance, and resourcing of family and other sources of informal support.

The network characteristics and later-life experiences of older people with intellectual disabilities mean that their informal support networks are vulnerable to loss and disruption. Accommodation options that are flexible and can adapt to an aging person's changing needs must be developed to tackle the issue of residential mobility and the resultant fracturing of networks and dislocation from acquaintances and community. Alternatively, major challenges confronting service providers are the preservation of networks and maintenance of friendships if change of residence, day activity location, or retirement occurs. However, an essential precursor to preservation of ties is that service personnel and family members begin to recognize the existence and value of the friendships that people with intellectual disabilities develop.

As people with intellectual disabilities grow older, they are increasingly likely to lack informal sources of primary care and to rely on formal services to fulfill this task. The nature and quality of this formal support may be a crucial determining factor of a person's informal support, particularly their friendships. Therefore, it is a concern that people in this group are particularly prone to living in restrictive residential settings that offer few challenges or opportunities. A major task confronting agencies is to counter the "ageist" expectations of our society that place limited expectations on the elderly and to ensure that services provide environments for older people that maximize opportunities for social interaction and friendship building and optimize development of their full potential.

The importance of informal support lies in its characteristics and the difficulty formal services have in replicating its functions and compensating for its absence. Characteristically, informal support is flexible and idiosyncratic and is often provided in the context of a lifelong commitment or a close relationship to the recipient, whereas formal services often lack these characteristics and are poor substitutes for some functions undertaken by informal sources. Formal services find it particularly difficult to replicate tasks vital to safeguarding quality of life, such as advocacy, monitoring well-being, and provision of emotional support, all of which require long-term commitment and flexibility. A challenge for the whole community is to ensure the development and delivery of optimal quality formal sources of primary care and other supports for older people with intellectual disabilities. However, the limitations of such services must be recognized. The greater challenge will be to foster the recognition, respect, and maintenance of informal support sources and provide resources and conditions that encourage and sustain their development. Formal and informal sources of support are both necessary and complementary for older people with intellectual disabilities to replace the care previously provided by their parents.

REFERENCES

Anderson, D., Lakin, K., Hill, B., & Chen, T. (1992). Social integration of older persons with mental retardation in residential facilities. *American Journal on Mental Retardation, 96*, 488–501.

Antonucci, T., & Akiyama, H. (1987). Social networks in adult life and a preliminary examination of the convoy model. *Journal of Gerontology, 42*, 519–527.

Ashman, A., Hulme, P., & Suttie, J. (1990). The life circumstances of aged people with an intellectual disability. *Australia and New Zealand Journal of Developmental Disabilities, 16*, 335–347.

Ashman, A., Suttie, J., & Bramley, J. (1993). *Older Australians with an intellectual disability* (Report to the Department of Health, Housing and Community Services, Research and Development Grants Committee). Brisbane, Queensland, Australia: University of Queensland, Fred and Eleanor Schonell Special Education Research Centre.

Baker, B.L., Seltzer, G.B., & Seltzer, M.M. (1977). *As close as possible: Community residences for retarded adults.* Boston: Little, Brown & Co.

Beange, H., & Taplin, J. (1996). Prevalence of intellectual disability in northern Sydney adults. *Journal of Intellectual Disability Research, 40*, 191–197.

Begun, A. (1989). Sibling relationships involving developmentally disabled people. *American Journal on Mental Retardation, 93*, 566–574.

Bigby, C. (1994). A demographic analysis of older people with intellectual disability registered with Community Services Victoria. *Australia and New Zealand Journal of Developmental Disabilities, 19,* 1–10.

Bigby, C. (1996). Transferring responsibility: The nature and effectiveness of parental planning for the future of adults with intellectual disability who remain at home until mid-life. *Journal of Intellectual and Developmental Disabilities, 21,* 295–312.

Bigby, C. (1997a). Later life for adults with intellectual disability: A time of opportunity and vulnerability. *Journal of Intellectual and Developmental Disabilities, 22,* 97–108.

Bigby, C. (1997b). In place of parents? The sibling relationships of older people with intellectual disability. *Journal of Gerontological Social Work, 29,* 3–21.

Bigby, C. (2000). *Moving on without parents: Planning, transitions, and sources of support for older adults with intellectual disability.* Baltimore: Paul H. Brookes Publishing Co.

Blacher, J. (1993). Siblings and out-of-home placement. In Z. Stoneman & P.W. Berman (Eds.), *The effects of mental retardation, disability, and illness on sibling relationships: Research issues and challenges* (pp. 117–141). Baltimore: Paul H. Brookes Publishing Co.

Brody, G.H., & Stoneman, Z. (1986). Contextual issues in the study of sibling socialization. In J.J. Gallagher & P.M. Vietze (Eds.), *Families of handicapped persons: Research, programs, and policy issues* (pp. 197–217). Baltimore: Paul H. Brookes Publishing Co.

Cicirelli, V. (1985). Sibling relationships throughout the life cycle. In L. L'Abate (Ed.), *The handbook of family psychology and therapy* (pp. 177–214). Homewood, IL: Dorsey Press.

Cicirelli, V. (1992). Siblings as caregivers in middle and old age. In J.W. Dwyer & R.T. Coward (Eds.), *Gender, families and elder care* (pp. 84–101). Thousand Oaks, CA: Sage Publications.

Community Services Victoria. (1992). *Services for older people with an intellectual disability* (research papers included). Melbourne, Australia: Author.

Connidis, I. (1994). Sibling support in old age. *Journal of Gerontology, 49,* S309–S317.

Edgerton, R. (1988). Aging in the community: A matter of choice. *American Journal on Mental Retardation, 92,* 331–335.

Engelhardt, J., Brubaker, T., & Lutzer, V. (1988). Older caregivers of adults with mental retardation. Service utilization. *Mental Retardation, 26,* 191–195.

Engelhardt, J., Lutzer, V., & Brubaker, T. (1987). Parents of adults with developmental disabilities: Age and reasons for reluctance to use another carer. *Lifestyles: A Journal of Changing Patterns, 8,* 177–184.

Finch, J., & Mason, J. (1993). *Negotiating family responsibility.* London: Routledge.

Gibson, J., Rabkin, J., & Munson, R. (1992). Critical issues in serving the developmentally disabled elderly. *Journal of Gerontological Social Work, 19,* 35–49.

Grant, G. (1986). Older carers, interdependence and the care of mentally handicapped adults. *Ageing and Society, 6,* 333–351.

Grant, G. (1987). The structure of care networks in families with mentally handicapped adult dependants. In P. Gutridge (Ed.), *Social work in action in the 1980s* (Occasional paper, University of Wales, Department of Social Theory and Institutions, pp. 24–48). Bangor, UK: University of Wales.

Grant, G. (1988). *Stability and change in the care networks of mentally handicapped adults living at home* (First report, University of Wales, Centre for Social Policy and Development). Bangor, UK: University of Wales.

Grant, G. (1989). Letting go: Decision making among family carers of people with mental handicap. *Australia and New Zealand Journal of Developmental Disabilities, 15,* 189–200.

Grant, G. (1993). Support networks and transitions over two years among adults with mental handicap. *Mental Handicap Research, 6,* 36–55.

Grant, G., & McGrath, M. (1990). Need for respite care services for caregivers of persons with mental retardation. *American Journal on Mental Retardation, 94,* 638–648.

Grant, G., McGrath, M., & Ramcharan, P. (1995). Community inclusion of older adults with learning disabilities: Care in place. *International Journal of Network and Community, 2*(1), 29–44.

Griffith, D., & Unger, D. (1994). Views about planning for the future among parents and siblings of adults with mental retardation. *Family Relations, 43,* 221–227.

Hand, J. (1994). Report of a national survey of older people with lifelong intellectual handicap in New Zealand. *Journal of Intellectual Disability Research, 38,* 275–287.

Hand, J., & Reid, P. (1989). Views and recollections of older people with intellectual handicaps in New Zealand. *Australia and New Zealand Journal of Developmental Disabilities, 15,* 231–240.

Heller, T., & Factor, A. (1988). *Development of a transition plan for older adults with developmental disabilities residing in the natural home* (Public Policy Monograph Series No. 37). Chicago: University of Illinois at Chicago.

Heller, T., & Factor, A. (1991). Permanency planning for adults with mental retardation living with family caregivers. *American Journal on Mental Retardation, 96,* 163–176.

Hogg, J., & Moss, S. (1993). The characteristics of older people with intellectual disabilities in England. In N. Bray (Ed.), *International review of research in mental retardation* (Vol. 19, pp. 71–92). New York: Academic Press.

Hogg, J., Moss, S., & Cooke, D. (1988). *Ageing and mental handicap.* London: Croom-Helm.

Janicki, M., & Seltzer, M. (Eds.). (1991). *Aging and developmental disabilities: Challenges for the 1990s* (Proceedings of the Boston Roundtable on Research Issues and Applications in Aging and Developmental Disabilities). Washington, DC: American Association on Mental Retardation, Special Interest Group on Aging.

Johnson, C., & Catalano, D. (1981). Childless elderly and their family supports. *Gerontologist, 21,* 610–618.

Kahn, R., & Antonucci, T. (1980). Convoys over the life course: Attachment, roles, and social support. In P. Baltes & O. Brim (Eds.), *Life-span development and behavior* (pp. 253–286). New York: Academic Press.

Kaufman, A., Adams, J., & Campbell, V. (1991). Permanency planning by older parents who care for adult children with mental retardation. *Mental Retardation, 29,* 293–300.

Kearney, G., Krishnan, V., & Londhe, R. (1993). Characteristics of elderly people with a mental handicap living in a mental handicap hospital. A descriptive study. *British Journal of Developmental Disabilities, 39,* 31–50.

Krauss, M. (1990, May). *Later life placements: Precipitating factors and family profiles.* Paper presented at the 114th annual meeting of the American Association on Mental Retardation, Atlanta, GA.

Krauss, M., & Erickson, M. (1988). Informal support networks among aging persons with mental retardation. A pilot study. *Mental Retardation, 26,* 197–201.

Krauss, M., Seltzer, M., & Goodman, S. (1992). Social support networks of adults with mental retardation who live at home. *American Journal on Mental Retardation, 96,* 432–441.

Krauss, M., Seltzer, M., Gordon, R., & Friedman, D. (1996). Binding ties: The roles of adult siblings of persons with mental retardation. *Mental Retardation, 34,* 83–93.

Kropf, N. (1994). *Older parents of adults with developmental disabilities: Issues for practice and service delivery.* Paper presented at the Young Adult Institute 15th Annual International Conference on Developmental Disabilities, New York City.

Lakin, K., Anderson, S., Hill, B., Bruininks, R., & Wright, E. (1991). Programs and services received by older persons with mental retardation. *Mental Retardation, 29,* 65–74.

Landesman-Dwyer, S., & Berkson, G. (1984). Friendship and social behavior. In J. Wortis (Ed.), *Mental retardation and developmental disabilities: An annual review* (Vol. 13, pp. 129–154). New York: Plenum Publishing Corp.

Litwak, E. (1985). *Helping the elderly: The complementary roles of informal networks and formal systems.* New York: Guilford Press.

Lobato, D. (1983). Siblings of handicapped children: A review. *Journal of Autism and Developmental Disorders, 13,* 347–364.

McGrath, M., & Grant, G. (1993). The lifecycle and support networks of families with a mentally handicapped member. *Disability Handicap and Society, 8,* 25–41.

Moss, S., Hogg, J., & Horne, M. (1989). *Residential provision and service patterns in a population of people over the age of 50 years and with severe intellectual impairment. A demographic study of older people with mental handicap in Oldham Metropolitan Borough* (Part 2). Manchester, UK: University of Manchester, Hester Adrian Research Centre.

Nahemow, L. (1988). *The ecological theory of aging as it relates to elderly persons with mental retardation.* Paper presented to the Ninth Congress of International Association for the Scientific Study of Mental Deficiency, Dublin, Ireland.

Prosser, H. (1989). *Relationships within families and the informal networks of older people with severe intellectual impairment (mental handicap): A demographic study of older people with mental handicap in Oldham Metropolitan Borough* (Part 3). Manchester, UK: University of Manchester, Hester Adrian Research Centre.

Prosser, H., & Moss, S. (1996). Informal care networks of older adults with intellectual disability. *Journal of Applied Research in Intellectual Disabilities, 9,* 17–30.

Richardson, A., & Ritchie, J. (1989). *Letting go: Dilemmas for parents whose son or daughter has a mental handicap.* Milton Keynes, England, UK: Open University Press.

Roberto, K.A. (1993). Family caregivers of aging adults with disabilities. A review of the caregiving literature. In K.A. Roberto (Ed.), *The elderly caregiver: Caring for adults with developmental disabilities* (pp. 3–21). Thousand Oaks, CA: Sage Publications.

Seltzer, G., Begun, A., Seltzer, M., & Krauss, M. (1991). Adults with mental retardation and their aging mothers: Impacts of siblings. *Family Relations, 40,* 310–317.

Seltzer, G., Finlay, E., & Howell, M. (1988). Functional characteristics of elderly persons with mental retardation in community and nursing homes. *Mental Retardation, 24,* 213–217.

Seltzer, G.B., Begun, A., Magan, R., & Luchterhand, C.M. (1993). Social supports and expectations of family involvement after out-of-home placement. In E. Sutton, A.R. Factor, B.A. Hawkins, T. Heller, & G.B. Seltzer (Eds.), *Older adults with developmental disabilities: Optimizing choice and change* (pp. 123–140). Baltimore: Paul H. Brookes Publishing Co.

Seltzer, M. (1985). Informal supports for aging mentally retarded persons. *American Journal of Mental Deficiency, 90,* 259–265.

Seltzer, M., Krauss, M., Choi, S., & Hong, J. (1996). Midlife and later-life parenting of adult children with mental retardation. In C. Ryff & M. Seltzer (Eds.), *The parental experience in midlife* (pp. 459–492). Chicago: University of Chicago Press.

Seltzer, M., & Seltzer, G. (1985). The elderly mentally retarded. A group in need of service. In G.S. Getzel & M.J. Mellor (Eds.), *Gerontological social work practice in the community* (pp. 99–120). New York: Haworth Press.

Seltzer, M., Seltzer, G., & Sherwood, C. (1982). Comparison of community adjustment of older vs. younger mentally retarded adults. *American Journal of Mental Deficiency, 87,* 9–13.

Seltzer, M.M., & Krauss, M.W. (1993). Adult sibling relationships of persons with mental retardation. In Z. Stoneman & P.W. Berman (Eds.), *The effects of mental retardation, disability, and illness on sibling relationships: Research issues and challenges* (pp. 99–115). Baltimore: Paul H. Brookes Publishing Co.

Seltzer, M.M., & Krauss, M.W. (1994). Aging parents with co-resident adult children: The impact of lifelong caregiving. In M.M. Seltzer, M.W. Krauss, & M.P. Janicki (Eds.), *Life course perspectives on adulthood and old age* (pp. 3–18). Washington, DC: American Association on Mental Retardation.

Seltzer, M.M., Krauss, M.W., & Heller, T. (1991). Family caregiving over the lifecourse. In M.P. Janicki & M.M. Seltzer (Eds.), *Aging and developmental disabilities: Challenges for the 1990s* (Proceedings of the Boston Roundtable on Research Issues and Applications in Aging and Developmental Disabilities, pp. 3–24). Washington, DC: American Association on Mental Retardation, Special Interest Group on Aging.

Simeonsson, R.J., & Bailey, D.B., Jr. (1986). Siblings of handicapped children. In J.J. Gallagher & P.M. Vietze (Eds.), *Families of handicapped persons: Research, programs, and policy issues* (pp. 67–77). Baltimore: Paul H. Brookes Publishing Co.

Skeie, G. (1989). Contact between elderly people with mental retardation living in institutions and their families. *Australia and New Zealand Journal of Developmental Disabilities, 15,* 201–206.

Smith, G., Fullmer, E., & Tobin, S. (1994). Living outside the system: An exploration of older families who do not use day programs. In M.M. Seltzer, M.W. Krauss, & M.P. Janicki (Eds.), *Life course perspectives on adulthood and old age* (pp. 19–38). Washington, DC: American Association on Mental Retardation.

Suelze, M., & Keenan, V. (1981). Changes in family support networks over the life cycle of mentally retarded persons. *American Journal of Mental Deficiency, 86,* 267–274.

Sussman, M. (1985). The family life of old people. In R. Binstock & E. Shanas (Eds.), *Handbook of aging and the social sciences* (2nd ed., pp. 415–449). New York: Van Nostrand Reinhold.

Todd, S., Shearn, J., Beyer, S., & Felce, D. (1993). Careers in caring: The changing situation of parents caring for offspring with learning difficulties. *Irish Journal of Psychology, 14,* 130–153.

Walmsley, J. (1996). Doing what mum wants me to do: Looking at family relationships from the point of view of adults with learning disabilities. *Journal of Applied Research in Intellectual Disability, 9,* 324–341.

Walz, T., Harper, D., & Wilson, J. (1986). The aging developmentally disabled person: A review. *Gerontologist, 26,* 622–629.

Wenger, C. (1987). *Relationships in old age: Inside support networks* [3rd report of a follow-up study of old elderly people in North Wales]. Bangor, UK: University of Wales, Centre for Social Policy Research and Development.

Zetlin, A. (1986). Mentally retarded adults and their siblings. *American Journal of Mental Deficiency, 91,* 217–225.

I

Essay

Aging

Achieving a Broader View

Nancy Breitenbach

The International Year for Older Persons 1999 provided a prime opportunity to ensure that older people with intellectual disabilities were included in people's understanding of increased life expectancy as it is enjoyed around the world. Given the breadth of their networks and their scale of operations, international organizations such as Inclusion International are in a unique position to track the issue of aging on a worldwide level. But before such organizations can achieve a broader view, they must develop an adequate sense of perspective. Three objectives must be kept in mind: 1) maintain a global view, 2) maintain a universal view, and 3) maintain a comprehensive view.

A GLOBAL VIEW

It is a very human failing to examine the immediate vicinity and consider that what one sees as representative of the rest of the world. A global view implies consistently looking farther, searching beyond our "natural" frontiers toward the neighboring state, the neighboring country, the next continent, across the ocean. It means accepting (even relishing) diversity and, above all, acknowledging that we do not know everything and that everything that we do know is relative.

To illustrate this point, accounts of longevity regarding people with intellectual disabilities come largely from developed countries. As a result, we tend to believe that most people with disabilities as well as most older people live in these same countries

71

and that the norm for life expectancy is 70–80 years. A global view obliges us to revise our thinking because

- Only 40% of people age 60 years and older live in developed countries
- Approximately 65% of the 600 million people with disabilities (some 60 million of whom have intellectual disabilities) live in developing countries
- Life expectancy is increasing throughout the world, but it is not as great for the majority of people as one might think: 62 years for men, 66 years for women.

When one compares extremes, the contrast is striking. The average life expectancy in Japan, Canada, France, Sweden, and Switzerland for the two sexes is 79–80 years, whereas the average in Sierra Leone, Malawi, Uganda, Rwanda, and Zambia is only half that: 38–43 (Yearbook of Labour Statistics, 1997).

What this means is that people with disabilities who live in developed nations are, in fact, a minority and that only a small percentage among all of the peoples of the world has the privilege of reaching what Westerners now consider "old age"—that is, 75 years or older. To be even clearer, the accomplishments of which Europeans and North Americans are so proud (e.g., the fact that in Northern Ireland, 22% of people with Down syndrome are age 40 years or older) represent more than what millions of ordinary people can reasonably hope for.

How many of the "older people" around the world have disabilities? This is extremely difficult to answer for a number of reasons. The cutoff point at which people are counted as "older" varies from country to country. Accountability depends not only on survival but also on local definitions and criteria of disability. In Austria, for example, where in 1976, 21% of the country's population was presented as having a disability, events in the first half of the 20th century had marked indelibly that country's demographic composition. Moreover, administrative choices included as "impaired" older people who had lost certain functions as a result of aging.

Very small percentages in developing countries, conversely, probably reflect high mortality rates among people with disabilities. But their disappearance also could be explained otherwise: Once they have reached adulthood, many are simply lost from sight—the men working in the community as unskilled laborers, the women making their contribution as wives and mothers. Inasmuch as they lead ordinary lives, they are not "disabled" and there is no reason to count them.

But to be frank, we honestly do not know. Many poor countries do not have resources available for collecting information. They have enough difficulty funding basic services such as nutrition and education programs.

In developing countries, are people who have an intellectual disability living longer lives, as do those in highly developed regions? Given worldwide statistics on infant mortality, coupled with figures concerning disability in general, researchers presume that few children born with intellectual disabilities survive. In fact, the BBC recently announced that in Africa, only a fraction of children who are born with intellectual disabilities survive to reach the age of 5 years, much less maturity. Yet we hear from the field echoes like this report from India:

Family A: Parents aged 73 and 75 years. Their child aged 50 years could not stand on his own feet but dragged himself on the floor. His speech was also not clear. He required help in self-care, and could not be left alone except for a very short time. The parents were too old and weak to physically help the child. Their other three children, being married and settled away from home, do not provide any support or help in a crisis. (Chen et al., 1987)

I myself encountered in French Polynesia a man with multiple disabilities who had spent 40 years on the floor of his parents' hut. So there *are* older people with intellectual disabilities out there. It is time to have a more substantiated picture of the long-term fate of adults with intellectual disabilities.

A UNIVERSAL VIEW

One may ask, "If it is so different everywhere from what is familiar to us, then what could we possibly have in common with people who live in other countries?" A universal view means going beyond ethnocentricity. The passage involves abandoning the perception of the world as "we here, they over there" and associating oneself with the entire human community as "all of us are in the same boat." A universal view also means taking on a multicultural approach; not everyone lives or thinks as we do, nor should they be expected to. It is a matter of teasing out shared issues and developing a sense of solidarity.

What is comparable between East and West? North and South? Should one compare population profiles, for example? Imagining that from one country to another we all deal with the same disability groups is misleading. Even within a same-language community (much less communities with differing languages), the labels used do not necessarily cover the same populations. Relative proportions vary: Developed countries may have many people with cerebral palsy, spina bifida, and Down syndrome, for instance, whereas less developed countries may have few of these people but large numbers marked by the after-effects of maternal malnutrition, deprivations, or illnesses in early childhood. As an example, the World Health Organization estimated that in 1997, some 16.5 million people were experiencing significant brain damage as a result of iodine deficiency disorder and that their numbers were concentrated in eight countries representing 54% of the world's population: Bangladesh, Brazil, China, India, Indonesia, Nigeria, Pakistan, and the Russian Federation.

Does it help to compare services? Not much. In any given country, service provision is the long-term product of traditions, belief systems, and economic and human resources. Inevitably, these vary a great deal from one country to another, and the resulting services vary accordingly. Thus, lining up one system against another is like comparing carrots to oranges because they are the same color. International comparisons often founder in detail and lead to implicit contests in which value judgments prevail. They tend to be a sterile exercise.

The best route is to pinpoint life situations that clearly are associated with aging. In all cultures, certain dilemmas spark recognition. Parents throughout the world are asking the following types of questions:

- *"What will happen after we are gone?"* This question is the key to future planning. For the first time in history, mothers and fathers are recognizing that, contrary to what they had been led to believe, they will probably depart first. In some developed countries, the question already may be current. But in others, for instance in a number of African nations, it is only now beginning to be formulated.
- *"After we are gone, how will (s)he cope?"or, more specifically, "How will (s)he feel about our having disappeared?"* The question of bereavement with regard to people with intellectual disabilities is a new one because formerly the parents were most likely to be bereaved. But no matter how grief is expressed from one country to another, it is a human reaction that everyone understands.

- *"In the meantime, how will we cope?"* I mentioned earlier two Indian and Polynesian families that have managed to keep their sons with severe disabilities alive for 40–50 years. Such families can be found in every country of the world where life expectancy, both for parents and their offspring with disabilities, has increased and where family care continues to be the norm. This illustrates that caregiving is no longer a matter of a few years (because the child was not expected to live very long) but of entire lifetimes, and brings out widespread issues such as social isolation, poverty, and ill health in elderly caregivers. Everywhere, the question being posed is, "To what degree do elderly family caregivers receive adequate health care, support, and so forth to help them continue to care for their aging offspring with intellectual disabilities?"

A COMPREHENSIVE (IF NOT TO SAY INCLUSIVE) VIEW

Aging affects us all. As a result of the greater life expectancy of individuals with intellectual disabilities, decisions about their future will have to be made, and no one should be left out when it comes time to make them. In the decision-making triangle, researchers and policy makers have tended to take their place in one corner of the plane and people in more direct contact with the dependent person (meaning parents and professionals) faced them from the other corner. The person with an intellectual disability often found him- or herself at the apex of the triangle, pointed toward the bottom: the "object" of the benevolent efforts of the others who made the decisions (elderly people often find themselves similarly disempowered). The new longevity of people with intellectual disabilities (coincident with the self-advocacy movement) has produced a shift in the triangle's position so that no one is clearly at the bottom. All parties are in a position to give their opinion.

I submit that the issue of "old age for people with intellectual disabilities" is a golden opportunity to change the image of these people: instead of being perceived as eternal children (not only because of their "mental age" but because, in the past, few outlived their childhood, or if they did, they spent their adulthood hidden away in backyards or behind institutional walls), people with intellectual disabilities are now seen as potential adults, people with enough time before them to learn the skills they need to function capably in society and sufficient life experience to be able to make mature decisions. They now have years enough to grow gray hair and to take on the image of wisdom that goes with silvered temples.

The new generation is being consulted more and more with regard to their preferred lifestyle. But when their future is at stake, older people with intellectual disabilities (including the "walking wounded," who have spent their lives behind the walls of institutions) may not have the same opportunities with regard to consultation as the younger generation that has had the benefit of self-advocacy training.

Some of our old folks may require a lot of encouragement before they dare express their wishes. But others already know exactly what they want, as witnessed in this account from New Zealand:

When an IHC team reached Lake Alice in mid 1988, Pat Donnellan was waiting. He wasn't on the list of about 20 patients rated by the hospital as a candidate for the community. Ironically, he had been there too long, was seen as perhaps too old at 61 to readjust. What the system was saying was: We have institutionalized him so well he can't survive without us. That certainly wasn't the way Pat saw it. An IHC bus was to carry the listed patients on a tour of the houses they would share. When it filled up outside Lake Alice, Pat Donnellan was sitting determinedly in the front seat. There was no way he was going to get out of that bus. Regardless of what the list said. Pat reckoned that his day had come and he was going out. And when the bus stopped at the Wainuiomata house, Pat got out and boasted, "That's where I am going to live." ("The Lost Life of Pat Donnellan," 1990)

Ageism is so strong that the negative images attached to old age can taint our actions. Literature is full of information about the downward slide. The famous Frenchman André Maurois wrote in a moment of pessimism, "Old age is the feeling that it's too late." But Pat Donnellan is proving Maurois wrong. As long as the people we fight for are here on God's earth, there's still time for them to live.

REFERENCES

Chen, C.C., Fraser, A.S., Lyen, K.R., Oon, D., Tan, D., & Wong, M.K. (1987, November). *Intellectual disability: Perspectives and challenges. Proceedings of the 8th Asian Conference on Mental Retardation.* Singapore: Asian Federation for the Mentally Retarded (AFMR).

The lost life of Pat Donnellan. (1990, May). *North and South,* quoted in Inclusion International (1998). *Extended Lives—Extended Opportunities.*

Yearbook of Labour Statistics. (1997). Geneva: International Labour Office.

II

WORKING WITH FAMILIES, CAREGIVERS, AND OTHERS WHO PROVIDE SUPPORTS

The intricacies of working with families or family-based organizations define this section. We begin with a second contribution from Bigby, whose chapter extensively reviews the complexities of parental planning for the future, exploring its several goals and multiple beneficiaries, and examines the various facets involved in planning to ensure the well-being of adults who may outlive their parents by a generation or more. Her commentary identifies the tensions and conflicts that planning may elicit. The second part of Bigby's chapter relates the outcome of a major qualitative study undertaken by the author on the effectiveness of *key person succession plans,* which are defined by the nomination of another to replace the parents' role in overseeing well-being. The potential of such plans to ensure a smooth transition and long-term security and to be responsive to the unforeseen contingencies during postparental care is contrasted with other forms of planning.

People with developmental disabilities from diverse cultures and their families historically have been underrepresented among those who receive services from formal service providers. There are concerns that available formal services are designed for, rather than by, "multicultural" families. In countries built by immigration, successive cultural groups have alternately been in the minority and then in the majority. *Multiculturalism* refers to the diversity of cultures that are in any one locale and the need to have the majority population be sensitive to the needs and differences of the groups that are in the minority. Thus, McCallion and Grant-Griffin in Chapter 6 bear witness to the often striking differences between the mainstream of a locality and its individual members. They maintain that existing services rarely respect or build on the strengths offered by cultural values and beliefs and by the variety of natural supports in the family and community. In this regard, McCallion and Grant-Griffin present a model for more culturally competent practice that responds to critical caregiving and cultural issues and includes collaboration with locally based multicultural agencies. Their chapter concludes with implications drawn for agency workers, administrators, and policy makers.

Berkobien and Davis in Chapter 7 report how developmental disabilities agencies can organize and provide targeted services to families of older adults. The authors reflect on the experiences of a national, voluntary advocacy organization as it tries to bring together the different actors in a locality to set the agenda for disability services. Their work with coalition development within several states and their approach to helping older families in their communities provide the context for how organizations can become competent coalition builders. Their chapter focuses on the various positive and challenging aspects of coalition building between local developmental disabilities and aging agencies, the unique services that the project's model sites developed, and the current status of these initiatives.

In Chapter 8, Clark and Susa describe the use of a structured approach that is designed to encourage families with older parents and adult sons or daughters with developmental disabilities to anticipate and plan for their futures together. The family futures planning approach relies on an educational intervention that is based on stages of change that move participating families into developing and implementing futures plans. Simultaneously, this approach encourages the collaboration of providers from both the aging and the developmental disabilities service systems to support the continued clarification and actual realization of family goals. The authors identify the challenges in this approach, including resistance to change on the basis of personal and family histories and behavior patterns, as well as of ideological, political, and economic barriers in the services system.

Ansello and Coogle examine in Chapter 9 the roles of aging adults with lifelong disabilities and family caregivers in achieving their own rights. The authors reference the "rights and responsibilities equation" in describing a professional/consumer advocacy council (PCAC) model that they helped institute in Virginia. The PCAC's composition, leadership, purpose, and operating principles served to facilitate the involvement of consumers and families in activities that enrich their own lives while benefiting others. The authors use this chapter to substantiate how the components of such a model contributed to successful advocacy in one state and to offer guidance in applying it to other situations.

In the concluding chapter of this section, Kultgen, Harlan-Simmons, and Todd consider the shift from a "services oriented" paradigm to a "community supports" approach to planning. Their use of a person-centered strategy is designed to foster membership in a range of community networks. Their chapter articulates the methods of community building through illustration of a number of strategies that can be employed by "community builders" to connect older adults with lifelong disabilities to their communities. These strategies can involve the recasting of historic "staff–client" relationships into new designs whereby individuals are introduced to roles and activities in the community and are encouraged to choose freely among them and connect with members of the community. Kultgen, Harlan-Simmons, and Todd note that community builders work one to one with individuals as unobtrusively as possible as they facilitate opportunities for connection to and inclusion in community networks. The authors state what resources may be needed to actualize community membership for adults with developmental disabilities and define some of the barriers to and successes of this approach.

Last, an essay by Ansello relates the efforts of a statewide advocacy council, composed of aging individuals with lifelong disabilities, family caregivers, agency staff, and others, that advocated for a greater goal that drew in rather than competed with other advocacy groups. He demonstrates how system advocates can have an effect on a state legislature and how a specific piece of legislation, the Caregivers Investment Bill, not only became a reality for the citizens of the Commonwealth of Virginia but also substantiated a philosophy for meaningful involvement of aging individuals and their families.

5

Models of Parental Planning

Christine Bigby

It is not a normative expectation that elderly parents will plan for the future care of their adult children (Heller & Factor, 1991), nor is this an issue dealt with by the mainstream gerontological literature. However, planning by aging parents for the future care of their adult child with intellectual disability is increasingly seen as a fundamentally important task. As Smith, Tobin, and Fullmer noted, "Because older parents of adults with mental retardation are increasingly likely to be survived by their offspring, they must make permanency planning arrangements" (1995, p. 487). Parental planning has diverse goals and multiple beneficiaries. Adequate planning, it is supposed, can avert the crisis of an ill-prepared transition from parental care, ensure longer-term security and stability of the person with intellectual disability, and forecast future service demands (Heller & Factor, 1988a, 1988b; Kaufman, Adams, & Campbell, 1991). The process of planning also has been suggested as psychologically important to elderly parents to resolve unfinished business (Grant, 1989; Heller & Factor, 1991; Kaufman, 1989; Kaufman et al., 1991; Smith & Tobin, 1989, 1993, 1994).

Planning is conceptualized in various ways but is usually seen to comprise three areas: guardianship, financial, and residential provisions (Heller & Factor, 1991; Seltzer & Seltzer, 1992; Smith & Tobin, 1994; Smith et al., 1995; Wood, 1993). Planning is generally seen as straightforward: "Proper planning includes making financial and guardianship arrangements and finding appropriate placements" (Heller & Factor, 1988b, p. 2). However, planning also can be conceptualized as a complex dynamic process whereby plans must be sufficiently flexible and adaptable to meet the changing residential, financial, and legal requirements of an adult who may survive his or her parents by 30 or 40 years

(Kaufman et al., 1991; Seltzer & Seltzer, 1985). With this in mind, Seltzer and Seltzer (1985) suggested that planning may not achieve a secure, permanent residential situation but may be important to ensure that family members remain involved with the person with intellectual disability and monitor the quality and appropriateness of services.

Freeling and Bruggeman (1994) suggested that planning involves the notion of guaranteed care and that a plan encompassing all life areas should be made jointly by the person with intellectual disability, his or her parents, and professionals, and include a guarantee of services by the local political authority. In Australia, for example, parental planning also has been used as a mechanism, whether desirable or otherwise, to promote cost sharing of future care between parents and the state (Community Services Victoria, 1988, 1992; Sach & Associates, 1991; Victorian Department of Health & Community Services, 1995a).

The first part of this chapter reviews research studies that have explored the reasons, nature, extent, obstacles, and motivations for parental planning. Central themes to emerge are the reluctance of parents to make concrete plans and the dilemmas and difficulties that confront parents and service providers if they do embark on the planning process. Despite the focus on the critical importance of planning, its outcomes, effectiveness, and whether parental expectations are met have not been well researched or documented. The latter part of the chapter addresses this deficit and focuses on the efficacy of an informal-based planning model derived from the author's own retrospective study of parental planning.

EXTENT AND NATURE OF PLANNING

Richardson and Ritchie (1986, 1989) suggested that parents of adults with intellectual disabilities hold three categories of attitudes toward planning: avoidance, ambivalence, and active planning, of which avoidance is the most common. Most studies of planning show that only between one third to one half of parents make concrete plans for future care of an adult with intellectual disability who is living at home (Campbell & Essex, 1994; Cooke, cited in Hogg, Moss, & Cooke, 1988; Freedman, Krauss, & Seltzer, 1997; Goodman, 1978; Grant, 1989; Heller & Factor, 1991; Kaufman et al., 1991; Krauss, 1990; Mulcahey, 1986). Financial planning is the most common type of planning that is undertaken. Smith, Fullmer, and Tobin (1994) suggested that planning is not a simple act occurring at one point but has five stages, ranging from no discussion to definite plans.

Some families may not move along the full continuum and plans may remain implicit, comprising informal agreements or understandings between family members (Heller & Factor, 1991; Kaufman et al., 1991). Some plans are never formalized and may not even be discussed with the family members who are expected to be involved in future care (Goodman, 1978; Richardson & Ritchie, 1986, 1989). The formulation of plans may not involve a discussion of alternatives with the person concerned (Gold, 1987; Richardson & Ritchie, 1986, 1989; Wood, 1993). For example, Smith and Tobin (1989) found that parents paid little attention to the wants of the adult with an intellectual disability and, when preferences were known, if they were incompatible with parental attitudes, they were sometimes disregarded. In contrast, however, Heller and Factor (1991) found that most families who had made concrete plans for a future residential placement had discussed these decisions with their adult child with intellectual disability and other children.

A quantitative analysis of parental planning can be misleading because of the different ways in which plans are conceptualized. For example, Gold (1987) discovered that many elderly parents (2 out of 3) had applied for future placement of their adult child in residential accommodation and that this could indicate a high level of residential planning. But only 10% of the sample had any intention of ever taking up residential care, and these "plans" often represented multiple applications made long ago. Some families formulate several plans representing a series of back-ups or different views among family members about the future. For example, Krauss, Seltzer, Gordon, and Friedman (1996) found that, in about one quarter of families where a sibling expected to co-reside with a brother or sister with an intellectual disability, the parent also placed the person's name on a waiting list for residential accommodation. Similarly, inconsistencies between family plans and perceptions of the future were found in a study by Griffith and Unger (1994). In their study, a higher proportion of siblings expressed a willingness to act as caregiver in the future than was reflected in parental expectations and encapsulated in plans. Plans and expectations may also change over time; for example, Grant (1988) found that during a 2-year period just more than half the parents in his study changed their preference for future care.

Parental Expectations of Future Care

The preferences expressed in plans, by parents, for the future care of their adult child with intellectual disability are generally evenly split between continued family care, primarily by siblings, and residential placement (Grant, 1989; Heller & Factor, 1991; Wood, 1993). Card (1983) found that an exceptionally high proportion of parents (80%) expected the statutory social services to provide accommodation for their child in the future. This may, however, be a result of the inclusion of younger parents with adolescent children in the study.

Sometimes, plans distinguish between the provision of direct and indirect care. Parents are more likely to expect a family member to provide indirect care for the adult with intellectual disability by, for example, overseeing their well-being, than to expect a relative to provide hands-on support (Bigby, 1996; Goodman, 1978; Krauss, 1990). Many of these parental expectations resemble the theoretical propositions derived from Litwak's (1985) model of informal care and the conceptualization of indirect informal care suggested by Sussman (1985). These types of expectations are usually informally based, although in some instances they may involve formal guardianship arrangements. Legal arrangements vary among local governmental entities. In Victoria, Australia, for example, the nature of guardianship legislation precludes the anticipatory appointment of a guardian for an adult with intellectual disability (Carney & Tait, 1997).

Findings consistently show that, although elderly parents make plans, they want to continue in their role of primary caregiver for as long as possible (Card, 1983; Goodman, 1978; Grant, 1989; Heller & Factor, 1991; Kaufman et al., 1991; Krauss, 1990; Richardson & Ritchie, 1986, 1989). This will inevitably impinge on the implementation and effectiveness of plans, because services such as residential situations may not be immediately available on demand and plans may need to be made a number of years prior to implementation.

Parental plans value protection and permanency rather than developmental opportunities. Instead of looking toward increased independence for their adult son or daughter in the future, parents seek residential accommodation to duplicate the care and protection that they have provided at home. Parents also want to select a residential situation where their adult child can remain for the rest of his or her life (Card, 1983; Gold, 1987). Griffin and Bennett (1994) found that when parents discussed planning in a group, they generally emphasized security, attaining peace of mind, and a safe, secure situation as most important to them. However, Brubaker and Brubaker (1993) suggested that the greatest concern that parents have regarding the future is the adult child's social and emotional well-being rather than his or her residential or financial needs.

Factors Affecting Planning

Most studies have found an association between the use of formal services and both the parental propensity to make plans and an expected reliance on formal services rather than other family members for future care. This suggests that use of services may lead to a greater knowledge of options and more trust in the quality of formal services (Essex, Seltzer, & Krauss, 1997; Grant, 1989; Heller & Factor, 1991; Seltzer, Krauss, & Heller, 1991; Smith & Tobin, 1993; Smith et al., 1994; Wood & Skiles, 1992). The decision to plan is multifactorial and has been associated with caregiver characteristics, stressors, and resources (Essex et al., 1997; Heller & Factor, 1991; Seltzer & Krauss, 1994). For example, behavior problems of the adult with intellectual disability, many unmet needs, and small support networks are positively associated with planning, whereas age of the caregiver is negatively associated (Essex et al., 1997). Smith and his colleagues (1995) constructed a model incorporating many of these factors, demonstrating the complexity of factors involved in parental planning decisions.

The choices and options that plans contain often emerge from the social context of care. Grant (1989) found that when continued family care was chosen, caring was generally judged to be trouble-free, with little involvement by professionals, and a supportive network, made up predominantly of kin, was in place. In contrast, families who expected to rely on formal services for future care had fewer kin supports and were more involved with professionals (Smith & Tobin, 1989).

Obstacles to Planning

Despite the suggested benefits of comprehensive planning, many parents do not undertake this task. Reasons for this vary but are often based on the perception that the process of planning is emotionally challenging for parents, logistically complex, and confronts professionals with difficult ethical issues. The most common reasons proposed for low levels of parental planning are that parents lack information about service options or that they are either distrustful of, or dissatisfied with, formal services (Card, 1983; Gold, 1987; Grant, 1988; Heller & Factor, 1988b; Kaufman et al., 1991; Kropf, 1994; Smith & Tobin, 1989; Smith et al., 1995).

Having to formulate a plan forces parents to come to terms with issues such as their own aging and mortality. They also may have to deal with the tension between a desire to continue caregiving and their anxiety about future care (Kropf, 1994; Seltzer & Ryff, 1994; Smith & Tobin, 1993; Smith et al., 1994). Strong bonds of interdependency often exist between parents and their adult child with an intellectual disability, and the process of planning and making decisions to relinquish care requires parents to balance their own needs and desires with the rights and needs of their adult child (Grant, 1986).

The types of future care parents want for their offspring may conflict with the values and options preferred by professionals in the specialist service system. When formal services are involved, a clash of values between parents and professional workers may be an obstacle to working effectively with older parents to develop plans. Research has noted that workers feel anger and frustration with elderly parents regarding their failure to make plans and parental protective attitudes toward their adult child are perceived as having jeopardized the growth and development of the person with intellectual disability (McCallion & Tobin, 1995; Smith & Tobin, 1993).

The role of formal services in encouraging and assisting parents to engage in planning has been the focus of discussion and service development (Bigby, Ozanne, & Gordon, 2000; Eloura Homes, 1995; Lehmann & Roberto, 1993; Smith & Tobin, 1993, 1994; Victorian Department of Health & Community Services, 1995a). Smith and Tobin (1994) suggested that social workers should act as both teachers and therapists with older parents, assisting them to confront the issues and providing information about possibilities. A comprehensive model of practice for work with older families has been developed by Kaufman (1989). Most programs suggest that any intervention around planning with elderly parents should be long term, family focused, and involve support and sensitivity to the psychosocial needs of all members of the family constellation.

However, the nature of formal services systems may create systemic obstacles to parental planning. These include an emphasis on short-term interventions that make it difficult to undertake the long-term work with parents that is required to gain parental trust and confront complex issues. Inadequate linkages between specialist and generic service systems and poor knowledge of other systems by staff also may be an obstacle to planning (Smith & Tobin, 1994; Victorian Department of Health & Community Services, 1993). A lack of concrete alternatives that can be offered to parents, particularly concerning residential situations, may mean that parents see planning as pointless. Backlogs are often the norm in many jurisdictions. For example, in Victoria, 3,030 people were waiting for a supported residence in 1994 (Victorian Department of Health & Community Services, 1995b), and Hayden and DePaepe (1994) reported that some 200,000 individuals with developmental disabilities were waiting for services in the United States at the time of their study.

The effect of resources on the outcomes of planning is highlighted by the longitudinal study of older caregivers undertaken by Seltzer and her colleagues (Essex et al., 1997; Seltzer et al., 1991). Findings suggested a poor fit between parental planning and service system resource decisions. Essex et al. (1997) found that residential placement occurred in emergency situations when caregiving was no longer tenable. Factors that precipitated low-level parental planning (e.g., adding the person's name to a local service residential waiting list) were not synonymous with factors that led to residential placement. Two possible explanations are suggested, both of which indicate planning may be less efficacious than anticipated. Either the service system is only responsive to emergencies and allocation of resources is based on urgency rather than on systematically planned for and foreseen need, or alternatively, parents turn down offers of help with a residential option, refusing to implement plans and relinquish care until absolutely necessary.

Planning Issues

Few researchers have raised questions about the appropriateness of parents formulating plans that resemble detailed blueprints for the future of their adult child with intellectual disability. However, Grant (1988) suggested that contemporary ideologies and values reflected in the service system may challenge previously taken-for-granted rights of parents to decide the future pattern of care. Edgerton, although not discussing planning directly, implied its restrictiveness when he noted that

> The lives of mentally retarded people who live with their parents or residential care providers are over determined; one might say because not only is their present day organized, arranged and regimented by other people, so is tomorrow and the future. (1994, p. 56)

Adults who remain at home and make the transition from parental care in their 40s and 50s have perhaps 20 or 30 years of their life ahead of them. Designing and implementing a plan to determine the course of their lives in the postparental care phase is a difficult task. Many contingencies must be dealt with. This phase of their lives may be characterized by instability and change; individual characteristics such as health status may vary, other skills may develop or decline, and social and service contexts may alter because of changes in the circumstances of family and friends or organizational policies (Bigby, 1996, 1997a). Although some changes may be foreseen, their impact cannot be accurately predicted. Other changes, perhaps unexpected, can be difficult for which to plan. Later life also is a period in which many adults with intellectual disabilities experience considerable personal development and increased autonomy, and may demonstrate more personal competence than at any other time in their lives (Bigby, 1997a; Edgerton, 1994). Attempting to identify a plan, particularly one that involves a suitable and desired residential situation for the rest of their adult child's life, may not be realistic for some parents. It may be argued that it is inappropriate, particularly in view of the lack of consultation that sometimes occurs, the later-life development that is yet to be experienced, and the risk of locking someone into an environment that may become inappropriate or be more restrictive than warranted.

AN INFORMAL MODEL OF PLANNING

The balance of this chapter draws on the findings of a retrospective study of parental planning and explores a model of parental planning that has the potential for flexibility and responsiveness to deal with the contingencies of the postparental care phase (Bigby, 1996, 2000). The study focused on the nature and success of parental planning for those who remained at home well into their middle-age years. Rather than parents, those with a stake in the plans, that is, the person with intellectual disability, their siblings, and other relatives, were the informants. Their memories, perceptions, and interpretations were relied on to describe the nature of planning undertaken by parents. Formal documents, such as wills, trusts, and family trees, sometimes supplemented memories. Experiences that were had since leaving parental care were used to consider the implementation and success of plans.

Parental Attitudes Toward Planning

Most parents have an enormous sense of responsibility and concern about the future care of their adult child with intellectual disability. Recognizing the difficulties inherent in making plans, some parents, fearful of their child's not being adequately cared for, express a desire that their adult child should die before they do. Some parents reduce their anxiety by becoming involved in establishing services that are required to ensure that their plans come to fruition. For example, one older woman's sister said, "Dad supported the day center with the establishment of a community residence and he expected my sister to live there. Once the residence was open, although my sister still remained at home, Dad had a peace of mind about the future." For parents who envisage that one of their other children will replace them as a primary caregiver, anxieties about the future may be reduced as children reach a stage in their life course at which providing care for their brother or sister with intellectual disability is feasible. For example, one man's mother had planned for his sisters to provide care for him. The mother became more relaxed about the future as her daughters' own children married and caring for their brother became a more realistic option for his sisters.

Parental Planning Models

Most parents undertake some form of planning, ranging from vague expectations to comprehensive blueprints. Plans are defined as ideas or arrangements that concern the care of their adult child with intellectual disability when parents have died, are incapacitated, or chose to cease being the primary caregiver. Their plans are either explicit or implicit. *Explicit plans* contain written or discussed ideas and concern financial support, supervision, or residential and care arrangements for the future. *Implicit plans* are expectations held by parents about future care that have not been formally discussed. Arrangements made at short notice, as a response to immediate or impending circumstances by either a parent or another person, are not seen as plans but as transition management issues.

Within this broad conceptualization, four types of plans are explored: implicit key person succession plans, explicit key person succession plans, residential plans, and financial plans. Key person succession plans are the most predominant. Financial and residential plans are usually made in conjunction with each other or with a key person succession plan (for detailed information on planning combinations, see Bigby, 1996, 2000).

Key Person Succession Plans   Key person succession plans are characterized by the planned transfer of responsibility for overseeing the well-being of the person with intellectual disability to some other person or people. The tasks specified in the plan vary from being highly prescribed to vague and open ended. When tasks are specified, supervision, oversight, and monitoring of service provision and administration of financial affairs are more common than direct provision of care.

In such plans, the sibling is most frequently nominated as the person to take on responsibility. When there is more than one sibling, particular expectations are often placed with each. Other people with a long-standing relationship to the family are sometimes nominated, particularly when there are no siblings or poor intrafamily relationships exist. One mother's plan involved a minister who was a friend of the family. He said, "The parents asked me to be the executor of the will and they charged me as it were to keep a roof over their son's head, and that when he died the property be given to his brothers or his brother's children."

Implicit Key Person Succession Plans   Implicit key person succession plans are generally not discussed; that is, they are composed of the unspoken expectations that parents hold of others about the roles they will assume in the future. The expected roles are usually vague but focus on oversight of well-being. This type of plan is, however, made up of more than just hopes. The nominated person is usually strongly aware of the parental expectations, which they implicitly accept. In one sense, these plans are minimalist; in another sense, they may portend enormous responsibility. The following are two examples of people for whom implicit key person succession plans were made.

> Nadia's sister, Julie, said that her mother had not needed to talk to her or plan for the future. It had just been accepted that the family and she, in particular, would provide care for Nadia. There were no formal agreements, and it had not even been talked about. Nadia herself said that her mother had never talked to her about what would happen when she died, but she believed that her mother may have talked to Julie about keeping an eye on her.

Ada's aunt, who had lived next door to Ada and her parents for many years and was now caring for Ada, said that her sister had never spoken openly to her about assuming responsibility for Ada. She went on to say, "I think she just took it for granted. We are Christians, you know. We believe in God and the Lord Jesus Christ, and I think she just knew the Lord would look after her and that I would fill in. We just more or less took it for granted, I think."

Explicit Key Person Succession Plans   Explicit key person succession plans have a similar defining characteristic: the nomination of another person to take responsibility to oversee the well-being of the person with intellectual disability. However, unlike implicit plans, these are discussed with the nominated person or written into a formal document, such as a will, and are frequently made in conjunction with residential or financial plans. An example of an explicit key person succession plan made in conjunction with a financial plan is the following:

Nora's brother said, "Dad certainly talked to me about the future plans for Nora. My wife and I would be responsible for her. He never expected us to take her into our own home. There was no doubt whatsoever when Dad died and we read the will. He had written that things would come to us that I would be responsible for Nora." He had said, "Your love and attention will be given to Nora during her lifetime."

The type of care that parents hope will be provided in the future is sometimes discussed, but more often is left as a general direction for the nominated person to follow rather than formulated into a more detailed plan. A good example of a plan that contained few details for implementation is the following:

An older man's sister said, "Mother always had this thing that you couldn't take Harry to live with you; that it was important to keep him in his own home. Mother's wishes regarding what would happen to Harry were made clear, but no plans were made for putting this into operation."

In contrast, another woman's parents made an explicit detailed key person succession plan in conjunction with a detailed residential and financial plan:

Her brother said, regarding his parent's plans for her, that "Part of the deal was that I had a whole of life situation in the family home on the understanding that when they were no longer able to look after her I would look after Madge. That was with Mutual Trustees. Just look after her well-being and to oversee. That was done in conjunction with an aunt of mine. My parents built and supplied a house to my aunt for that purpose. Part of the deal that my parents made with my aunt was that they would be co-trustees for Madge. In return for that my parents gave her the land and the money to build a house next door to the family home. I would live next door to Madge, on the other side, and supervise Madge and the other person living with her."

Residential Plans   Residential plans are usually more concrete and detailed than key person succession plans and are made in conjunction with another type of plan. They may involve a number of activities, such as the parents' placing their offspring's name on a waiting list, organizing his or her move to supported accommodation, or arranging support for continued living in the community. Preferences for future living situations expressed in these plans usually fall equally between generic aging services, specialist disability services, and informal support in the community.

Parents who plan for their adult child to live in specialist disability accommodation such as group homes, community residencies, or apartments are often involved with voluntary parent associations that have built or planned residential facilities. Where parents plan for their adult child to move to a generic age service, such as a retirement complex, they also may plan to move to the complex themselves and negotiate for their child to remain there after their death. For example, neither Jim nor his mother had a close relationship with his two siblings. Jim's mother negotiated with a church organization to build a house on an empty block of land in a retirement complex and leave the house and her estate to the church. In return, they would ensure Jim was provided with a place to live and support for the rest of his life. Other types of planned residential arrangements usually involve residing with a family member, volunteer, or paid co-resident. For example, Madge's plan, mentioned previously, involved a co-resident moving into the family home.

Financial Plans   Parents usually make financial plans in conjunction with another sort of plan. These are generally fairly simple and usually involve a will that leaves all or part of the estate to the older person, sometimes with another family member as a trustee. Alternatively, wills may leave the estate to siblings with an expectation that they will use part of it for the benefit of the older person. For example, the plans made by one father included a financial, residential, and key person succession plans.

> *Amy has a brother and two sisters. One of them, Gayle, has always had a close relationship with both Amy and her parents, and it was always accepted that she would look after Amy in the future. While he was still fit, Amy's father paid for an extension to be built onto Gayle's house to provide an extra bedroom and bathroom for Amy to use in the future. In his will, Amy's father left Gayle more than her expected share of his estate, some of which was to be held in trust by her for Amy.*

Implementing Parental Plans

Despite having made plans, most parents want to continue to care for their children with disabilities for as long possible, envisaging that their plans will not be implemented before absolutely necessary. Several factors explain their reluctance to relinquish care. A deep bond and a degree of interdependence develops between parents and their adult child in later life. As parents age, the degree of support they provide is often matched by support received from their adult child, leading to a finely balanced reciprocal care situation. For example, one mother's health deteriorated in the years before her death and she relied on her son to do much of the shopping and other domestic tasks. The son's sister said, "My mother didn't make any plans for John while she was alive, she needed him." Another older man's brother referred to the interdependence between his mother and brother by saying, "She was as dependent on George as he was on her. It was a knife-edge situation."

Plans and Transition   Parents who care for middle-age children may continue caring until they are forced to give up through death or incapacity. Despite this, the process of transition is rarely a sudden event and more often a gradual process that is managed informally. As parents become frail or incapacitated, close relatives, usually their children, become more involved in their care. These relatives may also be the same ones as those nominated in key person succession plans. Consequently, as well as caring for their parent, they gradually step in, assuming responsibility for both the direct care and organization of future care of their sibling with intellectual disability. Their close involvement clearly facilitates the process of transition. Typically, they foresee the necessity to confront and deal with the transition from parental care, cope with the current contingencies of the situation, investigate options, and make arrangements that avert crisis and inappropriate short-term placement. The example of one woman who took a proactive role in organizing alternative care for her brother is typical of someone nominated in a key person succession plan:

> *Brendan and his mother moved to live near his sister, Lois, after his father's death. In the years that followed, his mother's health deteriorated and she began to lose her sight. Lois gradually became more involved in managing her mother's and Brendan's household and in providing care for Brendan. After several years, as her mother's sight became more impaired, Lois found it increasingly difficult to care for both her mother and Brendan. Lois wanted her mother to move in with her family but knew they would be unable to cope with Brendan as well. She said, "I knew my mother would not leave her house while Brendan was there. So I made appointments to see some specialist disability services. My mother didn't know. I started the ball rolling and eventually they found Brendan a place. I had to put him in a community residence. My mother couldn't do it, it was too upsetting for her."*

Initially, all types of plans are successfully implemented: the expectations they encapsulate are reflected in both the process and the outcome of the transition from parental care. If residential and financial plans exist, they often provide a blueprint for those nominated in key person succession plans, making their task easier and more specific. Alternatively, the role of key people in organizing nonparental care compensates for the lack of more detailed or residential planning by parents.

A link between the existence and implementation of a key person plan per se and facilitation of transition is not always easy to establish. It is not clear, for instance, whether people nominated in key person succession plans would manage the transition because of their close relationship to the family, despite the plans' existence. It seems, however, that key person succession plans forewarn and prepare those nominated for their expected role in transition, make their involvement more proactive, and increase their willingness to intervene and to take preventive action before a crisis develops.

Long-Term Stability and Security

The postparental care phase is characterized by substantial change, which often triggers unpredictable residential moves (Bigby, 1997a). The formulation and initial implementation of a residential plan is not always associated with the achievement of residential stability. Almost one third of the arrangements put in place by residential plans are subsequently altered, and the length of time since transition is the only factor associated with stability. The longer people are out of parental care, the more likely they are to experience residential mobility (Bigby, 1996, 2000). Residential plans alone cannot procure long-term stability because they cannot take into account unforeseen contingencies. For example, one mother, after many years of involvement in a voluntary association, secured a place for her son in their hostel, where she expected him to remain permanently. Several years after her death, in accordance with the policy of their major funder, the organization changed its policies. This resulted in relocating the more able residents, including her son, to small, dispersed community residences. Another example of what can go wrong with residential plans is indicated in the following scenario:

After her mother's death, Madge remained at home with a co-resident in accord-
ance with her parent's plans. Her brother who lived next door provided supervision
for them on a daily basis. Madge was an incessant talker and several successive
co-residents found her very difficult to live with. They did not stay long, and new
co-residents were hard to find. When a place became vacant at a group home
attached to the specialist day center Madge attended, her brother arranged for her to
move there, despite his aunt's concern that this was not what Madge's mother had
wanted or planned. In retrospect, her brother believed that the move was the best
decision he had ever made. Madge remained at the group home for 12 years, spend-
ing some weekends with her brother. Toward the end of this time, Madge developed
some obsessive behavior and medical problems that posed management problems at
the group home. After a period in the hospital, she went back to the home, but staff
found it progressively harder to supervise her. She began to get up in the night and,
at times, was unsteady on her feet. Her brother's offer to pay for additional supervi-
sory staff was rejected. Staff suggested she move to a nursing home. Without her
brother's knowledge, staff arranged for Madge to be assessed by an Aged Care
Assessment Team who considered her inappropriate for a nursing home. Twelve
months elapsed during which time the group home staff continued to press for her
transfer. Eventually, she was reassessed as "barely eligible" for nursing home care,
so her brother moved her to a private hospital to give him some time to look around
for a suitable nursing home. He was still not convinced that she needed nursing
home care but could not find an appropriate alternative. Finally, when she was 58,
he gave up and had her admitted to a nursing home.

This one family's experiences illustrate both the fallibility of residential plans and the fundamental necessity and importance of a key person succession plan that ensures a committed individual is available to negotiate with formal services.

In contrast to residential plans, fewer expectations contained in key person succession plans go awry. As well as facilitating transition, nominated key people retain a vital ongoing involvement in the life of the person with intellectual disability. They maintain regular contact and take responsibility for overseeing their well-being, which involves tasks such as financial management, decision making, negotiation, coordination, mediation with services, monitoring services, supervision, and sometimes primary care. Roles are usually performed in consultation with the older person and in response to their capacity. A critical role is negotiation with the formal service system on which reliance is placed for provision of primary care. The existence of key people means that unforeseen contingencies in a person's life can be dealt with and informal advocacy is readily available (Bigby, 1997b, 2000).

CONCLUSIONS

If parental plans are to be effective, they must have several facets. Initially, plans must facilitate the transition from parental care and the immediate support needs that follow. In the longer term, plans should aim to procure security and stability. To fulfill these aims, planning cannot be a "one-off" task that confronts parents, but must be regarded as a continuing process throughout the postparental care phase, ensuring that optimal outcomes and adaptations are achieved as an individual ages and a multiplicity of life changes occur. Key person succession plans that center on the nomination of another person to replace the parental role of oversight of well-being may not appear to be very thorough, because arrangements to ensure well-being are largely left to the nominated key person. However, their critical features are flexibility and responsiveness, and they have enormous potential to meet the various facets required for successful planning. They provide a mechanism in the form of a key person to organize and plan the detailed provision of primary care and relationships with formal services.

Although key person succession plans are unspecific and remain informal, the relatively smooth nature of transition suggests their efficacy in this facet of planning. Despite parents continuing to care until the last minute and failing to make comprehensive or concrete plans, the sudden crisis transition and urgent requests to services for assistance and placements that figure so often in discussions and anecdotes of transitions occur only rarely. By mandating the intervention of a key person less emotionally involved than parents, these plans relieve parents from confronting the challenges of making detailed transition arrangements that often involve difficult choices and conflicting values and needs. They avoid a need for more concrete residential plans and perhaps also counter the conservatism of parents by handing decisions to key people with different, and perhaps less protective, attitudes. They do not tie adults with intellectual disabilities into the particular visions of their parents and earlier times. Instead, they allow for new opportunities to be created and expectations about potential that parents have not foreseen.

Key person succession plans also have advantages in the second aspect of parental planning. They rarely go awry. Nominated key people, with their open brief, can be responsive to unexpected changes that occur. These plans do not achieve stability but provide the security of an advocate to negotiate service provision and ensure that the interests of the older person with intellectual disability are foremost in decisions made about aspects of their life. Key person succession plans effectively ensure the continued availability of informal support in the lives of older people with intellectual disabilities. By means of key person succession plans, parents can negotiate commitments to provide care from a range of distant relatives or friends who would not normally be expected to take on such a role. The tasks required of those nominated in plans suits their characteristics, requiring long-term commitment but not proximity or the daily face-to-face contact that the direct provision of care requires.

Key person succession plans acknowledge that planning is an ongoing task faced by key people as they deal with changes that occur to individuals and their environments. Key person succession plans may fail when key people die and are not replaced or when they do not act in the best interest of the older person. It could be argued that the responsibility for these failures might lie with the formal service system. It may be incumbent on these formal services to seek out and nurture replacements, as well as to monitor and challenge decisions made by informal network members. The plans do, however, have the potential to deal with one of these contingencies. Just as parents have done, many key people plan for their own mortality and can nominate a successor who will ensure that this role will continue to be performed.

Building a supportive informal network with a key person may be as important as securing appropriate housing. The nature and efficacy of key person succession planning indicate ways in which planning may be fostered. Adopting a social network approach toward planning assistance to elderly parents may be useful. Such an approach can broaden the focus of intervention from parents and seek out and involve members of the person's broader informal support network. People nominated in key person succession plans may find such discussions less emotionally challenging than would parents who tend to avoid confronting these issues. Drawing them into the discussion of plans also may facilitate the involvement of the adult with intellectual disability in future care arrangements. Equipping potential key people with a knowledge of formal service systems, later-life opportunities, and the developmental potential of adults with intellectual disabilities in the pre–transition-planning stage on an individual or group basis is also an important strategy.

REFERENCES

Bigby, C. (1996). Transferring responsibility: The nature and effectiveness of parental planning for the future of adults with intellectual disability who remain at home until mid-life. *Journal of Intellectual and Developmental Disabilities, 21,* 295–312.

Bigby, C. (1997a). Later life for adults with intellectual disability: A time of opportunity and vulnerability. *Journal of Intellectual and Developmental Disabilities, 22,* 97–108.

Bigby, C. (1997b). When parents relinquish care: Informal support networks of older people with intellectual disability. *Journal of Applied Research in Intellectual Disabilities, 10,* 333–344.

Bigby, C. (2000). *Moving on without parents: Planning, transitions and sources of support for older adults with intellectual disability.* Baltimore: Paul H. Brookes Publishing Co.

Bigby, C., Ozanne, E., & Gordon, M. (2000). *Facilitating transition: An evaluation of pilot case management programs for older carers of adults with intellectual disability.* Melbourne, Australia: Department of Human Services.

Brubaker, E., & Brubaker, T. (1993). Caring for adult children with mental retardation. Concerns of elderly parents. In K.A. Roberto (Ed.), *The elderly caregiver: Caring for adults with developmental disabilities* (Sage Focus Editions No. 160, pp. 51–61). Thousand Oaks, CA: Sage Publications.

Campbell, J., & Essex, E. (1994). Factors affecting parents in their future planning for a son or daughter with developmental disabilities. *Education and Training in Mental Retardation and Developmental Disabilities, 29,* 222–228.

Card, H. (1983). What will happen when we've gone? *Community Care, 28,* 20–21.

Carney, T., & Tait, D. (1997). *The adult guardianship experiment: Tribunals and popular justice.* Leichhardt, New South Wales, Australia: The Federation Press.

Community Services Victoria. (1988). *Interim report: Accommodation for intellectually disabled people who are currently living at home with older parents.* Melbourne, Australia: Author.

Community Services Victoria. (1992). *The planned care approach: Future partnerships in residential care for people with intellectual disabilities.* Melbourne, Australia: Author.

Edgerton, R. (1994). Quality of life issues: Some people know how to be old. In M.M. Seltzer, M.W. Krauss, & M.P. Janicki (Eds.), *Life course perspectives on adulthood and old age* (pp. 53–66). Washington, DC: American Association on Mental Retardation.

Eloura Homes. (1995). *Report on family support program.* Melbourne, Australia: Author.

Essex, E., Seltzer, M., & Krauss, M. (1997). Residential transitions of adults with mental retardation: Predictors of waiting list use and placement. *American Journal on Mental Retardation, 101,* 613–629.

Freedman, R., Krauss, M., & Seltzer, M. (1997). Aging parents' residential plans for adult children with mental retardation. *Mental Retardation, 35,* 114–123.

Freeling, B., & Bruggeman, R. (1994, October). *Guaranteed care: Progress in South Australia.* Paper presented at the joint National Conference of the Association for the Study of Intellectual Disability and the National Council on Intellectual Disability, Perth, Western Australia, Australia.

Gold, M. (1987). *Parents of the adult developmentally disabled.* New York: Brookdale Center on Aging.

Goodman, D. (1978). Parenting an adult mentally retarded offspring. *Smith College Studies in Social Work, 48,* 209–234.

Grant, G. (1986). Older carers, interdependence and the care of mentally handicapped adults. *Ageing and Society, 6,* 333–351.

Grant, G. (1988). *Stability and change in the care networks of mentally handicapped adults living at home* (First report). Bangor, UK: University of Wales, Centre for Social Policy and Development.

Grant, G. (1989). Letting go: Decision making among family carers of people with mental handicap. *Australia and New Zealand Journal of Developmental Disabilities, 15,* 189–200.

Griffin, T., & Bennett, K. (1994, October). *Peering into the future: Focus group interviews with parents who have a child with an intellectual disability.* Paper presented at the joint National Conference of the Association for the Study of Intellectual Disability and the National Council on Intellectual Disability, Perth, Western Australia, Australia.

Griffith, D., & Unger, D. (1994). Views about planning for the future among parents and siblings of adults with mental retardation. *Family Relations, 43,* 221–227.

Hayden, M.F., & DePaepe, P. (1994). Waiting for community services: The impact on persons with mental retardation and other developmental disabilities. In M.F. Hayden & B.H. Abery (Eds.), *Challenges for a service system in transition: Ensuring quality community experiences for persons with developmental disabilities* (pp. 173–206). Baltimore: Paul H. Brookes Publishing Co.

Heller, T., & Factor, A. (1988a). *Development of a transition plan for older adults with developmental disabilities residing in the natural home* (Public Policy Monograph Series, No. 37). Chicago: University of Illinois at Chicago.

Heller, T., & Factor, A. (1988b). Permanency planning among black and white family caregivers of older adults with mental retardation. *Mental Retardation, 26,* 203–208.

Heller, T., & Factor, A. (1991). Permanency planning for adults with mental retardation living with family caregivers. *American Journal on Mental Retardation, 96,* 163–176.

Hogg, J., Moss, S., & Cooke, D. (1988). *Ageing and mental handicap.* London: Croom Helm.

Kaufman, A. (1989). Social work services for elderly persons with mental retardation: A case example. *Social Work in Health Care, 14,* 67–80.

Kaufman, A., Adams, J., & Campbell, V. (1991). Permanency planning by older parents who care for adult children with mental retardation. *Mental Retardation, 29,* 293–300

Krauss, M. (1990, May). *Later life placements: Precipitating factors and family profiles.* Paper presented at the 114th annual meeting of the American Association on Mental Retardation, Atlanta, GA.

Krauss, M., Seltzer, M., Gordon, R., & Friedman, D. (1996). Binding ties: The roles of adult siblings of persons with mental retardation. *Mental Retardation, 34,* 83–93.

Kropf, N. (1994, April). *Older parents of adults with developmental disabilities: Issues for practice and service delivery.* Paper presented at the Young Adult Institute 15th Annual International Conference on Developmental Disabilities, New York City.

Lehmann, J., & Roberto, K.A. (1993). Current and future service needs of aging individuals with developmental disabilities living with relatives. In K.A. Roberto (Ed.), *The elderly caregiver: Caring for adults with developmental disabilities* (Sage Focus Editions No. 160, pp. 108–125). Thousand Oaks, CA: Sage Publications.

Litwak, E. (1985). *Helping the elderly: The complementary roles of informal networks and formal systems (Perspectives on Marriage and the Family).* New York: Guilford Press.

McCallion, P., & Tobin S. (1995). Social workers perceptions of older adults caring at home for sons and daughters with developmental disabilities. *Mental Retardation, 33,* 153–162.

Mulcahey, M. (1986). *Life without parents: What will happen to the mentally retarded adult.* Unpublished doctoral dissertation, Vanderbilt University, Nashville.

Richardson, A., & Ritchie, J. (1986). *Making the break: Parents perspectives on adults with mental handicap leaving home.* London: King Edward's Hospital Fund.

Richardson, A., & Ritchie, J. (1989). *Letting go: Dilemmas for parents whose son or daughter has a mental handicap.* Milton Keynes, England, UK: Open University Press.

Sach & Associates. (1991). *The housing needs of people with disabilities* (National Housing Strategy discussion paper). Canberra: Australian Government Publishing Service.

Seltzer, M., & Krauss, M. (1994). Aging parents with co-resident adult children. The impact of life-long caring. In M.M. Seltzer, M.W. Krauss, & M.P. Janicki (Eds.), *Life course perspectives on adulthood and old age* (pp. 3–18). Washington, DC: American Association on Mental Retardation.

Seltzer, M., & Ryff, C. (1994). Parenting across the lifespan: The normative and non-normative cases. In D.L. Featherman, R.M. Learner, & M. Perlmutter (Eds.), *Life-span development and behavior* (Vol. 12, pp. 1–40). Mahwah, NJ: Lawrence Erlbaum Associates.

Seltzer, M., & Seltzer, G. (1985). The elderly mentally retarded: A group in need of service. In G.S. Getzel & M. Mellor (Eds.), *Gerontological social work practice in the community* (pp. 99–120). Binghamton, NY: Haworth Press.

Seltzer, M., & Seltzer, G. (1992). Aging in persons with developmental disabilities: A social work perspective. In F. Turner (Ed.), *Mental health and the elderly: A social work perspective* (pp. 136–160). New York: Free Press.

Seltzer, M., Krauss, M., & Heller, T. (1991). Family caregiving over the lifecourse. In M.P. Janicki & M.M. Seltzer (Eds.), *Aging and developmental disabilities: Challenges for the 1990s* (The proceedings of the Boston Roundtable on Research Issues and Applications in Aging and

Developmental Disabilities) (pp. 3–24). Washington, DC: American Association on Mental Retardation, Special Interest Group on Aging.

Smith, G., Fullmer, E., & Tobin, S. (1994). Living outside the system: An exploration of older families who do not use day programs. In M.M. Seltzer, M.W. Krauss, & M.P. Janicki (Eds.), *Life course perspectives on adulthood and old age* (pp. 19–38). Washington, DC: American Association on Mental Retardation.

Smith, G., & Tobin, S. (1989). Permanency planning among older parents of adults with lifelong disabilities. *Journal of Gerontological Social Work, 114,* 35–59.

Smith, G., & Tobin, S. (1993). Case manager's perceptions of practice with older parents of adults with developmental disabilities. In K.A. Roberto (Ed.), *The elderly caregiver: Caring for adults with developmental disabilities* (Sage Focus Editions No. 160, pp. 146–173). Thousand Oaks, CA: Sage Publications.

Smith, G., & Tobin, S. (1994). Practice with older parents of developmentally disabled adults. In T.L. Brink (Ed.), *The forgotten aged: Ethnic, psychiatric and societal minorities* (pp. 59–77). Binghamton, NY: Haworth Press.

Smith, G., Tobin, S., & Fullmer, E. (1995). Elderly mothers caring at home for offspring with mental retardation: A model of permanency planning. *American Journal on Mental Retardation, 99,* 487–499.

Sussman, M. (1985). The family life of old people. In R. Binstock & E. Shanas (Eds.), *Handbook of aging and the social sciences* (2nd ed., pp. 415–443). New York: Van Nostrand Reinhold.

Victorian Department of Health & Community Services. (1993). *Review of placement of eligible aged clients into aged care facilities.* Melbourne, Victoria, Australia: Author.

Victorian Department of Health & Community Services. (1995a). *Options for older families.* Unpublished service proposal, Melbourne, Victoria, Australia.

Victorian Department of Health & Community Services. (1995b). *Report to the Hon. Michael John, M.P., Minister for Community Services of the Intellectual Disability Services Taskforce.* Melbourne, Victoria, Australia: Author.

Wood, B. (1993). Planning for the transfer of care: Social and psychological issues. In K.A. Roberto (Ed.), *The elderly caregiver: Caring for adults with developmental disabilities* (Sage Focus Editions No. 160, pp. 95–108). Thousand Oaks, CA: Sage Publications.

Wood, J., & Skiles, L. (1992). Planning for the transfer of care. Who cares for the developmentally disabled adult when the family can no longer care? *Generations, 16,* 61–62.

6

Redesigning Services to Meet the Needs of Multicultural Families

Philip McCallion and Lucinda Grant-Griffin

Consistent with the changing demographics of the United States, the number of care-giving families from minority cultures is growing (Aponte & Crouch, 1995). Limited attention has been paid, however, to families from diverse cultures caring for family members with developmental disabilities. This chapter draws on experiences gained in locating older family caregivers from African American, Chinese American, Haitian American, Hispanic/Latino, Korean American, and select Native American communities, developing locally based resources and agencies for people with developmental disabilities within those communities, and responding to the newly identified needs of multicultural grandparent caregivers. Recommendations are offered for practitioners to develop more culturally aware practices, for administrators to develop cultural capacity, and for policy makers to consider more family- and community-friendly approaches.

BACKGROUND

Disabilities can and do occur in all cultural groups. However, people of diverse cultures with developmental disabilities and their families appear to be underrepresented among those enrolled for services with public developmental disabilities agencies (Grant-Griffin, 1995). This also has been found in the limited family-based research that is available. For example, in a study comparing African American with European heritage family caregivers of people with developmental disabilities, Heller and Factor

97

(1988) found that African American parents were somewhat less likely to use formal services or to plan for out-of-home placements.

Little is known about the effectiveness of service programs for people from diverse cultures when they do seek formal services (Toseland & McCallion, 1997). The representation of people from diverse cultures in samples of studies to date has usually been so small that separate analyses are not fruitful. However, there are indications that people from diverse cultures are less likely to participate in service programs, because they have economic, religious, transportation, and insurance barriers to participation, they do not feel welcome in the locations where the interventions are offered, or the intervention is simply not designed to meet their needs (Henderson, Gutierrez-Mayka, Garcia, & Boyd, 1993; McCallion, Janicki, & Grant-Griffin, 1997). However, where concerted efforts have been made to develop interventions that assist people from diverse cultures, participants have been located and have reported benefits from participation (see, e.g., Henderson et al., 1993; Minkler, Driver, Roe, & Bedeian, 1993).

Taken together, these findings and a myriad of anecdotal reports suggest that there are many reasons for low usage of formal services by family caregivers from a variety of cultural groups. This chapter argues that the development of services that demonstrate awareness of the role of culture in families will result in families gaining access to the services they need. Also, the development of new services that build on cultural strengths and greater use of a community's own local agencies will greatly assist access to and use of needed services.

Culture represents the values, beliefs, customs, behaviors, structures, and identity by which a group of people defines themselves (Axelson, 1999). All families are influenced by the values of the dominant culture in a society. This includes pressures to relinquish ethnic values and behaviors for those of the majority culture, which is also called acculturation (Aponte & Barnes, 1995). However, the families considered in this chapter continue to be influenced by their own cultures, including African American, Latino, Native American, and other traditions and values. They are multicultural families in the sense that they preserve values from their own ethnic identification, live within the dominant culture, and deal with conflicts inherent in participating in more than one culture. This will be the intended meaning of "multicultural family" as used in this chapter.

INFLUENCE OF CULTURE ON FAMILY CAREGIVING AND THE FAMILY'S WILLINGNESS TO USE FORMAL SERVICES

Three sets of assumptions have often been inappropriately used to justify not targeting services to people with developmental disabilities from diverse cultures and their families. The assumptions are that 1) families from diverse cultures prefer to use family, cultural, and community-based supports rather than formal services; 2) the role of culture in the day-to-day lives of families from diverse cultures has diminished and does not need to be considered; and 3) families from diverse cultures can be accommodated by existing agencies and services.

Preference for Family, Cultural, and Community-Based Supports

Some investigations of low usage of formal interventions by family caregivers from diverse cultures have noted a greater reliance on filial piety, greater availability of extended family supports, suspicion of formal structures, and cultural beliefs that a person should take care of his or her own (Lockery, 1991; Sakauye, 1989; Sung, 1995). A person's culture—the values, beliefs, customs, behaviors, structures, and identity by which a group of people define themselves (Axelson, 1999)—does appear to be an important influence on his or her willingness to use services. However, other investigators warn of the dangers in stereotyping families by assuming that identification with a particular culture means strict adherence to a specific set of beliefs and practices (Gratton & Wilson, 1988). Also, the experience of historic discrimination for all, legal status concerns for some, and the foreignness of services that have been developed for, rather than by, the communities to be served may be more important reasons for why families from diverse cultures choose not to use formal services. Such factors make many multicultural families, including those needing help, wary of formal services and poorly informed of what is available (Gratton & Wilson, 1988; Johnson, 1995; Lockery, 1991). Lower levels of use and reliance on community support does not mean that more formal assistance may not also be needed.

Diminishing Importance of Culture

Certain mediators make it increasingly difficult to discern the role of culture and encourage some people to believe that culture is no longer important. For example, one mediator of the impact of culture is migration (Aponte & Barnes, 1995). No matter how strong the value to rely on extended family members, geographic distance may make such reliance impossible. There may be few family members available, and regular contact between family members may be reduced. A similar mediator is generation. There are often different emphases on cultural values between older and younger members of a family, and between those who recently immigrated and those who are two and three generations removed from that experience.

The existence of mediators means that there is no one cultural profile for families from diverse cultures. This often causes workers, administrators, and policy makers to miss the significance of culture, or argue that its impact is overrated or declining over time. Yet, the impact of mediators on cultural adherence is rarely linear. It is possible to find a third-generation young man or woman reclaiming cultural values abandoned by their peers, and people from diverse cultures of all generations and ages adhering to select cultural practices that they have identified as core values (Johnson, 1995; Lockery, 1991). Far-flung family supportive networks have also been found among some diverse, caregiving families (McCallion et al., 1997):

> An African American woman living in New York City, who was caring for her mother, sister with a disability, and two children, suddenly died. Various components of the service system placed the mother in a nursing home, her sister in a group home, and the two children in foster care. Meanwhile, word of mouth had informed members of her extended family in South Carolina of her death. They in turn contacted a cousin in Chicago who agreed to assume the caregiving responsibilities and moved to New York City to do so. It took her 3 months to reunite the traumatized family.

Culture has an impact on caregiving and on the use of services, but its effects may be difficult to discern and may vary across families. Rather than be dismissed, the impact of culture should be assessed, family by family, if culturally competent interventions are to be initiated.

Incorporating Diverse Families into Existing Agencies

There have been growing efforts by existing agencies to reach out to families from diverse cultures with mixed results. Using staff, usually paraprofessionals, drawn from diverse communities, outreach to churches and civic groups, and public service announcements, agencies have attempted to draw families from diverse cultures into their existing programs and to establish satellite offices in their communities. Concerns have been raised about the seriousness of the agencies' commitments to diverse communities and insistence that everyone can be fitted into existing program and service models.

There also has been a failure to recognize the strengths offered by locally based multicultural agencies or to involve them in the expansion of services to underserved populations. Such agencies have always existed. Some are church based, whereas others are fraternal in nature. Many offer a combination of social, cultural, and human services. Most of their funding is raised within the community they serve. They serve locally based cultural communities where no services have been offered to that population, existing services are not appropriate, or a cultural community's language and customs make gaining access to formal services difficult. They are also

1. Easily accessed because they are close by, do not require appointments, and have longer hours of operation than other agencies
2. Seen by families as more nurturing, supportive, and likely to understand cultural concerns
3. More likely to see culture as an intervention facilitator than an intervention barrier
4. Based on empowerment approaches, helping families to change their environment, rather than looking at families for the source of the presenting problems

The following vignette illustrates the important role that these agencies play:

> Mr. D. is an immigrant from Jamaica. He is the primary caregiver to his daughter who has mild mental retardation and her two children, both of whom the public school has classified as having severe mental retardation. Mr. D. has been the primary caregiver since his wife left in 1992. Although active in his church, Mr. D. feels isolated and alone. Although he acknowledges that the school has sent him information, Mr. D. has little understanding of the rights of his grandchildren to an appropriate education. He says that he has difficulty reading and understanding the materials he has received from the school. This may be related to Mr. D's not having renewed his glasses for at least 5 years. He says he does not have time to go for new glasses because he has no one to look after his daughter who has no day program and is at home all day. His activities have also been limited since his quadruple bypass in 1993.
>
> Mr. D. is concerned about the education his granddaughters are receiving and about what the future will hold for his daughter and granddaughters when he is no longer able to care for them. However, he has been reluctant to accept services from agencies because he is suspicious that their intent is to take his child and grandchildren away. Finally, he agreed to talk to the director of a local multicultural agency, who he knew from the church he attends. Gradually, he was persuaded to accept respite services, and a worker from the agency accompanied him to his granddaughters' individualized education program (IEP) meetings. Staff at the agency report that he requires a lot of persuasion to try new things, but Mr. D. has begun talking about plans for the future of his family.

Multicultural service agencies have not been part of the traditional services network because meeting the needs of families from diverse cultures has not been a funding or policy priority. Underfunding has meant that multicultural agencies have had difficulty in supporting the professional staff expected by funders and regulators, existing agency administrators have resisted sharing resources, and service systems have only recently switched from personal responsibility perspectives that multicultural agencies did not share to emphasizing empowerment approaches that they do (Iglehart & Becerra, 1996). Service priorities are now being established for greater inclusion of people from diverse cultures in service delivery. Locally based multicultural agencies have the advantage of a long history of serving their own population, and of cultural competence in mediating between cultural imperatives and desires and the realities of available services. They have the potential of being the primary deliverer of services for their communities and of being a resource for other agencies seeking to serve those communities. Not every family prefers receiving services from their community's own agencies, but many do. Multicultural agencies are an underused resource.

Data Collection and Culturally Competent Approach Development

In 1993, the Administration on Aging (AoA) funded a series of demonstration projects across the United States to identify and demonstrate best practices for outreach and services for aging caregivers of people with developmental disabilities (Janicki, McCallion, Force, Bishop, & LePore, 1998). One such demonstration was funded in New York State. One of the project's objectives was to identify and implement outreach and service approaches likely to be successful in multicultural communities. Activities related to this objective were aided by supplementary funding from the Multicultural Professional Development Institute (MPDI) operated by New York State Office of Mental Retardation and Developmental Disabilities. MPDI served as the primary development, support, and resource vehicle in New York for the development of services for people from diverse cultures with developmental disabilities and of locally based resources to deliver those services. Some of the activities begun by the AoA project and sustained by MPDI were continued in an initiative funded by the Joseph P. Kennedy, Jr., Foundation designed to serve multicultural grandparents.

As part of the project's activities, focus group meetings were convened involving a total of 83 family members, service providers, and community leaders from African American, Chinese American, Haitian American, Hispanic/Latino American, Korean American, and select Native American communities. Data also were gathered from outreach and service delivery efforts that affected more than 50 multicultural family caregivers and from interviews with 25 multicultural providers and families attending a training conference sponsored by MPDI. Overall, many families from a variety of cultures identified core cultural values around what is disability, who is the family, and the cultural values that the family viewed as important. Such core values did influence willingness to use services. For example, where family values and attitudes caused them to "hide" the person with a disability, willingness to accept services appeared lowest. Participants also indicated that important family operations were culturally driven—who provides care, how the family makes decisions, what family members expect from one another, and what supports families receive from friends and community. Failure by workers to understand and work within a family's cultural roles around decision making was frequently highlighted by families as a major barrier to accepting services. Levels of adherence to cultural values also varied greatly by age, generation, and availability of family and community supports (McCallion et al., 1997). These findings led to the development of a "culturally competent service approach" for social workers and other case managers. It was developed as a means for workers to demonstrate a desire to understand the unique impact of culture on each family and to begin a process of building trust. The underlying premise of this approach is that the first step in planning for truly individualized services is an understanding of how culture and acculturation affects a particular family and its caregiving. The project activities also resulted in recommendations for administrators and policy makers.

Culturally Competent Service Approach

First Steps: Building Trust   Agency workers often have information and resources that enable them to make a difference in the lives of people with developmental disabilities and their families. Therefore, workers are often surprised when their help is rejected or when families are fearful or suspicious of their intentions. Families often attribute much of the conflict to workers' insensitivity of cultural concerns and to a lack of recognition of the need to build trust sufficiently that families are comfortable discussing cultural and family issues with them. They will argue that workers are rarely open to family structures and ways of caring that are different from their own. Given this, workers need to recognize that they are working with families, not just the presenting family members. Just as important, workers should avoid stereotyping family members by virtue of their gender, or society's, or even their own culture's expectations. Workers also must be open to recognizing that different values and structures may mean that a variety of services are warranted.

Many workers fail to get beyond the front door with multicultural families independent of the family's need for services. Often, this is because the worker fails to observe valued ways of approaching families and communities, addresses the wrong family member, fails to include key family members, offers unwanted as opposed to needed services, or appears not to offer appropriate respect to the family members. This can occur unintentionally or because workers insist that families conform to agency or worker expectations. Speaking with co-workers or members of local cultural organizations before approaching a family of a different culture about how to gain access to the community and approach families and to get information on cultural "do's and don'ts" can help to avoid these problems, shows respect, and begins a process of building trust that is more likely to result in families accepting needed services.[1]

Second Steps: Culturally Competent Practice   A thorough understanding of the role of culture and acculturation in an individual family caregiving situation, and its implications for delivering services to meet the family's needs, involves consideration of the following dimensions of cultural adherence: 1) how disability is perceived, 2) who is the family, 3) who provides care, 4) how the family makes decisions, 5) what family members expect of each other, 6) what supports families receive from friends and community, 7) why the family moved, 8) cultural values important to family members, 9) families' willingness to accept services from outside the family, 10) the family's first language, and 11) families' concerns about service providers.[2]

How Disability Is Perceived   There are many different ways that families might view a disability and the person who has a disability. Many families struggle not only with their own beliefs about disability, but also with how others perceive the disability and parents of children with disabilities. In some cultures, disability represents such a shame that families hide the person to such an extent that it appears that there are no

---

[1]An important resource on approaches to initial contacts with multicultural caregivers is Grant-Griffin (1995).

[2]A description of how these 11 cultural issues were arrived at can be found in McCallion et al. (1997).

people with disabilities in that community. In other cultures, the person with a disability is an active participant in family and community life. Workers need to understand how disability is perceived within the family and the community they identify with because it is likely to influence both the level of services needed and a family's willingness to accept those services.

Who Family Members Are   It is not always obvious who makes up a particular family. We often think of family as those people who either live in the household or individuals who are close blood relatives. However, some households encompass three and four generations, including cousins, siblings, and in-laws, expanding the number of available relatives who may provide care. For other families, some of those same relatives are available locally, or even live at some distance, and yet still participate in caregiving. There are also families where no other relatives are available to assist, and some families where other relatives living in the same household are not willing to provide care. Furthermore, some family members critical to caring and decision making might not be immediately recognizable as instrumental family members, for example, a sister-in-law from a marriage that is now over or a friend who has become part of the household. Other family members become involved only when they are needed. Finding out about family members and understanding their roles often requires both the building of trust and willingness by agency workers to commit time and resources to this effort.

Who Provides Care   The primary caregiver is usually the mother of the person with a disability. However, other family members provide significant levels of support and influence decisions. In some households, the majority of caregiving responsibility may have been transferred to a sibling or another younger relative, while the aging mother still receives the respect of the primary caregiver. Grandparents and other family members are also increasingly assuming caregiving responsibilities. In other households, there are additional people with chronic illnesses and related disabilities who also need care. In such households, the person with a developmental disability is often someone who provides care rather than someone who receives it. A focus by the worker on the "needs" of the person with a developmental disability risks not recognizing and respecting that person's independence, fails to recognize the family's other important caregiving responsibilities, and excludes important family members from services planning.

If workers focus exclusively on one or two family members or make assumptions about roles and needs of family members, they risk disrupting important family relationships. Consequently, their help will be rejected, even by the family members they have targeted for help. Understanding the roles of various family members in caregiving is an important task for workers.

How the Family Makes Decisions   Related to the need to understand who provides care is the need to explore how families make decisions about caregiving and other matters. Workers must recognize that families' decision-making processes are often different from their own approaches. For example, some families give a lot of weight to a particular family member's opinion, such as a father or a grandparent, even when that opinion proves to be a barrier to services or future planning and when that person appears to minimally contribute to completing caregiving tasks or lives in a different household. Other families may feel isolated from extended family members, even those who live close by or in their own household, and make all decisions alone. Workers who do not take the time to understand and respect long-established decision-making processes risk having their help rejected.

What Family Members Expect of Each Other   Native American families told us that they expected their other sons and daughters to take over caregiving responsibilities, but acknowledged that economic realities forced those sons and daughters to leave the local area and traditional ways. Chinese American families explained that acculturation of younger family members and reduced availability of extended family members meant that their hopes of support in their own old age would likely be unfulfilled. Haitian families talked about the importance of supporting other family members even in the face of acculturation and scattered family networks. Services were also sometimes refused by the families with whom we talked because acceptance of outside help was seen as assisting other family members to shirk their responsibilities to the family. Workers need an understanding of a caregiver's need for family support, expectations of support, support actually received, and conflicts that result when expectations are unfulfilled. The service plan must be designed to include and encourage valued family supports rather than replace them.

Support that Families Receive from Friends and Community   How families feel about receiving help and how much help they receive from friends and neighbors varies widely. For some families, help from friends, neighbors, churches, and culturally based social and service organizations can be particularly useful and is often a contributor to their caregiving success. Other caregivers may be disappointed that more help is not received. Others may not seek and will not accept help from their friends or community. Before offering the assistance of formal services, a worker should determine the extent of help received from community and friends, the availability of such support, and the caregiver's willingness to accept such help. Where support from friends and community is available and caregivers want to use such assistance, workers should offer formal services that supplement, but do not replace, this help.

Why the Family Moved   Families caring for a person with a developmental disability may have moved from another country to the United States, from small towns or rural areas to large cities, and from urban areas to the suburbs or rural areas. Reasons for such transitions include to find greater tolerance, to escape shame and labeling, to find more appropriate services, or to "hide" the person with a disability. For workers, understanding the reasons for a move can help to clarify a family's willingness to accept services, as well as their fears and concerns.

Importance of Cultural Values to Family Members   The importance of cultural traditions and values should never be assumed for any family or any family member. Adhering to traditional values is often the key reason for seeking and receiving informal family and community support. However, adherence can also present barriers to the acceptance of formal services because those services are not part of the traditional way of doing things. Some families may experience conflicts and disappointments when adherence to cultural values varies among key family members. Workers should seek to understand key values around aging, disability, and caregiving common to the culture with which the family identifies. They should then explore the family's level of adherence to those cultural values, and the conflicts and disappointments caused by variations in adherence among family members and key community members.

Families' Willingness to Accept Outside Services   Many families who acknowledge a specific cultural identity express a preference to receive services within their own community. They cite the following advantages: reduced language and access problems, fewer fears of formal service providers, services that are more familiar, and services offered that are more likely to respect their traditions. Other families more willingly accept services from agencies not of their cultural community. To better serve families who are more comfortable with receiving services from within their own communities, workers need to develop supportive alliances with workers within their own agencies and at locally based community agencies who share the family's cultural background.

Family's First Language   In addition to the barriers posed by workers' use of professional jargon and abbreviations, many families report increased difficulty in accessing services because English is not their first language. Many informational materials are written in English only, and many workers are only English speakers. Because of this, many families may know little about available services, and language difficulties exacerbate the situation. Most service agencies rely on neighbors, other family members, and even children as mediators for non–English-speaking family members. This is a situation that many families are not comfortable with, particularly because much personal information has to be shared. At the other end of the continuum, families with a good command of English complain of patronizing workers shielding them from information in the mistaken belief that they will not understand. Workers can build trust and develop more effective interventions if they 1) ask families about preferred interpreters, 2) learn basic greetings in the caregiver's language, and 3) form cooperative relationships with workers within their own agencies and at locally based community agencies who share the caregiver's primary language.

Family's Concerns About Service Providers   Families have many concerns about dealing with formal service providers: whether they will provide the services they need; what the quality of those services will be; if they ask for one service, will they be required to accept other services they do not want; and will their asking for services be used to justify removing the person with a disability from the home. Family members often feel judged by professionals, particularly by professionals from another culture. Families are concerned that information given to the agency will be used for other purposes. For example, traditional practices in their homes and family living arrangements that include large numbers of people may be misinterpreted and allegations of improper care may be reported to police, housing, and social welfare agencies. Use of formal agencies can also attract attention from other agencies such as the U.S. Immigration and Naturalization Service, independent of the family's actual legal status (Hominik, 1998). Workers should recognize that these are legitimate concerns and concentrate on building trust. In particular, workers should clarify why information is needed and with whom it will be shared. Workers should ensure that promised services are delivered and explain the implications, if any, of accepting particular services. Living arrangements, customs, and lifestyles also should not be judged by workers simply because they are different from their own.

CONCLUSIONS

Consideration of the 11 dimensions of cultural adherence can lead to a fuller understanding of the impact of disability and caregiving on each family, who needs to be involved in decision making, what types of services are more likely to be welcomed, and how the delivery of services should proceed. The comfort level of family members toward trusting and cooperating with service workers also will increase, making the successful realization of service plans more likely. In doing so, administrators must consider whether current agency networks are sufficient or appropriate to reach out to and serve multicultural families. For example, lacking staff speaking families' primary languages is an important barrier, as is agency networks' not including agencies based in and operated by multicultural communities. Increasing cultural competence within existing agencies and including multicultural agencies as part of the services network should serve to expand access, ensure that needed services are delivered, and help in creating service models and approaches that better meet the needs of people of multicultural backgrounds. Steps that administrators can undertake to increase their agencies' cultural capacity are noted in Table 1. Contacts with cultural communities and locally based multicultural agencies must begin with respect and with a desire to establish truly collaborative relationships. Also, a commitment is

Table 1. Specific steps administrators can undertake to increase their agencies' cultural capacity and sensitivity

Acknowledge that the agency has failed to extend services to all cultural and ethnic groups.

Identify and involve consumer, family, and community representatives from underserved groups in discussions about how to extend and modify services.

Establish a priority to extend services to cultural groups that are underrepresented among those individuals whom the agency serves.

Communicate to staff, board members, and other constituencies that increasing the level of services to cultural groups that are underrepresented among those whom the agency serves is a priority.

Identify the cultural groups within the agency's catchment area and their actual and potential service needs.

Determine the existing level of cultural competence within the agency specific to the cultural groups within the agency's catchment area; for example, does the agency have staff who are members of the cultural group(s) that the agency serves or who speak the cultural group's primary language?

Recognize barriers to serving the identified cultural groups.

Take steps to address identified gaps in the agency's cultural competence and to remove barriers to extending services. These steps might include the following:

- Ask consumers, families, and community leaders to identify gaps in staff members' cultural competence and barriers to extending services and to suggest solutions.
- Assess the need among agency staff for cross-cultural training related to the cultural groups within the agency's catchment area.
- Ensure that cross-cultural training is provided to all staff members and that assessment of cross-cultural competence is a component of staff members' performance evaluations.
- Establish relationships with cultural agencies within the catchment area that might offer training, interpreter services, and service alliances.

Promote the development of disability services expertise in local cultural agencies if those agencies previously have not served people with developmental disabilities.

Identify community leaders, people with developmental disabilities, and family members from cultural groups within the agency's catchment area to serve on the agency's boards and advisory groups.

Establish goals to increase outreach and services to members of cultural groups within the agency's catchment area, and regularly assess goal achievement and consumer satisfaction with the services offered.

Promote the use of culturally competent practices among the agency's employees.

Work with other service providers, multicultural agencies, and schools in health and human services disciplines to develop

- Valid and reliable assessment instruments for ethnically diverse populations
- Culturally appropriate treatment modalities
- Cultural competence training packages for staff
- Evaluation strategies to assess the incorporation and refinement of culturally competent approaches

needed from administrators to pursue these steps to increase cultural capacity over the long term.

There also are opportunities for policy makers to participate in the promotion of culturally competent practice. For example, in the course of our study, it emerged that the view of future planning among multicultural families challenged existing policy emphases on planning for independence and future transitions for the individual with a developmental disability. Also, participating multicultural families pointed out that services offered to one individual in the family, the person with a developmental disability, was often detrimental rather than helpful when the family had other more pressing concerns for which it needed assistance.

A significant concern for policy makers is that the emphasis in contemporary developmental disabilities services systems is on person-centered planning, a technique that was developed with little input from multicultural communities. It is suggested that the emphasis on this "one-culture" technique needs reexamination as developmental disabilities agencies begin to expand services to include more varied cultural communities within their catchment areas. Person-centered planning focuses on the individual's development of personal relationships, positive roles in the community, and skills for self-empowerment. Six principles underpin this approach:

1. Develop services based on the person's choices, interests, and dreams rather than fitting the person into existing services.
2. Plan and provide no more services than are needed and provide services that are meaningful, functional, and build on the person's strengths and abilities.
3. Help the person access community resources such as jobs, housing, and friends and move away from segregated services.
4. Coordinate services around the life of the person instead of the needs of staff and programs.
5. Recognize abilities in neighbors, co-workers, families, and ordinary citizens to teach skills, form relationships, and support participation.
6. Form a diverse group of people willing to know, value, and support the person.

These principles further empowerment for people with developmental disabilities, and empowerment strategies are appreciated in multicultural communities (Iglehart & Becerra, 1996). However, in the pursuit of those principles, workers, administrators, and policy makers often emphasize the needs of individuals over families, and even present individual and family needs as different, setting up conflicts with diverse communities who place high value on the family and unity with the family structure. This is not appreciated and discourages service participation. Person-centered planning was conceived around values that did not consider the importance that some cultures place on the integration of the person with a developmental disability within the broader family structure and assignment of decision making to one or more key senior members of the family or kin group. These cultural variations in family orientation and decision-making need to receive serious consideration.

In addition, the inclusion of multicultural agencies in service networks in a context of declining resources requires initiatives to target resources to such agencies, fiscal incentives to promote the development of cultural providers, greater cooperation and collaboration between agencies, and flexibility to initiate culturally competent approaches rather than require standardized strategies. The development of such initiatives must be informed by input from the communities to be served, rather than be designed for them as is the case with many existing services. Achieving this also will require policy makers to commit to greater representation of cultural communities on advisory and policy-making bodies.

REFERENCES

Aponte, J.F., & Barnes, J.M. (1995). Impact of acculturation and moderator variables on the intervention and treatment of ethnic groups. In J.F. Aponte, R.Y. Rivers, & J. Wohl (Eds.), *Psychological interventions and cultural diversity* (pp. 19–39). Needham Heights, MA: Allyn & Bacon.

Aponte, J.F., & Crouch, R.T. (1995). The changing ethnic profile of the United States. In J.F. Aponte, R.Y. Rivers, & J. Wohl (Eds.), *Psychological interventions and cultural diversity* (pp. 1–18). Needham Heights, MA: Allyn & Bacon.

Axelson, J.A. (1999). *Counseling and development in a multicultural society* (3rd ed.). Pacific Grove, CA: Brooks/Cole.

Grant-Griffin, L. (1995). *Best practices: Outreach strategies in multicultural communities.* Albany: New York State Office of Mental Retardation and Developmental Disabilities.

Gratton, B., & Wilson, V. (1988). Family support systems and the minority elderly: A cautionary analysis. *Journal of Gerontological Social Work, 13,* 81–93.

Heller, T., & Factor, A.R. (1988). Permanency planning among black and white family caregivers of older adults with mental retardation. *Mental Retardation, 26,* 203–208.

Henderson, J.N., Gutierrez-Mayka, M., Garcia, J., & Boyd, S. (1993). A model for Alzheimer's disease support group development in African-American and Hispanic populations. *Gerontologist, 33,* 409–414.

Hominik, D. (1998). *Immigration policies and practices on persons with mental retardation and related disabilities.* Washington, DC: United States International Council on Mental Retardation and Developmental Disabilities.

Iglehart, A.P., & Becerra, R.M. (1996). Social work and the ethnic agency: A history of neglect. *Journal of Multicultural Social Work, 4*(1), 1–20.

Janicki, M.P., McCallion, P., Force, L., Bishop, K., & LePore, P. (1998). Area agency on aging outreach and assistance models for households with older carers of an adult with a disability. *Journal of Aging and Social Policy, 10*(1), 13–36.

Johnson, T.W. (1995). Utilizing culture in work with aging families. In G. Smith, S.S. Tobin, B.A. Robertson-Tchabo, & P. Power (Eds.), *Strengthening aging families: Diversity in practice and policy* (pp. 175–202). Thousand Oaks, CA: Sage Publications.

Lockery, S.A. (1991). Family and social supports: Caregiving among racial and ethnic minority elders. *Generations, 15,* 58–62.

McCallion, P., Janicki, M.P., & Grant-Griffin, L. (1997). Exploring the impact of culture and acculturation on older families caregiving for persons with developmental disabilities. *Family Relations, 46,* 347–357.

Minkler, M., Driver, D., Roe, K.M., & Bedeian, K. (1993). Community interventions to support grandparent caregivers. *Gerontologist, 33,* 807–811.

Sakauye, K.M. (1989). Ethnic variations in family support of the frail elderly. In M.Z. Goldstein (Ed.), *Family involvement in treatment of the frail elderly* (pp. 65–106). Washington, DC: American Psychiatric Press.

Sung, K.-T. (1995). Measures and dimensions of filial piety in Korea. *Gerontologist, 35,* 240–247.

Toseland, R.W., & McCallion, P. (1997). Trends in caregiving intervention research. *Social Work Research, 27,* 154–164.

7

Coalitions as Forces of Change and Support

Rick Berkobien and Sharon Davis

With the aging of individuals with developmental disabilities and their families, local agencies have assumed support roles that reveal the need for the developmental disabilities systems to coordinate access to community services designed for the general aging population, referred to generically as the aging network. This chapter describes some approaches to developing local collaborations initiated by several local chapters of The Arc. The first part describes chapter experiences in building coalitions as well as those that can be designed to conduct outreach to families of aging individuals with intellectual disabilities. This is followed by a model for coalition building that can help integrate older people with developmental disabilities into general aging services. Last, examples of The Arc's state chapter coalitions are described.

NEEDS OF FAMILIES AND AGING
ADULTS WITH INTELLECTUAL DISABILITIES

Coordination of services between the developmental disabilities system and the aging network will assist in meeting needs of aging individuals with intellectual disabilities as well as their families. Aging individuals with intellectual disabilities traditionally have not been included in the community's general aging services. In addition, there are many two-generation older families in which parents in their 70s and 80s are still caring for sons or daughters with an intellectual disability. As these parents become frail, many find themselves increasingly isolated and unable to meet their own needs and those of their children. Many do not know about available services and how to gain access to the aging or intellectual disabilities service systems. When a crisis occurs in the family, the consequences can be devastating for the family and for the person with an intellectual disability. Local agencies often learn of these families only after the parent has been hospitalized, after the parent has died, or when a crisis worker gets involved with some aspect of the family's problems (Adlin, 1993). Too often, no plans have been made for the son or daughter with a disability. Suddenly, the agency is asked to find housing and arrange supportive services for the family member who is left behind.

Other families come to the attention of agencies when the frail older parent is referred to an aging agency for assistance. The aging agency typically lacks the information and/or the resources to assist the person with an intellectual disability and calls on local intellectual disabilities agencies for help. The following example of a family referred in this manner illustrates a common situation.

> *After his wife's death, an 80-year-old father became the primary caregiver for his 55-year-old son with an intellectual disability. Father and son did not have close relationships with any other family members or neighbors on whom they could call for assistance. The father's health was deteriorating, as were his personal grooming and hygiene skills. His son was neither involved with an agency for a day program nor on a waiting list for residential services. The son was not getting the training or supports he needed, and at the same time the father was experiencing increased stress at the realization that his son was unprepared to live on his own. There was no plan in place for the son after the father died. They both needed assistance from an agency that could coordinate services to meet the father's current needs and could assist with planning for the son's future after the father was no longer able to provide care.*

As the previous example illustrates, the most common living situation for adults with an intellectual disability is with the family (Heller & Factor, 1993). According to Janicki (1993), many of these families may be unknown to service providers as they have kept their children at home and have not been involved with any human services agencies. The Wingspread Conference Report on Aging and Lifelong Disabilities concluded that two-generation older families are becoming the rule for people with lifelong disabilities who are living at home with their families (Ansello & Rose, 1989). This sentiment was echoed through many of the concerns raised during the myriad mini-White House Conferences on Aging held during 1994 and 1995 (see Janicki, 1995, 1999, for issues arising from these meetings) and is reflected in the Policy Statement on Aging promulgated by the board of directors of The Arc of the United States, a national organization on mental retardation[1] (1997).

Despite the recognition that aging people with intellectual disabilities can and should be included in regular aging services, barriers that prevent inclusion still exist. These range from attitudes of aging network providers and developmental disabilities providers to issues of information, communication, financial, programmatic, and an array of other obstacles (Janicki, 1993). In most states, these providers have kept services for individuals who are aging separate from services for individuals with devel-

---

[1]The term *mental retardation* is the official term approved for use by The Arc in its constitution and by-laws.

opmental disabilities. Although federal standards call for unencumbered access to senior centers by adults with disabilities, many senior citizens' centers are still apprehensive and unknowledgeable about serving people with disabilities in their centers (Rinck, Naragon, & Shollenberger, 1996). Furthermore, aging individuals with developmental disabilities tended to be served less frequently by these centers than individuals with other types of disabilities. One approach to ameliorating the problems faced by two-generation older families, as well as to supporting inclusion of older individuals with intellectual disability, is for a community agency to engage in advocacy and coalition building to achieve coordination of aging and developmental disabilities services and supports to meet the needs of both parents and children.

ROLE OF AGING AND DEVELOPMENTAL DISABILITIES SERVICE SYSTEMS

The aging network is the system of federal, state, and local agencies, organizations, and institutions that are responsible for serving and/or representing the needs of older people, typically age 60 and older (National Association of State Units on Aging, 1985). In most states, the aging network comprises state and local government agencies as well as a large variety of community services provider agencies. Funding is provided under the Older Americans Act of 1965 (PL 89-73) and is passed from the federal level by the Administration on Aging to the state units on aging, or to state agencies for the aging, for distribution to the area agencies on aging (AAA) and local service providers. Funds at the state and local levels are also provided by state and local governments.

The developmental disabilities system refers to the many agencies, both private and public, that plan, coordinate, administer, offer, or finance services for people of all ages who have intellectual disabilities and related developmental disabilities. Because program funding comes from various sources (primarily state government and private resources), the developmental disabilities system is a much looser network than the aging network and does not depend on funds that are dispersed under a specific national statute. Many states do, however, rely on funds under the federal Medicaid program for financing residential, day, and support services.

In the United States, the publicly funded service delivery system for individuals with intellectual and/or developmental disabilities and adults who are older operates from a centralized and, too often, bureaucratized system. When states rely on federal Medicaid funding for services, they also must cope with federal regulations and oversight, which emanate from the federal government to states and, in turn, flow from the states to local agencies. Although public agencies are given much autonomy in providing various services, bureaucratic processes often force them to develop services that are designed more to comply with regulations than to meet individual consumer needs. Approval from several levels of administrators and grappling with policies and paperwork are often necessary before such agencies can initiate new services.

Conversely, decentralized or "grass roots" voluntary organizations, such as chapters of The Arc, can be instrumental in effectively establishing new services such as aging and developmental disabilities coalitions (Turner, 1994). *Grass roots* refers to a group or organization that is established by and consists of local community members and is not directly initiated or funded by government or public dollars (although it may receive some public funds in exchange for providing services). These organizations are often separately incorporated and governed by a board of directors. Some of these groups are affiliated with their respective state chapters and a national headquarters, but the national organization's governance, including the adoption of policies and changes in bylaws, must be approved by vote of local chapter delegates. As such, local groups retain much decision making and have considerable autonomy in providing advocacy and services based on local community need in terms of how they may initiate new efforts. Unlike centralized, publicly funded agencies, they are basically unencumbered by superfluous and hierarchical policies.

The role and mission of the grass roots organization in the community often reinforce the group's involvement in coalitions and may aid in the success of such a venture. These organizations normally maintain active and ongoing relationships within their "disability community"—the formal or informal network of disability groups and social service provider. Networking can assist in establishing necessary contacts when building coalitions and help keep community organizations abreast of issues that have an impact on the community's disability groups. Grass roots organizations are often composed of parent and consumer members who may play a governing role with the organization. Localized governance helps ensure that the organization feels "ownership" in both the organization and the community it serves, and thus helps ensure that it stays committed to the goals that a coalition sets to improve its community.

COALITION BUILDING TO PROVIDE SUPPORTS

Coalitions can be an effective way to bridge systems for meeting community needs, especially those affected by aging and developmental disabilities. A coalition can be defined as a group of organizations working together in a common effort for a common purpose to make more effective and efficient use of resources (National Association of Area Agencies on Aging [AAA], 1992). Coalitions tend to bring together unlike organizations within an informal structure and can effectively work toward expanding resources to people who need them. Collectively, the member agencies in a coalition can help meet local community needs that a single agency cannot address. Furthermore, effective coalitions can work to create new supports. Starting and maintaining a coalition is similar to starting and maintaining a committee where there is a need and people who are interested in finding a solution. A core group can lead the planning process. Davis and Berkobien (1994) noted that there are a number of critical tasks that should be undertaken in planning for a coalition:

- *Defining the coalition's purpose:* What will the coalition attempt to accomplish? It is important to know the particular needs of families in the community. Data should be gathered on the basis of existing needs assessments in the community or on the group's experiences in dealing with families in crisis to describe unique needs that the coalition can address.
- *Defining the community:* What will be the target area? Will the coalition serve the geographical area covered by the group, or will coalition activities serve a more restricted or a broader area? Kutza and Scannell (1993) suggested thinking small geographically when planning a community coalition.
- *Determining who should be members of the coalition:* Which agencies and organizations should be represented? Who are community leaders? Who is knowledgeable and committed to getting things done? Who would have a personal interest in the coalitions purpose?
- *Selecting a facilitator:* Who will make sure things get done? This person is key in obtaining commitment to goals of the coalition by its members. Who will be designated to facilitate beginning activities of the coalition? Should this person be "neu-

tral," a non–service provider as suggested by some coalition experts? What qualities should the coalition's facilitator have? Will a facilitator be encouraged to emerge from the group after the initial phases of the coalition process?

- **Recruiting members:** To be effective in recruiting members to the coalition, it is important to know just what another agency is and what it does. Face-to-face meetings with staff from other agencies and organizations to acquire information about others and to discuss the vision for the coalition are valuable. Strategies should be developed for selling potential coalition members on ideas of organizing a coalition around needs of two-generation, older, at-risk families.

THE ARC'S ROLE AS AN AGENT OF CHANGE

The Arc of the United States is a grass-roots organization with approximately 1,000 chapters located in a variety of communities across the United States. Its 140,000 members are people with intellectual disabilities and related developmental disabilities, parents and other family members, and friends of people with intellectual disabilities and professionals who work with them. Chapters of The Arc provide and/or advocate for services and supports to meet the needs of people with intellectual disabilities and their families. The Arc has been involved in aging and developmental disabilities coalition building at the national, state, and local levels. Six such local coalitions were developed through a demonstration project funded by the U.S. Administration on Aging. Others, such as the successful, long-term coalitions independently spearheaded by the Oneida-Lewis chapter of New York State Arc (NYSARC), The Arc of Pennsylvania, and The Arc of California, are examples of naturally evolving coalitions. All of these organizations and their respective coalitions also have engaged in state-level coalition building to support local coalition building and worked to initiate changes at the state level. What follows is a cursory examination of the efforts undertaken by these state and local models in coalition-building activities. These efforts are described in terms of steps undertaken or components necessarily put in place during their efforts to establish a coalition. Described also are the obstacles that these coalitions faced, as well as some of their accomplishments.

The Arc's Eldercare Project

Between 1992 and 1994, The Arc engaged in a 17-month federally funded project to demonstrate various ways in which chapters could actively help build coalitions to coordinate services and supports for two-generation older families. Six chapters of The Arc participated in the project that served to link aging and developmental disabilities services agencies and other organizations that provide needed supports and services to older families. Selected to represent geographical diversity (i.e., area of the nation and population density), the chapters participating in the demonstration were located in Alabama, California, Illinois, Pennsylvania, North Carolina, and Rhode Island. Although the chapters' models and approaches varied depending on the needs of families, available resources, and organizational capabilities, the coalitions and activities formed by the demonstration sites addressed these five core activities: 1) outreach to locate elderly families that were at risk for losing their independence, 2) assistance to caregivers in planning for the future needs of the family member with an intellectual disability, 3) identification of currently needed services and appropriate referrals for both caregivers and individuals with intellectual disabilities, 4) advocacy on behalf of families to assist them in obtaining needed and desired services, and 5) documentation of unmet needs and advocacy for developing and funding needed services.

The national demonstration project was carried out to identify what would work and under what conditions when the common goal was conducting outreach and assisting older families and caregivers. Each of the sites faced different problems in building coalitions, and each provided valuable "lessons learned" information for replication of coalition-building efforts when helping older families is the goal. As this national demonstration project involved a limited number of experiences across the United States and was conducted within communities of varying demographic character, the findings from each site may not necessarily be indicative of what another coalition might experience in an area with similar demographic distinctions. However, what was observed in evaluating the site experiences was telling.

Overall, rural chapters in The Arc's project had more difficulty with creating coalitions because of a lack of transportation and having to travel long distances to attend meetings, and dispersed and fewer services (meaning fewer participants) were often barriers to effective service provision. Rural sites also noted that rural families were characteristically more self-reliant and often were inclined to shun assistance from formal organizations, particularly if they were associated with the government. Agencies in these areas found that they needed to respect the wishes of these families and were often restrained when trying to conduct outreach. Conversely, coalition sites in urban and suburban communities found that many other agencies also were interested in eldercare issues and, in certain cases, that they were able to join groups that were already addressing problems. The demonstration sites collectively identified a number of barriers that were common in nearly every community. These included little, if any, previous collaboration between the aging and developmental disabilities systems and residual histories of developmental disabilities agencies providing services in segregated environments. Furthermore, when it came to coalition organizational efforts, the following often seemed like major obstacles: 1) conflicting demands on staff in other activities, which precluded most site demonstration coordinators from spending as much time on coalition building as they would have liked; 2) lack of sufficient time to nurture the development of a coalition, as the 9- to 12-month period allowed by the project was too brief to expect all coalitions to be fully functioning; and 3) in some areas, lack of interagency statements of collaboration at the state agency level to support coalition building at the community level.

After the conclusion of the demonstration project, the participating chapters were asked what they learned from their individual coalition-building experiences. Davis and Berkobien summarized the range of perceptions about the lessons learned:

Leadership and support from the state level are vital to the success of community coalition building. An interagency agreement or pact that acknowledges the need to serve people and families who cross the eligibility guidelines and that spells out the joint responsibilities would be most helpful. The aging and developmental disabilities networks need to be able to understand clearly the benefits and advantages of coalition building.

Coalition building is a process that takes time, care, and nurturing. Professionals tend to be more outspoken and hurried than family members in the group. It is important to take time to cultivate family participation and listen carefully to their needs. Also, members need to plan an active role in the group so that they can feel ownership of the goals and activities. Small committee work with specific projects can help get members actively involved. (1994, pp. 24, 26–27)

The most significant lesson learned in this process was how very many people are concerned about eldercare issues and how little has been done to address the issues. The lack of coordination between services agencies generally was painfully evident, as was the isolated place that developmental disabilities services have created for themselves, making it all the more difficult to meet the needs of people when those needs move outside the singular realm of developmental disabilities. Funding and training on providing optimal services and supports for aging people with developmental disabilities was a clearly determined major need. An equally important need was for a significant investment in training to assist aging parents in planning for the future for their adult children with development disabilities and, most important, avoiding "quick-fix placements" of their family member after a major crisis. As a further planning need, demonstration site participants noted a need to begin addressing retirement issues for aging people with developmental disabilities. Having each of the participating sites use a variation of a coalition-building method showed that professionals in the aging services network have many of the same unresolved issues that were observed among professionals in the developmental disabilities services network. It was evident that both systems are more alike than unlike.

Oneida-Lewis Aging and
Mental Retardation/Developmental Disabilities Coalition

The Oneida-Lewis chapter of NYSARC was instrumental in forming the Oneida County Aging and Mental Retardation/Developmental Disabilities Coalition. Conceived in 1987, this coalition bridged various networks of advocacy groups, service provider, and key officials in developmental disabilities, aging, and related areas (Bishop, VanDerhoof, & Lucchino, 1992; Janicki, 1992). The coalition formed an effective network of agencies to identify needs of aging individuals with developmental disabilities and work on filling service gaps. As a result, the coalition helped member agencies to develop an array of inclusive services for aging individuals with developmental disabilities and address a number of new goals, such as outreach to assist families in future planning. Coalition members outlined the methodical process they used to form their growing and evolving coalition. The Oneida County Aging and Mental Retardation/Developmental Disabilities Coalition identified three steps in their developing and maintaining a successful coalition: 1) identifying a need and a goal, 2) adopting a process to develop a goal and outcomes and meet needs, and 3) institutionalizing outcomes into a community network.

In the mid-1980s, The Oneida-Lewis chapter recognized that a growing number of individuals—more than 40%—served by the chapter were older than 55 years. These individuals were living in the community and experiencing many of the same age-related problems that other older adults were. The chapter recognized that their staff and other professionals were not trained to work with aging individuals with developmental disabilities and that current service providers for aging people without disabilities in the county were either not aware of or not trained to serve these individuals. Recognizing this need, the Oneida County Developmental Disabilities Network (the precursor to the Oneida County Coalition), which included the Oneida-Lewis chapter of NYSARC, formed a planning committee that met, clarified these needs, and agreed on the following goal: to avoid duplication of services for people with developmental disabilities by better utilizing available community resources among developmental disabilities, aging, and related service systems.

With local needs identified and a working goal in place, the planning committee began a coalition-building process that included pulling together a broader alliance, establishing a final goal for a coalition, and developing outcomes and tasks. The planning committee recognized the need for a diverse coalition that would represent the needs of the community's developmental disabilities and aging constituencies. The planning committee also realized that "turf" issues between these two systems might exist, so an initial step was to choose a coalition facilitator who had minimal vested interest in either group—someone who could be neutral between developmental disabilities and aging systems. They chose a facilitator from the local college's institute on gerontology, who was aware of issues of both systems and respected by both as a leader in their respective areas. Next, the planning committee identified and invited a number of member agencies and individuals to form a core group made up of people who would remain stable within the coalition throughout its existence. These included consumers and individuals from services directly affected by the needs, developmental disabilities agencies, health service providers, administrators, and representatives of other public and private agencies. Prospective coalition members then received information on the reason for the meeting, including a short concept paper describing the needs, how the needs were identified, a proposed goal, reason for a coalition, and a list of planning group members.

At the first meeting, held at the local college (a neutral site), the facilitator introduced the concept paper as a working draft. He invited coalition members to refine the working goal into a final goal, decide outcomes for the new coalition, and identify tasks to accomplish these outcomes. Participants were encouraged to discuss these needs and goals and the types of subcommittees necessary to address these areas. Some of the initial subcommittees developed by the coalition included those on education, policy, integration, teleconferencing, special events, public relations, funding/grant writing, and long-range planning. For all subsequent meetings, the coalition decided to ensure that all of its activities would be task oriented and include reports with subcommittee activities, time lines for completion, and steps needed to complete outcomes. The coalition also focused on outcomes that were dynamic—realizing that they may change—and recognized that these should be both measurable and realistic. The Oneida County Coalition identified the following outcomes on the basis of the need and goals that it established:

- Better cross-network understanding, with a common terminology between the two systems
- Integration of aging individuals with developmental disabilities into the community
- Better community understanding of the needs of aging individuals with developmental disabilities
- Increased options for all older people in the county
- Staff in both networks trained to provide support for both people who are aging and those with developmental disabilities

The Oneida County Coalition adopted a planning strategy that includes planning in stages of 1, 3, and 5 years, and its subcommittees annually report on their activities in achieving outcomes related to these stages. Collectively, coalition members examine these outcomes to determine whether the time lines are still realistic, what has been completed, and what needs to be adjusted. The coalition members then define further tasks on the basis of outcomes linked to achieve the coalition's goals and, if needed, form new subcommittees around each set of additional tasks. Early in the coalition process, the coalition provided its community with a report of the needs, goals, resources, gaps in resources, and identification of barriers by means of a press conference in which the report was released to help educate the community. Coalition activities and milestones were included in the press conference and circulated widely within the coalition's area.

Over the years, the Oneida County Coalition has become an integral part of its community. Its lifetime is contingent on a number of factors, primarily the continued interest of its members and the tasks still to be accomplished. The coalition has become an institution in its community but still is aware that it must attend to factors that add to the success of such an initiative. For example, the coalition remains administratively separate from any organization that provides direct services to people who are older or who have developmental disabilities. It is not housed within any of the organizations that are members of the coalition. It maintains its own mailbox, letterhead, and other components to help it maintain its own identity. In addition, the coalition was not formed on the basis of dedicated funding, a factor that often creates dependency and, if funding stops, may cause a coalition to cease or undergo turmoil. The coalition, however, recognized that if coalition activities were successful, various funding sources could be considered to underwrite coalition activities.

STATEWIDE AGING AND DEVELOPMENTAL DISABILITIES COALITIONS AND TASK FORCES

Chapters of The Arc have been and are active at the statewide level in coalition building between developmental disabilities systems and aging systems. Working in concert with many of their respective local chapters and members, statewide chapters support local community coalitions, are catalysts for initiating statewide systems changes, and can provide a "spark" for local communities in forming local aging and developmental disabilities coalitions. Two examples of effective state chapter involvement as change agents in aging and developmental disabilities are the activities of The Arc of Pennsylvania Older Adults Committee and The Arc of California Task Force on Aging. Both of these entities have been in existence for several years and are outgrowths of recognizing needs at the statewide level. Although they share different histories and vary in structure, both have activities and accomplishments in common, including the following:

- Serving as a clearinghouse for related materials and providing information and referral
- Lobbying for necessary funding
- Hosting and conducting training
- Serving on statewide aging-related committees and task forces to remind them about aging people with developmental disabilities
- Providing state, national, and international visibility to aging and developmental disabilities activities
- Joining with (and often being the catalyst for) their public developmental disabilities agencies and aging agencies to address specific needs of aging people with developmental disabilities and their families
- Stimulating the growth of regional and local aging and developmental disabilities coalitions

Statewide coalitions and task forces can be a natural extension of local community activities, ranging from developing further coalitions to helping initiate specialized services for aging people with developmental disabilities and their families (Janicki, 1993). As communities initiate local coalitions or as existing coalitions evolve and grow, they may want to explore forming statewide coalitions as a way to address statewide issues and/or to help network local coalitions.

CHALLENGE OF CONSUMER INVOLVEMENT IN COALITIONS

Historically, professionals have controlled the development and operation of services for people with intellectual disabilities and their families. However, there is now a recognition that adults with disabilities provide much-needed knowledge, insights, and other contributions to services and supports and that self-determination should be the organizing principle behind these kinds of efforts. The system for individuals with disabilities and their families should actively include individuals and families in the planning, administration, and oversight of this system, including involvement in aging and developmental disabilities coalitions. Coalitions, including many of those highlighted in this chapter, have reported challenges in getting consumers (i.e., individuals with developmental disabilities and family members) actively involved (Parkinson & Howard, 1996). When such people join and attend meetings, there have then been additional challenges to ensure that they actively participate (or are given the opportunity to participate) and remain involved in activities. There are a number of factors that may challenge the recruiting and retaining of consumers for coalitions. Some of these factors include the following:

- There are few adults who have the time or energy to contribute to (yet another) committee or activity. Organizations tend to overuse certain parents or individuals with disabilities, and many families lack the time to volunteer.
- People who have been active for years on various boards and committees may feel physically and mentally drained. They may feel that others need to contribute their time and energy.
- Some adults may lack knowledge or believe that they lack knowledge of the topics being addressed in the coalition. They may feel intimidated around degreed professionals whom they perceive as being "the experts."
- Some professionals may believe that people with disabilities or family members lack the skills and abilities to contribute to a coalition and consciously or unconsciously convey this attitude toward consumer participants.
- People with disabilities or family members may distrust or be hostile toward professionals who they believe do not understand what it is like either to have a disability or to be the parents of someone with a disability. Professionals may feel such consumers lack understanding of or sensitivity to the role of services systems.
- Coalition work may require a basic understanding of meeting protocols and how coalitions operate. Consumers, especially individuals with intellectual disabilities who do not have experiences in this area, may have difficulties and frustrations in effectively contributing to and feeling a part of the coalition milieu.

To address some of these potential problems and actively involve consumers in coalitions, organizers of coalitions should consider the barrier to participation caused by holding coalition meetings in the middle of the day, which may preclude people who work from attending meetings. To overcome this problem, meetings should be scheduled at different times, including some evenings, and on different days. Some consumers also may have difficulty with transportation, so locating the meeting near a transportation line or even arranging for a car pool may help ensure better attendance.

To ensure representation at coalition meetings, do not turn just to consumers who are or have been involved in other volunteer activities. Instead, ask these individuals whether they could recommend others who they believe would be effective participants, especially those who may not currently be involved in other activities. Explain to them what the coalition is about, and stress the importance of including a diversity of thought and experience in the coalition process. A coalition works most effectively when it includes the insights and knowledge of professionals as well as of parents and individuals who have disabilities. It also will be most responsive if it defines its goals to be consistent with the needs of its target group and if those needs have been articulated by consumer representatives to the coalition.

Coalition goals should be emphasized clearly at the first meetings and, if necessary, discussed periodically as the coalition evolves. If a consumer member expresses concern about lacking knowledge or expertise, offer to provide materials about the issues or even to meet to discuss what the coalition may be doing and review key issues. A parent may be surprised at how much he or she really does know about aging and developmental disabilities issues, even without having a professional degree. At the first meeting of the coalition, stress to all participants that a coalition will be most effective if it embraces diversity (including people from the community's various or predominant ethnic minority groups). Coalitions should also freely explore differences of opinions and encourage participants to disagree with one another. Open communication should be reinforced during meetings. If someone believes that another participant lacks understanding of what it is like to be a consumer or a professional, encourage participants to talk about their experiences. Everyone is capable of gaining new insights. Many people with developmental disabilities have never had the opportunity to learn and hone their skills in this area. Consider providing to consumers specific training on the basics of being in such a role, possibly by asking a consumer to pair with a person who has more experience, as a way of mentoring.

CONCLUSIONS

This chapter briefly examines the nature of developing coalitions that focus on aging and developmental disabilities from the perspective of a national advocacy association. It notes that community-based organizations for people with developmental disabilities, ranging from advocacy groups to direct service provider, can play a major role in meeting a broad spectrum of needs around aging and developmental disabilities. These organizations have been and remain advocates for local aging and developmental disabilities services, lobbyists for statewide systemic change, catalysts for and active members of local aging and developmental disabilities coalitions, operators of specialized services for aging people with developmental disabilities, and organizers and coordinators of other local and statewide efforts for these individuals and their families. When they coalesce into working coalitions, their influence and effectiveness generally multiplies, they have more of a role in educating their community, and they can be more vocal and pronounced change agents.

REFERENCES

Adlin, M. (1993). Health care issues. In E. Sutton, A.R. Factor, B.A. Hawkins, T. Heller, & G.B. Seltzer (Eds.), *Older adults with developmental disabilities: Optimizing choice and change* (pp. 49–60). Baltimore: Paul H. Brookes Publishing Co.

Ansello, E.F., & Rose, T. (1989). *Aging and lifelong disabilities: Partnership for the twenty-first century.* Palm Springs, CA: Elvirita Lewis Foundation.

Bishop, K., VanDerhoof, A., & Lucchino, R. (1992). Oneida County Aging and Mental Retardation/Developmental Disabilities Coalition. In M.P. Janicki (Ed.), *Integration experience casebook: Program ideas in aging and developmental disabilities* (pp. 18–21). Albany: New York State Office of Mental Retardation and Developmental Disabilities.

Davis, S., & Berkobien, R. (1994). *Meeting the needs and challenges of at-risk, two-generation, elderly families.* Silver Spring, MD: The Arc of the United States.

Heller, T., & Factor, A.R. (1993). Aging family caregivers: Support resources and change in burden and placement desire. *American Journal on Mental Retardation, 98,* 417–426.

Janicki, M.P. (1993). *Building the future: Planning and community development in aging and developmental disabilities* (Rev. ed.). Albany: New York State Office of Mental Retardation and Developmental Disabilities.

Janicki, M.P. (1995). Summary of major White House Conference on Aging recommendations with developmental disabilities as topic: Challenges through the year 2000 and beyond post–White House Conference. In *Proceedings of the Second North Dakota National Conference on Aging and Disabilities* (pp. 24–25). Minot: Minot State University, North Dakota Center for Disabilities.

Janicki, M.P. (1999). Public policy and service design. In S.S. Herr & G. Weber (Eds.), *Aging, rights, and quality of life: Prospects for older people with developmental disabilities* (pp. 289–310). Baltimore: Paul H. Brookes Publishing Co.

Janicki, M.P. (Ed.). (1992). *Integration experience casebook: Program ideas in aging and developmental disabilities.* Albany: New York State Office of Mental Retardation and Developmental Disabilities.

Kutza, E.A., & Scannell, A.V. (1993). *Community eldercare coalitions: Or, how your community can help you if you'll let it.* Portland, OR: Portland State University.

National Association of Area Agencies on Aging (AAA). (1992). *Handbook on coalition building.* Washington, DC: U.S. Department of Health and Human Services, Administration on Aging.

National Association of State Units on Aging. (1985). *An orientation to the Older Americans Act* (Rev. ed.). Washington, DC: Author.

Older Americans Act of 1965, PL 89-73, 42 U.S.C. §§ 3001 *et seq.*

Parkinson, C.B., & Howard, M. (1996). Older persons with mental retardation/developmental disabilities. *Journal of Gerontological Social Work, 25*(1–2), 91–103.

Rinck, C., Naragon, P., & Shollenberger, D. (1996). *Interface between aging and disabilities* (NCOA Rep. No. 1). Kansas City: University of Missouri–Kansas City, Institute for Human Development.

The Arc of the United States. (1997). *Policy statement on aging.* Silver Spring, MD: Author.

Turner, K.W. (1994). Modeling community inclusion for older adults with developmental disabilities. *Southwest Journal on Aging, 10*(1/2), 13–18.

8

Promoting Personal, Familial, and Organizational Change Through Futures Planning

Phillip G. Clark and Connie B. Susa

The aging of adults with developmental disabilities has created unique challenges for them and their families, especially in situations in which older parents may question what will happen to their son or daughter when they can no longer provide the care and supports required by their adult child. Encouraging future-directed planning by these families is an important first step toward giving them greater control over options and choices for the futures of both generations. For example, issues involving financial supports, living arrangements, and work or retirement opportunities can be more effectively addressed through advance planning than when faced with crisis situations that necessitate rapid responses. Similarly, supporting these families with programs and services from both the aging and the developmental disabilities service systems can promote more effective collaboration and communication between them, in keeping with emerging national trends. This service coordination can ensure a more complete and satisfactory response to the entire family's needs rather than to those of only one individual or generation.

This chapter is drawn from the experiences of the Family Futures Planning Project, supported in part by Grant No. 90AM0678 from the Administration on Aging, U.S. Department of Health and Human Services, Washington, D.C. Grantees undertaking projects under government sponsorship are encouraged to express freely their findings and conclusions. Points of view or opinions do not, therefore, necessarily represent official Administration on Aging policy.

121

However, encouraging such planning by individuals and families, as well as increased collaboration on the part of service providers from different systems, is not without substantial perils and pitfalls. Older parents who have spent their lifetimes caring for an adult son or daughter with a developmental disability do not readily relinquish the roles and responsibilities that they have spent so many years acquiring, even if it means giving their adult child more of the independence and control that he or she will need for the future. Similarly, service systems that have operated independently and with a fixed set of assumptions about their respective roles do not easily begin to collaborate and work with a new set of guidelines to meet the needs of two generations. Moreover, vested economic and political interests can oppose organizational change in the direction of more autonomy, community participation, and control for individuals and families as service consumers.

These were the challenges facing the Rhode Island Family Futures Planning Project, which developed an extensive educational program to empower caregiving families to think, feel, and act in new ways to overcome the dilemmas that prevented them from engaging in planning. Using an intervention based on core values supporting community involvement, respect, and competency, participants were encouraged to move along a continuum of behavior change to assume increased control over their lives and to achieve their life goals. Similarly, service providers and professionals were challenged to work together more closely in the support of these family goals and, as a result, to change their own knowledge, feelings, and actions related to interagency collaboration and the empowerment of families.

This chapter explores both the theoretical framework and the practical implications of this project in the hope that the lessons learned from it will help others avoid some of the pitfalls and problems we encountered. Throughout this discussion, emphasis is placed less on the description of the program and more on its implications for understanding the strategy of futures planning and how to implement it. To accomplish this goal, the chapter is divided into four sections. First, the unique issues facing individuals and families in undertaking planning are summarized, based on research and the experience of other programs. Second, a description of the conceptual framework and the actual processes of family futures planning is presented, including a brief summary of the methods and products developed in our program. Third, the major findings and results of the Family Futures Planning Project are summarized. These include especially the implications of personal, familial, and organizational change. Finally, how to apply the lessons about change learned from this project—particularly to human services system contexts—is explored, and recommendations are made about future directions for program and policy development.

PROBLEMS FAMILIES FACE: UNIQUE NEEDS AND ISSUES IN PLANNING

Of particular interest to service providers from both the aging and developmental disabilities networks are families in which older parents provide daily care and supports to adult sons or daughters with developmental disabilities. What will happen to the son or daughter when the parent(s) can no longer provide the assistance needed to keep him or her at home? Professionals from both the aging and the developmental disabilities fields are increasingly faced with the challenge of meeting the needs of these two-generation older families (Davis & Berkobien, 1995; Roberto, 1993; Smith & Tobin, 1989).

Many of these families are "hidden" from the service system because they are fearful or suspicious of it or are unaware of services for which they might qualify. It is not uncommon for them to "emerge" when a crisis—such as the illness or death of a parent—occurs. Research has confirmed the observations of service providers that these families do not plan for contingencies or future residential placements (Carswell & Hartig, 1979; Heller & Factor, 1988; Roberto, 1993; Wood & Skiles, 1992; see also Chapters 4 and 5). Related to making no plans are such factors as the denial of aging by the parents, not having other children who can provide assistance to their parents or the sibling with a developmental disability, not using resources and services for the adult son or daughter, and not using peer support groups.

Other research has stressed the impact of caregiving on the aging parents (Englehardt, Brubaker, & Lutzer, 1988). The parents are apt to be coping with the growing limitations imposed by their own physical aging at the same time as they are faced with the chronic and periodic stress of caregiving. Overall, as the parents struggle to meet both their own needs and the needs of their adult son or daughter, their problems are compounded. For such families, there may seem to be no place to turn for assistance in meeting their unique and interrelated needs.

Moreover, the problems facing parents and adult sons or daughters in long-term planning are complex and potentially psychologically distressing. The parents must deal with the emotional issues of relinquishing care and grapple with choices about finances, guardianship, and living arrangements. Research has indicated that parents are frequently paralyzed into inaction because of compelling dilemmas in caregiving decision making in which there are no totally satisfactory solutions (Grant, 1990). Many are inextricably caught in nets of interdependence, ambivalence, and indecision. Service providers similarly must both assist the family in making "permanency plans" and work to ensure that the service system is prepared to manage the increased demand for services that is inevitable in the future. In an era of shrinking resources and "doing more with less," this may pose real dilemmas for providers—not to mention their having to deal with their own biases and vested economic or political interests in keeping the service system unchanged.

Today's practitioners often have neither training nor guidelines to assist individuals and families in this process (Smith & Tobin, 1993). Although increased attention has been given to developing interventions for the older adult son or daughter with a developmental disability, the design of family-based programs that involve both the aging parents and the son or daughter has been virtually ignored. It is clear that both generations have related but unique needs that must be addressed clearly and creatively. Moreover, collaborative interventions may have the advantage of being both more effective and more efficient by avoiding duplication and overlap.

Reports and recommendations have highlighted the need for developing both systematic analyses of the issues facing these older caregivers (Roberto, 1993) and innovative programs for these families (Davis & Berkobien, 1995). In line with this emerging need, family futures planning can be an important model for intervention with these families. It focuses on both practical issues and guiding values that can provide direction for these families as they struggle with what can and should happen for both generations in the future.

CONCEPTS AND METHODS OF FAMILY FUTURES PLANNING

Family futures planning was designed to bring together the aging and the developmental disabilities service systems to support families with older parents and adult sons or daughters with developmental disabilities and to empower these families to take more control over their lives by envisioning the kind of future they want and to begin laying the groundwork for achieving it. The primary goal is to assist families in planning for future decisions they will have to make regarding lifestyle choices when the parents (or other family caregivers) are no longer able to provide supports and assistance. A secondary goal is to improve communication and collaboration between the aging and the developmental disabilities service systems to support the families' planning needs and processes.

Guiding Concepts

Family futures planning is based on three different yet interrelated concepts: personal futures planning, service quality outcomes, and the stages of change model. Having these concepts as guiding principles and approaches is extremely important, as they help to define the overarching values and mission of the method—themes to which program staff and participants may have to return in the face of conflict or opposition from agencies or programs that are resistant to change.

Personal Futures Planning   Personal futures planning, or person-centered planning, originated by Mount and her colleagues (e.g., Mount, 1991, 1992, 1994; Mount & Zwernik, 1988), is a methodology designed primarily for individuals with developmental disabilities to guide their creating and attaining positive future goals. Emphasis is placed on establishing a process to develop a positive future—a vision—of what life for the person with a disability could be like. The individual's personal past and present life—including likes, dislikes, and relative strengths—are reviewed and summarized. The emphasis, however, is on describing his or her life in positive terms, without the *deficit* and *deficiency* terminology that is typically used by professionals and formal service systems. Moreover, the vision of the future is not based on or limited by available services or programs. Individuals are encouraged to create a future that is unhindered by present resources, restraints, and restrictions.

Once this vision is articulated, attaining it is made possible and sustained by circles of support: family members, friends, neighbors, and others who come together around the person with a disability to provide informal supports and assistance. Members of the circle may provide ideas, information, or actual services to help the individual maintain his or her chosen life. Circles of support may grow larger or smaller and otherwise change their focus or direction as the needs and life of the person with the disability evolve and develop.

Service Quality Outcomes   Family futures planning also is guided by five core values, or "service quality outcomes," originally developed by O'Brien and O'Brien (1992), that can be applied equally to both the aging and the developmental disabilities service systems. These values help to give focus and structure to the futures planning process, in which they are explicitly addressed to aid families in developing their goals and plans. In addition, they help to provide important guiding values to drive change in the thinking of families and service providers alike, who are frequently trapped in the "old ways" in which choices and decisions are guided by existing programs and resources. Thus, these values help program participants visualize new ways of thinking about the lives and futures of both the adult sons or daughters with developmental disabilities and their older parents—furthering the sense of connectedness between the aging and developmental disabilities service systems.

Briefly, the following describes the family futures planning values, or core quality service outcomes:

Sharing places: Maintaining or increasing the presence of persons with disabilities in community environments; using generic services wherever possible; and interacting with others, including those of all abilities and ages

Making choices: Controlling the directions that the lives of people with disabilities take by having them express their interests and preferences and by learning what is needed to ensure that their decisions will be based on sound information

Increasing respect: Building a positive reputation for people with disabilities through valued social communication, roles, and associations; ensuring that they stand up for themselves when the need arises; and developing opportunities for them to serve in giving roles

Improving skills: Lifelong learning by people with disabilities of things that make a difference; building on their interests and other areas of strength; using adaptive equipment and modern technology to solve problems; and using skills where they make the most sense

Building relationships: Increasing the number and quality of social interactions of people with disabilities, having the assurance that others care about them, and using natural supports in the community

Stages of Change Model   Because family futures planning ultimately is about changing individual, familial, and organizational behaviors, it requires an innovative conceptual framework for thinking about the process of change. Research has indicated that changing behavior occurs in stages that are predictable and orderly (Prochaska, Norcross, & DiClemente, 1994; Prochaska & Velicer, 1997; Prochaska, Velicer, et al., 1994). Applying this principle helps to develop new insights into the family futures planning process.

Change as a progression through stages—rather than as a simple "either-or" situation—suggests very different approaches to the development of educational programs. Many health and human services professionals who design programs to change people's behavior express dismay at the difficulty of recruiting large numbers of participants who "stay with the program" and finish it. Not only is this difficult, but it is even more challenging to determine whether there is any real impact of the knowledge or skills attained by participants on their long-range behavior change and the retention of some new form of behavior. The reason for these difficulties is that for a particular behavior, only approximately 20% of any large group is actually ready for action in changing that behavior. Most large-scale information programs reach only this small percentage of people, and of this group fewer than 5% actually complete the program. This yields a very low "impact rate" and generally a disappointingly high relapse rate (Prochaska, Norcross, et al., 1994; Prochaska, Velicer, et al., 1994).

In contrast to this action-oriented approach, the stage model of behavior change is based on a sequence of stages along a continuum of decision-making readiness to initiate a new behavior (see Table 1). Central to this model is a balance in decision making based on a comparison of the perceived positive and negative aspects (pros and cons) of a new behavior. People who are in the Action and Maintenance stages have a decisional balance that favors the pros, those in the Precontemplation stage have a balance weighted toward the cons, and those in the Contemplation and Preparation stages tend to fall in the middle. The model also suggests that there are processes of change— cognitive and social or interpersonal action strategies—that move individuals toward greater readiness to change and ultimately into action and maintenance. Programs that

Table 1.   Stage model of behavior change

Stage	Readiness to initiate new behavior
Precontemplation	Not active and not intending to change
Contemplation	Not active but considering a change
Preparation	Intending to take action in the very near future
Action	Initiating a new behavior
Maintenance	Sustaining the change over time
Relapse	Returning the behavior to Precontemplation/Contemplation

are tailored to address each participant "where they are" in the process of change will be more successful than those that are "shotgun" in their approach.

Project Products and Processes

To achieve its goals of fostering the development of intergenerational futures plans for the families it served, the Family Futures Planning Project put the previously discussed concepts into action and developed an extensive set of materials and methods, which were pilot-tested and revised over three successive "waves" of program implementation. What was learned at each stage was incorporated into successive drafts of the written products and the methods they embodied. The published project materials[1] embodying family futures planning principles use a "building" or "construction" metaphor to represent the nature of the process needed for long-term change (see Table 2). For the families that participated in the program, there were four basic components to the family futures planning process: recruitment, education, planning, and supports.

Recruitment   Potentially interested families in our pilot project were recruited by fliers posted at senior centers and community agencies that serve families with members with developmental disabilities. Press releases were prepared for distribution to local newspapers, and announcements were posted in the newsletters of service agencies in the community. These explained the purposes of our program and what it offered to participating families; a telephone number was given for more information. We also relied heavily on service providers that were based at the cooperating agencies to identify families that they knew or with which they worked and that might benefit from the program and to make personal contact with the family to encourage their participation. This personalized approach was often more effective, because it was based on a relationship of trust that had already been established with the family.

The families in the initial pilot phases of our program typically were composed of parents in their 60s and 70s, with adult sons or daughters in their 30s and 40s. However, we did not establish an age eligibility criterion for program participation, and some families were younger than these ages.

Education   Many programs have provided informational workshops for individuals with developmental disabilities or their families. The Family Futures Planning Project, however, informed both older caregivers and their son or daughter with a developmental disability, melding the perspectives of both generations around the common theme of having a vision for the future and acquiring the knowledge and skills to plan for and achieve it. As indicated previously, the first six workshops in our program were based largely on the nuts-and-bolts topics that provide basic background

---

[1]Copies of these materials may be ordered from the Program in Gerontology, White Hall G-15, The University of Rhode Island, Kingston, RI 02881. Telephone: (401) 874-2689; Fax: (401) 874-2061; e-mail: aging@uri.edu.

Table 2.   Products for family futures planning assistance

Drafting a Blueprint for Change: The Coordinator's Manual

The Coordinator's Manual provides background on family futures planning—
including guiding concepts and values—and a detailed, step-by-step set of
directions on how to run an actual program using the model developed in Rhode
Island.

Gathering the Materials: The Curriculum Guide

The Curriculum Guide presents an outline and detailed, step-by-step lesson plans
for 11 workshops on topics determined to be essential to the futures planning
process. The first six are content-oriented, and the last five are process-based.
The first series is open to all participants who are generally interested in the core
issues involving planning, whereas the second series is intended only for those
willing to make a commitment to the longer-range planning process.

Topics for the first six workshops:

Introduction to the program and its values and vision
Housing options
Estate planning
Home- and community-based supports
Work and getting a job
Health care: access and information

Topics for the last five workshops:

Confronting dilemmas based on fears, frustrations, and feelings
Empowering parents to let go of caregiving roles and relationships
Self-advocacy for people with developmental disabilities
Beginning to draft a blueprint and plan for the future
Developing and maintaining a family support network

Building Your Dream: The Family Handbook

This manual is structured around the themes and topics of the curriculum outlines
included in *Gathering the Materials.* Each session includes an outline and all the
handouts and worksheets assigned for it. Thus, each family member has a
complete set of all project materials, bound and complete.

The Toolkit: A Resource Guide

This directory of resources encompasses both print and program materials generally
related to the field of aging and developmental disabilities, including major
national publications and resources in this area. In addition, materials specific to
each session in the curriculum outline are presented. How to order these
resources—including names, addresses, and telephone numbers of suppliers—is
also included.

information considered essential for developing a plan; these have become fairly commonplace in educational workshops of this type. These workshops were held weekly in
the community or all-purpose room of one of the community agencies—either a senior
center or a center for people with developmental disabilities—that were cooperating
with the Family Futures Planning Program. The second series, however, emphasized
the internal psychological processes and social environments that can enhance or
weaken the family's ability to begin a planning process. These workshops were open to
the smaller number of families that were willing to make a real commitment to the planning process—typically six to eight families per center. These families met weekly with
program facilitators in a smaller conference room at the community site.

Planning   Distributed at each educational workshop was at least one personal
worksheet, which helped family members think about and record how the information
from that particular session could relate to their own lives. Some worksheets gave a

structure for organizing factual information; others asked for interests and personal styles of participants. Some actually began to develop goals, and one helped participants to identify and think about how to overcome barriers to achieving their plans. Taken together, these worksheets created a foundation for bringing a positive vision of the future to pass.

Near the end of the planning phase in our program, process facilitators (trained and paid by the project) were introduced to the families. These people had been taught to build on strengths and to focus on community-based options in helping families establish meaningful plans. Together with the participating families, they wrote the actual plans to serve as a "blueprint for change." The intent was to create an extended planning process that kept participants from simply reacting to the problems of the moment and that empowered them to seek a more desirable future based on possibilities. These facilitators met with the families in their homes at times that were convenient for the families and provided basic background information that was essential for developing a plan.

Supports   In our pilot project, the formal planning facilitators provided one type of support for families; but, by its very nature, paid support is limited. Families that came to know one another well over the 2½-month training period also began to provide encouragement and, at times, more tangible supports to one another. Most important, throughout the training series, references were constantly made to people within each participating family's natural circle of friends and relatives who could be called on to help in specific areas—to network in locating jobs, for example, or as advocates to provide legal or moral support.

The project continued to give families an understanding of how a support network might be organized to continue with problem solving in their progress toward the goals they had set. One special person was invited by each family to the last informational workshop to "catch the vision" and to learn how his or her commitment might maintain a more formal support network to help family members achieve their goals. Finally, each family had the opportunity to bring their identified helpers together to create a support network. Those who reached out for help, either in the creation of an ongoing support network or simply to ask for help in achieving a discrete goal, made the greatest progress toward attaining their ideal futures.

WHAT FAMILY FUTURES PLANNING TEACHES ABOUT CHANGE AND BARRIERS TO CHANGE

Family futures planning is really about change: changing individual and family behavior in developing a plan for the future and changing the ways in which human services agencies and providers work together and think about their mission. Unfortunately, there often are barriers to effecting change in individuals, families, and service systems. This project afforded us the opportunity to gain insight into what these forces are in the fields of aging and developmental disabilities.

Barriers to Change in Families and Service Providers

Both families and service providers face a significant array of barriers to change, embodying personal, social, economic, and political factors.

Families   Families in our project identified a number of barriers to planning for the future:

- We do not want to think about our illness or death.
- We are not sure that the services will meet our desires.

- We assume that others will provide, if the need arises.
- My son (or daughter) contributes at home.
- None of us welcomes change, in general.
- I overprotect my daughter (or son).
- I always procrastinate.
- I am unsure of legal procedures and costs.

Conversely, participating parents also identified reasons for undertaking the planning process:

- Change is inevitable for all of us.
- We have more control of the outcomes now and can design our own system.
- We gain peace of mind.
- We can make changes gradually, easing the transition for our son (or daughter).
- It will be less of a burden to future caregivers because we can help them now.
- Resources may diminish with time.
- Decisions made in crisis may result in taking what is available, not what is best.
- We would like the same freedom from caregiving that other older parents enjoy.

Previous research has identified a number of dilemmas faced by families whose children with developmental disabilities are making the transition into young adulthood (Thorin, Yovanoff, & Irvin, 1996). These dilemmas also held true for families that were participating in family futures planning. Additional analysis revealed that other dilemmas were embedded in the barriers to and rationales for planning that participating older people had identified. The first five dilemmas listed next are adapted from the previous research; the remaining two are derived from the statements of our participants:

- Families want a worry-free present but also a worry-free future.
- Families want others to manage daily supports for their adult sons or daughters, but they want to influence the design of those supports themselves.
- Families enjoy the many benefits of having their sons or daughters live at home, but they want freedom from their many caregiving responsibilities.
- Families want the security of continued sameness, but they want to be prepared for necessary change.
- Families can provide security for both generations by remaining close, but they can also provide security by facilitating separation.
- Families recognize that procrastination frees them from decision making but that, at the same time, it robs them of decision making.
- Families believe that commitment to a plan is scary but that failure to secure a plan also is scary.

Wanting good outcomes in each dilemma but believing that they are incompatible creates cognitive dissonance in these families—an uncomfortable state of maintaining conflicting thoughts, feelings, or behaviors. The status that older families have maintained for years is inaction out of fear that any movement will result in their losing one of the two desired outcomes or states.

Service Providers   Similar to families, some service providers may have a long history of "doing things a certain way," as well as a vested economic or political interest in maintaining the status quo. Change is seen as potentially threatening, so providers may become defensive and suspicious of the motivations of those who present a "new vision" of interagency collaboration and partnership with families. For these reasons, it can be extremely difficult for administrators and staff to recognize that there is a different way of thinking about the needs of the families they serve and how best to meet them—let alone actually change the ways in which they work and provide services. For example, a senior center may not want to open its doors to an older person with a developmental disability "because they are so different from the other people who attend our center, and they just wouldn't fit in." Or an agency for people with developmental disabilities may want only to recommend a group home environment for its participants because it benefits financially from having its group homes full.

Stages of Change

The stage model is helpful in understanding change at both the individual and family levels and at the provider agency and organizational system levels. When family futures planning was first developed, it was conceptualized as a series of educational workshops that would give participants the knowledge and skills they needed to develop a futures plan for their family—and then they would actually "go out and do it." Instead of families clamoring for our program and eager to start the planning process as soon as possible, we found parents extremely conflicted over what to do about the present and the future, ambivalent over whether to do anything at all, and caught on the horns of the compelling dilemmas outlined previously. Similarly, we expected to find service providers eager to provide supports to families that clearly needed their assistance. Instead, we often found agencies threatened by "something new and different" and reluctant to get involved in a project that might jeopardize their own programs or place greater strain on already overworked staff. An application of the stages of change model helped us in understanding these potential barriers to our program's mission and goals, and it suggested some possible strategies for coping with them.

Individuals and Families   It was soon realized that the original design of an educational workshop series dealt too much with just the intellectual, or "thinking," aspects of change and that the emotional, or "feeling," dimensions had to be addressed as well. Moreover, rather than conceptualizing the program as a series of six to eight workshops that would end in the development of a futures plan, we started thinking about planning as an ongoing process—with a slow progression through different stages or levels of readiness for action, and occasionally with relapse and regression. In other words, planning is a multidimensional set of behaviors—not a simple "either/or" dichotomy. For this reason, sustaining a "forward direction" of planning behavior can be a real challenge. Conversely, success should also be recognized, even if only "consciousness raising" about the need for and issues associated with planning and making choices has been achieved. For example, some participating families did not continue with the project to the point that they actually completed a futures plan, but project staff knew that, for the first time, the parents and their son or daughter had actually started talking about each other's hopes, dreams, fears, and concerns. This was counted as success!

The vast majority of families recruited by the Family Futures Planning Project were in the stage of contemplation for planning for their futures. Precontemplators did not attend the workshop series. Because this was not a research project, we did not systematically assess each person's stage of readiness for futures planning, nor did we objectively monitor their progression through stages as the process unfolded. However, we did note in general that moving participants from contemplation through preparation into action proved to be difficult and challenging—participating parents frequently knew they should do something, but they were too caught in an emotional ambivalence fueled by the psychosocial dilemmas mentioned previously. They had the "thinking" part down well, but the "feeling" dimension prevented the behavioral outcomes associated with actually doing something about planning for the future.

In the Family Futures Planning Project, specific materials and processes were developed for individuals and families at different stages. Materials emphasizing the advantages of planning were developed for those in earlier stages of change, whereas acquiring skills on how to develop social supports was more relevant to families closer to action. Specific examples of the kinds of program materials and methods targeting participants at different stages are outlined in Table 3. At each step along the way, participants were supported, encouraged, and invited to keep progressing along a course that would more effectively prepare them for a future of their own vision and choosing. The process was envisioned as an "uphill" one, because clearly it required perseverance, energy, and stamina. Yet the program showed, at each step along the way, the advantages of planning over the lack of it.

Provider Agencies and Organizational Systems   As both people with developmental disabilities and parent caregivers grow older in greater numbers, it makes increasing sense to develop strong linkages between the aging and developmental disabilities service systems. Family futures planning focuses on the challenge of encouraging greater collaboration between these two service networks. Unfortunately, there are many barriers to achieving greater linkages: federal legislation that has established different administrative structures, programs, and funding streams; eligibility requirements; differences in training of program staff; client and community perceptions; and resistance to change based on vested political and economic interests.

The Family Futures Planning Project addressed these barriers by emphasizing input and collaboration from both "sides" of the service systems throughout the development of the workshop series and with the support of interdisciplinary service teams as part of the piloting process. Organizational change came to be understood as changing the individuals within those organizations. This change also was conceptualized

Table 3.   Stage-related program materials and methods targeted at participants

Contemplation
    Educational workshop series
    Handouts of reprints and references
    Family and resource manuals
    Personal histories of participants

Preparation
    Small-group discussions and exercises
    Peer and staff sharing of success stories
    Values clarification exercises and worksheets
    Planning process workshops

Action
    Making a family futures plan
    Verbal affirmations and celebrations
    Setting up informal support opportunities
    Establishing a circle of support

as a gradual process, requiring consciousness raising about the issues, gradually increasing involvement and "buy in" from agency staff, and ultimately—we hoped—not just acceptance of "our program" but actual identification of agency staff with "their program."

For example, as the workshop series was designed, one speaker from the aging side of the topic and one from the developmental disabilities side were recruited as co-presenters. This led to the development of a paired and interconnected presentation on the specific topic for that week. This type of collaboration was found in the workshop on employment opportunities, in which a representative of the Supported Employment Program of the American Association of Retired Persons (AARP) collaborated with the employment and work specialist of the Rhode Island University Affiliated Program—supported by funds from the U.S. Administration on Developmental Disabilities. Discovering that they shared a lot in common—for example, a reliance on similar philosophies, approaches, and materials—these staff members learned so much from each other and collaborated so closely in the development of their team-taught workshop that there was a complete integration of both the aging and the developmental disabilities perspectives.

More important, after the workshop series, the AARP project director had an inquiry about an older person with a developmental disability, associated with a regional Arc program in the state, who qualified and was interested in receiving training through the AARP-sponsored employment project. The AARP staff person's reaction was different from what she reported it would have been before her participation in the Family Futures Planning Project. She said, "Let's try it and see what happens. Now that I'm aware of the issues and similarities between the two systems, I'm more willing to work with the developmental disabilities programs."

Similarly, in developing family futures planning, three successive phases, or "waves," of pilot testing the model and the written materials were implemented. At each stage, a community agency from the aging network was paired with one from the developmental disabilities side as the "host" agencies to collaborate on the development of the workshop model, review methods from previous pilot phases, and provide input into the design of written materials. The attempt was to meld the perspectives, approaches, materials, and professional insights from both fields to achieve a "unified" program directed toward the needs and concerns of both parent and adult child generations.

In this process, some exciting developments occurred. Many of the agency staff from the two different service systems had never actually met each other, let alone worked together. An occasional telephone call to consult on a particular case or to gather information was the extent of the contact. Truly working together on a common project, with a collaborative mission, created tangible enthusiasm among some of the agency staff members. An example of such systemic change occurred after the completion of the Family Futures Planning Project. One of The Arc community centers that had participated in our program helped to bolster dwindling participant numbers at a local senior center by transferring some of their attendees to this center from the aging services side. This action helped to maintain the senior center's viability at a time when its programs and attendance were under scrutiny by budget-minded administrators. This outcome is precisely what was hoped would be achieved by family futures planning: greater coordination and collaboration between the aging and the developmental disabilities systems.

CONCLUSIONS

The implications of this project for educational programs specifically and policy development generally in the emerging aging and developmental disabilities field are significant. They fall into the following categories: futures planning as a process, not an outcome; the importance of developing and improving consumer-driven service systems; and the challenge of fostering increased collaboration between the two service networks.

Futures Planning as a Continuum and a Process

Many educational programs targeted toward individuals or families presume a positive impact. The assumption is that if people receive important information, they will act on it and change their behavior accordingly. As discussed previously, family futures planning represents a new approach to developing educational materials and methods that "meet participants where they are" on a continuum of stages of change. Such a model recognizes that different individuals and families are at different points in their readiness to accept change and make plans for the future.

Overall, the Family Futures Planning Project was successful in raising the awareness of individual and family participants about the importance of and need for change—and in achieving some successes in actual behavior change. However, the difficulty of changing long-standing behaviors cannot be underestimated, and the recognition that change is a constant process is very important. As discussed previously, the project originally assumed that families would eagerly participate in its programs, develop concrete and written plans, and then proceed to implement them in a logical and rational way. Instead, we learned that planning is a continual process rather than a neatly defined endpoint. Grappling with the dilemmas, risks, and problems confronting families that try to change requires constant support and long-term encouragement from both informal and formal support networks.

In developing the Family Futures Planning Project, we encountered many disappointments and a few pleasant surprises. For example, one participating older parent had an extensive background in the field of developmental disabilities and seemed particularly concerned about her son's future. However, despite her intellectual knowledge about the issues, she was never able to come to grips with the emotions and feelings involved in establishing the plans needed for her son's future and became inactive by the end of the program. In contrast, one older mother entered the program with a very limited and specific goal for her daughter, and her only purpose in joining the project was to enlist our help in achieving it. During the course of her participation, however, she changed dramatically, acquiring a new philosophy about community participation for her daughter. At the end of the program, she was pursuing this new goal with the same enthusiasm and commitment that she had originally for a much more limited and traditional goal for her daughter's living arrangements.

One implication of this insight into the process of change is that futures planning by families must be supported by programs that are staffed with trained personnel who are familiar with the planning principles and methods required to move families toward their vision of a desirable future. In our program, we found that such people were not easy to recruit or train. At the same time, however, the emphasis in such programs must be on the empowerment of the family to move beyond the paralysis created by dilemmas and conflicts between competing personal goals and familial outcomes. The emotional grip of these conflicts must be broken by emphasizing the advantages of planning and by providing the social support necessary to sustain families over the potentially long course represented by this process. After our development of the family futures planning model in Rhode Island, we were fortunate to have major components of the program assimilated into the on-going family support training efforts sponsored by the University Affiliated Program in our state, which now uses many of the educational materials and methods we designed and piloted.

Importance of Developing Consumer-Driven Service Systems

Models of consumer empowerment within the fields of aging and developmental disabilities are beginning to emerge (Cohen, 1988). They emphasize the importance of giving the client or consumer ultimate control over decision making and resource use. Beginning within the disabilities community in general and specifically within the community living movement, these models have important implications for those working within the aging network as well (Clark, 1995).

Ideological changes in how services are conceptualized need to occur. Increasing the power of families to choose and shape services and supports they define to be helpful and needed—rather than trying to fit what professionals define to be individual needs to predetermined services, programs, and options—is a crucial step. Many families believe that their futures are defined by what is available—rather than by what could be built, developed, or invented by a collaborative of progressive individuals, families, and providers working together to achieve a vision in which all people are respected as an integral part of their community. These beliefs must now be changed.

The conscious inclusion in the Family Futures Planning Project of the five O'Brien quality service outcome values placed the program squarely at the forefront of this effort to transform the system from its current professionally dominated and defined mode, in which needs are determined by professionals and services are defined in terms of which needs they meet. This problem-based and deficit-driven system needs to change if the aging and developmental disabilities fields are to be successful in collaborating in the future. For example, the barriers established within families that receive services from both systems—but do so independent of each other—only reinforce that the systems operate on principles that are not user friendly. Many of these issues were also explored in the 1995 White House Conference on Aging and led to the development of specific recommendations on their being addressed (White House Conference on Aging, 1996).

However, the efforts made by the Family Futures Planning Project on a systemwide basis to bring about such changes were not particularly successful. The usual effort expended by agency staff when a grant is funded to "rise to the occasion" was evident, and we did get willing involvement by several knowledgeable and committed staff members. However, we also were keenly aware in many cases of the lack of support by agency leadership, who may have had vested political or economic interests in avoiding major changes in how their program operated or in the guiding vision it articulated for its services. For example, centers for people with developmental disabilities that sponsored sheltered workshop–type programs or group home living arrangements were threatened by the message of the Family Futures Planning Project to seek work opportunities and housing in the larger community. The O'Brien principles (O'Brien & O'Brien, 1992), which we promoted, were clearly perceived as a threat to those vested in the status quo. Even the major initial primary sponsor of the Family Futures Planning

Project never went public with a strong endorsement of what we were attempting to do, because—we reasoned—they could not afford to move too quickly beyond their constituencies in the state.

Challenges of Increased Collaboration Between Two Service Networks

It is apparent from the experience of the Family Futures Planning Project that significant change must be made in the funding and operational methods that are in place in the aging and developmental disabilities networks if they are to continue to develop linkages with each other. Demonstration projects and models are a good start, but more fundamental changes will have to be made for true collaboration to become a reality. This development creates significant conceptual and value-based dilemmas, as well as very real practical service issues. The debate between categorical and general services is at the very center of this controversy. For example, should services be established on age-based criteria or simply on the presence of a certain defined level of impairment?

In addition, the training of service providers and professionals in the aging and developmental disabilities fields will have to become coordinated and, possibly, merged into one unified career track. This will take time and effort. The Family Futures Planning Project developed a model of grass roots collaboration between service providers at the front lines of delivery, but such an initiative will have to become more institutionalized in the development of the education and training structures needed to sustain it into the future. This will require reshaping educational career tracks, academic curricula, and faculty expertise and collaboration. At the very least, greater emphasis will have to be placed on the importance of interdisciplinary education and the development of opportunities for students from different disciplines to learn to work together collaboratively across the aging and disabilities fields (Clark, 1996).

As discussed previously, our project was able to "point the way" as a demonstration, but long-term change is difficult to achieve in a 2-year period that comes to a close when the grant support ends. Other, larger institutional changes also must come about in the service and educational sectors if sustained change is to be achieved. For example, as a result of the Family Futures Planning Project, a course on aging and developmental disabilities was proposed at the university for training students in this new field. However, it was not recommended for approval by the departmental curriculum committee because no new resources could be made available to cover the increased faculty time for this new course—at a time when existing faculty were already stretched to the limit to cover current curriculum requirements. Once again, innovative and interdisciplinary efforts tend to be difficult to sustain when resources are limited.

In summary, change is not always easy when it requires the modification of long-standing patterns of individual, familial, or organizational behavior. There may be emotional, social, institutional, and systemic forces that make change difficult and lengthy. However, the Family Futures Planning Project demonstrated that thinking about change as a continuum or process can be helpful in recognizing that small steps taken can, over time, lead to overt and recognizable progress. Especially with regard to the kinds of changes necessary to support futures planning by families, both top-down and bottom-up strategies are essential—both to empower families to take more control over their lives and to provide the systemwide incentives to spur the educational and programmatic changes that are the core of increased collaboration across service system boundaries. Overall, probably the most important change must be ideological: the acceptance of the values supporting enhanced respect, choice, community involvement, skills, and social relationships that underlie what makes life worthwhile for people of any age or ability. Without the shared vision provided by these values, any kind of change will be difficult.

REFERENCES

Carswell, A.T., & Hartig, S.A. (1979). *Older developmentally disabled persons: An investigation of needs and social services.* Athens: Georgia Retardation Center, University of Georgia.

Clark, P.G. (1995). Quality of life, values, and teamwork in geriatric care: Do we communicate what we mean? *Gerontologist, 35,* 402–411.

Clark, P.G. (1996). Learning from education: What the teamwork literature in special education can teach gerontologists about team training and development. *Educational Gerontology, 22,* 387–410.

Cohen, E.S. (1988). The elderly mystique: Constraints on the autonomy of the elderly with disabilities. *Gerontologist, 28*(Suppl.), 24–31.

Davis, S., & Berkobien, R. (1995). *Meeting the needs and challenges of at-risk, two-generation, elderly families.* Silver Spring, MD: The Arc of the United States.

Englehardt, J.L., Brubaker, T.H., & Lutzer, V.D. (1988). Older caregivers of adults with mental retardation: Service utilization. *Mental Retardation, 26,* 191–195.

Grant, G. (1990). Elderly parents with handicapped children: Anticipating the future. *Journal of Aging Studies, 4,* 359–374.

Heller, T., & Factor, A. (1988). Permanency planning among black and white family caregivers of older adults with mental retardation. *Mental Retardation, 26,* 203–208.

Mount, B. (1991). *Person-centered planning: A sourcebook of values, ideals, and methods to encourage person-centered development.* New York: Graphic Futures.

Mount, B. (1992). *Personal futures planning: Promises and precautions.* New York: Graphic Futures.

Mount, B. (1994). Benefits and limitations of personal futures planning. In V.J. Bradley, J.W. Ashbaugh, & B.C. Blaney (Eds.), *Creating individual supports for people with developmental disabilities: A mandate for change at many levels* (pp. 97–108). Baltimore: Paul H. Brookes Publishing Co.

Mount, B., & Zwernik, K. (1988). *It's never too early, it's never too late: An overview of personal futures planning.* St. Paul, MN: Metropolitan Council.

O'Brien, J., & O'Brien, C.L. (1992). *Framework for accomplishment.* Atlanta, GA: Responsive Systems Associates.

Prochaska, J.O., Norcross, J.C., & DiClemente, C.C. (1994). *Changing for good: The revolutionary program that explains the six stages of change and teaches you how to free yourself from bad habits.* New York: William Morrow & Co.

Prochaska, J.O., & Velicer, W.F. (1997). The transtheoretical model of health behavior change. *American Journal of Health Promotion, 12,* 38–48.

Prochaska, J.O., Velicer, W.F., Rossi, J.S., Goldstein, M.G., Marcus, B.H., Rakowski, W., Fiore, C., Harlow, L.L., Redding, C.A., Rosenbloom, D., & Rossi, S.R. (1994). Stages of change and decisional balance for twelve problem behaviors. *Health Psychology, 13,* 39–46.

Roberto, K.A. (Ed.). (1993). *The elderly caregiver: Caring for adults with developmental disabilities.* Thousand Oaks, CA: Sage Publications.

Smith, G.C., & Tobin, S.S. (1989). Permanency planning among older parents of adults with lifelong disabilities. *Journal of Gerontological Social Work, 14,* 35–59.

Smith, G.C., & Tobin, S.S. (1993). Practice with older parents of developmentally disabled adults. *Clinical Gerontologist, 14,* 59–77.

Thorin, E., Yovanoff, P., & Irvin, L. (1996). Dilemmas faced by families during their young adults' transitions to adulthood: A brief report. *Mental Retardation, 34,* 117–120.

White House Conference on Aging. (1996). *The road to an aging policy for the 21st century.* Washington, DC: Author.

Wood, J.B., & Skiles, L.L. (1992). Planning for the transfer of care: Who cares for the developmentally disabled adult when the family can no longer do so? *Generations, 16,* 61–62.

9

Activating
Consumers and Families

Edward F. Ansello and Constance L. Coogle

The fullest participation in community living by aging adults with lifelong disabilities requires the involvement of others. This is at the heart of the Developmental Disabilities Assistance and Bill of Rights Act of 1975 (PL 94-103). Often, family members such as parents and siblings have enabled individuals with developmental disabilities to reach late life, sometimes with the additional help of community-based agencies, sometimes without it. Although each individual's circumstances and community supports are different, the key players in community support are the aging individual, the caregiving family, and community-based agencies. The likelihood is that all three will be involved at one point or another in the meaningful aging of the person with lifelong disabilities.

Birth cohort and the individual's particular developmental disability seem to influence involvement by others. For instance, those currently near 55 or 60 years of age or older tend, more than their younger counterparts, to have grown up and older without as much benefit from enlightened legislation intended to improve education, employment, and socialization skills. Their parents' courage and initiatives as caregivers and advocates made the difference. Often, when the parents' efforts eventually produced legislation and the bureaucracies and services that accompany it, they continued on their own without agency involvement. Ohle (1999) documented the lifelong, determined independence of a sample of parents of now-aging children with Down syndrome, an independence forged by the unresponsiveness of the medical and other support systems during their children's youth. At the same time, individuals whose developmental disabilities do not include substantial cognitive involvement have a greater likelihood of having learned to become self-advocates in adulthood and to have left their caregiving families behind.

The discussion that follows assumes that growing older in community environments requires supports and that these are most effective when all three sets of players are engaged in producing the supports. The discussion refers to general principles and expectations for partnerships involving adults with disabilities and family caregivers, as well as to specific experiences with a forum for this engagement called, imperfectly, the Professional/Consumer Advocacy Council (PCAC). In this instance, *professional* is used broadly to include service providers, educators, planners, health care practitioners, and others, whereas *consumer* encompasses both the adult with developmental disabilities and the caregiving family members and friends. Consumers can be professionals, of course, so the terms are used somewhat loosely.

RIGHTS AND RESPONSIBILITIES EQUATION

Advocates have championed the "rights" of older people with lifelong disabilities. These are said to include the right to an array of services; the right to a favorable image; the right to nonsegregated life experiences; the right to a "normalized," if not a normal, life; and so forth. The inextricable linkage between rights and responsibilities, however, has not always been so well applied. Securing the rights of older people with lifelong impairments, indeed, the rights of adults of any age with disabilities, is the responsibility of these individuals themselves. One acknowledges the impressive accomplishments that determined advocates have made on behalf of others whose disabilities have compromised their capacity to achieve these rights on their own. Disabilities- and aging-related advocates have fought for and won unprecedented rights in the arenas of education, health care, employment, transportation, and elsewhere. At the same time, one also must acknowledge that adults with lifelong disabilities are often left out of the very advocacy process meant to benefit them.

Securing rights and exercising responsibility require a dialogue among all of the parties affected by their practice: agencies, families, and the individuals themselves. An enterprise that aims to improve community supports for aging adults with lifelong disabilities that does not include these adults in a meaningful way is effectively a monologue. The concept of community integration of individuals with developmental disabilities logically requires the exercise of participation and choice. Not every aging adult with developmental disabilities is able to participate meaningfully; in some instances, such as substantial intellectual disability, most cannot. However, demonstration projects have repeatedly "uncovered" aging adults with lifelong impairments who have been living in the community their entire lives without the awareness of any human services agency. These adults, in family contexts or on their own, have been exercising choices and making decisions. Their aging and the aging of their caregiving families create a special urgency that they be integrated into the processes that set policy and practice that affect growing old with lifelong impairments. The caregiving parents cannot live forever. Plans must be made for continuation of care. The incapacity or loss of caregiving parents may drastically increase the scope and number of decisions that must be made regarding an aging adult with disabilities, and this adult should be involved in the process.

At the same time, individuals with lifelong impairments who are in their 30s or 40s (and who may well express characteristics of older people) are likely to have benefited from national legislation such as mainstreaming education and personal support services that enable them to live in the community relatively, if not absolutely, on their own. They tend to be more experienced in self-advocacy. Yet, overall, they and other aging adults with lifelong disabilities and family members who are caregivers participate infrequently in the responsibility half of the rights and responsibilities equation. Often, it is not because of lack of desire to do so.

Improving the community living of aging adults with lifelong impairments requires the combined efforts of the three principal partners in the community: the relevant organizations and agencies, from those affiliated with disabilities- and aging-related systems to others such as health, social services, protective services, recreation, and religion; the family caregivers, including parents, siblings, spouses, and others; and the individuals with disabilities. The interplay of these three groups should substantiate a fundamental commitment to the "assisted autonomy" (Chapter 1; see Moody, 1992) of the person with lifelong disabilities. Whenever feasible, policies considered, programs planned, and issues advocated reflect an awareness that all of these efforts are aimed at assisting the individual to be as autonomous as possible, exercising choices and making decisions for oneself. Autonomy in this context refers to a negotiated or assisted process involving others.

INTEGRATED MODEL

The Partners I, II, and III Projects in Maryland and Virginia, funded over the course of a decade by the Administration on Aging, sought to improve the community living of older adults with developmental disabilities through a range of initiatives that focused on agency staff, family caregivers, and the older adults. Partners III operationalized a plan for intersystem cooperation between the aging and developmental disabilities networks that incorporates the values and the most effective practices of the previous Partners Projects and of several others on aging and disabilities that the team had completed. The values include basing care coordination and choices on the preferences of the older person with a developmental disability, strengthening the abilities of family caregivers of these older adults to continue appropriate care, improving the expertise of agency staff relative to issues of aging with developmental disabilities, and engaging all of the parties—individuals, family caregivers, and agency staff—in the conduct of activities that relate to services for older adults with developmental disabilities. These proven features form the Integrated Model of Services for Older Adults with Developmental Disabilities.

The Integrated Model of Services for Older Adults with Developmental Disabilities reflects the experience that, for intersystem cooperation that benefits older adults with lifelong disabilities to occur, three basic ingredients are necessary: 1) some formal means of collaboration for ongoing communication between the systems; 2) strategies for outreach to older adults with developmental disabilities and informal caregivers (family and friends) who provide community-based assistance; and 3) methods of building the capacities of formal providers of assistance, informal providers, and older adults with lifelong disabilities to identify and use appropriate resources that maximize the community functioning of these older adults. Central to each of the three basic ingredients is the involvement of older people with disabilities and of family caregivers. The philosophy behind their involvement is instrumentality—that is, being agents in actions rather than simple recipients. In practice, the Integrated Model of Services for Older Adults with Developmental Disabilities operationalizes "consumer-agents" and "caregiver-agents" in the collaboration, outreach, and capacity-building activities.

Aging individuals with lifelong impairments and, when present, their family caregivers also put flesh to the conviction that the most productive intersystem cooperation occurs when there are both top-down and bottom-up commitments to this cooperation. *Top-down* refers both to the top of the administrative hierarchies in the systems involved and to the larger geographical focus where the initiative takes place. In Partners III, this translates to the state-level directorships of the public aging and developmental disabilities administrations, in the first instance, and to the state of Maryland and the commonwealth of Virginia, as opposed to a municipality or county, in the second. *Bottom-up*, in contrast, refers both to the lower end of the administrative hierarchies and to the more localized geographical focus; this encompasses service delivery and the municipality or county, respectively. Pointedly, the Partners III Project's Integrated Model of Services for Older Adults with Developmental Disabilities seems most effective when consumer-agents and caregiver-agents are involved at both top-down and bottom-up directions. They were key to successfully implementing the model in each of Partner III's five local applications. Certainly, the literature repeats the mantra that consumers need to be involved locally, especially when the issues at hand affect them personally and immediately (Browning, Rhoades, & Crosson, 1980; Pederson, Chaikin, Koehler, Campbell, & Arcand, 1993; Valentine & Capponi, 1989). Equally as important is meaningful participation by aging adults with lifelong disabilities and by family caregivers in activities that affect them less personally and less immediately, such as policy formulation, curriculum development, and legislative processes.

In Partners III, one of the principal instruments for involving aging adults and family caregivers is the PCAC. Conceptually and, for the most part, in practice, the PCAC serves in the broad, top-down role. Since 1995, it has helped to influence policy on personal assistance services, advance pilot projects to integrate older adults with developmental disabilities into community senior centers, offer statewide cross-training workshops, develop expositions of the latest assistive technology, and pass legislation to provide financial grants to family caregivers of people with disabilities, while also becoming over time a forum for PCAC members to discuss, sometimes to vent, the most personal of concerns.

In the discussions that follow, unless otherwise noted, *PCAC* will be used as a generic term to refer to community-based groups composed of the three principal players needed to improve the community living of aging adults with lifelong impairments, namely, relevant organizations and agencies, family caregivers, and the aging adults themselves. The principles outlined by Stroud and Sutton (1988) for working with groups are appropriate general guidelines for the conduct of PCAC meetings and activities. Those who initiate the councils are committed to developing the strength and independence of the others involved. The initiators refrain from assuming the roles of leader or co-leader and consciously avoid unduly influencing discussions. Suggestions are limited and offered only after others have had ample chance to contribute. The initiators may make the group aware of the steps involved in problem solving, but arriving at solutions becomes part of the self-direction of each member. The general principles help to establish a foundation of partnership among those in the PCAC, which fosters a sense of ownership among members and discourages passive dependence on the professionals. Not the least of the consequences of such partnerships is a strengthened sense of empowerment gained from working toward a greater good.

ADVOCACY, SELF-ADVOCACY, AND EMPOWERMENT

One of the PCAC's most important roles is to lead consumers and families into advocacy that results in benefits beyond themselves. Advocating for the greater good can help build connection to the larger community while strengthening the skills and personal contacts they may need for resolving their own challenges. Advocacy is a reflection of the rights and responsibilities equation in action. There are a number of exemplary programs and models that have been developed with these purposes in mind (Fawcett et al., 1994; Wolfe, Ofiesh, & Boone, 1996; Zirpoli, Hancox, Wieck, & Skarnulis, 1994).

As adults with lifelong disabilities age, they may be exercising control over their lives for the first time or they may be experiencing changes in their ability to maintain the relative independence they have achieved. In the first instance, some individuals with disabilities have only recently ceased receiving institutionalized services, which has sometimes meant paternalistic, relatively inflexible, and largely residential care—caring manifested as control. Service delivery systems have "placed persons with disabilities and their families in passive roles with few opportunities to express their needs, review alternatives, and make decisions regarding their own future" (Zirpoli, Wieck, & McBride, 1989, p. 125). Others have spoken for them. They have been viewed in terms of functional or perceived limitations rather than as individuals who, if given appropriate support, could speak and decide for themselves. This view has decreased their value in the eyes of others and has decreased their self-esteem. Some adults with lifelong disabilities have worked to achieve high levels of independence only to find these threatened by diminishing strength, decreased reserve capacity, or new impairments brought on by growing older. Extraordinary accomplishments have been attained with subsequently extraordinary costs, as in postpolio syndrome.

Advocacy, including self-advocacy, when fully realized, reinforces a larger sense of community, puts individuals in control of their own lives, and transforms service system personnel into effective facilitators. These improvements can help older adults with lifelong disabilities to initiate or regain control over their lives. Ultimately, advocacy can simplify access to services while decreasing the size and cost of the service system.

When aging adults with lifelong disabilities and their primary caregivers assume the responsibility of coordinating services, they essentially take on the role of case managers. To do so, however, requires preparation. They need to be aware of the community resources available to them. Education that helps them navigate the service system can be invaluable. The PCAC, whose membership includes representatives of community agencies, can serve as a catalyst for information about available resources, contact people, a variety of consumer-oriented training topics and where to obtain them, and so forth. The PCAC can empower families and consumers within the council and outside.

The PCAC also can increase participants' and others' knowledge about particular advocacy strategies and efforts. Individuals and families can learn to speak assertively, to ask the right questions in the right way, and to communicate more effectively with service providers. They can be encouraged to participate more fully in community activities, make informed choices, and plan for the judicious use of community services. Parental caregivers can be assisted in "letting go" and fostering independence; consumers can learn valuable problem-solving and decision-making techniques.

The PCAC can facilitate the involvement of consumers and families in the planning of coordinated community services. Pederson et al. (1993) described the role of facilitators in encouraging consumer participation on boards and committees. They also enumerated the specific attitude, knowledge, and skills-training competencies that are required for meaningful involvement. When aging adults with developmental disabilities and family caregivers become knowledgeable about how public decisions are made, they can be forthright in ensuring that their rights are respected. By learning about the related laws and legal responsibilities that are mandated, families and consumers can play a role in governance at the state and local levels. Unlike earlier efforts that tended to focus on "providing information about the content of the law rather than on how to effectively access the system in order to receive services mandated by law" (Zirpoli, Hancox, Wieck, & Skarnulis, 1989, p. 163), the PCAC can help to ensure that consumers and families apply their knowledge to make services more accessible. The Partners in Policymaking program in Minnesota (Zirpoli et al., 1994) may serve as a model for PCACs that seek to engage their members and others in the community in the broader decision-making processes.

Yet another vital role for any PCAC is that of instigator of support initiatives that enable older adults with lifelong disabilities to contribute their time and services to other adults in need of assistance. This theme, championed by the 1987 Wingspread Conference on Aging and Lifelong Disabilities (Ansello & Rose, 1989), underlies a potent dimension of consumer empowerment. That aging adults with developmental disabilities seldom transcend the categorization of "care recipient" is a misfortune that denies them the opportunity to experience the sense of worth in helping others and denies others the gifts they may need (Ansello & Roberto, 1993). Stroud and Sutton (1988) suggested using volunteer assistants to expand the opportunities for gaining access to community activities. Employing consumers who already have been integrated into the community as voluntary peer facilitators would simultaneously accomplish the goals of consumer empowerment and engagement. It has been suggested that a major challenge facing researchers in geriatrics is to conceptualize models in which older people with developmental disabilities have a valued status as contributing members of society (Dossa, 1990).

The independent living movement views the provision of services as a means of reaching the goals of involvement and engagement (Cohen, 1992). It is apparent that activating collaborations of aging adults with lifelong disabilities, family caregivers, agency staff, and others serves these goals as well. The state-level self-advocacy training program initiated as a consequence of the Partners in Policymaking project (Zirpoli et al., 1994) resulted in the development of enduring support networks and friendships. Similarly, the self-empowerment efforts of PCACs may be conceived as activities that secondarily result in greater socialization. Relatively few adults with mental retardation have social relationships with individuals who do not have intellectual disabilities (Edgerton, 1989). Structured opportunities for social engagement typically have been segregated. Stroud and Sutton (1988), however, discussed how volunteers can be instrumental in combating social isolation. By modeling appropriate social behavior, volunteers from the community can help adults with lifelong disabilities improve their conversational style and acquire needed social skills. This is a common strategy used by agencies (e.g., The Arc). Conversely, when individuals with disabilities themselves are engaged as peer volunteers, both parties can make social advances.

PROFESSIONAL/CONSUMER ADVOCACY COUNCILS IN PARTNERS III

Hoping that its history and continuity might offer suggestions for activating aging adults and caregivers, we discuss the PCAC in Virginia in some detail. The statewide

PCACs were formed in Maryland and Virginia as part of the federally funded Partners III project. Besides representation from the two state units on aging and the Developmental Disabilities Planning Councils, the PCACs are composed of older adults with lifelong disabilities, family caregivers, and community-based professionals from the aging and developmental disabilities networks.

The group has organized and defined itself over time. It first came together in 1995 as a result of an invitation from Virginia's Commissioner on Aging, who urged top-down responsibilities (i.e., to review the policy issues and obstacles to service coordination identified in Partners II; see Coogle, Ansello, Wood, & Cotter, 1995) and to serve as an advisor to the since-completed Partners III Project. Although the PCAC's focus has evolved since then, several principles of operation remain; some were present at the outset, others have revealed themselves over the years. These principles have helped the PCAC to endure and to succeed. They include 1) a committed core membership and leaders to serve as the spark; 2) a common understanding of language and territory in disabilities and aging; 3) meetings that are mutually convenient, regular, and appropriately paced; 4) a practical purpose; and 5) activities that are relevant to the membership.

Composition and Leadership

The composition of a PCAC or any collective that seeks to activate consumers and families is certainly a critical issue in the early stages, but it also should be an ongoing concern. A periodic assessment can reveal where there are gaps in participation or when additional organizations should be represented. As the activities of the group change, it is reasonable and advantageous to adjust the membership. The Virginia PCAC has, of some 2 dozen members, a core of approximately 12–15 regulars, almost half of whom are individuals with lifelong disabilities. The other half is a mix of agency staff members and gerontologists. Three or four family caregivers participate episodically. The consumers are in their 40s, 50s, and 60s; most have cerebral palsy. The agency professionals represent a range of environments from adult day care to rehabilitative services to state agency staff members. Whereas the participation of the state unit on aging has been consistent and supportive, the area agencies on aging (AAAs) have been only transiently engaged in task-specific ways. Survey data suggest that the AAAs should be encouraged to conduct needs assessments and provide support for older caregivers of adults with developmental disabilities (Janicki, McCallion, Force, Bishop, & LePore, 1998; McCallion & Janicki, 1997). For a PCAC to influence the extent to which these families are targeted by the aging network's outreach and direct services efforts, the commitment from one or two AAA representatives is essential. The PCAC can influence the development of more consumer-centered approaches and consumer-directed services (Coogle et al., 1995), but for pervasive change to occur at the local and state levels, all of the relevant parties must be collaborating.

Janicki (1993) wrote of the irreducible need for someone to be the "spark" in collaborations. To commit to what will surely be a slow, haltingly progressive group process, someone who has not only the spark of enthusiasm but also the fortitude of endurance needs to step forward. At the same time, there is risk of a group's developing a cult of personality around its leader. So, the leader must be accepting and a team builder. The Virginia PCAC has been fortunate to have had two such leaders who initially served as co-leaders, an older experienced advocate who was formerly a caregiver and an attorney in his 40s who has relatively severe cerebral palsy with dyskinesia and spastic athetosis. He has continued as the group's leader after a life-threatening illness curtailed his co-leader's involvement.

Composition can be key to continuation of the PCAC. The involvement of all partners must be actively maintained. The activities of the PCAC, therefore, need to appeal to consumers, family caregivers, and professionals in the aging and developmental disabilities service systems. In a related vein, the results of the Partners III field projects indicate that achievement of consumer-based successes contributes to the longevity of collaborative planning groups. There needs to be some tangible benefit to older adults with lifelong disabilities and their families. In our experience, securing and maintaining the involvement of consumers and family members can be challenging (Ansello, Coogle, & Wood, 1997). The field projects report that the participation of family caregivers can be limited by time constraints and that the recruitment of aging individuals with more insular disabilities and of minority members can be exceedingly difficult.

Long-term continuity of the PCAC also requires maintenance of a balanced representation from both the developmental disabilities and aging services networks. Because aging service providers are only beginning to see older adults with developmental disabilities as part of their constituency, it may be difficult at first to engage them fully in the activities of the PCAC. Conversely, disabilities service providers, having noted the aging of their consumers, tend to see the advantages of cooperative planning and coordinated service provision. Yet neither sector likely appreciates the value of "precrisis," or preventive, planning and collaboration. They may not regard initiatives designed to activate aging consumers and families as particularly applicable to professional practice. Furthermore, it may be helpful to examine who is contributing most to the bridge building between systems and why construction is under way. We have heard some aging providers maintain that integrating older adults with developmental disabilities into aging programs and services compromises their own professional interests while benefiting their counterparts in the disabilities system. To the extent that aging-related professionals perceive an inequitable exchange, they are less likely to share the enthusiasm of disabilities service providers who regard the bridge as a way to enhance the independence and actualize the potential of aging individuals (Coogle, Ansello, & Wood, 1998).

The PCAC has the potential to be a powerful means of promoting intersystem collaboration. Its informal structure can provide significant opportunities for a gradual sensitivity training that is almost subliminal as those in the aging network come to recognize the capabilities of fellow members with developmental disabilities and learn to appreciate their wholeness as individuals.

Common Understanding

The PCAC's first agenda anticipated elements that have proved to be central to the group's continuity. The first item, after introductions and socializing, was a review of past projects and recommended practices in intersystem cooperation and the recommendations that flowed from them, and a review of the terminology and language used to describe impairments and determine eligibility for services. There is a remarkable difference between the aging and the developmental disabilities systems in their bureaucracies, funding streams, operations, culture, and language (Ansello & Rose, 1989). In the United States, the National Academy for State Health Policy identified 129 federal programs for people with disabilities in 1994, having 70 different definitions of eligibility, administered by 15 separate agencies (Scully & Snow, 1995). These reviews, in the first meeting of the PCAC, helped to establish a common language for discussions that followed.

One of the first tasks suggested by the PCAC's co-leader was the writing of a brief, internal "White Paper" to summarize the known status of older Virginians with developmental disabilities. It recapped numbers, living situations, and the disposition of agencies charged with responding to the needs of citizens with lifelong impairments. The concluding paragraph states,

> The key to responding to both the historical tendency toward treatment versus prevention and the current push to block-granting may be community action. Community-based groups that band together to identify capacities and needs among fellow community members can be effective in 1) identifying real-world priorities for governmental services, 2) organizing ways of sharing existing resources, and 3) developing creative approaches to using the local community's expertise and resources. If self-reliance is to be government's ultimate philosophy, then citizens need to take action. In order to achieve greater self-reliance while aging with lifelong developmental disabilities, family caregiving needs to be strengthened, self-advocacy must be reinforced, and the maze of bureaucracies with relevant services needs to be navigated, at least, if not trained and made more user friendly. (Ansello, 1993, p. 3)

Convenient, Appropriately Paced Meetings

Scheduling PCAC meetings that are mutually convenient as to time and place seems obvious. In fact, our experience with collective groups suggests that far too often "convenience" is unconsciously determined by the professionals. This was brought home to us painfully when we received an e-mail message from a PCAC member with a lifelong disability who said that he could no longer attend our 10:00 A.M. meetings, because with advancing age, he was too tired to continue his routine of rising at 5:00 A.M. to dress and have breakfast in time to meet the schedule of the transportation van for people with disabilities. We promptly rescheduled meetings to later in the day.

The Virginia PCAC meets only on Tuesdays or Thursdays because its leader has a personal assistant on those days. The group schedules its next meetings a month or more in advance so that members can arrange special transportation, such as adapted vans, or coordinate with family caregivers. The pace of the meeting itself can be an adjustment for some participants, especially the professionals without disabilities. One entrepreneurial aging professional, whose valuable contributions included suggesting the formation of a cerebral palsy and aging focus group to identify topics for a sponsored conference, ultimately dropped out of the PCAC because his business-like temperament was incompatible with the pace of meetings. Discussions are slower paced out of necessity. Several consumers have great difficulty speaking because of their disabilities. Words must be laboriously spelled out. Time regularly is taken for an individual's personal assistant to interpret what he is saying. The professionals in the PCAC have taken varying amounts of time to adjust to the speech and behavior patterns of their fellow members with lifelong disabilities. The result now, however, is that PCAC meetings have a rhythm of their own, a slower paced, expository style that encourages everyone to listen to one another, engendering a quality of mutual assistance.

Practical Purpose

The first meeting of the PCAC set in place another key to the group's continuity: its practical purpose. These professionals, adults with lifelong disabilities, and caregivers would henceforth meet to help formulate policy, train and educate others, monitor and lobby for legislation, and so forth. Advocacy that has a practical purpose helps to attract and retain members in a PCAC. In its first meeting, the Virginia PCAC created subcommittees with applied, verifiable purposes to coalesce the different backgrounds and expectations of a diverse group of individuals with disabilities, family caregivers, agency staff members, and others. The three subcommittees were Crisis Prevention, Interagency Coordination, and Aging and Developmental Disabilities Awareness. Each subgroup defined its practical goals and set to work to achieve them incrementally, reporting back to the full PCAC at its monthly meetings.

The Crisis Prevention subcommittee considered greater access to and use of assistive technology to be a means of averting crises in the daily lives of aging adults with lifelong disabilities (Ansello & Roberto, 1993; Justesen & Menlove, 1993; Parette, 1997; Wehmeyer, 1998). It wished to replicate a highly successful "gadgets and gizmos exposition" that one of the subawardees in the Partners III Project had conducted in Northern Virginia. The subcommittee drafted a grant proposal to the state's Assistive Technology System, which encouraged a full proposal. This proposal was submitted and funded with the Virginia Geriatric Education Center as fiduciary recipient of the award because the PCAC is not a legal entity.

The Interagency Coordination subcommittee sought to broaden membership in the PCAC. One of its pursuits, never fully realized, was to engage the AAAs in the PCAC process. Their limited participation might be attributable to the essentially top-down focus of the council. AAAs operate more locally. Nonetheless, some of them are responsible for sizable geographical regions and, of course, are the front line implementers of initiatives. Janicki and colleagues (1998) suggested that the AAAs should be targeted to conduct outreach and assistance to help these caregivers; they also should be encouraged to conduct local needs assessments (McCallion & Janicki, 1997). The PCAC can facilitate these aims more readily if representatives from the AAAs participate actively in the PCAC.

The Aging and Developmental Disabilities Awareness subcommittee set itself a highly unusual goal: to work to conceptualize, lobby for, and help pass legislation in the General Assembly of Virginia to assist family caregivers of relatives with disabilities financially. Together with a statewide coalition previously organized by the state commissioner on aging to support family caregivers, the subcommittee wrote a rationale for a tax credit bill, then met with a prominent legislator to solicit his patronage. The legislative processes that followed provided many hours of on-the-job training for the subcommittee in presenting arguments, testifying, and forming broad-based coalitions to lobby for passage. Over the course of four sessions of the General Assembly, the tax credit bill was fine-tuned, picking up extensive multigenerational grass roots support and broad bipartisan co-patronage. The subcommittee saw its practical goal, a bill modified in the 1999 session to become a grant fund rather than a tax credit (thereby benefiting caregivers with little or no taxable income), passed unanimously by both houses of the General Assembly and signed by the Governor (see Essay II).

Relevance to Members

The structure of the PCAC had evolved away from subcommittees while still retaining their practical purposes. The PCAC as a whole continues to monitor legislation and welcome new members. But having more members with cerebral palsy has shifted the application of the PCAC's energies. The council created the Cerebral Palsy and Aging Focus Group as a parallel entity and spun it off from the PCAC to provide a forum for aging adults with this lifelong disability. It has since been reintegrated into the PCAC, transforming its organizational culture.

Begun because of the concerns of the PCAC's leader, who was experiencing aging-related deterioration in his presumably "static" cerebral palsy, the Cerebral Palsy and

Aging Focus Group decided to host a regional conference on the most critical issues that affect the daily lives of people with cerebral palsy. Over the course of months, this Focus Group identified five topics that present them and their peers with ongoing challenges in their daily lives:

1. Health care, especially access to and the training of health care providers knowledgeable about the triangulation of their own specialties, aging, and developmental disabilities
2. Assistive technology, including both high- and low-technology devices
3. Independent living, including cost-benefit analysis of living independently, housing systems, and letting go from family caregiving scenarios
4. Social isolation and community integration, encompassing issues from gaining access to the tangible resources in the community to contending with the absence of the intangible, such as opportunities to meet or to date others
5. Sexuality, including reproductive health matters, erroneous beliefs of health care providers regarding the sexuality of aging people with lifelong disabilities, affection needs, and sex

The PCAC hosted a highly successful conference, "Aging with Cerebral Palsy: Meeting Everyday Needs," that addressed three of the focus group's practical issues: health care, assistive technology, and sexuality. It secured co-sponsorships, selected speakers, convened, and evaluated the event.

As it plans for a second conference, it is focusing on the socialization/isolation issue (Seltzer & Seltzer, 1985), investigating the quality and quantity of opportunities for interpersonal interactions, and searching for model programs that reduce social isolation. The issue resonates with the Cerebral Palsy and Aging Focus Group, which suggested it for the conference, and it may be especially important for older, as opposed to younger, adults (Seltzer & Seltzer, 1985). Later life for adults with lifelong disability is likely a time of increased vulnerability, loss, and disruption of social networks (Bigby, 1997). Maintaining a high quality of life during the transitions that occur as individuals age is particularly challenging (Hoge & Wilhite, 1997). As the PCAC members demonstrate in their own lives, as the number of older adults with developmental disabilities increases, there is a compelling interest in finding meaningful ways to integrate aging consumers into community recreation and leisure opportunities (Boyd, 1997). Earlier studies acknowledged that opportunities for socialization should be considered when activities that are more appropriate to retirement are substituted for vocational ones (Riddick & Keller, 1990; See, Ellis, Spellman, & Cress, 1990). Methods for fostering intimacy and maintaining companionship are equally important. The importance of facilitating meaningful relationships should be revisited as advocates seek more comprehensive approaches to addressing the everyday needs of aging people with lifelong disabilities.

The PCAC serves, as mentioned, a valuable top-down role in advocacy. At the same time, the group's longevity has nurtured the slow growth of a more personal, immediate aspect. The group's history together has cultivated the acceptance that allows self-disclosure. PCAC members with lifelong disabilities share problems that they are encountering with the health care system, and they seek answers. They recount their experiences with physicians, dentists, and others who have been inadequately prepared to deal with their aging- and disabilities-related problems. Sexuality and sexual dysfunction apparently stymie even the newest medical residents, who do not see individuals with disabilities as whole people with sexual needs. Together, the members of the PCAC seem to form a mutual support group, all the while continuing their work in advocacy for their peers across the state.

Further Professional/Consumer Advocacy Council Activities

The activities undertaken by the Virginia and Maryland PCACs offer suggestions for implementation of similar collaborations elsewhere, but they do not exhaust the need. There is a particular need for advocacy efforts that target low-income consumers and families, as well as those in medically underserved and rural areas. One needs assessment of rural older adults with developmental disabilities and their relatives, caregivers, or service providers indicates that transportation, hearing services, recreation/exercise, and older friends are high-priority issues (See et al., 1990). Other PCACs may want to work for legislative changes that preserve the rights of older adults with developmental disabilities—for example, the right to age in place. Perhaps the most fundamental area of focus for aging adults with developmental disabilities and their family caregivers is permanency planning.

Persuading consumers and families to develop a strategy for transferring care in the event of the primary caregiver's death is one of the most helpful activities that could be undertaken by any PCAC. The literature suggests that more than half of aging parents who are caring for adult children with mental retardation have not made residential plans (Freedman, Krauss, & Seltzer, 1997; Kaufman, Adams, & Campbell, 1991). This finding most likely extends to the other developmental disabilities as well. An estimated one half to one third of those who care for adults with developmental disabilities prefer future out-of-home placement (as opposed to continued home care by a family member) when they are no longer able to provide care themselves (Goodman, 1978; Heller & Factor, 1991; Roberto, 1988). There is some suggestion that older parents who do not make alternative plans because they fully intend to continue caring indefinitely for their offspring with mental retardation may experience special benefits, despite the threat of an uncertain future (Tobin, 1996). It may be that perpetual parenting permits the maintenance of a persistent sense of self when confronting age-associated losses. Having said this, the unexpected happens. Friday afternoon telephone calls to human services agencies bring news of family caregivers who have died or become incapacitated while still having the responsibility for another (Wood, 1993). PCACs can directly advocate for futures planning and promote awareness among consumers and families of the value of making alternative arrangements. They also may be able to influence the development of appropriate out-of-home placement plans by encouraging changes in related factors, such as use of formal and informal assistance (Black, Cohn, Smull, & Crites, 1985; Smith, Tobin, & Fullmer, 1995) or improving the level of parental social activities (Kaufman et al., 1991). The PCAC can facilitate permanency planning.

CONCLUSIONS

We have reviewed benefits to aging adults with lifelong disabilities derived from their involvement in collaborative groups where they, family caregivers, agency staff, and other professionals interact as partners. We have maintained that such groups, which we call PCACs, put into practice the rights and responsibilities equation and can contribute substantially to the aging individual's well-being. PCACs focus their collective attention on issues that transcend the members' personal and immediate needs to benefit the greater good. PCACs thereby operationalize a top-down approach to advocacy and empowerment. This differs from the more common support group and circle of support models in which the individual with lifelong disabilities is the center and object of attention.

We believe that an effective PCAC will, over time, not only generate initiatives with broad-based impact, such as strengthening the capacities of family caregivers and improving the resources available to aging adults with lifelong disabilities, but also produce benefits within the diverse individuals who constitute the PCAC. We have detailed the history of the Virginia PCAC created during the Partners III Project (1993–1996) but continuing meaningfully today. The Virginia PCAC is a rich font of practical lessons learned for activating consumers and professionals. Experience suggests some keys to continued productivity: a balanced membership and committed leadership; a shared language or common understanding of terminology, philosophies, funding streams, and operations of the aging and developmental disabilities systems; mutually convenient and appropriately paced meetings; practical, verifiable purposes for the group; and activities that are relevant to the lives and experiences of the members.

At the same time, we have learned that a top-down orientation has the promise of enriching the individual members of the PCAC in ways that are decidedly personal. PCACs tend to develop a special appreciation of the rhythms, restrictions, aspirations, and frustrations that each must live everyday, whether an aging adult, a family caregiver, an agency staff member, or a university gerontologist. To label this "sensitivity training" is too objectified a description; rather, the group process seems slowly to uncover the human within each participant.

REFERENCES

Ansello, E.F. (1993). *Aging with lifelong impairments: A background.* Unpublished paper, Virginia Commonwealth University, Virginia Center on Aging, Richmond.

Ansello, E.F., Coogle, C.L., & Wood, J.B. (1997). *Partners: Building intersystem cooperation in aging with developmental disabilities.* Richmond: Virginia Commonwealth University, Virginia Center on Aging.

Ansello, E.F., & Roberto, K.A. (1993). Empowering elderly caregivers: Practice, research, and policy directives. In K.A. Roberto (Ed.), *The elderly caregiver: Caring for adults with developmental disabilities* (Sage Focus Editions No. 160, pp. 173–189). Thousand Oaks, CA: Sage Publications.

Ansello, E.F., & Rose, T. (1989). *Aging and lifelong disabilities: Partnership for the twenty-first century.* Palm Springs, CA: Elvirita Lewis Foundation.

Bigby, C. (1997). Later life for adults with intellectual disability: A time of opportunity and vulnerability. *Journal of Intellectual and Developmental Disability, 22,* 97–108.

Black, M.M., Cohn, J.F., Smull, M.W., & Crites, L.S. (1985). Individual and family factors associated with risk of institutionalization of mentally retarded adults. *American Journal of Mental Deficiency, 90,* 271–276.

Boyd, R. (1997). Older adults with developmental disabilities: A brief examination of current knowledge. *Activities, Adaptation, and Aging, 21*(3), 7–27.

Browning, P., Rhoades, C., & Crosson, A. (1980). *Advancing your citizenship: Essays on consumer involvement of the handicapped.* Eugene, OR: Rehabilitation Research and Training Center in Mental Retardation.

Cohen, E.S. (1992). What is independence? *Generations, 16*(1), 49–52.

Coogle, C.L., Ansello, E.F., & Wood, J.B. (1998). Partners III: Bridge-building between the aging and developmental disabilities service networks: An integrated model of collaborative planning and service. *Southwest Journal on Aging, 14*(2), 69–78.

Coogle, C.L., Ansello, E.F., Wood, J.B., & Cotter, J.J. (1995). Partners II—Serving older persons with developmental disabilities: Obstacles and inducements to collaboration among agencies. *Journal of Applied Gerontology, 14,* 275–287.

Developmental Disabilities Assistance and Bill of Rights Act of 1975, PL 94-103, 42 U.S.C. §§ 6000 *et seq.*

Dossa, P.A. (1990). Toward social system theory: Implication for older people with developmental disabilities and service delivery. *International Journal of Aging and Human Development, 30,* 303–319.

Edgerton, R.B. (1989). Retarded people of adult years. *Psychiatric Annals, 19,* 205–209.

Fawcett, S.R., White, G.W., Balcazar, F.E., Suarez-Balcazar, Y., Mathews, R.M., Paine-Andrews, A., Seekins, T., & Smith, J.F. (1994). A contextual-behavioral model of empowerment: Case studies involving people with physical disabilities. *American Journal of Community Psychology, 22,* 471–496.

Freedman, R.I., Krauss, M.W., & Seltzer, M.M. (1997). Aging parents' residential plans for adult children with mental retardation. *Mental Retardation, 35,* 114–123.

Goodman, D.M. (1978). Parenting an adult mentally retarded offspring. *Smith College Studies in Social Work, 94,* 259–271.

Heller, T., & Factor, A. (1991). Permanency planning for adults with mental retardation living with family caregivers. *American Journal on Mental Retardation, 96,* 163–176.

Hoge, G., & Wilhite, B. (1997). Integration and leisure education for older adults with developmental disabilities. *Activities, Adaptation, and Aging, 21*(3), 79–90.

Janicki, M., McCallion, P., Force, L., Bishop, K., & LePore, P. (1998). Area agency on aging outreach and assistance for households with older carers of an adult with a developmental disability. *Journal of Aging and Social Policy, 10,* 13–36.

Janicki, M.P. (1993). *Building the future: Planning and community development in aging and developmental disabilities* (2nd ed.). Albany: New York State Office of Mental Retardation and Developmental Disabilities.

Justesen, T.R., & Menlove, M. (1993). Assistive technology education in rehabilitation counselor programs. *Rehabilitation Education, 7,* 253–260.

Kaufman, A.V., Adams, J.P., & Campbell, V.A. (1991). Permanency planning by older parents who care for adult children with mental retardation. *Mental Retardation, 29,* 293–300.

McCallion, P., & Janicki, M. (1997). Area agencies on aging: Meeting the needs of persons with developmental disabilities and their aging families. *Journal of Applied Gerontology, 16,* 270–284.

Moody, H.R. (1992). *Ethics in an aging society.* Baltimore: The Johns Hopkins University Press.

Ohle, C. (1999). *Medical experiences of families with adults with Down syndrome.* Unpublished master's thesis, Virginia Commonwealth University, Richmond.

Parette, H.P. (1997). Assistive technology devices and services. *Education and Training in Mental Retardation and Developmental Disabilities, 32,* 267–280.

Pederson, E.L., Chaikin, M., Koehler, D., Campbell, A., & Arcand, M. (1993). Strategies that close the gap between research, planning, and self-advocacy. In E. Sutton, A.R. Factor, B.A. Hawkins, T. Heller, & G.B. Seltzer (Eds.), *Older adults with developmental disabilities: Optimizing choice and change* (pp. 277–325). Baltimore: Paul H. Brookes Publishing Co.

Riddick, C.C., & Keller, M.J. (1990). Developing recreation services to assist elders who are developmentally disabled. *Activities, Adaptation and Aging, 15*(1–2), 19–34.

Roberto, K.A. (1988, December). *Caring for aging developmentally disabled adults: Perspectives and needs of older parents.* Final report presented to the Colorado Developmental Disabilities Planning Council, Greeley, CO.

Scully, D., & Snow, K.I. (1995). *Coordinating services with and for persons with disabilities: A challenge for state government.* Portland, ME: National Academy for State Health Policy.

See, C.J., Ellis, D.N., Spellman, C.R., & Cress, P.J. (1990). Using needs assessment to develop programs for elderly developmentally disabled persons in a rural setting. *Activities, Adaptation and Aging, 15*(1–2), 53–66.

Seltzer, M.M., & Seltzer, G.B. (1985). The elderly mentally retarded: A group in need of service. *Journal of Gerontological Social Work, 8,* 99–119.

Smith, G.C., Tobin, S.S., & Fullmer, E.M. (1995). Elderly mothers caring at home for offspring with mental retardation: A model of permanency planning. *American Journal on Mental Retardation, 99,* 487–499.

Stroud, M., & Sutton, E. (1988). *Expanding options for older adults with developmental disabilities: A practical guide to achieving community access.* Baltimore: Paul H. Brookes Publishing Co.

Tobin, S.S. (1996). Non-normative old age contrast: Elderly parents caring for offspring with mental retardation. In V.L. Bengtson (Ed.), *Adulthood and aging: Research on continuities and discontinuities* (pp. 124–145). New York: Springer Publishing Co.

Valentine, M.B., & Capponi, P. (1989, June). Mental health consumer participation on boards and committees: Barriers and strategies. *Canada's Mental Health*, 8–12.

Wehmeyer, M.L. (1998). National survey of the use of assistive technology by adults with mental retardation. *Mental Retardation, 36*, 44–51.

Wolfe, P.S., Ofiesh, N.S., & Boone, R.B. (1996). Self-advocacy preparation of consumers with disabilities: A national perspective of ADA training efforts. *Journal of The Association for Persons with Severe Handicaps, 21*, 81–87.

Wood, J.B. (1993). Planning for the transfer of care: Social and psychological issues. Older caregivers of family members with developmental disabilities: Changes in roles and perceptions. In K.A. Roberto (Ed.), *The elderly caregiver: Caring for adults with developmental disabilities* (Sage Focus Editions No. 160, pp. 95–107). Thousand Oaks, CA: Sage Publications.

Zirpoli, T.J., Hancox, D.H., Wieck, C., & Skarnulis, E. (1989). Partners in policymaking: Empowering people. *Journal of The Association for Persons with Severe Handicaps, 14*, 163–167.

Zirpoli, T.J., Hancox, D.H., Wieck, C., & Skarnulis, E. (1994). Partners in policymaking: The first five years. *Mental Retardation, 32*, 422–425.

Zirpoli, T.J., Wieck, C., & McBride, M. (1989). Case management: A new challenge for families. In M.H. Linz, P. McAnally, & C. Wieck (Eds.), *Case management: Historical, current, and future perspectives* (pp. 125–136). Cambridge, MA: Brookline Books.

10

Community Membership

Phyllis Kultgen, Jane E. Harlan-Simmons, and Jennie Todd

As we move into the 21st century, the "community supports paradigm" (Bradley & Knoll, 1990) continues to challenge the "services in segregated settings" approach to planning for people with developmental disabilities. The community-building strategy presented in this chapter reflects the community supports paradigm and, consistent with that ideal, makes use of person-centered techniques. Just as practitioners of community building who use person-centered methods cannot precisely delineate and routinize those methods, neither can those who work to support community membership. Just as person-centered methods originated at the edges of the system in a fuzzy outline (O'Brien, O'Brien, & Mount, 1997), so did efforts to build community membership. Consequently, the processes and steps for developing community membership, described in this chapter, form an approach that is unbound and flexible.

Early supporters of the community supports paradigm defined *community membership* as the intentional creation of relationships and social structures that extend the possibilities for shared identity and common action among people (O'Brien & O'Brien, 1996). The facilitators of the approach are described as "community builders." Briefly described, community builders take the time needed to discover the unique gifts, interests, and preferences of an individual before they introduce him or her to places within the community where he or she can realize identified interests. Community builders then seek natural supports for the focus person in the environments that she or he has chosen.

Portions of this chapter were originally developed for a paper presented at the 1997 annual meeting of the American Association on Mental Retardation in New York City.

The community-building process uses a person-centered approach. This process matches the focus person's expressed desires for community involvement with his or her preferences for activities within the community (Butterworth, Steere, & Whitney-Thomas, 1997). The strength of this strategy is that it can be applied across a span of age groups (Amado, Conklin, & Wells, 1990; Pearpoint, O'Brien, & Forest, 1993). In this chapter, we apply this approach to older adults and relate how the use of community builders can be used to accomplish community membership for older adults with developmental disabilities as they reach their retirement years. Thus, four general areas are covered in the chapter: 1) community membership as a lifestyle for older adults, 2) community builders as the means to recast historical staff–client relationships, 3) connecting older adults to the community and to community members, and 4) commentary on required resources and barriers to and successes of the community-building approach. The applications of the approach of community bridge building, as exemplified by a variety of strategies and techniques used by community builders, are presented in Sections II–IV. We use our experiences at the Indiana University's Center for Aging Persons with Developmental Disabilities (CAPDD)[1] to provide a framework for the applications of the model, particularly as it is applied to means of creating relationships. Qualitative aspects of a successful community builder are offered in the last section.

COMMUNITY MEMBERSHIP AS A LATE-LIFE LIFESTYLE

Community membership and participation may be considered a late-life lifestyle for all mature adults. How does community membership as a lifestyle for older adults in the general population differ from the lifestyle that many older adults with developmental disabilities experience? As the latter begin to tire of employment, work activities, or other structured activity programs, they may find themselves in "retirement programs" that mimic the activities of a senior services or center site prevalent in the general population. Often, this type of day program is maintained at the same site as a previously attended sheltered work/prevocational environment so that individuals "travel on their preretirement schedules to their former places of employment" (Sutton, Sterns, & Roberts, 1992, p. 64).

Retirement—or even part-time retirement—can be a dreaded transition for an employed individual with a lifelong disability (Cotten & Laughlin, 1989) when that person has little understanding of what retirement means. For example, when several older adults with a developmental disability, who serve as advisors to the CAPDD's What is Retirement? Project, were asked to describe retirement, their responses reflected a common theme. "Retirement is when you do nothing and sit around waiting to die." Although some of the adults were unemployed because there was a lack of appropriate employment in the area in which they lived, employment rather than structured group activities was the preference of all but one individual.

How did this erroneous conception of retirement arise? As the issue of retirement is addressed in Chapter 11, only a brief speculative answer to this question is proposed here. Most of us unknowingly prepare for retirement in one way or another all of our lives. We develop hobbies and activities during our life span that may, in turn, be pur-

[1]The Indiana University's CAPDD staff project was supported by Grant No. OHD 90 DD291-02 from the U.S. Administration on Developmental Disabilities. This project ran for approximately 2 years and helped 14 older adults who were living both in group living environments and with their families experience new activities and explore their wants and desires. These experiences form the basis for the work of this chapter.

sued with greater intensity when we retire. Many adults save for retirement, and those who do not save have at least a minimal Social Security income that may allow them to partake of some favored retirement activities. In many instances, older adults with developmental disabilities who have not had typical family lives and who have lived in specialized housing programs with other similar adults seldom have had the experience of planning for retirement or enjoying avocational interests. Many have spent so much time "practicing" how to work and/or developing values around work that possible avocational-oriented hobbies and interests that lie beyond the workplace may be underdeveloped and untapped. This broad generalization points out the need for many older adults with disabilities to play "catch up" in the development of interests that could be pursued in their older age. A community membership approach, along with dedicated community builders, can be used to help older adults in such situations experience the game of catch up. Put another way, the community building strategy provides preparation for retirement and participation in a life resembling a more typical active retirement found among age-peers in the general society.

COMMUNITY BUILDERS AS A MEANS TO RECAST THE HISTORIC STAFF–CLIENT RELATIONSHIP

How does a community builder introduce an older individual to a variety of roles and activities within the community, facilitate choices among those activities, and then help the individual to enrich his or her social relationships? A partial answer is found within the philosophy behind community building. The assumptions and beliefs that underlie the philosophy are introduced next, then the philosophical principles of the approach follow.

Assumptions and Beliefs

Although community membership is a fluid, unfinished process, the beliefs and assumptions behind community membership for older adults with a developmental disability are somewhat fixed. Next, three of those assumptions or beliefs are formulated and illustrated by case example.

Assumption 1: Years of repression do not destroy talents and abilities. The older adult (even after long periods of experiential deprivation as a result of institutionalization in private or public facilities, nursing homes, or other sheltered environments) will usually be able to tap abilities and talents long repressed. Harry's story underscores the point.

> *Harry has been frequently reminded of the limitations with which he has been labeled throughout his 50 years and sometimes says, "I was born with Down syndrome, so I can't do that." However, he will readily admit that he is proud of his spotless apartment, decorated with university sports insignia, and is excited that he rides his new mountain bike to and from work during milder weather.*

Assumption 2: Issues of double jeopardy are recognized. Older adults with disabilities may face the double stigma of "handicappism" and "ageism" (Janicki, 1997). "Perhaps nowhere else is the issue of heightened jeopardy more appropriate than when discussing today's elders who happen also to be mentally retarded" (MacDonald & Tyson, 1988, p. 256). Although the contributors to this chapter are optimists and are not overly concerned with the possibility of double jeopardy, exposing individuals to stigma is avoided whenever possible.

*When a minister was asked about opportunities for volunteer work for an older
individual at his church, he responded, "After all, we all love children, no matter
what. But an older adult with disabilities—isn't there a better place for him?"
No further contact on behalf of an older adult was made to either the minister or
his congregation.*

Assumption 3: No one is too old for community membership. Declining physical
and mental vigor is another issue that may separate the practice of community membership for older adults from community participation by younger individuals. Adults
experience changes in eyesight and hearing, in the musculoskeletal system, in the cardiovascular system, and in the central nervous system as they age.

> A reduction in the speed with which older people can react and move has substantial sig-
> nificance for all aspects of their life. It takes longer to complete physical tasks, which means
> that fewer tasks can be accomplished in a day. . . . [Thus the] societal pressure to hurry can
> be socially intimidating to older people, discouraging them from active involvement in
> community activities. (Spirduso, 1995, p. 186).

If the previous assumption holds true for older adults in general, then there is little reason to doubt that those aging individuals with disabilities will be aware, at some level,
of reduction in reaction time and experience societal pressures to hurry.

> *John takes his time in everything he does. He walks at a slow pace, takes his time
> to make up his mind, and, in short, would be a challenge to a community builder
> or anyone without a lot of patience. John continually responds to challenges with
> the comment, "Too old," or, "Gettin' old."*

However, the rates of physical and cognitive changes and the consequent reductions in reaction time vary so much among older adults that it is important to look at
each person as an individual, letting each one set his or her own pace. A fundamental
belief is that all older adults with disabilities can benefit from community participation
and membership and that no one should be denied the opportunity because of age.

Philosophy of Community Building

Community building is about making people fade into the ordinary life of work, living,
and playing. First, it is important to guide a person toward situations in which he or she
will be seen as competent and as someone who has something to offer (rather than as a
recipient of services) and in which he or she will be treated as an ordinary person, without labels and stereotyped preconceptions. Consequently, a staff member who is accustomed to performing the role of teacher and behavior manager must relinquish his or
her position of authority and be on equal terms with the focus person. "Distinctions
between staff and clients and family members and ordinary citizens dissolve as the
familiar patterns of interaction that maintain them shift, and people discover new possibilities for shared action" (O'Brien & O'Brien, 1996, p. 80). The traditional staff–client
relationship is based in part on control. This new interaction is built on collaboration
(Lovett, 1996). Ducharme and Beeman (1991) described it as "walking with" a person—
that is, a partnership. We accept where the person is; go at his or her pace; and maintain a stance of commitment, presence, and responsiveness.

> *For years, Margie struggled unsuccessfully to counteract the weight problem and
> associated health problems that her doctor believed could consign her to a nursing*

home. She stopped going to Weight Watchers group meetings and was refused ongoing nutritional counseling by dietitians, who judged her to be uncooperative in her dietary habits. The community builder attempted to support her by facilitating exercise opportunities and providing access to recipe ideas and advice from fellow diabetics. No substantial weight loss occurred, and she continued to eat high-fat foods, such as bacon cheeseburgers. The community builder decided, nevertheless, that "walking with" Margie meant accepting her, weaknesses and all, while at the same time continuing to remind Margie of the consequences of her actions and supporting her to adopt a more healthful lifestyle.

Another principle of the philosophy is that the community builder should be as invisible as possible in the assistance that he or she provides. Obtrusive support can discourage assistance and involvement from ordinary citizens. Harry's experience is instructive here.

Exploring a local fitness center, Harry's community builder decided not to answer all of Harry's questions about how to use the weight-lifting equipment. As a result, Harry successfully solicited help from others who were exercising near him.

"Getting-to-Know-You" Process

Before community support can become a reality, the community builder must get to know the person so that, together, they can create a vision for a desired life in the community. No one, however, can get to know a person by means of a narrowly defined reputation, including a thick file of "information" about diagnoses, identified areas of deficits, strategies to reach habilitation goals, incidents of behavior difficulties, and so forth. To discover the person behind a label requires spending a considerable amount of time, one to one, in a large variety of contexts outside of a service agency.

The process is not one of merely checking what a person says they want and then hunting for it in the community. It often seems to be a process of accompanying, encouraging and directly assisting the person to discover interests and possibilities by trying things with someone who gives them . . . a sense of safety and confidence." (O'Brien & O'Brien, 1996, p. 105)

John, at the age of 60, has spent years in a confined environment. Leaving the nursing home in which he lived and just taking a ride in a car seemed to be all that he, at first, desired. Continued frequent contact with John revealed a love of "Big Band" music and the desire to make music. Listening to a volunteer band of older men with his community builder, John revealed that he had once played the bongo drums. Introductions to the band members and leader, facilitated by the community builder, has provided John with the opportunity to sit in with the group on several occasions.

John's story represents some of the pitfalls and bumps that occur along the road toward community membership. After using four different community builders over a period of 3 years, members of the community-building project are still figuring out and making best guesses as to his interests. In addition, there are still no natural supports or any new unpaid people in his life. This example is given here to remind the reader that building community can be exhausting and, at times, discouraging work in spite of its long-term rewards.

Looking for Clues to the Person's Interests and Wants

What are some of the contexts outside an agency in which a community builder can interact with and listen for clues as to possible interests and dreams of the person being served? Places that help us get to know a person are those that allow spontaneous social interaction, those that offer opportunities for nonverbal participation, and those associated with the individual's past. When they are explored without preconceptions, unexpectedly helpful information emerges. Social encounters happen in parks, which are frequented by dog walkers, pets, and children. Clerks and wait staff in small, friendly, not-too-busy establishments are more inclined to interact. Visits to a shopping mall may turn up someone whom the focus person has known previously.

> *When Bernie, who lives in a nursing home, walked through the mall, his enthusiastic attempts to interact with babies in strollers provided a clue to previously unarticulated interests. With the discovery of this interest, Bernie now works as a volunteer in the local YMCA child care center.*

Nonverbal activities may provide clues in getting to know people who communicate conversationally, as well as people who do not. Visiting tactile or interactive exhibits at museums, petting animals, going to a greenhouse, getting one's hair done, trying weight-lifting equipment, and listening to music with headphones at stores and libraries are examples of varied excursions that can be undertaken with little need for spoken communication.

For older adults, locations that are connected to memories are particularly helpful. These locations may help the community builder become acquainted with forgotten skills or aspects of the older adults' lives that were particularly enjoyable.

> *When Margie visited the county historical museum, she shared a childhood reminiscence of being allowed to whittle wood in her father's workshop. Picking up on this clue, her community builder decided to acquaint her with woodworking classes offered by the local arts center.*

Even rides in a car can reveal untapped capacities.

> *When Bernie pointed at all of the construction sites he passed as he drove around town with his community builder, the community builder knew that it would make sense to investigate related activities in which Bernie could get involved. Bernie has since, in the days he does not spend at the child care center, taken up woodworking with a fellow woodworker from the community and has also become a volunteer with Habitat for Humanity.*

In the initial period of community building (the getting-to-know-you stage), it is helpful to allow for spontaneity. Although the community builder makes plans around specific experiences that he or she wishes to introduce, the focus individual should be allowed to take the lead whenever possible. Spontaneity coupled with serendipity is a powerful combination.

> *A trip to a baseball game with Harry was expected to confirm Harry's apparent preference for sports, but it also revealed an unexpected talent for dancing, which*

was demonstrated in the bleachers as a show of team support. Harry has since par-
ticipated in jazzercise activities at the YMCA.

Developing a Vision

During the getting-to-know-you phase, the community builder learns firsthand about
the person's strengths and preferences by spending time in a multitude of community
contexts. Some time also should be spent talking with family members or others who
have known the person in the past. It is particularly important to find out about periods when things went well. Having kept a journal or log is useful, as is having recorded
an ongoing list of "things that work" and "things that don't work."

> *For Nina, things that work included opportunities for conversation, singing along*
> *with hymns, humor, walking on an outdoor track, ice cream, and listening to bird*
> *calls. Things that don't work included having to be quiet when others are talking,*
> *bingo, unfamiliar environments, and new situations.*

With the information gathered during the first phase, one can begin to organize
and define the vision. One useful resource is an adaptation of a capacity inventory, a
tool developed by Mount (1995). Unlike traditional client files, this descriptive inventory focuses on positive attributes that can form the basis of new relationships and valued community roles. A capacity inventory takes into account likes and dislikes,
strengths to play up, social identities that are important to the individual, preferred
environments, skills and interests, and dreams for the future. These elements are then
distilled into a few brief statements that describe the capacities of the focus person.

> *A capacity inventory completed for Harry identified his love of social interaction*
> *and performing, his musical and dance skills, his fondness of sports and the local*
> *university campus, and the importance of his religious beliefs and independence.*

Of course, there are many other effective ways to formulate a vision, including the
various person-centered planning processes that bring together a group that is dedicated to identifying what the person wants and how to get it (e.g., see Mount &
Zwernik, 1988; Pearpoint et al., 1993). It is important to realize that a person's capacities or gifts need not be extraordinary talents. Snow defined a gift as "anything you
have or do which allows for a meaningful interaction with at least one other person"
(1995, unpaginated). Therefore, she said, difference itself is something that can be
offered to others: "Walking is a gift and not walking is also a gift; knowing how to dress
is a gift and not knowing how to dress is a gift" (Snow, 1992, p. 110). Often, the best
clues to what we do well are things we enjoy or appreciate the most. Personal experience, both good and bad, can also form the basis of gifts.

> *Tim, a man who was unhappy living in a group home and now enjoys living in a*
> *rented apartment, helped a woman who wanted to leave a nursing home make*
> *informed decisions about her future living arrangements.*

Once free of traditional roles, adults who are touched by community membership
activities often portray themselves by role descriptors such as carpenter, artist, potter,
student, dancer, apartment renter, "Y" member, and volunteer or by successes they
have experienced, such as having been able to host a party, present a handmade gift,

bestow a surprise bouquet of flowers, make a speech, send Christmas cards with personal news, advocate for others, or deliver meals. Making a contribution of aspects of ourselves is deeply satisfying to many of us, yet it is likely that older people with life-long disabilities have had few chances to be on the giving end. They have been seen as needing "help," as perhaps unable to give at all. When we have gotten to know individuals and had opportunities to discover their hidden talents and interests and when we begin to glimpse their aspirations, we are ready for the next stage of the community membership process—building connections to particular groups and locations and facilitating possibilities for genuinely reciprocal relationships.

CONNECTING OLDER ADULTS TO THE COMMUNITY AND TO COMMUNITY MEMBERS

Getting connected is the next logical step toward community membership. Here we explore the community for actual sites and activities in which the focus person will contribute and enjoy meaningful participation. Through this community exploration, the community builder comes in contact with a diverse group of people, environments, and activities and discovers ways in which an individual can "be positioned" in valued roles and contribute to community life. Some hints for locating activity sites of interest to the participant have been given in the preceding section. A long-time community resident who also works as a community builder may have no difficulty in finding sites where interests can be pursued, but someone new to the job and new to the community may need suggestions as to how to locate sites that match participant interests.

Possible Community Sites

Places for community connection are boundless. They are in neighborhoods, clubs, organizations, churches, business groups, and civic organizations. They are everywhere, and often they are very ordinary places. Most communities have a resource guide that maps out all associations, clubs, organizations, and networks (e.g., in Bloomington, Indiana, the county library has a resource guide that is available to the public). All communities have libraries, churches, and parks, all of which are excellent resources. Libraries also offer meeting rooms to outside groups. The librarian can provide a list of organizations and meetings. Churches also offer a variety of activities, such as Bible groups, men's groups, women's groups, youth groups, choirs, nurseries, sports leagues, and potlucks (dinners to which each participant brings a food dish). Parks provide a variety of league activities, nature walks, bicycling, and meeting places.

The Internet is another resource that offers local community calendars (e.g., the state of Indiana hosts the HoosierNet, which provides an array of activities spanning a 2-month period). It also provides a listing of volunteer opportunities. City or neighborhood newspapers are a source of current events and local happenings. Almost all newspapers publish community calendars, announcements, and news about local groups and organizations. These papers will also report upcoming community affairs, club meetings, sporting events, and civic function rallies as well as advertise volunteer positions.

Community guides or bridge builders are important allies in creating opportunities for "community space" and discovering places of hospitality. Community guides are the community leaders, the business owners, the politicians, the "locals," and the active community members. Guides can help with introductions and making the right connections. Many times, all a community builder has to do is ask.

Behavior need not be an impediment to community connection. When introducing the idea of community building for mature adults, the issue of "difficult behavior" may arise. A way to move forward and take the focus off this issue is to ask, "Where would this behavior be less likely to occur, and where, if this behavior occurs, will it be most likely to be accepted?" For instance, if you, as a community builder, are supporting someone who has a great deal of energy, likes to keep moving, and speaks with a loud voice, then a library or painting class might not be a good match. However, an aerobics class, an auction barn, certain sporting events, a dance club, and/or landscape work would be a good match.

It also is critical that the right questions be asked about the behavior in question (Carie, 1995). For example, one could ask, "How do we get George ready for community?" Alternatively, one could also ask, "What supports can we give George to enable him to participate in community?" Instead of asking, "How do we 'protect' the community from Nina?" we should ask, "What places will be most effective in helping Nina to maximize his gifts and talents?" And, instead of asking, "How can we keep Bernie from being disruptive?" we should ask, "What activities would keep Bernie interested all morning?"

Strengthening Relationships with Longtime Community Members

The final stage of building or cultivating relationships on behalf of another person can be compared to cultivating a garden. One plants the seed, nurtures, watches, and waits patiently in hopes of a fruitful bounty. In cultivating connections on behalf of another person, using a tool such as a relationship map (Harlan, Todd, & Holtz, 1998) is helpful. This map incorporates the concept of Snow's (1994) circle of support/friends and work from Mount and Zwernik (1988). One may think of the map as a complex of six relationship clusters: intimate friends and relatives, good friends, circles of participation (people affiliated with places in the community where the focus person is engaged as a participant or volunteer), paid support persons, distant but valued friends, and change agents (people who have supported a major positive transition in the individual's life). The focus person's name appears in the center of the clusters. As the map is filled in, ideas for strengthening present relationships and nurturing new ones are generated. The map also suggests avenues that the focus person can take to reciprocate, and it gives a sense of direction for next steps. The following story illustrates the dynamics of some of the relationship clusters.

> Tina and Tim were co-workers and over the course of a year became very good friends. Tim shared with Tina the frustration and sadness he was experiencing in his living situation, a group home, and that he wanted help to make a change. He wanted to live in his own apartment. Tina encouraged Tim to pursue his dream, and he began sharing his story with other co-workers, unknowingly soliciting their help. Tim, Tina, and several others formed the beginning of a circle of support, which 3 years later still functions but in a different capacity. Shortly after the inception of the circle, Tina accepted another job; however, her relationship with Tim and her commitment to see him in his own apartment did not wane. Tina was a change agent as well as an intimate friend.

The degree to which friendship and social supports develop will depend on a combination of attentive listening, thoughtful strategy, persistent support, and simply good luck. Thus, one never stops hoping for a fruitful bounty from the seeds of friendship planted and nourished.

CONSTRUCTING AND SUPPORTING A COMMUNITY-BUILDING APPROACH

A major purpose of this chapter is to stimulate interest in the community-building strategy by describing benefits to older adults with developmental disabilities who are involved in their community. A description of the implementation of the approach and the resources needed is an additional aim. A discussion of barriers encountered and successes achieved completes our objectives.

Needed Resources

Because the flexible approach depicted in the two preceding sections was made possible through a demonstration grant, costs of implementation for a community agency can only be estimated. In what follows, we offer our best guess of the numbers of hours needed to train community builders as well as the work time commitment needed to connect an individual to the community. A brief discussion of funding sources that can be used by community agencies to make community connections possible is also included.

Hours of Training Needed   The CAPDD staff has recently implemented the community membership approach at the community agency level by offering intensive technical assistance to selected provider agencies in Indiana. Preliminary results from this effort suggest that the task of training direct care professionals is facilitated by a number of factors. First, potential community builders are usually those who have attended a number of training events on the philosophy of community membership. As a supplement to training, the potential community builder may talk to and observe other professionals who are experienced community builders. Project staff members who are acting as community builders need to travel both of these paths. Not surprising, experience has shown that the most effective community builders are those who are deeply committed to the full inclusion of people with a disability.

Reviewing the characteristics of successful community builders reveals that those characteristics needed to be successful in the task of building community connections are also the factors that allow quick absorption of training techniques. As the brief case examples presented in the second section suggest, community builders are risk takers, creative and flexible, and capacity focused (able to see limitless opportunities for participation). In addition, they are able to look at apparent failures as learning experiences and move on. Successful community builders are good listeners, have the ability to recognize and appreciate small successes, and are comfortable with people from all walks of life. Several hours per week over a period of 4–6 weeks may be all the initial training time needed for people who possess the personal qualities discussed previously. The real learning takes place while playing the role rather than during the period devoted to learning about the role.

Work Time Commitment   How much time is needed to connect an individual to the community? The answer to this question is difficult for reasons best illustrated by the variety of personalities that seek community membership, for example:

> *Tim is an outgoing and extremely gregarious man who can make friends easily. His gifts also include an ability to play the card game euchre "with the best of them," to express himself artistically, and to take chances. After his community*

builder became thoroughly acquainted with Tim, community connections were relatively easy to facilitate for him. He now takes public transportation to the Older Americans Center, where he is a welcome member of the euchre group. Tim lives in a rented apartment by himself where he relaxes, entertains friends, and is the host to meetings of his circle of support. He has traveled far—from working in a sheltered workshop and living in a group home with few friends to a 20-hours-per-week job he has held for 3 years and to his own apartment with many friends—in a relatively short time (2–3 years). However, the few hours per week needed to support Tim are counterbalanced by the many hours spent with John. The latter still has not found his niche in the community.

Fourteen individuals participated in our community membership demonstration project over a period of 2 years. All were in the community exploring options for varying lengths of time. Three of the individuals dropped out of the project: One individual moved; another became too frail, in the opinion of his guardian and residential provider, to continue; and a third—living at home—decided that he preferred the security of his "familiar environment." Six of the remaining individuals are fully or somewhat connected to their community, four still need some limited project support, and one has yet to find any substantial source of community support. Limited support means 1–2 hours per week. For the participant still seeking community membership, 2–3 hours per week, at the minimum, are required.

On average, we estimate that we contributed approximately 10 hours per week per person for the individuals who participated in the demonstration. Initially, approximately 4 of those hours were spent on the telephone seeking out activity sites that matched the participants' expressed interest, transportation opportunities, and the recruitment of community members for social support. Five to six hours per week were spent with the participant in the community. Time expenditure ebbs and flows with a lot of up-front time at the beginning of the focus person's participation in the community and less time spent as she or he "gets connected."

Perhaps measuring the cost-effectiveness of the approach only as to work time expended is impossible. One should withhold judgment about cost-effectiveness until the successes are weighed against the limitations of the approach. Judgments of families and people with disabilities about the quality of their lives before and after life in the community should be a measure of success in weighing effectiveness.

Funding Sources   Funding sources for supports to people with developmental disabilities vary widely across the United States. Consider a flexible use of categorical dollars or a creative use of discretionary funds in instances in which designated funding streams for community supports are lacking. For example, if a human services or provider agency is committed to community building "from the top down," then that agency will find ways to arrange one-to-one community connections for its service provider. One way to accomplish this for individuals who live with their families is to use monies set aside for respite (Stumpner, 1998). For those interested in community connections, time spent in the community with a respite worker may be more satisfying than time spent at home with a respite worker. Federal resources, such as Medicaid waiver dollars, are another source. Community building for individuals who live in congregate environments may be accomplished through community-focused individual habilitation plan goals.

The long-term solution to lack of funding for community-building efforts lies in policy changes at the system level that encourage person-directed funding. Conversion from program-directed services to person-directed services at the provider-agency level is also needed. Demonstration of successful efforts to connect individuals with developmental disabilities to their communities could be one way to stimulate change at both the policy and provider-agency levels.

Barriers to and Successes of the Community-Building Approach

Barriers that may impede provision of community membership for older people with developmental disabilities may include 1) the extensive staff time needed to find natural supports for individuals who have no families, 2) the inability of some residence programs to invest resources for community participation for individuals with developmental disabilities who live in their facilities, 3) the resistance to change expressed by guardians of some of the participants, and 4) lack of transportation to community participation sites and congregate residences that may not be centrally located. Solutions to potential transportation problems include soliciting rides through bulletin boards and newspaper ads, using public transportation, and requests to friends.

Factors that affect successes include 1) the introduction of individuals with little previous experience of community to an often rich and varied community life, 2) the acquisition of natural supports by some of the participants, and 3) functional advances coinciding with community experiences among most of the participants. Success is not limited to individuals who are considered to be "high functioning." For example, we observed that Bernie, who had been labeled by some as "less functional," dramatically improved his verbal skills as well as gained woodworking and child care skills.

Acquiring new identities, new interests, new friends, and new places to live; being seen as competent; and being valued by family all are outcomes that can be experienced by participants in a community membership effort. For example, Tim's family doubted that he could live outside a group living site and now proudly visits him in his own apartment. Judy's experiences with life in the community prompted her to request a move from a nursing home to a community residence. Bernie's delight with the gain of a male friend from the community produces broad smiles as he describes their "good times" together. Successes both large and small are worthy of celebration. Having people in the community know another person by name rather than by label and save a new friend a seat at the senior center card table are joyous marks of the journey.

In summary, community involvement means that older adults with developmental disabilities, for the first time in their lives, can have a range of new experiences and participate in such activities as volunteer grandparenting, studying and playing musical instruments, working as volunteers in the community food kitchen, making and selling woodcraft items, playing card games, participating in reading literacy classes, taking art classes at a community arts center, and learning country line dancing. They can do this in partnership with community builders whose aim is to engage them in community membership. On their way to active, full participation, participants are learning that opportunities for social relationships go beyond those provided only by paid services personnel and families.

REFERENCES

Amado, A., Conklin, F., & Wells, J. (1990). *Friends: A manual for connecting persons with disabilities and community members.* St. Paul, MN: Human Service Research and Development Center.

Bradley, V.J., & Knoll, J. (1990). *Shifting paradigms in services to people with developmental disabilities.* Cambridge, MA: Human Services Research Institute.

Butterworth, J., Steere, D.E., & Whitney-Thomas, J. (1997). Using person-centered planning to address personal quality of life. In R.L. Schalock (Ed.), *Quality of life: Application to persons with disabilities* (Vol. 2, pp. 5–23). Washington, DC: American Association on Mental Retardation.

Carie, M. (1995). *Developing community connection: Assisting individuals with disabilities to fully participate in the community.* Bloomington, IN: Institute for the Study of Developmental Disabilities.

Cotten, P.D., & Laughlin, C.S. (1989). Retirement: A new career. *American Association on Mental Retardation, Aging/MR Interest Group Newsletter, 3*(3), 13.

Ducharme, G., & Beeman, P. (1991, Spring). Perspectives. *Communitas Communicator,* 2–3.

Harlan, J., Todd, J., & Holtz, P. (1998). *A guide to building community membership for older adults with disabilities.* Bloomington, IN: Institute for the Study of Developmental Disabilities.

Janicki, M.P. (1997). Quality of life for older persons with mental retardation. In R.L. Schalock (Ed.), *Quality of life: Application to persons with disabilities* (Vol. 2, pp. 105–115). Washington, DC: American Association on Mental Retardation.

Lovett, H. (1996). *Learning to listen: Positive approaches and people with difficult behavior.* Baltimore: Paul H. Brookes Publishing Co.

MacDonald, M.L., & Tyson, P. (1988). Decajeopardy: The aging and aged developmentally disabled. In J.L. Matson & A. Marchetti (Eds.), *Developmental disabilities: A life-span perspective* (pp. 256–291). Philadelphia: Grune & Stratton.

Mount, B. (1995). *Capacity works: Finding windows for change using personal futures planning.* New York: Graphic Futures.

Mount, B., & Zwernik, K. (1988). *It's never too early. It's never too late: A booklet about personal futures planning.* St. Paul, MN: Metropolitan Council.

O'Brien, C.L., O'Brien, J., & Mount, B. (1997). Person-centered planning has arrived . . . or has it? *Mental Retardation, 35,* 480–484.

O'Brien, J., & O'Brien, C.L. (1996). *Members of each other: Building community in company with people with developmental disabilities.* Toronto: Inclusion Press.

Pearpoint, J., O'Brien, J., & Forest, M. (1993). *PATH: A workbook for planning positive futures.* Toronto: Inclusion Press.

Snow, J. (1992). Giftedness. In J. Pearpoint, M. Forest, & J. Snow (Eds.), *The inclusion papers: Strategies to make inclusion work* (pp. 109–110). Toronto: Inclusion Press.

Snow, J. (1994). *What's really worth doing and how to do it: A book for people who love someone labeled disabled (possibly yourself).* Toronto: Inclusion Press.

Snow, J. (1995, May). *Untitled.* Presentation at a staff colloquium at the Institute for the Study of Developmental Disabilities, Indiana University, Bloomington.

Spirduso, W.W. (1995). *Physical dimensions of aging.* Champaign, IL: Human Kinetics.

Stumpner, S. (1998, March). *Possible funding sources for community building.* Presentation at a staff colloquium at the Institute for the Study of Developmental Disabilities, Indiana University, Bloomington.

Sutton, E., Sterns, H.L., & Roberts, R.S. (1992). Retirement for older persons with developmental disabilities. *Generations: Journal of the American Society on Aging, 16*(1), 63–64.

II

Essay

Legislative Advocacy

The Caregivers Investment Bill

Edward F. Ansello

In a good story, one probably should not tell the ending first, but this story's ending—success in obtaining legislation to benefit family caregivers of relatives with disabilities—is the motivation for this essay. Reaching this ending required, among other plot details, building a broad coalition of advocates that included aging adults with lifelong disabilities and family caregivers; maintaining steady interaction with and support from legislators; and, perhaps above all else, persisting toward the goal, even when bureaucrats, political dynamics, and chance dealt obstacles to progress.

This is the story of advocating for a $500 tax credit for family caregivers for three sessions of the General Assembly of Virginia and receiving a $500 grant fund for them during the fourth. Although the end result is not exactly what was originally intended, in significant ways it is a greater triumph. That this story does not turn out the way it was planned is one of the lessons of building coalitions to advocate, even when powerful legislators are not involved. Advocacy is invariably interwoven with politics. Just the arena changes. Sometimes it is the neighborhood; sometimes it is the nation. In the present story, the principals advocated for a similarly perceived greater good, a benefit to families. This drew disparate groups together. Family caregiving of relatives with disabilities is the underrecognized foundation of long-term care. At the same time, families provide this ongoing care to relatives of every age. Advocating for some financial assistance for family caregivers, then, transcends age-group advocacy issues such as those that may pit advocates for children against those for older adults and allows the convergence of various age-group and disabilities advocates into a common cause.

The following sections relate the steps taken in Virginia to obtain a legislated program of financial assistance for family caregivers that we called the Caregivers Investment Bill. We offer a rationale for recognizing family caregivers and assumptions behind a legislated program of financial assistance. A synopsis of our experiences in the first session of the General Assembly conveys, I hope, the combination of exuberance and disappointment that may well typify many advocacy efforts in the early stages. The lesson is to continue. There follow highlights of the ups and downs of the next 3 years that led to unanimous passage by the House and Senate of the Caregivers Grant Program and its signing into law by the governor.

FAMILY CAREGIVING AND DISABILITIES

The "gift of time" (Ansello, 1992), or the many added years of life expectancy that are typical in the developed nations, has meant that individuals with early-onset disabilities (e.g., intellectual disability, polio) are surviving to later life in unprecedented numbers and, at the other end, that individuals are living long enough to experience late-onset disabilities (e.g., Alzheimer's disease, poststroke aphasia) that were relatively rare in the past. We are, increasingly, experiencing what Ansello and Rose (1989) called "the intersection of aging and disabilities." Kunkel and Applebaum (1992) projected a substantial increase near-term in the numbers of older adults with functional disabilities in the United States. These researchers offered four projection models for the combination of mortality and disability: 1) constant (present trends continue), 2) longer life/lower disability, 3) longer life/higher disability, and 4) moderately longer life/moderately higher disability. Their projections show that even under the most favorable scenario (i.e., longer life and lower disability), the number of older adults with functional disabilities will increase from 5.1 million to 9.4 million by 2020, not including those with lifelong developmental disabilities. At the same time, most people with disabilities choose to live in and be a part of their communities and neighborhoods. Clearly, it is time to reinforce the family as a principal agent in supporting the community choice of people with disabilities.

Reinforcing family caregiving can take a variety of forms: supportive services such as respite and home chores, assistive technology, more broadly available training in such caregiving-related topics as medication management and conflict resolution, and so forth. Moreover, the delivery place for such interventions can be the caregiver's home, the workplace, or some community environment. In Virginia, a number of us chose to attempt to reinforce family caregiving by providing recognition and modest financial relief for caregivers who are taxpayers. We undertook a legislative strategy to enact a $500 tax credit, the Caregivers Investment Bill.

Two entities played the leadership role in this initiative: 1) the Statewide Coalition for the Support of Family Caregivers, which was begun in late 1991 under the inspiration of then-Commissioner Thelma Bland of the Virginia Department for the Aging (VDA) and which had a membership of 20, mostly professionals in aging and human services, and 2) the Partners III Project, a multiyear project (1993–1996) on aging and developmental disabilities, supported by the U.S. Administration on Aging, that tested its Integrated Model for intersystem cooperation in Maryland and Virginia and that includes to this day the professional/consumer advocacy council (PCAC).

ASSUMPTIONS BEHIND A TAX CREDIT OR GRANT

Advocating for a tax credit reflected not only our conviction that a credit provides more monetary benefit than a tax deduction but also that a tax credit means that the beneficiary is a bona fide taxpayer; this is a potentially important consideration during fiscally conservative times when meritorious initiatives might be dismissed as "giveaways." That a grant fund for caregivers, not a tax credit, was ultimately passed by the General Assembly reflects several developments over the course of our continued advocacy. These include the following: 1) Legislators came to see that family caregiving of dependent relatives is a means of achieving what most people want, legislators included, which is to grow older in their own communities; 2) legislators recognized that strengthening family caregiving makes economic sense, as our fiscal impact analyses demonstrated that revenues returned to caregiving taxpayers might be expected to delay use of more costly state-financed Medicaid long-term care services; 3) those who were advocating for assistance to family caregivers represented diverse interest groups that were united on this particular issue, including young and middle-age adults with lifelong disabilities who lived in the community without the help of family caregivers; 4) we demonstrated to everyone who would listen the win–win politics of supporting the bill (e.g., fiscal prudence, support for families), so conservatives, moderates, and liberals could find reasons to vote for its passage; 5) the emergence of another powerful legislator on the Senate side of the General Assembly to "carry" the bill as others had been doing for years on the House side; and, finally, 6) the recognition during the last days of the 1999 session, when conflicting bills passed by the House and Senate were being harmonized by the joint conference committee, that a Caregivers Grant Fund could better benefit the very poor who had paid little or no taxes and hence would receive little or no tax credits.

The initiative for a tax credit or grant for family caregivers, known to us as the Caregivers Investment Bill, may serve as a prototype for similar efforts elsewhere to support family caregivers. This initiative incorporates several assumptions. First, a tax "credit" in a given amount is a direct benefit to the taxpayer in that amount. A tax "deduction," conversely, is a benefit whose net savings to the taxpayer will be mitigated by the taxpayer's overall tax return, including his or her income bracket. So, a $500 tax deduction might produce a true benefit of only $140 for the caregiver whose adjusted gross income is subject to a 28% tax levy. Second, we all know that a $500 tax credit or grant will not be an incentive to take up the tasks of family caregiving. Motivations for caregiving lie elsewhere. However, we believe that a tax credit or grant is a fitting recognition by the state of the vital role that families play in the long-term care process. This recognition may be incentive to some caregivers to continue their care. Third, a tax credit or grant is a form of investment by the state in one of the principal means of sustaining long-term care. It is not a giveaway any more than investing taxpayers' dollars in the form of Medicaid payments to nursing homes is a giveaway. Fourth, reinforcing family caregiving is good economics.

For some time, it has been common understanding that for every person in a nursing home, there are two, three, or four living in the community with similar levels of impairment. Simply put, the longer a family continues caring for a member with functional limitations, the longer the care recipient remains out of more costly alternatives. Inasmuch as the state, through Medicaid, is the main supporter of nursing home care throughout the United States, outnumbering "private pay" care substantially, the state may save many times its tax credit or grant in avoided Medicaid nursing home expenses. Fifth, an effort to obtain a tax credit or grant for family caregivers can be launched in a reasonably brief time and can be successfully concluded within a manageable number of sessions of the state legislature. To do so requires 1) broad-based coalition building among groups of advocates, 2) finding legislators with both compassion for the issues and power in the political process to sponsor the appropriate legislation, and 3) a small number of individuals to monitor the daily ups and downs of the bill, from obtaining co-patrons to testifying to committees.

CAREGIVERS INVESTMENT BILL: FIRST SESSION

Knowing what we do now about legislative advocacy might well have improved our initial prospects. In 5 months, we crafted the language of the first bill and secured legislative co-patrons, and the bill was launched on the seas of politics. Not surprising, it foundered. But the lessons of the first session of Virginia's General Assembly forged the practices that ultimately succeeded.

Our immersion in legislative advocacy began on October 3, 1995, when Bill Peterson proposed to the Statewide Coalition for the Support of Family Caregivers (SCSFC) that it consider some form of tax benefit for family caregivers. Amidst considerable discussion, I suggested the term "caregivers investment" to connote prudent action by the commonwealth rather than revenue giveaway. SCSFC chose to work with the PCAC, which itself was a statewide group fathered by the Partners III Project on aging with developmental disabilities. Both groups decided that the tax benefit would be "disability-based and targeted to all age groups." By the end of the month, Bryan Lacy (a middle-age attorney with cerebral palsy) and MaryEllen Cox (an older family caregiver), co-leaders of the PCAC, had convened the council to debate tax deductions versus tax credits, study the language of House Bill (H.B.) 1215 newly introduced in the U.S. Congress for a tax deduction for care of ancestors, and adopt several priorities for actions by the PCAC, including the Caregivers Investment Bill. Four weeks later, both the SCSFC and the PCAC concluded that a tax credit would probably benefit low-income caregivers more, because they are unlikely to file the more complicated tax returns with itemized deductions. By the end of November, Lacy and Cox had convened a subcommittee of the PCAC, supplemented by Peterson and Jim Payne of the SCSFC, and we began drafting an outline for a possible bill: rationale, eligibility, how it differs from current law, and fiscal impact. The core of the tax credit would be caring for someone with disabilities. Aging, youth, family, and disabilities networks would have common cause. A month later, I met with Delegate Frank Hall, a long-time friend of aging issues and a senior member of the General Assembly. He offered critical insights to me, a novice, on how different political factions might view this bill, and he encouraged the groups to orient the tax credit toward older care recipients to facilitate passage, for "the elderly have a powerful voice in Virginia politics" and a restricted focus on older citizens would reduce the fiscal impact or lost tax revenue of the bill.

The SCSFC members chose to reemphasize the age-irrelevant nature of the sought-after tax credit and proposed income bracketing to reduce the bill's fiscal impact. Delegate Hall agreed to introduce an age-neutral, income-bracketed tax credit for caregivers of family members with disabilities. During the first week of the 1996 session of the General Assembly (January 15–22), MaryEllen Cox and I visited legislators in their offices to explain the bill. We secured co-patron signatures from 24 delegates and 12 senators, and Delegate Hall (D) introduced our bill, H.B. 1519. Unexpectedly, Delegate Wilkins (R) introduced H.B. 1269 with identical language. The bills specified that the care recipient must have two or more impairments in activities of daily living and must not be receiving Medicaid-reimbursed long-term care services. Senator Woods requested that corroboration of impairment level be obtained by the taxpayer through testing with the Uniform Assessment Instrument (UAI), a lengthy and potentially expensive screening test. Our advocates solicited the opinions of government agencies regarding the bill.

I met with the executive director and staff of the Virginia Department of Medical Assistance Services (DMAS), the agency that is responsible for Medicaid, to explain the bill and obtain DMAS's official position. They suggested changes in the fiscal impact draft and noted that Virginia's share of Medicaid community-based long-term services average $7,900 and nursing home costs average $14,000–$20,000 a year. They supported the bill. Shortly, the Department of Taxation informed Delegate Hall verbally of its negative tax position regarding his bill. In the absence of detailed projections on taxpayers who were eligible for the credit, the Department of Taxation was wary. MaryEllen Cox reported that the Leadership Council on Aging will not support a bill that requires that confirmation of level of impairment be made through the UAI as it is perceived to be too costly. I began to confer with the Department of Taxation on fiscal impact, never having previously attempted to carry out the detailed estimate they require. In the 1996 session, the House Finance Committee narrowly failed (10–12) to "report" or pass our bill.

LESSONS LEARNED FROM THE CAREGIVERS INVESTMENT BILL

The work of advocacy became more sophisticated. After the 1996 session ended, Delegate Hall addressed the Annual Meeting of the Virginia Coalition on Aging. In a stirring keynote speech on grass-roots advocacy, he devoted all of his remarks to the Caregivers Investment Bill as an exemplar. He encouraged us to continue. The next month, he attended the new Ad-Hoc Coalition that we had organized with a broad range of advocacy groups from various developmental disabilities, health care, aging, Alzheimer's, and so forth. He urged us to "actively engage the media." We worked smarter, but the unexpected still managed to happen. In the 1997 session of the General Assembly, our broadened group of advocates canvassed legislators' offices on behalf of the bill. Delegate Hall filed the Caregivers Investment Bill together with Delegate Wilkins as chief co-patron and with 74 additional co-patrons whom we had solicited. Just as the full House Finance Committee was poised to "report" (i.e., pass) the caregivers tax credit that its own subcommittee had endorsed, the Richmond newspaper headlined dire warnings of a $58 million deficit in state funding of the state employees' health insurance program. The House Finance Committee tabled all tax credits. The deficit subsequently proved ephemeral.

In the 1998 session, the House Finance Committee reported that year's caregivers tax credit, as did the full House, which, in turn, conveyed the bill to the Senate. However, the senator in Senate Finance who had championed the bill in previous sessions and who had chaired the Finance Committee now co-chaired the committee with a member from the opposition party, as a result of power-sharing arrangements brokered after the previous November's elections. The co-chair looked disapprovingly on tax credits.

We learned to refine our presentations to 1 minute on the run and 3 minutes in testimony as the upper limits of legislators' sustained attention. We improved the quality of our estimates of fiscal impact, as the PCAC and other sources gathered more data on the prevalence of disabilities caregiving and as we understood better what the Department of Taxation required for the analyses of proposed legislation that it provided legislators. We learned to learn how to "do" legislative advocacy. Before the 1999 session of the General Assembly, we met with Senator Walter Stosch to request that he introduce in the Senate a parallel version to the Hall-Wilkins Caregivers Investment Bill in the House. He introduced, instead, a variation on the theme—that is, a grant fund with a defined annual appropriation rather than a projected fiscal impact on tax revenues. In 1999, four bills were introduced on the House side, one of which would have limited tax credits to caregiving of older adults with impairments. In true democratic fashion, what emerged from the 1999 session was a blend of House versions into the Senate's.

In late February 1999, the Virginia General Assembly, with both House and Senate concurring, unanimously passed the Virginia Caregivers Grant Program, one of two different tacks advocated by our Caregivers Ad-Hoc Coalition in the 1999 session. Signed by the governor shortly thereafter, it creates a program of $500 grants to Virginia family caregivers who have adjusted gross incomes up to $50,000 annually and who provide care to relatives of any age with two or more impairments in activities of daily living. Care recipients may live with the caregivers, on their own, or anywhere in the community except nursing homes or assisted living facilities. The fund is administered by the Virginia Department of Social Services (VDSS). We advocates who lobbied so long for passage of the bill constituted an advisory group to VDSS over the course of 1999 to write the policies for administering the program.

LESSONS LEARNED IN LEGISLATIVE ADVOCACY

Success, like failure or any intense endeavor, can crystallize one's focus. There seem to be a number of keys that help to obtain a satisfactory outcome to this type of greater good advocacy. The following does not exhaust this list, but it does contain what we found to be prominent:

1. *Public awareness:* There needs to be a fairly regular, if not steady, output of essays, newspaper editorials, interviews, public addresses, and related activities to sustain both the public's and the legislators' awareness of the issue. This is where coalitions shine; they divide the load. Members of the Ad Hoc Coalition ghost wrote essays for legislators on the value of families and family caregiving, answered telephone inquiries, and photocopied supportive articles for distribution. The awareness campaign, however, must contain hard facts about numbers of people in need, numbers to be helped, and the cost of the help or fiscal impact on the state's revenue stream. One-page fact sheets and talking points prove invaluable. For example, legislators tuned in when we testified that a $500 tax credit or grant will buy (we used "will" rather than "would" to convey the inevitability of the bill's passage) 25–26 weeks of home-delivered meals from an Area Agency on Aging in Virginia or 2 months of once-a-week full-day visits by home health aides.

2. *Constant contact with legislators:* Visiting legislators during the General Assembly is valuable for communicating facts and lobbying for a bill, but seeing them when not in session—for example, during the summer or fall—may be more effective. The press on their time is less, and they tend to be more expansive in their opinions of the proposed bill. We first obtained chief patronage of a Senate version of the Caregivers Investment Bill, to parallel a House version, after meeting with the Senator in his home office in August.

3. *Accumulate advocates:* From the outset, the advocates of the Caregivers Investment Bill rejected age-specific restrictions. The bill might have faced an easier run had it oriented the tax credit toward care of older adults with disabilities. Then again, it might not have, and it would most probably have set advocacy groups against each other. By the time the Virginia Caregivers Grant Program was passed, the caregivers initiative had been endorsed by more than 3 dozen different advocacy groups. These included the Virginia chapters of the Alzheimer's Association, the American Association of Retired Persons, the National Alliance for the Mentally Ill, and the National Association of Retired Federal Employees, plus many state-specific groups.

4. *Legislative platforms:* Groups experienced in legislative advocacy are often pulled in many directions in attempting to respond to worthy needs. They prioritize their responses by developing their legislative platforms. They may endorse dozens of initiatives, but they will likely list on their platforms only the top three or four issues that they are most committed to seeing enacted. It is important to get on their platform.

5. *Eggs in different baskets:* In legislative advocacy, it is prudent to have one's proposed legislation traveling through both House and Senate simultaneously rather than to depend on one version to be passed and conveyed to the other house for its consideration. With bills on parallel tracks, it means that there are different sets of chief patrons to watch over them, and if a bill is derailed on one side, that on the other might still be passed and conveyed. Multiple bills mean, of course, that advocates may sometimes have to be testifying before different committees at the same time.

6. *Meetings to monitor and respond:* To be effective, advocates need to meet frequently and regularly to monitor the progress of what they are championing and to divide among themselves responsibilities for responding to difficulties or opportunities. This is especially pertinent during the relatively brief periods when many legislative bodies are in session. We found that weekly Thursday noon meetings were almost not frequent enough to monitor various pieces of aging-related legislation progressing through the General Assembly. Aside from legislative advocacy, advocates concerned about advancing most any agenda need to be together frequently.

7. *Feedback from disinterested parties:* Advocates can delude themselves when surrounded by like-minded people. Objectivity may suffer, obstacles may not be seen, and support may be overestimated. Explaining one's position to disinterested parties can be a sobering lesson, but it can reveal deficiencies in goals and in the strategies and tactics to reach the goals. It can be a humbling experience to seek others' opinions, but it strengthened our process.

CONCLUSIONS

Adults with lifelong disabilities; family caregivers of relatives with developmental or late-onset disabilities; elected officials; representatives from several systems of human services, such as aging, health, social services, and disabilities; educators; and others worked together successfully to gain passage of legislation to assist family caregivers financially, with the aim of strengthening their capacities to continue their care. Success required four sessions of Virginia's General Assembly over the course of 3½ years. This seemingly lengthy time, however, must be compared with all of the time when no such assistance existed.

Professionals in the gerontology and developmental disabilities fields can be particularly valuable and effective in the legislative arena. They can apply their knowledge in this practical environment to improve the status of people with disabilities and of family caregivers who often play critical roles in their lives. In the process of legislative advocacy, professionals can translate extant research on family caregiving or lifelong disabilities to policy makers, assist policy makers in crafting appropriate legislative responses, conduct economic analyses and fiscal impact studies, and help to advance the passage of proposed legislation by educating legislators in informal meetings or in committee testimony.

REFERENCES

Ansello, E.F. (1992). Seeking common ground between aging and developmental disabilities. In E.F. Ansello & N.N. Eustis (Eds.), *Aging and disabilities: Seeking common ground* (pp. 9–24). Amityville, NY: Baywood Publishing Co.

Ansello, E.F., & Rose, T. (1989). *Aging and lifelong disabilities: Partnership for the twenty-first century.* Palm Springs, CA: Elvirita Lewis Foundation.

Kunkel, S.R., & Applebaum, R.A. (1992). Estimating the prevalence of long-term disability for an aging society. *Journal of Gerontology: Social Sciences, 47,* S253–S260.

III

MAKING EVERYDAY COMMUNITY LIVING WORK

Adapting community systems to the needs and perspectives of people with disabilities is the theme of Section III. As organizations and communities mobilize to provide supports to people with lifelong disabilities and to enable them to become active agents in their own communities, we need to know more about the dynamics of adaptation and facilitating change. In this section, we have assembled several contributions that focus specifically on making community involvement work to the benefit of adults with developmental disabilities. In Chapter 11, Sterns, Kennedy, Sed, and Heller appraise several areas of daily living where later-life planning would benefit individuals with developmental disabilities, especially when they are intimately part of the planning process. The authors discuss a curriculum that they conceptualized, implemented, and tested to help in this function.

In much the same vein, Mughal articulates in Chapter 12 sound health promotion and disease prevention principles, offering guidelines for enhancing the quality of life of older adults with intellectual disabilities who live in community settings. Mughal maintains that nutrition screening can detect warning signs of malnutrition or health problems, facilitate assessment and appropriate intervention, and help continue or enhance functional independence and the quality of life of vulnerable individuals. She emphasizes the importance of regular nutrition screening as a vital health promotion strategy for older adults with disabilities in community settings. She provides a range of topics of relevance to the nutritional assessment of people with lifelong disabilities, particulars of screening and intervention, and general principles to prevent or alleviate nutritional problems. Issues arise with regard to applying commonly used standards for body weight and obesity. In an appendix, she includes an overview of nutrition screening tools that the public, community workers, and health professionals can adapt to their needs.

In Chapter 13, Simon-Rusinowitz and her colleagues relate the status of cash and counseling, a model of structuring and financing support services. It is an alternative support strategy for aiding adults with disabilities to obtain services that maintain independent living. The authors report the results of telephone interviews conducted in Florida to assess the preferences of adults with developmental disabilities for a cash option versus traditional services. The survey, a first of its kind to assess this population's interest in a cash option, identified the characteristics of adults and surrogate decision makers who may wish to participate in a cash and counseling option for day-to-day supports for community living. Also explored are methods for developing communication and social marketing materials. Commentary also is provided on information that is essential to educating participants about the cash option so that they can make informed decisions on whether to choose a consumer-directed option or stay in traditional financing programs.

Hutchings, Olsen, and Ehrenkrantz remind us in Chapter 14 that as people with developmental disabilities age, it becomes necessary to ensure that their home environments meet their needs while providing the supports necessary to maintain them in the community. Because older people can move from the high to the low end of the functional abilities spectrum in a relatively short period of time, environments for older people with and without preexisting disabilities should be designed with maximum flexibility to adapt to these changing needs. Whereas unsafe environments can promote dependency and increase feelings of alienation and dissatisfaction, a home that is safe, supportive, and homelike and that includes opportunities for growth and stimulation can enhance an individual's sense of competency, independence, and self-worth. This chapter outlines modifications that can be made to existing homes, as well as to new home designs, to achieve these goals while retaining a homelike quality.

Davies, Davies, and Sheridan, in Chapter 15, deal with a variety of asset problems and solutions associated with housing and services for aging people with disabilities, particularly individuals with developmental disabilities. Housing and services for people with disabilities pose a dilemma at any age. However, having experienced a lifetime of limited financial and diminishing natural supports as they age, many older people with lifelong disabilities are left with a lack of choices, dignity, and self-determination. The authors propose a model that brings together the several facets and resources of an individual's life into a comprehensive plan. The foundation of this plan is the premise that the whole asset picture—the person, the family, the state disability agency, other government agencies, and local community supports—is greater than the sum of its parts. They posit that completing this plan ensures that the person with the disability will have security, financial stability, and choices in housing and services as he or she ages.

Henry, Keys, and Factor in Chapter 16 describe value-based job analysis, a method for providing a foundation for human resource management in human services agencies, and apply it to agencies that serve older adults with lifelong disabilities. Value-based job analysis incorporates core organizational values in the process of recruitment, selection, socialization, training, and evaluation of staff, thus making core values central to the organization's human resource activities. This chapter describes the process of value-based job analysis, provides examples from applications of the method, and states how agencies can incorporate progressive values into their organizational cultures.

Finally, Wang's essay reviews the relative statuses in Taiwan of people with disabilities and those of advanced age. She shares her perceptions of a series of governmental initiatives for citizens with lifelong disabilities. Wang notes the evolution of mandates for services and the unanticipated impact of these mandates on local governments and citizens without disabilities. Her perceptive analysis illustrates not only the idiosyncrasies of Taiwanese public policy but also the universality of issues that adults with lifelong disabilities face as they age.

11

Later-Life
Planning and Retirement

Harvey L. Sterns, Elizabeth A. Kennedy, Chad M. Sed, and Tamar Heller

Later-life planning involves making decisions regarding the direction of one's future. Beyond individual constraints, it is limited only by the options considered and the goals set. Later-life planning is most frequently thought of under the broad category of retirement planning (Atchley, 2000; Ekerdt, 1995). Issues that most typically are associated with retirement planning include finances (e.g., Social Security benefits, pensions) and health-related expenses (e.g., Medicare/Medicaid, insurance premiums). The retirement preparations of people in the general population also focus on new roles that they may adopt (e.g., volunteer, student) and on new ways of spending their increased free time (e.g., traveling, joining health clubs, engaging in more family- and home-based activities; Taylor & Shore, 1995). Planning for the various aspects of retirement has been shown to be significantly related to greater life satisfaction and better adjustment to the retirement process (Sterns, Matheson, & Park, 1997). This is particularly true when life goals are used to augment the transition from work to retirement (Robbins, Lee, & Wan, 1994). In addition, Richardson (1993) reported that being an active, involved participant in the planning and decision making regarding retirement was related to greater life satisfaction and better health during retirement. Later-life planning for people with intellectual disabilities or other developmental disabilities can have similar positive

This chapter was funded in part by the U.S. Department of Education, Office of Special Education and Rehabilitation Services, National Institute on Disability and Rehabilitation Research Grant No. H133B30069.

results. This chapter discusses several areas of daily living in which later-life planning would benefit individuals with developmental disabilities, especially when they are intimately part of the planning process. Furthermore, we report on a later-life planning curriculum that has been implemented and tested.

PERSON-CENTERED LATER-LIFE PLANNING
FOR ADULTS WITH DEVELOPMENTAL DISABILITIES

Person-centered later-life planning for adults with developmental disabilities places the person for whom future plans need to be developed at the center of the decision-making processes. It incorporates many of the tenets of later-life and retirement planning in the general population. One important tenet is that "successful" transitions into new life phases are largely a product of informed and active planning. A second major tenet concerns the rights of the individual to choose, control, and direct his or her life decisions throughout the life course, including the retirement period.

For both people in the general population and adults with developmental disabilities, older adulthood presents its own special challenges. Older adults may experience declines in physical abilities, increased risk for disease, chronic illnesses, and other health problems. There may be transitional adjustments related to work and retirement that may be coupled with concurrent changes in family and social roles. Individuals may experience a sense of impending personal mortality as occurrences of death and loss involving family and friends increase (Adlin, 1993).

This is not to suggest that this phase of the life span consists solely of negative, degenerative life events but rather to point out that adaptation is a lifelong process (Seltzer, 1993). As articulated most clearly by Baltes and Graf (1996), a life-span perspective of older adulthood involves both multidirectionality (i.e., stability, growth, and decline) as well as plasticity (i.e., modifiability and improvement). A large amount of literature on older adult learning and training interventions supports these ideas. Given appropriate considerations, the capacities of older adults can be significantly modified and may even reach a skill level comparable to that of younger adults (e.g., Salthouse, 1985; Sterns & Sanders, 1980).

In line with a life-span development orientation, person-centered later-life planning incorporates an ecological perspective of empowerment (Rappaport, 1987). According to Rappaport (1987), empowerment involves individuals' gaining a sense of mastery and control over their lives and becoming more connected to their communities. Positive consequences of greater individual empowerment include increased well-being, more positive affect, enhancement of problem-solving abilities, and greater maintenance of positive behavior changes (Brickman et al., 1982; Heller, Factor, Sterns, & Sutton, 1996).

In regard to person-centered later-life planning for adults with intellectual disabilities, empowerment is accomplished by enhancing the decision-making abilities of these individuals by providing information, skills training, and opportunities to experience new options and make informed choices (Heller et al., 1996). Successful intervention requires the involvement of families, professionals, and caregivers who have learned how to help adults with developmental disabilities identify, implement, and understand their life choices. They often need support and decision-making opportunities.

Development and implementation of a person-centered approach to later-life planning require an orientation that endorses the potential for both growth and change throughout the life cycle. It is believed that, given the appropriate skills, abilities, and support, individuals will make the most of opportunities presented to them. However, unlike members of the general population, adults with intellectual disabilities often are not provided the opportunities for hands-on decision making and goal setting (e.g., Sutton, Sterns, & Park, 1991). Many families of individuals with intellectual disabilities fail to make long-term plans for their loved one for such important life events as guardianship and financial security (Essex, Seltzer, & Krauss, 1997; Freedman, Krauss, & Seltzer, 1997). Families that do make long-term plans typically do not involve the individuals for whom the plan is created (Heller & Factor, 1993). Rarely is information regarding retirement and/or later-life options made available to older adults with intellectual disabilities, and even more rarely is preretirement education provided (Sutton, Sterns, & Roberts, 1992).

Successful adaptation to many of the developmental tasks of older adulthood can be assisted through thoughtful planning for later-life events. Although some aspects of later-life and retirement planning may differ between older adults in the general population and those with intellectual disabilities, these two groups do share many similar issues and concerns. A key point of emphasis is that limited cognitive and/or adaptive behavior skills do not negate the possibility for later-life development but, rather, delineate the approach that such planning should take.

ISSUES IN WORK AND RETIREMENT: DIFFERENCES AND SIMILARITIES

Retirement for older people with intellectual disabilities may present a different picture from that in the general population simply because the two groups differ in their work experiences. Although practices vary from state to state, the majority of older adults who have participated in the broader developmental disabilities system since the 1970s have experienced only sheltered work.

Most Americans with developmental disabilities achieve an income level far below the average American worker's and depend primarily on income support programs for stable income (Fujiura & Yamaki, 1997). Among the estimated 756,000 adults with developmental disabilities who received employment services nationally in 1991, 45% worked in sheltered environments, 25% were provided non–work-oriented services alone, and only 30% were employed in regular work environments (McGaughley, Kiernan, McNally, Gilmore, & Keith, 1994).

Before the deinstitutionalization movement, employment for people with developmental disabilities who lived at home was uncommon. Employed individuals who lived in institutions tended to hold jobs that were limited to in-service or agricultural tasks related to the functioning of the environment (Sutton et al., 1991). The net result has been that older adults with intellectual disabilities had significantly different work histories from adults in the general population. The predeinstitutionalized older worker experienced work as a necessity to keep his or her place of residence in operation. The postdeinstitutionalized older worker is more likely to have worked in a day program. This work experience may be affected by extraneous events such as "downtime" for lack of work or closure of the facility as a result of inclement weather.

The ability to retire also differs between the two groups. In many states, the retirement age for people with developmental disabilities ranges between 55 and 60 years. For example, Ohio state law defines the retirement option as being at age 55 (Ohio Rev. Code § 5123:2-2-06 [Anderson 1999]; Sutton, Sterns & Park, 1993). This is in contrast to the generally expected retirement age of 65 (age 66 in 2009 and age 67 in 2027) for the general population under the Social Security Act of 1935 (PL 74-271) and the Social

Security Amendments of 1983 (PL 99-499). The use of a younger retirement age has been based on the assumption that some adults with developmental disabilities experience more rapid age-related declines. There is some evidence of earlier age-related declines for people with Down syndrome (Hawkins & Eklund, 1994; Zigman, Seltzer, & Silverman, 1994), cerebral palsy (Arcand, 1996; Brown, Bontempo, & Turk, 1991), and more severe forms of intellectual disability (Eyman & Borthwick-Duffy, 1994).

The amount of contact that retirees have with their former employers also differs between the two groups. Workers who do not have disabilities may maintain limited contact with their former workplace but, for the most part, focus most of their energies on experiences in new or expanded arenas. In contrast, many workshop retirees return to their former workplace on a daily basis. Many individuals have the opportunity to engage in part-time or phase-down work and/or to participate in alternative (i.e., retirement) programs. Alternative work programs most frequently offered include outings to places within the general community (e.g., the mall, fast food shops) and/or trips, crafts, music, and exercise. Activities such as dance, health care education, and volunteer work may also be available but are not typical to the programs of most centers.

As an example, the state of Ohio's developmental disabilities services system has formally recognized that alternative-to-work programming is both useful and necessary. A 1990 statewide investigation of the retirement practices of individuals with intellectual disabilities in the Ohio developmental disabilities services system indicated that of the 1,500 respondents ages 55 years or older, slightly more than 80% reported working either full or part time. Of those individuals, approximately 50% reported involvement in some form of alternative programming on either a full- or part-time basis at their respective services centers or in community-based senior centers (Sutton et al., 1991). However, in many cases, the alternative programming is directly affected by service agency priorities and associated funding and staffing limitations (Sutton et al., 1992).

Similarities do exist in the retirement experiences of individuals in the general population and those with developmental disabilities. For example, for both groups, the workplace is a main source of social support and interaction, which directly affects life satisfaction. The importance of being a productive, contributing member of American society is an ideal endorsed by both groups as well (Sutton et al., 1992). Retirement, however, causes a rift in one's social identity by changing the nature of one's role in society. It represents a transition to another phase of one's life, which one may or may not be completely prepared to make. As is similar to many older adults in the general population, two studies that addressed the retirement preferences of older adults with intellectual disabilities (Factor, 1989; Heller et al., 1996) found that many of these adults preferred to continue working as long as possible and expressed the desire to obtain better paying jobs in the community.

RETIREMENT PLANNING FOR LATER LIFE

In addition to work and retirement, other areas in life are amenable to future planning among individuals with intellectual disabilities, including health-related behaviors, residency, leisure, volunteerism, and death and dying.

Health-Related Behaviors

Physical well-being in later life includes attention to proper nutrition and participation in an appropriate exercise program. Older adults with intellectual disabilities have the same basic nutritional requirements as older adults without intellectual disabilities. Like their counterparts in the general population, they must deal with the adverse effects of the aging process on their nutritional status (e.g., metabolic changes, decreased gastrointestinal function; Huber, 1985). Factors such as ignorance about the importance of good nutrition and limited decision-making power in food selections compound the problem (Heller et al., 1996). Person-centered later-life planning promotes nutritional health by educating older individuals with intellectual disabilities about proper nutrition and teaching them how to make optimal dietary choices.

The benefits of a regular exercise program on physical health among older adults in the general population are well documented (e.g., Spirduso & McCrae, 1990). However, even among older adults who practice health-promoting behaviors, performance of a regular exercise program often is not part of their routine (Hawkins, 1993). Exercise regimes may be especially important to older adults with developmental disabilities because obesity and cholesterol levels may often be higher than for the general population. This is mostly true for women and for adults who live in independent environments (Rimmer, Braddock, & Fujiura, 1994; Rimmer, Braddock, & Marks, 1995). Among adults with Down syndrome, Chicoine, Rubin, and McGuire (1997) found that nearly half of the women and nearly one third of the men had morbid obesity. Findings from the National Medical Expenditure Survey indicated that older adults who have intellectual disabilities and who live at home exercised less frequently than older adults in the general population (Anderson, 1997). However, it is not known to what degree individuals with intellectual disabilities have input regarding their physical activity regimes. Creating a person-centered exercise plan involves first providing information about exercise (e.g., its benefits, the different varieties, clothing worn, importance of warm-up/cool-down stretching) and then allowing the individual to make an informed choice that is compatible with his or her physical capabilities.

Residency

The most common type of housing arrangement for individuals with intellectual disabilities is family-based care (Anderson & Kloos, 1992). Most families voluntarily provide care, but when relocation becomes unavoidable, many families display anxiety, fear, and ambivalence about the proposed change (Essex et al., 1997; Heller & Factor, 1991). According to Bigby (see Chapter 5) and Freedman et al. (1997), among others, these negative feelings may result in the family's failing to make concrete plans for their loved one's future residence. Those who do plan often fail to discuss these plans with their son or daughter with intellectual disabilities and do not include his or her preferences when making the necessary arrangements.

In addition, although the current national trend is toward using smaller community living options for individuals with developmental disabilities, few states engage in collaborative planning and values-based planning when meeting the residential needs of older adults with intellectual disabilities (Martinson & Stone, 1993). As reported by Heller et al. (1996), personal preference in residence has been significantly related to life satisfaction, such that those who are not given a voice in relocation decisions typically report lower satisfaction levels. Person-centered later-life planning takes into account the individual residency preferences by presenting all possible (i.e., available and practical) housing arrangements.

Leisure

Leisure has many definitions but, in general, can be conceptualized as unobligated time in which the individual can exercise both personal choice and control (Hawkins, 1993). Choice concerns the type of activities pursued, whereas control centers on the frequency and duration of the desired activities. For older adults in the general population, leisure typically is reported as being positively related to life satisfaction; that is, older adults who report that they are satisfied with the quality of their leisure time generally report greater life satisfaction as well (Hawkins & McClean, 1993). Among older retirees, this relationship is particularly strong for older adults who maintain their sense of life purpose and meaning through a high level of goal-directed behaviors (Payne, Robbins, & Dougherty, 1991).

However, the research on leisure and life satisfaction among older adults with intellectual disabilities is noticeably scarce. One exception is a study conducted by Hawkins (1993), which examined the leisure patterns, preferences, and barriers to participation in two groups of older adults with intellectual disabilities (64 adults with Down syndrome and 64 older adults without Down syndrome). Results indicated that leisure participation and preference to increase participation in leisure activities were significantly related to perceived life satisfaction among the older adults without Down syndrome. They indicated greater preference to participate in more current activities as well as greater interest in initiating new activities. Hawkins suggested that one contributing factor to lower perceived life satisfaction among older adults with intellectual disabilities could be unfulfilled leisure preferences. As part of a person-centered later-life plan, leisure skills building, which incorporates abilities such as leisure awareness and leisure activity skills, could help circumvent this problem.

Volunteerism

Volunteerism among older adults has increased approximately 40% since the 1960s (Papalia, Camp, & Feldman, 1996). Reasons for this increase include a better educated older adult population that has more skills and is more motivated to contribute those skills altruistically to society, an increase in the social status of volunteerism, and a recognition that older adulthood can be a time of activity and involvement in the community. As Papalia et al. (1996) pointed out, the more older adults are seen in active, productive roles, the more likely society is to perceive them as useful and necessary members of that society. Volunteerism, then, becomes another vehicle by which to reduce ageism and encourage a more positive view of older adults (Chambre, 1993). Although a similar philosophy guides community/competitive employment practices among adults with intellectual disabilities (Catapano, Levy, & Levy, 1985), the opportunity to reduce negative stereotypes of individuals with intellectual disabilities through volunteerism has not received attention in the literature.

Volunteerism among older adults with intellectual disabilities is most often mentioned as a replacement activity when full-time work is reduced (e.g., Sutton, Sterns, et al., 1993) or as a leisure option (e.g., Hawkins, 1993); rarely is volunteerism addressed as an important activity in its own right. Harlow and Cantor (1996) reported that voluntary participation in community services leads to an increase in life satisfaction. A person-centered later-life plan with respect to volunteerism could potentially serve two functions. The first function is to help negate stereotypes faced by individuals who are also older adults. The second function is to increase life satisfaction levels by optimizing volunteer activities.

Death and Dying

The need for appropriate death education and bereavement counseling for individuals with intellectual disabilities has been recognized by many in the applied field (e.g.,

Deutsch, 1985; Kaufmann, 1994; Kloeppel & Hollins, 1989; Seltzer, 1985; Sterns & Kultgen, 1989). As in the general population, mortality rates have decreased and life expectancies have increased among individuals with intellectual disabilities (e.g., Factor, 1993). In simple terms, this has created a larger proportion of middle-age individuals who will live into older adulthood (Jacobson, Sutton, & Janicki, 1985). On a more complex level, this results in many more individuals with intellectual disabilities outliving parents and siblings who were their primary caregivers and facing their own mortality alone. In addition, the grief experiences (which accumulate with greater frequency with advancing age) of these individuals will not be limited to death and dying. Other life circumstances that may engender a sense of real loss include staff turnover, age-related declines in physical abilities, retirement, relocation, and issues associated with housing. As previously mentioned, planning related to these life events for most adults with intellectual disabilities does not happen, occurs only with the onset of a family crisis, (e.g., illness or death of a caregiver parent [Essex et al., 1997]), and/or makes no allowances for the individual's preferences (e.g., Ashman, Suttie, & Bramley, 1995; Freedman et al., 1997).

The belief that death should remain a taboo topic when dealing with individuals with intellectual disabilities is still expressed by many (e.g., Luchterhand & Murphy, 1998; Seltzer, 1993; Sterns & Kultgen, 1989). According to Deutsch (1985), reasons for this protectionist stance are numerous and may overlap. For example, family members may feel inadequate or uncomfortable discussing the subject. Parents may be reluctant to address the issues of their own death or may not know how to discuss death openly and appropriately with their son or daughter with a developmental disability. Staff and other caregivers may believe that death experiences are too stressful for individuals with intellectual disabilities whose ability to cope with everyday stressors may be compromised. Staff and caregivers may not see the need to include, educate, or support aging adults with intellectual disabilities who may face death, dying, and loss experiences. A common but erroneous assumption is that individuals with intellectual disabilities do not possess or are not capable of a mature understanding of the concept of death (Yanok & Beifus, 1993).

Research evidence disputes the notion that individuals with intellectual disabilities do not or cannot understand the concept of death (e.g., Kauffman, 1994; Sternlicht, 1980). Although few empirical studies have examined death understanding among individuals with intellectual disabilities (the majority of research consists of anecdotal reports), the overall findings do suggest that varying degrees of death awareness and understanding are present, even among those who have severe impairments (e.g., Lipe-Goodson & Goebel, 1983). However, what is missing from the literature is precise information regarding both the specific levels of comprehension of the concept of death and the factors that influence development of the death concept.

Person-centered later-life planning can be directed toward issues related to death, dying, and loss among older individuals with intellectual disabilities by focusing on education and empowerment. Although it is unclear whether an individual with immature death concepts can be taught a more sophisticated understanding of death, clearly more concrete aspects of death, dying, and loss such as grief, bereavement, and mourning are possible and necessary components. Individuals who receive this information are then better prepared to make informed decisions regarding their own mortality (e.g., type of funeral ceremony, distribution of personal effects) and are better able to recognize and work through grief and mourning experiences (see Chapter 22).

PERSON-CENTERED PLANNING FOR LATER LIFE:
A CURRICULUM FOR OLDER ADULTS WITH MENTAL RETARDATION

Heller et al. (1996) reported on a training program titled Person-Centered Planning for Later Life: A Curriculum for Older Adults with Mental Retardation (Sutton, Heller, Sterns, Factor, & Miklos, 1993), which was designed specifically for older adults with intellectual disabilities and their families and staff. The training curriculum included both a planning content component (later-life planning issues and options) and a planning process component (individual empowerment skills and abilities). Curriculum content included making choices; current and potential living arrangements; work options, including part-time, volunteer, and new work roles; health and wellness; use of leisure and recreational activities; use of informal and formal support; making action plans; participating in service planning meetings; and self-advocacy strategies. Heller et al. (1996) identified six specific goals that a later-life training curriculum should address. It should 1) increase knowledge of later-life options, 2) facilitate greater individual choices and participation in life decisions, 3) facilitate the setting of realistic goals, 4) maintain and increase wellness behaviors, 5) increase the participation in leisure and recreational activities (including community-based activities), 5) increase perceived life satisfaction, and 6) engage staff in greater encouragement of personal choice making among older adults with intellectual disabilities.

Heller and her colleagues (1996) evaluated the effectiveness of the curriculum as it related to the six goals. The evaluation involved 70 adult participants who had an intellectual disability, with ages ranging between 35 and 87 years (mean age, 57 years). One third of the participants lived with their relatives, one third lived in some type of formal residential environment, and the remainder resided in foster homes, lived independently, or lived semi-independently. Most of the participants were employed by local sheltered workshops. Those who were not employed were involved in some type of work activity, day activity, or supported job placement. The participants were divided into two groups: intervention or comparison/control. The adults in the intervention group received the curriculum instruction, which was composed of 17 training modules that incorporated small-group sessions using multiple, explicit learning methods. Each module focused on choices and decision-making skills. Joint involvement of staff, families, and individuals with intellectual disabilities in the decision process was highly encouraged. Participants were assessed both before training (pretests) and 6 months after training (posttests). The pre- and posttest assessments included measures of life satisfaction, leisure activity, social support, choices related to daily living, and curriculum content knowledge.

Heller et al. (1996) noted three significant outcomes. First, individuals who received the training curriculum demonstrated significantly improved knowledge of the skills and concepts contained in the curriculum as compared with the individuals in the comparison group. Specifically, improvements were seen in the topical areas devoted to leisure and recreation, work, retirement, volunteerism, and social support systems. Second, there was a significant increase in the leisure participation (i.e., volunteer activities) for the intervention individuals who lived at home. Third, the service planning meetings of individuals who received the training included significantly greater family involvement, more encouragement of individual participation, and more incorporation of the individual's desires in the written goals.

DEATH, DYING, AND LOSS

Although the training curriculum just described covers many important aspects of later life, it does not address the topic of death, dying, and loss. Appropriate death education among older adults with intellectual disabilities is a widely recognized need but often is not provided (e.g., Deutsch, 1985; Kauffman, 1994; Kloeppel & Hollins, 1989; Luchterhand & Murphy, 1998; Seltzer, 1985; Sterns & Kultgen, 1989). As a consequence, a new module addressing death, dying, and loss has been developed by Sterns, Kennedy, and Sed (2000). This module incorporates the same type of methodology as was used in the original curriculum. Module content addresses death understanding, issues related to loss, bereavement, mourning, grief reactions, death- and loss-related behaviors, and personal futures planning. The curriculum development was assisted by an ongoing research project that examined the impact of several cognitive development and socialization factors on the concept of death among older adults with intellectual disabilities. The findings from this research significantly assisted in fitting curriculum content to an appropriate level of death understanding and allowed for modifications in the curriculum based on individual death comprehension levels.

GOAL SETTING AND ACHIEVEMENT

In the general population, goal setting and achievement are important for effective adaptation to major life events, such as retirement. Payne et al. (1991) demonstrated that high goal–oriented individuals were more outgoing (e.g., sociable) and involved in their retirement process and adjustment than low goal–oriented individuals. It seems that goal-oriented behavior may help retirees maintain a sense of purpose and life direction.

The maintenance of purposeful behavior and directive behavior leads to a continuity in the adjustment to retirement. In a study on goal continuity and retirement adjustment Robbins et al. (1994) found that goal continuity increased life satisfaction in retirement. This study also found that social support increased goal continuity. These results are consistent with those of Payne et al. (1991), who indicated that social support was an important factor for satisfaction in the retirement adjustment. High goal–oriented individuals were found not only to be more sociable but also to believe that they had more social support than low goal–oriented individuals.

Research on goal setting and achievement among adults with intellectual and developmental disabilities is virtually nonexistent. However, goals are an integral part of the helping process. Personal goal setting and assessment can range from work-related goals (e.g., production output) to social behaviors (e.g., appropriate dating and dancing behaviors) to daily living skills (e.g., putting away one's coat, brushing one's hair). To date, the effects of goal setting and achievement on the life satisfaction and adjustment of older adults with lifelong disabilities have not been examined fully.

The relationships among goal continuity, social support, and goal achievement have received minimal attention. In one pertinent study, Heller et al. (1996) revisited 21 of the Later-Life Planning Training participants. These participants were assessed on the degree to which they attained their desired goals, as well as on the barriers and facilitators they encountered when attempting to attain them, some months after their original goal-setting exercises. The adults who were followed up had set 62 personal goals, the most frequent being in the domains of leisure (61%), living arrangements (20%), health and wellness (18%), academics (3%), and work (2%). Three years after setting these goals, approximately 21% of the participants had met or exceeded their goals; 32% had partially met their goals, and 47% had not meet their goals. The goals most likely to have been met were in the areas of leisure and health and wellness.

Heller et al. (1996) observed that support from staff and family was probably the most crucial aspect in helping the adults with intellectual disabilities meet their personal goals. These included organizing activities, accompanying them to the activities, and providing and arranging transportation. In several instances, changes in agency policy helped the participant meet his or her goals. For example, one residential facility changed the dietary menu to accommodate a participant's desire to eat less high-calorie food. When Heller et al. reviewed goal attainment failures, they found that major barriers included the expense of the activity chosen and unavailability of transportation. For example, many of the participants wanted to attend favorite sports events but could not afford to attend them because of the ticket costs. Heller et al. noted that if this process is to be used, once the goals are set and are realistic, agencies should provide help in overcoming barriers that may impede their attainment.

CONCLUSIONS

Person-centered later-life planning for older adults with intellectual disabilities ties together freedom, rights, and responsibilities. Within this framework, older adults with intellectual disabilities are given the knowledge necessary to make informed choices regarding the direction of their lives and the skills needed to implement those choices successfully. Support and guidance from families, caregivers, and staff allow self-expression and a sense of true personal autonomy to develop. Creating opportunities for older adults with intellectual disabilities to learn how to choose and how to evaluate their choices is one of the biggest challenges facing those who work in the intellectual and developmental disabilities services. However, as seen in the general population, the benefits accrued from being an involved, active participant in later-life and retirement planning should be similarly positive for the older adults with intellectual and developmental disabilities who engage in a well-developed planning process.

REFERENCES

Adlin, M. (1993). Health care issues. In E. Sutton, A.R. Factor, B.A. Hawkins, T. Heller, & G.B. Seltzer (Eds.), *Older adults with developmental disabilities: Optimizing choice and change* (pp. 49–60). Baltimore: Paul H. Brookes Publishing Co.

Anderson, D. (1997, April). *Health status and conditions of older adults with mental retardation.* Paper presented at the Eighth International Roundtable on Aging and Intellectual Disabilities of the International Association for the Scientific Study of Intellectual Disabilities, Chicago.

Anderson, D.J., & Kloos, E. (1992). Community integration of older people with developmental disabilities. *Journal on Developmental Disabilities, 1,* 16–26.

Arcand, M. (1996). *Cerebral palsy and aging: A report to adults with cerebral palsy and their families.* Madison: Wisconsin Council on Developmental Disabilities.

Ashman, A.F., Suttie, J.N., & Bramley, J. (1995). Employment, retirement, and elderly persons with an intellectual disability. *Journal of Intellectual Disability Research, 39,* 107–115.

Atchley, R.C. (2000). *Social forces and aging: An introduction to social gerontology* (9th ed.). Belmont, CA: Wadsworth.

Baltes, P.B., & Graf, P. (1996). Psychology aspects of aging: Facts and frontiers. In D. Magnusson (Ed.), *The lifespan development of individuals: Behavioral, neurobiological and psychosocial perspectives* (pp. 427–460). Cambridge, UK: Cambridge University Press.

Brickman, P., Rabinowitz, V., Karuza, J., Coates, D., Cohn, E., & Kidder, L. (1982). Models of helping and coping. *American Psychologist, 37,* 368–384.

Brown, C.M., Bontempo, A., & Turk, M. (1991). *Secondary consequences of cerebral palsy: Adults with cerebral palsy in New York State.* Albany: New York State Office of Mental Retardation and Developmental Disabilities.

Catapano, P.A., Levy, J.M., & Levy, P.H. (1985). Day activity and vocational program services. In M.P. Janicki & H.M. Wisniewski (Eds.), *Aging and developmental disabilities: Issues and approaches* (pp. 305–316). Baltimore: Paul H. Brookes Publishing Co.

Chambre, S.M. (1993). Volunteerism by elders: Past trends and future approaches. *Gerontologist, 33,* 221–228.

Chicoine, B., Rubin, S., & McGuire, D. (1997, April). *Health and psychological findings of the Adult Down Syndrome Center.* Paper presented at the Eighth International Roundtable on Aging and Intellectual Disability of the International Association for the Scientific Study of Intellectual Disabilities, Chicago.

Deutsch, H. (1985). Grief counseling with mentally retarded clients. *Psychiatric Aspects of Mental Retardation Reviews, 4,* 17–20.

Ekerdt, D.J. (1995). Retirement. In G.L. Maddox (Ed.), *The encyclopedia of aging: A comprehensive resource in gerontology and geriatrics* (2nd ed., pp. 819–823). New York: Springer Publishing Co.

Essex, L.E., Seltzer, M.M., & Krauss, M.W. (1997). Residential transitions of adults with mental retardation: Predictors of waiting list use and placement. *American Journal of Mental Retardation, 101,* 613–629.

Eyman, R.K., & Borthwick-Duffy, S.A. (1994). Trends in mortality rates and predictors of mortality. In M.M. Seltzer, M.W. Krauss, & M. Janicki (Eds.), *Life course perspectives on adulthood and old age* (pp. 93–108). Washington, DC: American Association on Mental Retardation.

Factor, A.R. (1989). *A statewide needs assessment of older persons with developmental disabilities in Illinois.* Chicago: University of Illinois at Chicago, Institute for the Study of Developmental Disabilities.

Factor, A.R. (1993). Translating policy into practice. In E. Sutton, A.R. Factor, B.A. Hawkins, T. Heller, & G.B. Seltzer (Eds.), *Older adults with developmental disabilities: Optimizing choice and change* (pp. 257–275). Baltimore: Paul H. Brookes Publishing Co.

Freedman, R.I., Krauss, M.W., & Seltzer, M.M. (1997). Aging parents' residential plans for adult children with mental retardation. *Mental Retardation, 35,* 114–123.

Fujiura, G.T., & Yamaki, K. (1997). An analysis of ethnic variations in developmental disability: Prevalence and household economic status. *Mental Retardation, 35,* 286–294.

Harlow, R.E., & Cantor, N. (1996). Still participating after all these years: A study of life task participation in later life. *Journal of Personality and Social Psychology, 39,* 1235–1249.

Hawkins, B.A. (1993). Leisure participation and life satisfaction of older adults with mental retardation and Down syndrome. In E. Sutton, A.R. Factor, B.A. Hawkins, T. Heller, & G.B. Seltzer (Eds.), *Older adults with developmental disabilities: Optimizing choice and change* (pp. 141–155). Baltimore: Paul H. Brookes Publishing Co.

Hawkins, B.A., & Eklund, S.J. (1994). *Aging-related changes for adults with mental retardation: Final report.* Bloomington, IN/Chicago: Indiana University/Rehabilitation Research and Training Center on Aging with Mental Retardation, Institute on Disability and Human Development, University of Illinois at Chicago.

Hawkins, B.A., & McClean, D. (1993). Delivering services to a diverse aging population: Challenges for the future [Leisure Today—Special Issue]. *Journal of Health, Physical Education, Recreation, and Dance, 64,* 31–34.

Heller, T., & Factor, A.R. (1991). Permanency planning for adults with mental retardation living with family caregivers. *American Journal of Mental Retardation, 96,* 163–176.

Heller, T., & Factor, A.R. (1993). Support systems, well-being, and placement decision-making among older parents and their adult children with developmental disabilities. In E. Sutton, A.R. Factor, T. Heller, B.A. Hawkins, & G.B. Seltzer (Eds.), *Older adults with developmental disabilities: Optimizing choice and change* (pp. 107–122). Baltimore: Paul H. Brookes Publishing Co.

Heller, T., Factor, A.R., Sterns, H.L., & Sutton, E. (1996). Impact of person-centered later life planning training program for older adults with mental retardation. *Journal of Rehabilitation, 16,* 77–83.

Huber, A.M. (1985). Nutrition, aging, and developmental disabilities. In M.P. Janicki & H.M. Wisniewski (Eds.), *Aging and developmental disabilities: Issues and approaches* (pp. 257–268). Baltimore: Paul H. Brookes Publishing Co.

Jacobson, J.W., Sutton, M.S., & Janicki, M.P. (1985). Demography and characteristics of aging and aged mentally retarded persons. In M.P. Janicki & H.M. Wisniewski (Eds.), *Aging and developmental disabilities: Issues and approaches* (pp. 115–142). Baltimore: Paul H. Brookes Publishing Co.

Kauffman, J. (1994). Mourning and mental retardation. *Death Studies, 18,* 257–271.

Kloeppel, D.A., & Hollins, S. (1989). Double handicap: Mental retardation and death in the family. *Death Studies, 13,* 31–38.

Lipe-Goodson, P.S., & Goebel, B.L. (1983). Perception of age and death in mentally retarded adults. *Mental Retardation, 21,* 68–75.

Luchterhand, C.M., & Murphy, N.E. (1998). *Helping adults with mental retardation grieve a death loss.* Philadelphia: Accelerated Development.

Martinson, M.C., & Stone, J.A. (1993). Small-scale community living options serving three or fewer older adults with developmental disabilities. In E. Sutton, A.R. Factor, B.A. Hawkins, T. Heller, & G.B. Seltzer (Eds.), *Older adults with developmental disabilities: Optimizing choice and change* (pp. 223–235). Baltimore: Paul H. Brookes Publishing Co.

McGaughley, M.J., Kiernan, W.E., McNally, L.C., Gilmore, D.S., & Keith, G.R. (1994). *Beyond the workshop: National perspectives on integrated employment.* Boston: Training and Research Institute for People with Disabilities.

Ohio Rev. Code § 5123:2-2-06 (Anderson 1999).

Papalia, D.E., Camp, C.J., & Feldman, R.D. (1996). *Adult development and aging.* New York: McGraw-Hill.

Payne, E.L., Robbins, S.B., & Dougherty, L. (1991). Goal directiveness and older adult adjustment. *Journal of Counseling Psychology, 38,* 302–308.

Rappaport, J. (1987). Terms of empowerment/exemplars of prevention: Toward a theory for community psychology. *American Journal of Community Psychology, 15,* 121–128.

Richardson, V.E. (1993). *Retirement counseling: A handbook for gerontology practitioners.* New York: Springer Publishing Co.

Rimmer, J.H., Braddock, D., & Fujiura, G. (1993). Prevalence of obesity in adults with mental retardation: Implications for health promotion and disease prevention. *Mental Retardation, 31,* 105–110.

Rimmer, J.H., Braddock, D., & Marks, B. (1995). Health characteristics and behaviors of adults with mental retardation residing in three living arrangements. *Research in Developmental Disabilities, 16,* 489–499.

Robbins, S.B., Lee, R.M., & Wann, T.T.H. (1994). Goal continuity as a mediator of early retirement adjustment: Testing a multidimensional model. *Journal of Counseling Psychology, 41,* 18–26.

Salthouse, T.A. (1985). Anticipatory processing in transcription typing. *Journal of Applied Psychology, 70,* 264–271.

Seltzer, G.B. (1985). Selected psychological processes and aging among older developmentally disabled persons. In M.P. Janicki & H.M. Wisniewski (Eds.), *Aging and developmental disabilities: Issues and approaches* (pp. 211–227). Baltimore: Paul H. Brookes Publishing Co.

Seltzer, G.B. (1993). Psychological adjustment in midlife for persons with mental retardation. In E. Sutton, A.R. Factor, B.A. Hawkins, T. Heller, & G.B. Seltzer (Eds.), *Older adults with developmental disabilities: Optimizing choice and change* (pp. 157–184). Baltimore: Paul H. Brookes Publishing Co.

Social Security Act of 1935, PL 74-271, 42 U.S.C. §§ 301 *et seq.*

Social Security Act Amendments of 1983, PL 99-499, 42 U.S.C. §§ 301 *et seq.*

Spirduso, W.W., & McCrae, P.G. (1990). Motor performance and aging. In J.E. Birren & K.W. Schaie (Eds.), *Handbook of the psychology of aging* (3rd ed., pp. 183–200). San Diego: Academic Press.

Sternlicht, M. (1980). The concept of death in preoperational retarded children. *Journal of Genetic Psychology, 137,* 157–164.

Sterns, H.L., Kennedy, E.A., & Sed, C.M. (1999). *Person-centered planning for later life: A curriculum for adults with mental retardation.* Akron, OH/Chicago: University of Akron, Research and Rehabilitation Training Center on Aging with Mental Retardation/University of Illinois at Chicago/Clearinghouse on Aging and Developmental Disabilities.

Sterns, H.L., & Kultgen, P. (1989). *Loss, death, and dying: A person-centered later life planning training program for older adults with mental retardation/developmental disabilities.* Unpublished manuscript, University of Akron, OH.

Sterns, H.L., Kennedy, E.A., & Sed, C.M. (2000). *Person-centered planning for later life: Death and dying: A curriculum for adults with mental retardation.* Chicago/Akron, OH: Clearinghouse on Aging and Development Disabilities, Rehabilitation Research and Training Center on Aging with Mental Retardation, Institute on Disabilities and Human Development, University of Illinois at Chicago and Institute for Life-Span Development and Gerontology, University of Akron.

Sterns, H.L., Matheson, N.S., & Park, L.S.S. (1997). Work and retirement. In K.F. Feraro (Ed.), *Gerontology: Perspectives and issues* (2nd ed., pp. 171–192). New York: Springer Publishing Co.

Sterns, H.L., & Sanders, R.E. (1980). Training and education of the elderly. In R.R. Turner & H.W. Reese (Eds.), *Life-span developmental psychology: Intervention* (pp. 307–330). San Diego: Academic Press.

Sutton, E., Heller, T., Sterns, H.L., Factor, A.R., & Miklos, S. (1993). *Person-centered planning for later life: A curriculum for adults with mental retardation.* Akron, OH/Chicago: University of Akron, Research and Rehabilitation Training Center on Aging with Mental Retardation/University of Illinois at Chicago/Clearinghouse on Aging and Developmental Disabilities.

Sutton, E., Sterns, H.L., & Park, L.S.S. (1991). *Retirement for older persons with developmental disabilities: The realities.* Cincinnati, OH: Research and Rehabilitation Training Center, Consortium on Aging and Developmental Disabilities.

Sutton, E., Sterns, H.L., & Park, L.S.S. (1993). Realities of retirement and pre-retirement planning. In E. Sutton, A.R. Factor, B.A. Hawkins, T. Heller, & G.B. Seltzer (Eds.), *Older adults with developmental disabilities: Optimizing choice and change* (pp. 95–106). Baltimore: Paul H. Brookes Publishing Co.

Sutton, E., Sterns, H.L., & Roberts, R. (1992, Winter). Retirement for older persons with developmental disabilities. *Generations,* 63–64.

Taylor, M.A., & Shore, L.M. (1995). Predictors of planned retirement: An application of Beers' model. *Psychology and Aging, 10,* 76–83.

Yanok, J., & Beifus, J.A. (1993). Communicating about loss and mourning: Death education for individuals with mental retardation. *Mental Retardation, 31,* 144–147.

Zigman, W.B., Seltzer, G.B., & Silverman, W.E. (1994). Behavioral and mental health changes associated with aging. In M.M. Seltzer, M.W. Krauss, & M.P. Janicki (Eds.), *Life course perspectives on adulthood and old age* (pp. 67–91). Washington, DC: American Association on Mental Retardation.

12

Health Promotion and Disease Prevention

Dawna Torres Mughal

People with intellectual disabilities often are more prone to health problems than the rest of the population because of gross obesity, hypertension, epilepsy, cerebral palsy, poor dental health, and an increase in levels of psychiatric morbidity (Evenhuis, 1999; Wells, Turner, Martin, & Roy, 1997). Other risk factors for coronary heart disease and stroke (elevated blood cholesterol level and low level of physical activity) are prevalent among people with intellectual disabilities (Wells et al., 1997).

The coexistence of intellectual disabilities and syndrome-specific morbidity compounds the complexity of health care needs. Feeding problems, polypharmacy, drug–nutrient interactions, metabolic abnormalities, and altered growth patterns put some people with intellectual disabilities at increased nutritional risk (American Dietetic Association [ADA], 1997b). Although older people are heterogeneous in both chronological age and functional status, as a group, because of their age and the physical, physiological, and psychosocial changes associated with aging, they are considered to be at risk for malnutrition and other health problems (White, 1991). Superimposing the multiple risk factors associated with aging on those of lifelong disabilities magnifies the risks for older adults with intellectual disabilities.

Because many older adults with intellectual disabilities are vulnerable, they can benefit from a prevention strategy, such as regular nutrition screening, to detect early warning signs of malnutrition. Nutrition screening, assessment, and intervention can preserve or improve functional status, decrease preventable illnesses and death, reduce health care cost, and enhance quality of life. For adults with intellectual disabilities to become healthier and better able to maintain their independence and dignity is consistent with the shift of the national health objectives to prevention as the foundation of health for all (U.S. Department of Health and Human Services [DHHS], 1996).

This chapter makes a case for nutrition screening as a vital health promotion strategy for older adults with intellectual disabilities who live in community environments. Topics include some of the major nutritional concerns of this group, which can benefit from a systematic program of nutrition screening, assessment, and intervention, and general principles to prevent or alleviate these concerns. Because many people frequently use body weight as a measure of health risk, issues with the application of commonly used "standards" to the assessment of older adults' body weight and obesity are discussed. Nutrition screening tools are included in Appendix A. Service providers, caregivers, and the individuals themselves can adapt the screening tools to their needs and resources. The appendixes also contain a number of other helpful resources. The goal is to encourage providers to integrate nutrition screening into their health promotion programs.

NUTRITION SCREENING AND ASSESSMENT: DEFINITIONS AND PURPOSES

Nutrition Screening

Nutrition screening is the process of identifying characteristics known to be associated with nutritional problems. It includes the collection of relevant data or risk factors and the interpretation of data for intervention or treatment. It determines the need for nutrition assessment (Posthauer et al., 1994).

Nutrition Assessment

Nutrition assessment, completed by a registered dietitian or dietetic technician, is a comprehensive approach to defining nutritional status. It includes the organization and evaluation of medical, nutrition, and medication histories; physical examination; anthropometric measurements; and laboratory data to declare a professional judgment (Posthauer et al., 1994).

Nutrition assessment is one of the two phases of medical nutrition therapy (MNT), defined as the use of nutrition services to treat an injury, illness, or condition. Treatment, the other phase of MNT, includes diet therapy, counseling, or use of specific nutrition supplements. MNT services can be provided in a variety of environments, including group and independent living environments (Posthauer et al., 1994).

NUTRITIONAL CONCERNS OF OLDER ADULTS WITH INTELLECTUAL DISABILITIES

Significant deviations in body weight (overweight or underweight) and unintended weight gain or loss are risk factors for poor nutritional status (Nutrition Screening Initiative [NSI], 1994). Although there are disagreements regarding the standards for assessing these deviations, when viewed in the context of other concurrent risk factors in older adults with intellectual disabilities, these deviations are "red flags" that call for assessment and intervention.

Obesity

Trends   Obesity, commonly known as excess body weight or fat, is a problem among some people with intellectual disabilities. Its clinical definition, using such measures as body mass index (BMI), is discussed later in this section. Results from health screens of 120 adults with intellectual disabilities in one study indicated that this group, as compared with the control group, was heavier as measured by BMI and less active (Wells et al., 1997). According to Wells et al. (1997), this finding confirmed the previously reported high prevalence of obesity among people with intellectual disabilities in both the United Kingdom and the United States. They concluded that people with intellectual disabilities have a higher prevalence of risk factors for coronary artery disease than does the general population. A study (Prasher, 1995) of 201 adults (16–76 years old) with Down syndrome revealed that 31% of the males were overweight and 48% had varying degrees of obesity as assessed by BMI. Gender- and residence-related differences in obesity were noted. A greater proportion of females than males had a more severe form of obesity. The prevalence of obesity was greater for adults living in the community than for those in large congregate care environments. It was highest for individuals who lived at home. The residence-related differences in obesity have implications for health promotion programs for people with intellectual disabilities who live in community environments as a result of deinstitutionalization and proactive inclusion initiatives.

Cause   The cause of obesity involves the interplay of genetic, metabolic, physiological, social, behavioral, and cultural factors (National Heart, Lung, and Blood Institute [NHLBI] Expert Panel, 1998). Whatever its cause may be, obesity results from chronic calorie surplus when intake exceeds expenditure. Diet and physical activity affect this balance. Inappropriate eating practices, limited mobility, lower-than-typical energy needs that are characteristics of certain syndromes (e.g., Prader-Willi syndrome, Down syndrome), and changes in body composition contribute to obesity (American Dietetic Association [ADA], 1997b). Two thirds of the reduction in energy needs in older adults has been attributed to decreased physical activity, and the remainder has been attributed to decreased basal metabolic rates. The decrease in lean body mass and increase in fat stores that occur with aging contribute to a reduction in basal metabolic rates (Ausman & Russell, 1999).

Measures of Obesity   Obesity is assessed using various methods. In clinical practice, two common measures, based on body weight for height, are percentage "ideal," or "desirable," body weight and BMI. Another physical measurement is waist circumference. Only a few weight standards for older adults exist (Ausman & Russell, 1999), and there are no standards for older adults with intellectual disabilities. Methods used to assess appropriate weights of people with Prader-Willi syndrome who live in group homes vary with different assessors (Hoffman, Aultman, & Pipes, 1992). Table 1 (see Appendix C[1]) summarizes three commonly used measures of weight status, acceptable values, and some practical advantages and sources of errors. Although controversies continue regarding the use of height-weight tables for determining optimal weights for older adults and special groups, there is a general agreement that excess weight is a risk factor for heart disease (NHLBI Expert Panel, 1998).

Percentage of Ideal, or Desirable, Body Weight   Calculation of an individual's percentage of ideal, or desirable, body weight (% IBW/DBW) uses reference height–weight tables such as the 1983 Metropolitan Life Insurance Company (MLIC) tables (see Table 2), the average height and weight tables for people age 65 years and older published by Master, Lasser, and Beckman (1960) (see Table 3), the Dietary Guidelines for Americans tables (USDA, 1995) (see Table 4), and another reference discussed here. The values for the 1983 MLIC tables are for young adults 25–59 years old; therefore, they may not be

---

[1]All tables in this chapter appear in Appendix C; all figures appear in Appendix A.

useful for older adults. Ham (1991) suggested using the Master and colleagues (1960) tables, with a note that these weights are average and possibly not ideal or desirable. Ham also recommended for adults age 65–70 years the age-specific tables (for 20- to 69-year-olds) developed by Andres (1985; see also Hazzard, 1999). These age-adjusted tables, which permit weight gain with increasing age, are applicable only to individuals who do not have medical conditions that are exacerbated by greater weight (Andres, 1985; Hazzard, 1999). A sample calculation of % IBW/DBW is provided in Appendix B. People who are 10%–20% heavier than their IBW are classified as overweight, and those who exceed their IBW by more than 20% are classified as obese. It is recommended that, despite the limitations of the tools, weights be measured regularly using consistent procedures (e.g., time of day, amount of clothing, scale) and recorded to assess changes over time (Mitchell & Chernoff, 1999).

Body Mass Index   As Table 1 in Appendix C shows, recommendations for upper and lower BMI cut-offs vary, indicating the need for better guidelines. Despite the variations, there is a general agreement that a BMI of 30 or higher indicates risk for all ages (Dwyer, 1991). The new federal evidence-based clinical guidelines on the identification, evaluation, and treatment of obesity state that BMI should be used to assess both overweight status and obesity (NHLBI Expert Panel, 1998).

There are no specific BMI standards for older adults with intellectual disabilities. The presence of co-morbidities such as hypertension, heart disease, and diabetes, which are exacerbated by overweight, should be considered in determining what is a desirable BMI. Desirable BMI values are individualized so that they are "realistic" or "reasonable" in the context of an individual's condition. For example, for people whose developmental disabilities are associated with low weight, BMI standards used in the diagnosis of anorexia may be more appropriate (Dietetics in Developmental and Psychiatric Disorders [DDPD] and Consulting Dietitians in Health Care Facilities Toolbox, 1998). For people with Prader-Willi syndrome, a realistic BMI for most would be between 27.8 and 31.0 for men and between 27.3 and 32.1 for women. Although these values are still classified as overweight, they are outside the obesity category and can be achieved by most individuals (Hoffman et al., 1992).

Waist Circumference   Positively correlated with abdominal fat content, abdominal girth is an independent predictor of risk factors and morbidity (NHLBI Expert Panel, 1998; Vanitallie, 1998). A larger-than-normal waistline indicates location of excess fat deposit in the upper body, which poses health risks. Waist circumference is an easy and practical tool for older adults with an intellectual disability or caregivers to use. As Table 4 shows, the federal guidelines (NHLBI Expert Panel, 1998) use the sex-specific values to detect increased relative risk (compared with risk at normal weight) for the development of obesity-related risk factors with most adults whose BMI is 25.0–34.9.

Prevention   Because nutrition in childhood and adolescence is a major determinant of obesity and blood cholesterol concentration (McGill, 1997), prevention efforts should begin early in life to avoid obesity. Food plans and physical activity should be individualized to support children's energy and nutrient needs for growth and development and to meet demands imposed by co-existing medical conditions.

Data indicate that the prevalence of overweight is increasing in the United States among children of preschool age from low-income families (Mei et al., 1998). Obesity occurs in children with meningomyelocele (Atencio, Ekvall, Openheimer, & Grace, 1992) and Down syndrome (Luke, Sutton, Schoeller, & Roizen, 1996) and is characteristic of Prader-Willi syndrome. Childhood obesity has been found to be a predictor of obesity in later years, such that 30%–80% of obese children become obese adults (Dietz,

1999). Data from the Bogalusa Heart Study indicated that more than 75% of the children consumed more fat, saturated fat, and cholesterol than is recommended (Nicklas, 1995). A study (Anding, Kubena, McIntosh, & O'Brien, 1996) on male and female adolescents reported that a large proportion of the individuals studied were obese and had cardiovascular fitness that was lower than average. Several had high blood cholesterol levels and hypertension. Given this picture, emphasis on integrating the Dietary Guidelines into school lunch programs and physical activity into schools' health agenda becomes more compelling, particularly for children with disabling conditions. Surveys have shown that many children have positive attitudes and behavior about food, nutrition, and physical activity, but the pursuit and maintenance of a healthy lifestyle should be a family affair (Borra, Schwartz, Spain, & Natchipolsky, 1995). Many children with disabilities, chronic conditions, and special health care needs are included in general education schools and can benefit from efforts of schools to serve healthful foods and promote regular physical activity.

Intervention   Treatment decisions and intervention plans should be based on a complete assessment of individuals and should include a maintenance plan and follow-up. The federal guidelines emphasize the importance of diet therapy, physical activity, and behavioral approaches. Diet therapy is designed to create a 500- to 1,000-kilocalorie deficit per day compared with the usual intake (NHLBI Expert Panel, 1998). For older adults, this goal translates to an allowance of 1,200–1,500 kilocalories for women and 1,500–1,800 kilocalories for men (Jensen & Rogers, 1998). Table 5 lists the nutritional characteristics of the National Cholesterol Education Program Step I diet (DHHS, 1993), the basis for the dietary recommendations of the federal guidelines. A new feature is the recommendation for calcium (1,000–1,500 milligrams per day). The diet is designed to reduce risks for high blood cholesterol and hypertension (Van Horn et al., 1998).

Hoffman and colleagues (1992) reported that, on the average, a 1,000-kilocalorie diet is appropriate for controlling weight of some group home residents with Prader-Willi syndrome when exposed to a controlled diet. Their survey results indicated that one third of the 106 residents had lost excess weight under these diet conditions. When 75% of the recommended dietary allowances (RDAs) have not been met, a vitamin and mineral supplement may be used. Increasing aerobic exercise and controlling access to food should be part of the weight control program. Guidelines for estimating calorie intake have been developed for certain syndromes. For example, for adults with Down syndrome, the formula is 40.9 kilocalories per inch for males and 36.3 kilocalories/inch for females (DDPD and Consulting Dietitians in Health Care Facilities Toolbox, 1998). For individuals with Prader-Willi syndrome, energy intake of 7–8 kilocalories per centimeter is recommended for weight loss and 10–14 kilocalories per centimeter is recommended for weight maintenance (Hoffman et al., 1992). A modest, initial weight loss of 10% of the baseline weight (or 1- to 2-pound weight loss per week in 6 months) is reasonable and achievable (NHLBI Expert Panel, 1998). The weight loss should be maintained for at least 6 months so that it becomes the usual body weight, and further weight loss can be attempted (Meisler & St. Jeor, 1996).

Reduced-calorie diets may be inadequate in nutrients and can cause nutrient deficiencies in older adults (NHLBI Expert Panel, 1998). Education regarding nutrition and monitoring weight changes to ensure that the weight loss is not due to medical conditions can help minimize the potential risks. Federal guidelines are less certain about the importance of treating overweight condition in older adults than in younger individuals. The older adults' motivation, the presence of obesity-related diseases, and the risks for a cardiovascular event should be evaluated before making a clinical decision of whether to treat (NHLBI Expert Panel, 1998). Medications should be reviewed for their effects on appetite and food intake. Psychotropic medications and alcohol abuse can alter appetite and food intake, which can cause unwanted weight gain or loss.

Obese hypertensive older adults with an intellectual disability may benefit from a nonpharmacologic approach. Results of the multicenter Trial of Nonpharmacologic Interventions on the Elderly (TONE) (Whelton et al., 1998) indicated that weight loss, through calorie reduction and physical exercise, reduced blood pressure and the use of medication in obese hypertensive participants. Hypertension affects an estimated 8%–18% of adults globally and approximately 50 million (one in four adults) in the United States (World Health Organization [WHO], 1995) and is prevalent in adults with intellectual disabilities (Wells et al., 1997). From 1988 to 1991, hypertension affected 54% of older adults ages 65–74 years in the United States who were not living in institutions (DHHS, 1994). It is a major contributor to cardiovascular diseases and stroke. Stroke is a leading cause of disability and expensive rehabilitation in middle-age and older adults (WHO, 1995).

Regular physical activity is an important part not only of weight-reduction programs but also of everyday living. It enhances both physical and psychosocial well-being. Federal guidelines recommend daily cumulative physical activity of 30 minutes or more of moderate-intensity activity on most and preferably all days. Everyday activities such as housecleaning, climbing stairs, swimming, gardening, and walking can be a part of the exercise program (NHLBI Expert Panel, 1998). Many frail older adults may be unable to achieve the recommended physical activity level. However, strength training can benefit them. Fiatarone et al. (1994) demonstrated that high-intensity, progressive strength training of the hip and knee extensors improved muscle strength and size in frail, older adults. These muscles were chosen for training because they affect functional mobility. The exercise group had improved habitual gait, velocity, stair climbing ability, and overall level of physical activity. The authors concluded that exercise training corrects muscle disuse and significantly improves functional mobility and overall activity. Evans and Cyr-Campbell (1997) observed similar results among 10 older adults who were frail and lived in institutions (mean age 90 ± 3 years) after 8 weeks of progressive resistance training. In this type of training, the resistance against which a muscle generates force is increased over time. It involves a few muscle contractions against a heavy load. The participants increased muscle strength by almost 180% and muscle size by 11%. Equipment for strength training can be simple weight-lifting devices such as Velcro-strapped wrist and ankle bags filled with sand or lead shot, or heavy household objects such as plastic milk jugs filled with water or gravel or food cans of various sizes. With proper training, older adults can use these devices in a strength training program that is tailored to their individual needs and capacities.

Anecdotal notes from health screens of adults with intellectual disabilities indicated that many individuals can follow dietary advice and have significant weight loss and can maintain the improvements for 6–9 months after stabilization, but this is not without a challenge. Wells and colleagues (1997) noted that physical activity seemed to be a difficult task; in their study, a smaller proportion (51.8%) of the individuals had done moderate, intense physical activity as compared with the control group (93.5%). Furthermore, Janicki and colleagues (1999) observed low rates of self-initiated physical exercise among adults with intellectual disabilities who were living in group homes.

To improve adherence to a physical activity program, Singh Fiatarone (1999) strongly recommended a comprehensive geriatric exercise prescription that includes the purpose of the exercise, dose, frequency, potential side effects, alternatives, and any interactions with nutritional or pharmaceutical preparations that the person is taking. Because the exercise needs of most aging adults are complex, she recommended referral to a qualified fitness instructor or a physical therapist and emphasized the importance of safety and medical risk assessment.

Maintenance Phase   Protocol for ensuring weight loss maintenance over time should be a part of the intervention program. The desired dietary changes and clinical outcomes achieved at immediate postintervention tend to return to baseline level when the participants have been away from the intervention program (Mughal, 1992). Monitoring, follow-up, and other social support help individuals maintain desired behavior changes (Mughal, 1992; NHLBI Expert Panel, 1998).

Commentary

Obesity and its associated morbidity affect the longevity and quality of life of older adults with intellectual disabilities perhaps more profoundly than they do the general population. Obesity further limits ambulation and exacerbates musculoskeletal disorders. Current federal guidelines use BMI and waist circumference measurements to identify obesity. For % IBW, height–weight tables for older adults may be used as references. Weight should not be based on self-reports because people tend to under report their weight (DHHS, 1996). All of these methods have limitations and should be considered in the context of other relevant information when setting an appropriate weight goal with the person. Despite their limitations, they are practical and convenient to use in a community environment. The intervention method of choice is nonpharmacologic, consisting of a therapeutic diet, physical activity, and behavioral approaches. Its success requires the person's motivation and an interdisciplinary effort of health professionals. There are no specific guidelines for special groups. For older adults with intellectual disabilities who are unable to achieve weight loss, prevention of further weight gain may be an appropriate goal. Follow-up, monitoring, and social support help the person achieve and maintain the desired outcome.

Involuntary Weight Loss and Underweight Condition

Percentage of Usual Body Weight   Significant unwanted weight loss is an important indicator of risk for malnutrition (White, Ham, Lipschitz, Dwyer, & Wellman, 1991). Significant weight loss is defined as 5% or more of usual body weight in 1 month, 7.5% or more in 3 months, or 10% or more in 6 months or involuntary weight loss of 10 pounds in 6 months (NSI, 1994). Many older adults with intellectual disabilities may not fit the standard for ideal or desirable weight. In the absence of medical complications, their own usual body weight may be the better standard for them, and maintaining a stable weight over a period of 6 months or more may be a more appropriate goal (Niedert, 1998).

Low Body Weight   Like excess weight, low weight for height increases risks for diseases and mortality (Andres, 1985; Hazzard, 1999; Meisler & St. Jeor, 1996). An older person who is 20% less than (or more than) desirable weight for height at a given age (considering loss of height as a result of vertebral collapse, kyphosis, or deformity) exhibits one of the indicators of poor nutritional status (White et al., 1991). Gray-Donald (1995) noted that older people in the lowest 15th percentile of the weight-for-height distribution have a higher mortality rate than do people of normal weight. Older people with the best functional status are in the middle weight-for-height distribution, the 15th–85th percentiles. Underweight not only affects functional status and general health but also may be related to the incidence of hip fracture. Many older adults with intellectual disabilities, especially at an advanced age, are likely to be underweight and undernourished.

Weight loss results when food intake chronically does not meet energy needs. Physiological stress imposed by infection and certain diseases increases energy requirement that the vulnerable person, because of poor food intake, may not be able to meet. Changes in taste and smell that occur with aging (Schiffman & Covey, 1984) as well as chewing and swallowing problems, inability to buy and prepare foods, diseases, medications, and neurologic and sensory impairments can affect food intake. Weight loss is frequently seen in people with depression, Parkinson's disease, Alzheimer's disease, dementia, and cerebral palsy. Refusal to eat among older adults who live in institutional and community care environments has been reported to be widespread (Marcus & Berry, 1998). Among nursing facility residents, weight loss can be associated with food intake that is half of or less than the food served during the previous 7 days, refusal of half or less of food replacement during the previous 7 days, and altered ability or desire to eat. Chewing problems, broken or missing teeth, swallowing problems, impaired vision, and reduced functional ability can alter the capacity or the desire to eat (Gilmore, Robinson, Posthauer, & Raymond, 1995).

Prevention Factors that cause involuntary weight loss should be identified and corrected to prevent decline in health and functional status. Providing the energy and nutrient needs of older adults who have multiple and concurrent risk factors is a challenge to caregivers. It requires working with qualified health professionals in the community to plan and implement the most appropriate intervention. Providing at meal- and snacktimes calorie- and nutrient-dense foods that meet the person's food preferences and tolerance, allowing adequate time for meals, promoting socialization, and providing encouragement and social support can increase food intake. Studies have shown that nutrition rehabilitation programs can help increase energy intake and weight of people with severe physical and developmental disabilities. If other activities are planned so that they do not interfere with snacktime, frequent snacks can also boost calorie intake (Hogan & Evers, 1997).

Loss of Height

Except for waist circumference, all of the measurements discussed so far require the appraisal of height. In many environments, height is often measured perfunctorily or not at all or is based on self-report. Height needs better attention and periodic assessment because loss of height is a sign of osteoporosis and may precede symptomatic osteoporosis by several years (Ham, 1991). Guidelines for estimating the height of a person who cannot stand straight are available (Chumlea, Roch, & Mukerjee, 1984; Niedert, 1998), as are guidelines for adjusting body weight for missing body parts (in cases of amputations) and for paralysis and quadriplegia (Niedert, 1998). Weight and height measurements are important for estimating the person's energy, protein, and fluid needs for maintenance or repletion. Measurement errors yield incorrect calculations and, therefore, inappropriate provision of energy and nutrients.

Commentary

Significant unwanted weight loss and low body weight for height are risk factors for poor nutritional status. They can be measured easily by family members or caregivers. Height should be measured as accurately as possible because a loss in height is an early sign of osteoporosis. Detecting these risk factors requires obtaining baseline and monitoring it for changes over time. Significant unintentional weight loss should be avoided in vulnerable individuals. Nutrition screening can identify people who are at risk for weight loss, help pinpoint the causes, and facilitate further assessment and intervention before serious health problems occur. Although objective measures and numbers are important, the key factors of seeing and hearing older adults with intellectual disabilities should not be overlooked. Many nutritional deficiencies have physical manifestations that can be detected by regular visual assessment.

Oral Health

Poor oral health, because it adversely affects food intake, is a risk factor for poor nutritional status (NSI, 1994). Oral problems include periodontal disease, taste dysfunction, dry mouth, gum hyperplasia, dental caries, loss of teeth, oral lesions, and orofacial pain. Oral health affects the type or the amount of foods consumed and therefore energy and nutrient intake. A national dental survey in 1987 showed that approximately 41% of older adults were edentulous, 88% had gingival recession, and 95% had periodontal attachment loss (Martin, 1999). Poor oral health is a global problem. The World Health Organization (1995) stated that 1.9 billion people had dental caries, 163 million had periodontal disease, and 13 million were edentulous. People with intellectual disabilities seem to be more susceptible to dental caries and gum diseases (Patterson & Ekvall, 1993). Many neuropsychiatric medications cause xerostomia (dry mouth), taste alteration, and gum hyperplasia. Oral health problems diminish diet quality and quantity as well as enjoyment of foods. A pattern of poor oral hygiene also contributes to periodontal disease and dental caries. For more information, see Chapter 18.

Prevention   As with other healthful practices, good oral health practices should start in early childhood. Good oral hygiene, avoidance of sweets, regular dental examinations, review of medications, and a well-balanced diet can help maintain good oral health. For existing problems, eating a balanced diet modified for appropriate texture and consistency can improve nutrient intake. Tender meats, fish, and poultry, dairy products, soft fruits and vegetables, and a variety of choices from the grain group can be included easily in a day's meals. Dietary modifications depend on specific problems. For example, dry mouth, taste changes, and sore mouth call for specific changes to counteract these conditions.

Dysphagia and Risk for Aspiration

Dysphagia, or difficulty in swallowing, occurs more often with aging and with neurologic impairments. It is not a disease itself but is caused by an underlying problem. Causes include stroke, multiple sclerosis, Alzheimer's disease, and other types of dementia. Uncorrected, it causes weight loss and contributes to aspiration pneumonia (Evans, White, Wood, Hood, & Bailey, 1998). Dysphagia and risk for aspiration should be evaluated by professionals with special training. Feeding and dietary interventions should be planned collaboratively with a qualified dietetics professional. In general, nutrition management includes modifying the texture and consistency of foods and liquids in order to promote safe swallowing, correcting other conditions (e.g., hiatal hernia, obesity) that increase the risk of gastroesophageal reflux, adjusting the timing and volume of meals and liquids to prevent gastroesophageal reflux, and avoiding foods that increase risk for choking and aspiration.

Dehydration

Because of age-related decline in thirst drive and reduced response to fluid deprivation, dehydration is common among older adults (Lipschitz, 1992). Dehydration also is common among people with intellectual disabilities, especially those who are frail, dependent on caregivers, and have cognitive and functional status impairments. People who are dependent on caregivers may be less likely to receive adequate fluids. The number and frequency of medications influence the amount of fluid the residents obtain during nonmeal feedings. Dehydration is a risk factor for pressure ulcers, especially among individuals who are immobile, undernourished, and underweight (Chidester & Spangler, 1997). It also can cause confusion and disorientation (Lipschitz, 1992). Because dehydration is life threatening, it should be prevented at all times. Fluid comes not only from water, beverages, and food but also from the individual's metabolic processing of food. Many conditions can affect water balance. Congestive heart failure and renal function impairment can cause fluid retention, and vomiting, diarrhea, fever, infection, and other physiologic stresses can increase fluid loss (Lipschitz, 1992). Also, diuretic therapy can induce abnormal fluid losses.

Prevention   A medical nutrition therapy protocol is available for fluid maintenance or prevention of dehydration (Vogelzang, 1999). Making water accessible in the living space and using cues or reminders can help ensure sufficient fluid intake. Caregivers should be alert to physical signs of dehydration. These include sunken eyes, hollow cheeks, stunned facial expression, dry mucous membranes, deep, gasping respiration, weak, rapid pulse, and skin that lacks elasticity (Whitney, Cataldo, & Rolfes, 1998). In general, water requirement is 30 milliliters per kilogram of body weight or 1 milliliter per kilocalorie consumed (Lipschitz, 1992). If the caloric intake of older adults with intellectual disabilities who are underweight is low, then fluid recommendation that is based on body weight or caloric intake will be unrealistically low. A fluid intake of 1,500–2,000 milliliters per day (i.e., six to eight 8-ounce glasses) is adequate for most older adults in most situations (Chidester & Spangler, 1997). A better way to estimate an individual's fluid needs is to use the following formula: 100 milliliters per kilogram for the first 10 kilograms of actual body weight, 50 milliliters per kilogram for the next 10 kilograms of actual body weight, and 15 milliliters per kilogram for the remaining kilograms of actual body weight (Chidester & Spangler, 1997; Lensen, 1998). This formula provides a minimum of 1,500 milliliters even for older adults with low body weight and adjusts for high weight, reflecting possible obesity (for increased fat mass in obesity, reduce the percentage of water content in the body composition) (Chidester & Spangler, 1997). Caregivers should monitor fluid intake and offer sufficient fluids to ensure adequate hydration.

Constipation

It is widely recognized that constipation is prevalent in older adults with intellectual disabilities (DDPD and Consulting Dietitians in Health Care Facilities Toolbox, 1998). The most common gastrointestinal complaint in the United States, it leads to approximately 2 million physician visits annually (Niedert, 1998). Constipation can be caused by low intake of food, fiber, or fluid, lack of physical activity; lack of regular schedule for elimination, medications, chronic laxative use, and hypothyroidism. Medications that are associated with constipation include antipsychotics (Haldol), anticonvulsants, and antidepressants (Tofranil) (Isaacs et al., 1997). The causes of constipation should be identified to rule out diseases such as diverticular disease and colon cancer, which can cause bowel habit changes. Chronic constipation can cause dependence on laxatives, fecal impaction, and obstruction. Chronic use of certain laxatives can cause fluid and electrolyte losses (Niedert, 1998).

Prevention   The best management of constipation is a high-fiber diet, liberal fluid intake, increased physical activity, and maintenance of a regular elimination schedule

(Niedert, 1998). Daily meals should contain 20–35 grams of fiber (ADA, 1997a). Fiber-rich fruits and vegetables and whole grain breads and cereals, especially wheat bran, should be emphasized. Fiber intake should be increased gradually to avoid gastrointestinal discomfort, and plenty of fluids should be consumed to soften the fiber as it passes through the intestinal tract (Whitney et al., 1998). Prunes and prune juice contain dihydroxyphenyl isatin, a natural laxative. This and other nonpharmacologic treatments should be tried before resorting to medications. To relieve resistant constipation, laxatives may be necessary. Acceptable bulking agents include cellulose, cellulose derivatives, and psyllium. A stool softener also may be used (Mahan & Escott-Stump, 1996).

Pressure Ulcers

Pressure ulcers are chronic wounds that occur on areas where pressure, shear, or friction impedes blood and nutrient supply, causing damage to the muscle and subcutaneous tissue (Fox, 1997). The best treatment for pressure ulcer is prevention. Older adults with intellectual disabilities who have pressure ulcers are at increased risk for medical complication and death. Prevention includes maintaining good nutritional status and hydration, conducting systematic skin inspection, avoiding pressures on bony prominences, improving mobility, and screening for nutritional and other preventable risk factors. Immobility or limited physical activity, fecal incontinence, altered mental status, older age, lower blood pressure, and higher body temperature are non-nutritional risk factors. Nutritional factors include inadequate calorie and protein intake, a poor score on the Braden Scale (Breslow & Bergstrom, 1994; see also Braden & Bergstrom, 1988, for details of the Braden Scale) (a risk assessment instrument that includes a nutrition component), possibly low serum albumin value, dehydration, and anemia (Niedert, 1998). Antikinetic drugs, such as antidepressants and sleeping pills, may also contribute to pressure ulcer development (Niedert, 1998). Nutrition therapy for pressure ulcers includes a diet high in protein (1.2 grams of protein per kilogram of actual body weight) and calories (1.5 times the energy required based on weight goal). It also includes adequate fluid and supplementation of vitamin C (120 milligrams or more daily) and zinc (15 milligrams daily) (Gilmore et al., 1995). The stage of the ulcer and the person's medical condition affect estimated needs. The goal of medical nutrition therapy is to promote healing, prevent infection, and maintain good nutritional status.

Commentary

Poor oral health, chewing and swallowing problems, dehydration, constipation, and pressure ulcers are risk factors for poor nutritional status. Eating problems adversely affect food intake and hydration, and dehydration and poor nutritional status predispose older adults with intellectual disabilities to the development of pressure ulcers. Pressure ulcer is a hypermetabolic condition which imposes high demand on energy and nutrient reserves. It is preventable.

Osteoporosis

Osteoporosis, which affects more than 25 million people in the United States, is the major underlying cause of bone fractures in postmenopausal women and older adults (National Institutes of Health, 1994). A global problem, it affected one in three women older than 50 years and caused approximately 1.7 million hip fractures in 1990 throughout the world (WHO, 1995). Osteoporosis is a reduction in bone mineral mass, which makes bones fragile. The bones break easily with a moderate degree of stress (Krall & Dawson-Hughes, 1999). Osteoporosis has been reported to have increased prevalence in community populations of young adults with intellectual disabilities (Center, Beange, & McElduff, 1998). Risk factors associated with low bone density in this group include small body size, hypogonadism, presence of Down syndrome in both males and females, low physical activity, and a high serum phosphate level in females (Center et al., 1998). Aging exacerbates this problem among people with intellectual disabilities, especially postmenopausal women. Loss of endogenous estrogen at menopause causes the initial acceleration of bone loss (Marcus, 1999). Bone fractures in people with intellectual disabilities are linked to the use of antiepileptic drugs, such as phenobarbital, phenytoin, and carbamazepine. Sun exposure, vitamin D content of the diet, and physical activity are also related to the incidence of fractures (Tohill, 1997). Morbidity after bone fractures is serious among the general aging population and is more serious among older adults with intellectual disabilities. Therefore, reducing the risk for developing osteoporosis is important. Table 6 lists some of the major risk factors for the development of osteoporosis, illustrating the multifactorial cause of this crippling disease and the need for comprehensive prevention and management.

Prevention   Preventing osteoporosis requires consideration of all factors (genetics, hormones, diet, and physical activity) that affect bone health (Marcus, 1999). Although many nutrients function as bone builders, the link between calcium (and its regulator, vitamin D) and bone health is so strong that these two nutrients are emphasized. Prevention should start at the pubertal growth spurt, when 60% of bone mass is deposited. Dietary calcium has greater influence on bone mass during this period than at any other time in life. When calcium nutritional status is low at this time, women do not seem to recover the loss (Marcus, 1999). Luke et al. (1995) indicated that half of the prepubescent children with Down syndrome who participated in their study had calcium intake of less than 80% of the RDA, and Unonu and Johnson (1992) noted that preschool African American children with Down syndrome ate inadequate amounts of dairy foods. These early dietary habits clearly set the stage for a health problem that brutally expresses itself in old age. If older adults with intellectual disabilities are unable to obtain calcium and vitamin D from diet alone, then they may benefit from supplementation to meet the recommended adequate intake (AI). The AI for calcium is 1,200 milligrams for older adults ages 51–70 years and older than 70 years, and the value for vitamin D is 400 international units (IU) for 51- to 70-year-olds and 600 IU for those older than 70 years (Yates, Schlicker, & Suitor, 1998). The benefit of regular weight-bearing physical activity to bone health is well documented (Marcus, 1999) and already has been discussed. Regular physical activity, individualized to a child's ability, should begin early in life. Results of a study of a large group of children with developmental disabilities who were receiving anticonvulsant therapy indicated that nonambulatory status, not anticonvulsant medication use, contributed significantly to the abnormalities in calcium, vitamin D, and bone status (Baer et al., 1997).

Besides adequate calcium and vitamin D status and regular weight-bearing exercise, sun exposure can help build healthy bones. Hollick (1999) recommended that older adults have 5–30 minutes of exposure of the hands, forearms, and face three times per week to a suberythemal amount of sunshine in the morning and afternoon during spring, summer, and fall. This exposure allows storage of extra vitamin D in fat for the winter months. He also recommended that older people protect themselves from the damaging effects of chronic exposure to sunlight by applying a sunscreen after short exposure to sunlight. The sunscreen should have a protection factor of at least SPF-15.

Commentary

Although osteoporosis has a multifactorial cause, older adults with intellectual disabilities can reduce their risk by maintaining good vitamin D and calcium status, participating in regular physical activity, having adequate energy intake to provide sufficient nutrients, maintaining healthy body weight to avoid frailty and thinness, and being subject to medication review to identify and monitor adverse effects of drugs on calcium and vitamin D. Postmenopausal women may benefit from estrogen replacement therapy.

Drug and Nutrient Interactions

It is widely recognized that older adults and people with intellectual disabilities, as a group, are heavy users of concurrent prescription and nonprescription medications. Age-related changes in the gastrointestinal tract, body composition, and liver and kidney functions can alter drug absorption, distribution, metabolism, and excretion of pharmacokinetics. They also can affect the sensitivity of target organs to the drugs or pharmacodynamics (Hemle, 1997). These changes increase older people's risks for adverse drug reactions. Poor nutritional status and concurrent use of multiple medications, especially on a long-term basis, further increase these risks. Adverse reactions include nutrient deficiency, toxicity, reduced drug efficacy, and changes in body weight (Blumberg & Couris, 1999). Many older adults with intellectual disabilities, because they use many medications concurrently on a long-term basis, are a high-risk group for adverse drug-drug and drug-nutrient interactions.

Table 7 shows selected neuropsychiatric medications and their effects on food intake, the gastrointestinal tract, and certain nutrients. Trying a nonpharmacologic approach first, if possible, and monitoring medications for adverse reactions and appropriate use are essential to the nutritional status and well-being of older adults with intellectual disabilities.

Commentary

Nutrition education fosters behavior change and is one of the factors that affect food choices (Porter et al., 1998). There are no studies on the nutrition knowledge of older people with intellectual disabilities or of their family members and caregivers. Schlenker (1998) noted that many older adults have limited knowledge of how food affects good health. For example, study participants (with type 2 diabetes) who participated in an education program for diabetes management had low preintervention mean diet knowledge scores despite the fact that the majority of them had had diabetes for several years (Mughal, 1992).

The barrage of conflicting nutrition messages from a variety of sources, including the media, family and friends, fitness professionals, and commercial operations, can confuse anyone and can be more confusing to older adults, especially those with intellectual disabilities. Older adults are concerned about their health and are vulnerable to food fads and quackery. Seeking a cure for various maladies, as a group, they are heavy users of vitamin and mineral supplements. For example, older men and women were reported to take 10 times the RDA of vitamin A (Ausman & Russell, 1999), yet it is known that excessive intake of vitamins A and D is toxic.

Older adults with intellectual disabilities and their caregivers can benefit from nutrition education tailored to their needs and abilities by qualified dietetics professionals. This education should focus on positive messages and be culturally relevant to the people's needs. Most people prefer messages that focus on what they should eat rather than on what they should not eat. Education programs tend to be more successful when they set behavior change as a goal, teach strategies for behavior changes, attempt to build health-enhancing environments, and include active involvement of both the person and the community (Porter et al., 1998). A needs assessment study of staff and residents in community-based homes for people with developmental disabilities suggested that helpful teaching methods for consumer education include ongoing one-to-one training and support, coincidental training, use of pictures and posters, and a reward program (Walter, Cohen, & Swicker, 1997).

Psychosocial factors influence food intake and nutritional status. Social isolation, which can be caused by health problems and disability, living arrangements, income or poverty, and inappropriate food choices that may be associated with poor nutrition knowledge, should be a part of the nutrition screening process. Many factors affect nutritional status, and malnutrition has many causes. Integration of the biopsychosocial factors can help service providers see the total picture of the human being. The picture portrays needs perhaps so complex that they can overwhelm the caregivers' and the providers' resources and sense of priorities. We propose that as a prevention strategy, regular nutrition screening and assessment and referral to appropriate health care and community resources become one of the top priorities. Malnutrition is expensive in terms of health care cost and human suffering. It is preventable.

REFERENCES

American Dietetic Association (ADA). (1997a). Position of the American Dietetic Association: Health implications of fiber. *Journal of the American Dietetic Association, 97,* 1157–1159.

American Dietetic Association (ADA). (1997b). Position of the American Dietetic Association: Nutrition in comprehensive program planning for persons with developmental disabilities. *Journal of the American Dietetic Association, 97,* 189–193.

Anding, J.D., Kubena, K.S., McIntosh, A., & O'Brien, B. (1996). Blood lipids, cardiovascular risks, obesity, and blood pressure: The presence of potential coronary heart disease risk factors in adolescents. *Journal of the American Dietetic Association, 96,* 238–242.

Andres, R. (1985). Mortality and obesity: The rationale for age-specific height-weight tables. In R. Andres, E.L. Bierman, & W.R. Hazzard (Eds.), *Principles of geriatric medicine* (pp. 311–318). New York: McGraw-Hill.

Atencio, P.L.F., Ekvall, S.W., Openheimer, S. & Grace, E. (1992). Effect of level of lesion and quality of ambulation on growth charts measurements in children with myelomeningocele: A pilot study. *Journal of the American Dietetic Association, 92,* 858–861.

Ausman, L.M., & Russell, R. (1999). Nutrition in the elderly. In M.E. Shils, J.A. Olson, M. Shike, & A.C. Cross (Eds.), *Modern nutrition in health and disease* (9th ed., pp. 770–780). Baltimore: Williams & Wilkins.

Baer, M.T., Kozkowski, B.W., Byler, E.M., Trahms, C.M., Taylor, M.L., & Hogan, M.P. (1997). Vitamin D, calcium, and bone status in children with developmental delay in relation to anticonvulsant use and ambulatory status. *American Journal of Clinical Nutrition, 65,* 1042–1051.

Blumberg, J.B., & Couris, R. (1999). Pharmacology, nutrition, and the elderly: Interactions and implications. In R. Chernoff (Ed.), *Geriatric nutrition: The health professional's handbook* (2nd ed., pp. 342–365). Gaithersburg, MD: Aspen Publishers.

Borra, S.T., Schwartz, N.E., Spain, C.G., & Natchipolsky, N.M. (1995). Food, physical activity, and fun: Inspiring America's kids to more healthful lifestyles. *Journal of the American Dietetic Association, 95,* 816–812.

Braden, B., & Bergstrom, N. (1998). Braden Scale. In K.C. Niedert (Ed.), *Nutrition care of the older adult: A handbook for dietetics professionals working throughout the continuum of care* (pp. 168–169). Chicago: American Dietetic Association.

Breslow, R.A., & Bergstrom, N. (1994). Nutritional prediction of pressure ulcers. *Journal of the American Dietetic Association, 94*, 1301–1304.

Center J., Beange, H., & McElduff, A. (1998). People with mental retardation have an increased risk of osteoporosis: A population study. *American Journal on Mental Retardation, 103*, 19–28.

Chidester, J.C., & Spangler, A. (1997). Fluid intake in institutionalized elderly. *Journal of the American Dietetic Association, 97*, 23–28.

Chumlea, W.C., Roch, A.F., & Mukerjee, D. (1984). *Nutritional assessment of the elderly through anthropometrics*. Columbus, OH: Ross Laboratories.

Committee on Diet and Health. (1989). *Diet and health: Implications for reducing chronic disease risks*. Washington, DC: National Academy Press.

Dietetics in Developmental and Psychiatric Disorders (DDPD) and Consulting Dietitians in Health Care Facilities Toolbox. (1998). A resource for dietetics professionals working with adults with developmental disorders/mental retardation in community-based programs. Chicago: Dietetic Practice Groups of the American Dietetic Association.

Dietz, W.H. (1999). Childhood obesity. In M.E. Shils, J.A. Olson, M. Shike, & A.C. Ross (Eds.), *Modern nutrition in health and disease* (9th ed., pp. 869–878). Baltimore: Williams & Wilkins.

Dwyer, J.T. (1991). *Screening older Americans' nutritional health: Current practices and future possibilities*. Washington, DC: Nutrition Screening Initiative.

Evans, W.B., White, J.L., Jr., Wood, S.D., Hood, S.B., & Bailey, M.B. (1998). Managing dysphagia: Fundamentals of primary care. *Clinical Reviews, 8*, 47–64, 69.

Evans, W.J., & Cyr-Campbell, D. (1997). Nutrition, exercise, and healthy aging. *Journal of the American Dietetic Association, 97*, 632–638.

Evenhuis, H. (1999). Associated medical aspects. In M.P. Janicki & A.J. Dalton (Eds.), *Dementia, aging, and intellectual disabilities: A handbook* (pp. 103–122). Philadelphia: Taylor & Francis.

Fiatarone, M.A., O'Neill, E.F., Ryan, N.D., Clements, K.M., Solares, G.R., Nelson, M.E., Roberts, S.B., Kehayias, J.J., Lipsitz, L.A., & Evans, W.J. (1994). Exercise training and nutritional supplementation for physical frailty in very elderly people. *New England Journal of Medicine, 330*(25), 1769–1775.

Fox, G.L. (1997). Pressure ulcers: An update for the primary care provider. *Physician Assistant, 21*, 80–89, 93–96, 101–104.

Gilmore, S.A., Robinson, G., Posthauer, M.E., & Raymond J. (1995). Clinical indicators associated with unintended weight loss and pressure ulcers in elderly residents of nursing facilities. *Journal of the American Dietetic Association, 95*, 984–992.

Gray-Donald, K. (1995). The frail elderly: Meeting the nutritional challenge. *Journal of the American Dietetic Association, 95*, 538–540.

Guigoz, Y., Vellas, B., & Garry, P.J. (1994). Nutritional assessment: A practical assessment tool for grading the nutritional state of elderly patients. *Facts and Research in Gerontology, 4*(Suppl. 2), 15–59.

Ham, R.J. (1991). Indicators of poor nutritional status in older Americans. In *Report of the nutrition screening: I. Toward a common view* (pp. 37–67). Washington, DC: Nutrition Screening Initiative.

Hazzard, W.R. (Ed.). (1999). *Principles of geriatric medicine and gerontology* (4th ed.). New York: McGraw-Hill.

Heaney, R. (1999). Bone biology in health and disease. In M.E. Shils, J.A. Olson, M. Shike, & A.C. Ross (Eds.), *Modern nutrition in health and disease* (9th ed., pp. 1379–1388). Baltimore: Williams & Wilkins.

Hemle K. (1997). Drug therapy in the elderly. *Physician Assistant, 21*, 34, 37–44, 48–56, 59–65.

Hoffman, C.J., Aultman, D., & Pipes, P. (1992). A nutrition survey of recommendations for individuals with Prader-Willi syndrome who live in group homes. *Journal of the American Dietetic Association, 92*, 823–830.

Hogan, S.E., & Evers, S.E. (1997). A nutritional rehabilitation program for persons with severe physical and developmental disabilities. *Journal of the American Dietetic Association, 97*, 162–166.

Hollick, M.F. (1999). Vitamin D. In M.E. Shils, J.A. Olson, M. Shike, & A.C. Ross (Eds.), *Modern nutrition in health and disease* (9th ed., pp. 329–342). Baltimore: Williams & Wilkins.

Isaacs, J.S., Cialone, J., Horsley, J.W., Holland, M., Murray, P., & Nardella, M. (1997). *Children with special health care needs: A community nutrition pocket guide*. Columbus, OH: Dietetics in Developmental and Psychiatric Disorders and Pediatric Nutrition Practice Group of the American Dietetic Association and Ross Products Division, Abbott Laboratories.

Janicki, M.P., Davidson, P.D., Henderson, C.M., McCallion, P., Force, L.T., & Dalton, A.J. (1999, August). *Health and disability status of adults with intellectual disabilities: Demographic and health indicators comparisons.* Paper presented at the National Conference on Health Statistics (Health in the Millennium: Making Choices and Measuring Impact), Washington, DC.

Jensen, G.L., & Rogers, J. (1998). Obesity in older persons. *Journal of the American Dietetic Association, 98,* 1308–1311.

Krall, E.A., & Dawson-Hughes, E. (1999). Osteoporosis. In M.E. Shils, J.A. Olson, M. Shike, & A.C. Ross (Eds.), *Modern nutrition in health and disease* (9th ed., pp. 1353–1364). Baltimore: Williams & Wilkins.

Lacy, L.L., Armstrong, L.L., Ingrim, N.B., & Lance, L.L. (1997). *Drug information handbook.* Hudson, OH: Lexi-Comp Inc. and American Pharmaceutical Association.

Lensen, P. (1998). Management of total parenteral nutrition. In A. Skipper (Ed.), *Dietitian's handbook of enteral and parenteral nutrition* (pp. 481–525). Rockville, MD: Aspen Publishers.

Lipschitz, D.A. (1992). Nutritional needs of the elderly: An approach to rational management. *Long Term Care Forum, 2,* 9–15.

Luke, A., Sutton, M., Schoeller, D.A., & Roizen, N.M. (1995). Nutrient intake and obesity in prepubescent children with Down syndrome. *Journal of the American Dietetic Association, 96,* 1262–1267.

Mahan, L.K., & Escott-Stump, S. (1996). *Krause's food, nutrition, and diet therapy* (9th ed.). Philadelphia: W.B. Saunders Co.

Marcus, E.L., & Berry, E.M. (1998). Refusal to eat in the elderly. *Nutrition Reviews, 56,* 163–171.

Marcus, R. (1999). Skeletal aging. In R. Chernoff (Ed.), *Geriatric nutrition: The health professional's handbook* (2nd ed., pp. 364–319). Gaithersburg, MD: Aspen Publishers.

Martin, W. (1999). Oral health in the elderly. In R. Chernoff (Ed.), *Geriatric nutrition: The health professional's handbook* (pp. 107–181). Gaithersburg, MD: Aspen Publishers.

Master, A.M., Lasser, R.P., & Beckman, G. (1960). Tables of average weight and height of Americans age 65 to 94 years. *JAMA: Journal of the American Medical Association, 114,* 658–662.

McGill, H.C. (1997). Childhood nutrition and adult cardiovascular diseases. *Nutrition Reviews, 55,* S2–S8.

Mei, Z., Scanlon, K.S., Grummer-Strawn, L.M., Freedman, D.S., Yip, R., & Trowbridge, F.L. (1998). Increasing prevalence of overweight among US low-income preschool children: The Centers for Disease Control and Prevention pediatric nutrition surveillance, 1993 to 1995. *Pediatrics, 101,* e12.

Meisler, J.G., & St. Jeor, S. (1996). Summary and recommendations from the American Health Foundation's Expert Panel on Healthy Weight. *American Journal of Clinical Nutrition, 63,* 474S–477S.

Metropolitan Life Insurance Co. (1983). 1983 Metropolitan height and weight tables for men and women. *Statistical Bulletin, 64*(1), 2.

Mitchell, C.O., & Chernoff, R. (1999). Nutritional assessment of the elderly. In R. Chernoff (Ed.), *Geriatric nutrition: The health professional's handbook* (2nd ed., pp. 382–415). Gaithersburg, MD: Aspen Publishers.

Mughal, D.T. (1992). *The relationships of diet-related knowledge and self-efficacy to dietary adherence among adults with non-insulin-dependent diabetes mellitus.* Unpublished doctoral dissertation, Pennsylvania State University, University Park.

National Heart, Lung, and Blood Institute (NHLBI) Expert Panel. (1998). Executive summary of the clinical guidelines on the identification, evaluation, and treatment of overweight and obesity in adults. *Journal of the American Dietetic Association, 98,* 1178–1191.

National Institutes of Health (NIH). (1994, June 6–8). NIH consensus statement on optimal calcium intake. *NIH Consensus Statement, 12*(4), 1–31.

Nicklas, T.A. (1995). Dietary studies of children: The Bogalusa Heart Study experience. *Journal of the American Dietetic Association, 95,* 1127–1133.

Niedert, K.C. (Ed.). (1998). *Nutrition care of the older adult: A handbook for dietetics professionals working throughout the continuum of care.* Chicago: American Dietetic Association.

Nutrition Screening Initiative (NSI). (1991). *Nutrition screening manual for professionals caring for older Americans.* Washington, DC: American Academy of Family Physicians (AAFP), American Dietetic Association (ADA), and National Council on Aging (NCOA).

Nutrition Screening Initiative (NSI). (1994). *Incorporating nutrition screening and interventions into medical practice: A monograph for physicians.* Washington, DC: American Academy of Family

Physicians (AAFP), American Dietetic Association (ADA), and National Council on Aging (NCOA).

Nutrition Screening Initiative (NSI). (1996a). *Keeping older Americans healthy at home: Guidelines. Nutrition programs in home health care.* Washington, DC: Greer, Margolis, Mitchell, Burns & Associates.

Nutrition Screening Initiative (NSI). (1996b). *Managing nutrition care in health plans.* Washington, DC: Greer, Margolis, Mitchell, Burns & Associates.

Patterson, B., & Ekvall, S.W. (1993). Down syndrome. In S. Ekvall (Ed.), *Pediatric nutrition in chronic diseases and developmental disorders: Prevention, assessment, and treatment* (pp. 149–156). New York: Oxford University Press.

Porter, P., Kris-Etherton, P., Borra, S., Christ-Erwin, M., Novelli, P., Foreyt, J., et al. (1998). Educating consumers regarding choices for fat reduction. *Nutrition Reviews, 56,* S75–S92.

Posthauer, M.E., Dorese, B.E., Foiles, R.A., Escott-Stump, S., Lysen, L., & Balogun, L. (1994). ADA's definitions for nutrition screening and nutrition assessment. *Journal of the American Dietetic Association, 94,* 838–839.

Prasher, V.P. (1995). Overweight and obesity amongst Down's syndrome adults. *Journal of Intellectual Disability Research, 39,* 437–441.

Ryan, C., Eleazer, P., & Egbert, J. (1995). Vitamin D in the elderly: An overlooked nutrient. *Nutrition Today, 30,* 228–233.

Schiffman, S.S., & Covey, C.E. (1984). Changes in taste and smell with age: Nutritional aspects. In J.M. Ordy, D. Harman, & R.B. Alfin-Slater (Eds.), *Nutrition in gerontology* (pp. 43–63). Philadelphia: Lippincott-Raven.

Schlenker, E.D. (1998). *Nutrition in aging* (3rd ed.). Boston: McGraw-Hill/WCB.

Singh Fiatarone, M. (1999). The geriatric exercise prescription: Nutritional implications. In R. Chernoff (Ed.), *Geriatric nutrition: The health professional's handbook* (2nd ed., pp. 366–381). Gaithersburg, MD: Aspen Publishers.

Stensland, S.H., & Margolis, S. (1990). Simplifying the calculation of body mass index for quick reference. *Journal of the American Dietetic Association, 90,* 856.

Tohill, C. (1997). A study into the possible link between anti-epileptic drugs and the risk of fractures in Huckamore Abbey Hospital. *Journal of Intellectual and Developmental Disability, 22,* 281–292.

U.S. Department of Agriculture (USDA), Agriculture Resource Service, Dietary Guidelines Advisory Committee. (1995). *Report of the Dietary Guidelines Advisory Committee in the dietary guidelines for Americans. Report to the Secretary of Health and Human Services and the Secretary of Agriculture.* Washington, DC: U.S. Department of Agriculture.

U.S. Department of Agriculture (USDA), Agriculture Resource Service, Dietary Guidelines Advisory Committee. (2000). *Report of the Dietary Guidelines Advisory Committee in the Dietary Guidelines for Americans: Report to the Secretary of Health and Human Services and the Secretary of Agriculture* (Available http://www.usda.gov/news/releases/2000/02/003/). Washington, DC: U.S. Department of Agriculture.

U.S. Department of Health and Human Services (DHHS). (1993, September). *Cholesterol education program: Second report of the Expert Panel on Detection, Evaluation, and Treatment of High Blood Cholesterol in Adults. Executive Summary (NIH Publication No. 90–3096).* Washington, DC: U.S. Department of Health and Human Services, National Institutes of Health.

U.S. Department of Health and Human Services (DHHS). (1994, July). *Working group report on hypertension in the elderly* (Publication No. 3527). Bethesda, MD: National Institutes of Health.

U.S. Department of Health and Human Services (DHHS). (1996). *Healthy people 2000: National health promotion and disease prevention objectives. Mid-course review and 1995 revisions.* Boston: Jones and Bartlett.

Unonu, J.N., & Johnson, A.A. (1992). Feeding patterns, food energy, nutrient intakes, and anthropometric measurements of selected black children with Down syndrome. *Journal of the American Dietetic Association, 92,* 856–858.

Van Horn, L., Donato, K., Kumanyika, S., Winston, M., Prewitt, E., & Snetselaar, L. (1998). The dietitian's role in developing and implementing the first federal obesity guidelines. *Journal of the American Dietetic Association, 98,* 1115–1117.

Vanitallie, J.B. (1998). Waist circumference: A useful index in clinical care and health promotion. *Nutrition Reviews, 56,* 300–302.

Vogelzang, J.L. (1999). Overview of fluid maintenance/prevention of dehydration. *Journal of the American Dietetic Association, 99* 605–611.

Walter, A., Cohen, N.C., & Swicker, R.C. (1997). Food safety training needs exist for staff and consumers in a variety of community-based homes for people with developmental disabilities. *Journal of the American Dietetic Association, 97,* 619–625.

Wells, M.B., Turner, S., Martin, D.M., & Roy, A. (1997). Health gain through screening coronary heart disease and stroke: Developing primary health services for people with intellectual disability. *Journal of Intellectual and Developmental Disability, 22,* 251–263.

Whelton, P.K., Appel, L.J., Espeland, M.A., Applegate, W.B., Ettinger, W.H., Kostis, J.B., Kumanyika, S., Lacy, C.R., Johnson, K.C., Folmar, S., & Cutler, J.A. (1998). Sodium reduction and weight loss in the treatment of hypertension in older persons: A randomized controlled trial of nonpharmacologic interventions in the elderly (TONE). *JAMA: Journal of the American Medical Association, 279,* 839–846.

White, J.V. (1991). Risk factors associated with poor nutritional status in older Americans. In *Report of nutrition screening I: Toward a common view* (pp. 5–36). Washington, DC: Nutrition Screening Initiative.

White, J.V., Ham, R.J., Lipschitz, D.A., Dwyer, J.T., & Wellman, N.S. (1991). Consensus of the Nutrition Screening Initiative: Risk factors and indicators of poor nutritional status in older Americans. *Journal of the American Dietetic Association, 91,* 783–787.

Whitney, E.N., Cataldo, C.B., & Rolfes, S.R. (1998). *Understanding normal and clinical nutrition* (5th ed., pp. 96–97, 128). Belmont, CA: Wadsworth.

World Health Organization (WHO). (1995). *The world health report 1995: Bridging the gaps. Report of the Director-General.* Geneva: Author.

Yates, A., Schlicker, S.A., & Suitor, C.W. (1998). Dietary reference intakes: The basis for recommendations for calcium and related nutrients, B vitamins, and choline. *Journal of the American Dietetic Association, 98,* 669–706.

Appendix A

Nutrition Screening
Process and Tools

Nutrition Screening Tools

The Nutrition Screening Initiative (NSI), a broad interdisciplinary effort led by the American Academy of Family Physicians, the American Dietetic Association, the National Council on Aging and many other organizations, has developed screening tools to promote efforts that will help improve the nutritional status and health of older adults. These screening tools can be adapted by physicians, home health programs, senior health care centers, and other agencies that have contact with older adults. They can also be adapted to other groups. NSI has developed guides for incorporating nutrition screening into medical practice (NSI, 1994), home care (NSI,1996a) and health plans (NSI,1996b). Several managed care organizations have included nutrition screening into their health plans (NSI, 1996b). The screening tools are the DETERMINE Your Nutritional Health Checklist (Figure 1), Level I Screen (Figure 2) and Level II Screen (Figure 3).

DETERMINE Your Nutritional Health Checklist

The checklist is designed to increase people's awareness of the nine early warning signs of malnutrition. DETERMINE is the mnemonic for Disease, Eating poorly, Tooth loss or mouth pain, Economic hardship, Reduced social contact, Multiple medications or drugs, Involuntary weight loss or gain, Need assistance with self-care, and Elder years, age above 80 (NSI, 1991).

This tool is written in simple language, easy to use, and can be easily completed by the older persons themselves or by their friends, family members, or caregivers. Testing of the checklist showed that it is a valid and reliable measure; that is, the higher checklist scores were linked to the poorest nutrient intake levels, and older adults with higher scores were shown to have increased risk for negative health episodes (NSI, 1994).

NSI (1996a) recommends that scores be placed in the following risk groups: Scores of 1 to 3 indicate low risk, 3 to 4, moderate risks, and 5 and higher, high risk. People in the low-risk group may be given information about health and educational programs and rescreened after one year. Those in the moderate risk group may be given educational materials on nutrition and health, and should be directed to nutrition and wellness programs and appropriate health professionals. They also can be linked to appropriate community services. They should be rescreened after three months. Older adults in the high-risk group need further assessment, using Level I Screen (Figure 2) or Level II Screen (Figure 3) (NSI, 1994).

Level I Screen

This tool (Figure 2) separates clients into category 1 and category 2. Those in category 1 have involuntary weight gain or loss (BMI above 27 or below 22). They should be referred to a physician or other qualified health professional for further assessment. Clients in category 2 have not had involuntary weight change but may have many risk factors and may benefit from preventive measures such as diet counseling, meals on wheels, and nutrition support. They should be screened at least yearly (NSI, 1994).

Level II Screen

This tool (Figure 3), which includes diagnostic parts and more detailed information, helps identify individuals with common nutrition problems such as obesity and protein-energy malnutrition, and conditions (depression and cognitive impairment) which can seriously affect nutritional status. It should be completed in collaboration with a physician or primary care provider (NSI, 1994).

Mini Nutritional Assessment (MNA)

MNA (Figure 4) has been reported to be a rapid and simple assessment tool which has been validated for older populations in free-living or long-term care environment. The Nestlé Research Center in Lausanne, Switzerland, and the University Hospital in Toulouse, France, developed this instrument for Clintec. Cross-validation indicated that the assessment tool was sensitive enough so that 70%–75 % of the subjects could be classified as well nourished or malnourished without further biochemical or clinical evaluation (Guigoz, Vellas, & Garry, 1994).

Commentary

Regular screening of older persons with intellectual disabilities can facilitate early assessment and intervention which will link them with appropriate community support services. These services include social services, oral health, mental health, medication use, nutrition education and counseling, and nutrition support (NSI, 1994). Preventive measures such as these clearly convey the heart of the Healthy People 2000 objectives. As the WHO report stated (1995, p 41), "It is important for the infrastructure to provide health promotion and disease prevention as an integral part of the services rather than only concentrating on curative medicine." Investing in prevention is a worthwhile investment in health. All people, including those with intellectual disabilities, have the right to healthy aging.

The warning signs of poor nutritional health are often overlooked. Use this checklist to find out if you or someone you know is at nutritional risk.

DETERMINE
Your
Nutritional
Health

Read the statements below. Circle the number in the "YES" column for those statements that apply to you or to someone you know. For each "YES" answer, tally the number in the box at the right. Enter the total nutrition score at the bottom of the "YES" column.

Statement	YES
I have an illness or condition that makes me change the kind and/or amount of food that I eat.	2
I eat fewer than two meals per day.	3
I eat few fruits or vegetables or milk products.	2
I have three or more drinks of beer, wine, or liquor almost every day.	2
I have tooth or mouth problems that make it hard for me to eat.	2
I don't always have enough money to buy the food that I need.	4
I eat alone most of the time.	1
I take three or more different prescribed or over-the-counter drugs per day.	1
Without wanting to, I have lost or gained 10 pounds in the previous 6 months.	2
I am not always physically able to shop for, cook for, and/or feed myself.	2
TOTAL	

Total Your Nutrition Score

If it's—

0–2   **Good!** Recheck your nutrition score in 6 months.

3–5   **You are at moderate nutritional risk.** See what can be done to improve your eating habits and lifestyle. Your local Office on Aging, senior nutrition program, senior citizens center, or Health Department can help. Recheck your nutrition score in 3 months.

6 or higher   **You are at high nutritional risk.** Bring this checklist the next time you see your physician, dietitian, or other qualified health or social services professional. Talk with one of these professionals about any problems you may have. Ask for help to improve your nutritional health.

Remember that warning signs suggest risk but do not represent a diagnosis of any condition.

Figure 1.   DETERMINE your nutritional health. (Reprinted with permission from the Nutrition Screening Initiative, a project of the American Academy of Family Physicians, the American Dietetic Association, and the National Council on Aging, Inc., and funded in part by a grant from Ross Products Division, Abbott Laboratories Inc.)

Level I Screen

Body Weight

Measure height to the nearest inch and weight to the nearest pound. Record the values below and mark them on the Body Mass Index (BMI) scale to the right. Then use a straight edge (ruler) to connect the two points and circle the spot where this straight line crosses the center line (body mass index). Record the number below.

Healthy older adults should have a BMI between 22 and 27.

Height (in):_____
Weight (lbs):_____
Body Mass Index:_____
(number from center column)

Check any boxes that are true for the individual:

☐ Has lost or gained 10 pounds (or more) in the past 6 months.

☐ Body mass index <22

☐ Body mass index >27

For the remaining sections, please ask the individual which of the statements (if any) is true for him or her and place a check by each that applies.

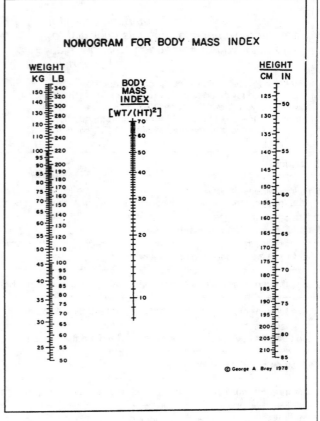

NOMOGRAM FOR BODY MASS INDEX

© George A Bray 1978

Eating Habits

☐ Does not have enough food to eat each day

☐ Usually eats alone

☐ Does not eat anything on one or more days each month

☐ Has poor appetite

☐ Is on a special diet

☐ Eats vegetables two or fewer times daily

☐ Eats milk or milk products once or not at all daily

☐ Eats fruit or drinks fruit juice once or not at all daily

☐ Eats breads, cereals, pasta, rice, or other grains five or fewer times daily

☐ Has difficulty chewing or swallowing

☐ Has more than one alcoholic drink per day (if woman); more than two drinks per day (if man)

☐ Has pain in mouth, teeth, or gums

(continued)

Figure 2. Nutrition Screening Initiative Level I Screen. (Reprinted with permission from the Nutrition Screening Initiative, a project of the American Academy of Family Physicians, the American Dietetic Association, and the National Council on Aging, Inc., and funded in part by a grant from Ross Products Division, Abbott Laboratories Inc.)

Figure 2.   *(continued)*

A physician should be contacted if the individual has gained or lost 10 pounds unexpectedly or without intending to during the past 6 months. A physician should also be notified if the individual's body mass index is above 27 or below 22.

Living Environment

☐ Lives on an income of less than $6000 per year (per individual in the household)

☐ Lives alone

☐ Is housebound

☐ Is concerned about home security

☐ Lives in a home with inadequate heating or cooling

☐ Does not have a stove and/or refrigerator

☐ Is unable or prefers not to spend money on food (<$25-30 per person spent on food each week)

Functional Status

Usually or always needs assistance with (check each that apply):

☐ Bathing

☐ Dressing

☐ Grooming

☐ Toileting

☐ Eating

☐ Walking or moving about

☐ Traveling (outside the home)

☐ Preparing food

☐ Shopping for food or other necessities

If you have checked one or more statements on this screen, the individual you have interviewed may be at risk for poor nutritional status. Please refer this individual to the appropriate health care or social service professional in your area. For example, a dietitian should be contacted for problems with selecting, preparing, or eating a healthy diet, or a dentist if the individual experiences pain or difficulty when chewing or swallowing. Those individuals whose income, lifestyle, or functional status may endanger their nutritional and overall health should be referred to available community services: home-delivered meals, congregate meal programs, transportation services, counseling services (alcohol abuse, depression, bereavement, etc.), home health care agencies, day care programs, etc.

Please repeat this screen at least once each year--sooner if the individual has a major change in his or her health, income, immediate family (e.g., spouse dies), or functional status.

These materials developed by the Nutrition Screening Initiative.

Level II Screen

Complete the following screen by interviewing the patient directly and/or by referring to the patient chart. If you do not routinely perform all of the described tests or ask all of the listed questions, please consider including them but do not be concerned if the entire screen is not completed. Please try to conduct a minimal screen on as many older patients as possible, and please try to collect serial measurements, which are extremely valuable in monitoring nutritional status. Please refer to the manual for additional information.

Anthropometrics

Measure height to the nearest inch and weight to the nearest pound. Record the values below and mark them on the Body Mass Index (BMI) scale to the right. Then use a straight edge (paper, ruler) to connect the two points and circle the spot where this straight line crosses the center line (body mass index). Record the number below; healthy older adults should have a BMI between 22 and 27; check the appropriate box to flag an abnormally high or low value.

Height (in):_____
Weight (lbs):_____
Body Mass Index
(weight/height²):_____

Please place a check by any statement regarding BMI and recent weight loss that is true for the patient.

☐ Body mass index <22

☐ Body mass index >27

☐ Has lost or gained 10 pounds (or more) of body weight in the past 6 months

Record the measurement of mid-arm circumference to the nearest 0.1 centimeter and of triceps skinfold to the nearest 2 millimeters.

Mid-Arm Circumference (cm):_____
Triceps Skinfold (mm):_____
Mid-Arm Muscle Circumference (cm):_____

Refer to the table and check any abnormal values:

☐ Mid-arm muscle circumference <10th percentile

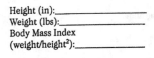

NOMOGRAM FOR BODY MASS INDEX

WEIGHT KG LB

BODY MASS INDEX [WT/(HT)²]

HEIGHT CM IN

© George A Bray 1978

☐ Triceps skinfold <10th percentile

☐ Triceps skinfold >95th percentile

Note: mid-arm circumference (cm) - {0.314 x triceps skinfold (mm)}= mid-arm *muscle* circumference (cm)

For the remaining sections, please place a check by any statements that are true for the patient.

Laboratory Data

☐ Serum albumin below 3.5 g/dl

☐ Serum cholesterol below 160 mg/dl

☐ Serum cholesterol above 240 mg/dl

Drug Use

☐ Three or more prescription drugs, OTC medications, and/or vitamin/mineral supplements daily

(continued)

Figure 3.   Nutrition Screening Initiative Level II Screen. (Reprinted with permission from the Nutrition Screening Initiative, a project of the American Academy of Family Physicians, the American Dietetic Association, and the National Council on Aging, Inc., and funded in part by a grant from Ross Products Division, Abbott Laboratories Inc.)

Figure 3.   *(continued)*

Clinical Features

Presence of (check each that apply):

- ☐ Problems with mouth, teeth, or gums
- ☐ Difficulty chewing
- ☐ Difficulty swallowing
- ☐ Angular stomatitis
- ☐ Glossitis
- ☐ History of bone pain
- ☐ History of bone fractures
- ☐ Skin changes (dry, loose, nonspecific lesions, edema)

Percentile	Men 55-65 y	Men 65-75 y	Women 55-65 y	Women 65-75 y
Arm circumference (cm)				
10th	27.3	26.3	25.7	25.2
50th	31.7	30.7	30.3	29.9
95th	36.9	35.5	38.5	37.3
Arm muscle circumference (cm)				
10th	24.5	23.5	19.6	19.5
50th	27.8	26.8	22.5	22.5
95th	32.0	30.6	28.0	27.9
Triceps skinfold (mm)				
10th	6	6	16	14
50th	11	11	25	24
95th	22	22	38	36

From: Frisancho AR. *New norms of upper limb fat and muscle areas for assessment of nutritional status. Am J Clin Nutr 1981; 34:2540-2545.* © 1981 American Society for Clinical Nutrition.

Eating Habits

- ☐ Does not have enough food to eat each day
- ☐ Usually eats alone
- ☐ Does not eat anything on one or more days each month
- ☐ Has poor appetite
- ☐ Is on a special diet
- ☐ Eats vegetables two or fewer times daily
- ☐ Eats milk or milk products once or not at all daily
- ☐ Eats fruit or drinks fruit juice once or not at all daily
- ☐ Eats breads, cereals, pasta, rice, or other grains five or fewer times daily
- ☐ Has more than one alcoholic drink per day (if woman); more than two drinks per day (if man)

Living Environment

- ☐ Lives on an income of less than $6000 per year (per individual in the household)
- ☐ Lives alone
- ☐ Is housebound
- ☐ Is concerned about home security

- ☐ Lives in a home with inadequate heating or cooling
- ☐ Does not have a stove and/or refrigerator
- ☐ Is unable or prefers not to spend money on food (<$25-30 per person spent on food each week)

Functional Status

Usually or always needs assistance with (check each that apply):

- ☐ Bathing
- ☐ Dressing
- ☐ Grooming
- ☐ Toileting
- ☐ Eating
- ☐ Walking or moving about
- ☐ Traveling (outside the home)
- ☐ Preparing food
- ☐ Shopping for food or other necessities

Mental/Cognitive Status

- ☐ Clinical evidence of impairment, e.g. Folstein<26
- ☐ Clinical evidence of depressive illness, e.g. Beck Depression Inventory>15, Geriatric Depression Scale>5

Patients in whom you have identified one or more major indicator (see pg 2) of poor nutritional status require immediate medical attention; if minor indicators are found, ensure that they are known to a health professional or to the patient's own physician. Patients who display risk factors (see pg 2) of poor nutritional status should be referred to the appropriate health care or social service professional (dietitian, nurse, dentist, case manager, etc.).

These materials developed by the Nutrition Screening Initiative.

MINI NUTRITIONAL ASSESSMENT
MNA™

Last name _____ First name _____ M.I. _____ Sex _____

Date _____ Age _____ Weight (in kg) _____ Height (in cm) _____ Knee height (in cm) _____

Complete this form by writing the numbers in the boxes. Add the numbers in the boxes and compare the total assessment to the Malnutrition Indicator Score.

ANTHROPOMETRIC ASSESSMENT

1. Body Mass Index (BMI) (weight in kg)/(height in m)^2 Points
   a. BMI < 19   = 0 points
   b. BMI 19 to < 21   = 1 point
   c. BMI 21 to < 23   = 2 points
   d. BMI ≥ 23   = 3 points   □

2. Midarm circumference (MAC) (in cm)
   a. MAC < 21   = 0.0 points
   b. MAC 21 ≤ 22   = 0.5 points
   c. MAC > 22   = 1.0 points   □ · □

3. Calf circumference (CC) (in cm)
   a. CC <31   = 0 points
   b. CC ≥ 31   = 1 point   □

4. Weight loss during the last 3 months
   a. Weight loss > 3 kg (6.6 lbs)   = 0 points
   b. Does not know   = 1 point
   c. Weight loss 1–3 kg (2.2–6.6 lbs) = 2 points
   d. No weight loss   = 3 points   □

GENERAL ASSESSMENT

5. Lives independently (not in a nursing home or hospital)
   a. No = 0 points   b. Yes = 1 point   □

6. Takes more than three prescription drugs per day
   a. Yes = 0 points   b. No = 1 point   □

7. Has suffered psychological stress or acute disease in the previous 3 months
   a. Yes = 0 points   b. No = 2 points   □

8. Mobility
   a. Bed- or chairbound   = 0 points
   b. Able to get out of bed or chair but does not go out   = 1 point
   c. Goes out   = 2 points   □

9. Neuropsychological problems
   a. Severe dementia or depression   = 0 points
   b. Mild dementia   = 1 point
   c. No psychological problems   = 2 points   □

10. Pressure sores or skin ulcers
    a. Yes = 0 points   b. No = 1 point   □

DIETARY ASSESSMENT

11. How many full meals does the patient eat daily?
    a. 1 meal   = 0 points
    b. 2 meals   = 1 point
    c. 3 meals   = 2 points   □

12. Selected consumption markers for protein intake
    - At least one serving of dairy products (milk, cheese, yogurt) per day?   Yes ___ No ___
    - Two or more servings of legumes or eggs per week?   Yes ___ No ___
    - Meat, fish, or poultry every day?   Yes ___ No ___
    a. If 0 or 1 yes   = 0.0 points
    b. If 2 yes   = 0.5 points
    c. If 3 yes   = 1.0 points   □ · □

13. Consumes two or more servings of fruits or vegetables per day?
    a. No = 0 points   b. Yes = 1 point   □

14. Has food intake declined over the past 3 months due to loss of appetite, digestive problems, or chewing or swallowing difficulties?
    a. Severe loss of appetite = 0 points
    b. Moderate loss of appetite = 1 point
    c. No loss of appetite   = 2 points   □

15. How much fluid (e.g., water, juice, coffee, tea, milk) is consumed per day? (1 cup = 8 oz)
    a. Less than 3 cups = 0.0 points
    b. 3–5 cups   = 0.5 points
    c. More than 5 cups = 1.0 points   □ · □

16. Mode of feeding
    a. Unable to eat without assistance   = 0 points
    b. Self-fed with some difficulty   = 1 point
    c. Self-fed without any problem   = 2 points   □

SELF-ASSESSMENT

17. Do they view themselves as having nutritional problems?
    a. Major malnutrition   = 0 points
    b. Does not know or moderate malnutrition   = 1 point
    c. No nutritional problem = 2 points   □

18. In comparison with other people of the same age, how do they consider their health status?
    a. Not as good   = 0.0 points
    b. Does not know   = 0.5 points
    c. As good   = 1.0 points
    d. Better   = 2.0 points   □ · □

ASSESSMENT TOTAL (max. 30 points)   □ · □

MALNUTRITION INDICATOR SCORE

≥ 24 points	Well nourished
17–23.5 points	At risk of malnutrition
< 17 points	Malnourished

Figure 4. Mini Nutritional Assessment (MNA™). (*Source:* Guigoz, Vellas, and Garry [1994]. Courtesy of Nestlé Clinical Nutrition, Deerfield, IL, copyright © 1994 by Nestec Ltd [Nestlé Research Center]/Clintec Nutrition Co.)

Appendix B

Sample Calculations

Sample Percentage Ideal Body Weight, or Percentage Desirable Body Weight, Percentage Weight Loss, and Body Mass Index Calculations

Given: Older adult male, age 65 years; height, 65 inches; current weight, 160 lbs.; usual weight, 170 lbs.; weight for height in Master and colleagues' (1960) tables, 146–156 lbs. (midpoint is 151 lbs.).

Weight measurement category	Sample calculation
Percentage desirable body weight (Current weight ÷ weight for height [in reference tables]) x 100	(160 lbs. ÷ 151 lbs.) x 100 = 1.05 x 100 = 105% (This is within "normal" range.)
Percentage weight loss (Usual weight – [Present weight ÷ usual weight]) x 100	$[170$ lbs. – 160 lbs.$]$ ÷ 170 lbs.) x 100 = (10 lbs. ÷ 170 lbs.) x 100 $\cong$ 6% weight loss Or determine the person's current body weight as a percentage of the person's usual body weight as follows: % usual body weight = (Current weight ÷ usual weight) x 100 = (160 lbs. ÷ 170 lbs.) x 94% (Current weight is 94% of person's usual body weight, a 6% weight loss.)
Body mass index (BMI) using two formulas BMI = Weight in kilograms ÷ height^2 (in meters) (National Heart, Lung, and Blood Institute, 1998) (*Note:* This calculation requires conversion of pounds and inches to metric units: 1 kg = 2.2 lbs., 1 inch = .0254 meters	72.72 kg ÷ 1.65 meters^2 = 72.72 kg ÷ 2.72 meters^2 = 26.7 (Note that this is the original formula.) BMI = (Weight in pounds ÷ Height^2 (in inches) x 705 (Stensland & Margolis, 1990) (160 lbs. ÷ 65 inches^2) x 705 = (160 lbs. ÷ 4,225 inches^2) x 705 = .03787 x 705 = 26.7 This is a modified formula that eliminates conversion of units of measure. The insignificant slight difference in calculated values is not shown because of rounding off.

Appendix C

Tables

Table 1. Commonly used measures of weight status and their interpretation

Measure	Acceptable values	Overweight	Obesity	Comments
Percentage (%) "ideal" body weight (IBW) or desirable body weight (DBW)[a] Compare the current body weight with the weight for height in reference "standard" (e.g., height and weight tables).	90%–109%	110%–120%	>120%	This measure does not distinguish fat weight from lean tissue. Kyphosis, loss of height, bent lower extremities, measuring techniques, the type of equipment used, inability to stand on the scale, and fluid retention are some of the sources of measurement errors.[b] Questions remain that the average weights in the reference tables are not necessarily the "desirable" or optimal weight for an individual.[c]
Body mass index (BMI)	23–28 (for 55- to 64-year-olds)[d] 24–29 (for 65-year-olds and older)[d] 22–27 (for 65-year-olds and older)[e]			BMI highly correlates with body fat proportion. Fluid retention and increased body mass will raise it.[c]
	18.5–24.9 (for adults)	25–29.9[f]	30–34.9 (Class I)[f] 35–39.9 (Class II)[f]	

Ratio of weight to
height
(squared)

Calculate BMI using either one of these formulas:

$$\frac{\text{Weight (in kilograms)}}{\text{Height}^2 \text{ (in meters)}}[f]$$

[Weight (in lb)/Height² (in inches)] × 705 (g)[g]
BMI can also be determined using a nomogram
(Level I Screen).

(continued)

Table 1.   *(continued)*

Measure	Acceptable values	Overweight	Obesity	Comments
Waist circumference Compare abdominal girth measurement with a reference standard. Use this with BMI to assess increased relative risk for developing obesity-related risk factors for most people with a BMI of 25–34.9				This measures the location of body fat in the abdominal area, a risk factor for obesity-related morbidity and mortality. With BMI of 25–34.9, the following values are high risk: Men: > 102 cm (40 in) Women: > 88 cm (35 in) The measurement is easy, convenient, and practical. As with the other measures, it should be used with other relevant information.[f]

[a]Mahan and Escott-Stump (1996).
[b]Mitchell and Chernoff (1999).
[c]Ham (1991).
[d]Committee on Diet and Health (1989).
[e]NSI (1994).
[f]NHLBI (1998).
[g]Stensland and Margolis (1990).

Table 2.   1983 Metropolitan Life Insurance Co. height and weight tables for men and women according to frame, ages 25–59

Men				
Height				
Feet	Inches	Small frame	Medium frame	Large frame
5	2	128–134	131–141	138–150
5	3	130–136	133–143	140–153
5	4	132–138	135–145	142–156
5	5	134–140	137–148	144–160
5	6	136–142	139–151	146–164
5	7	138–145	142–154	149–168
5	8	140–148	145–157	152–172
5	9	142–151	148–160	155–176
5	10	144–154	151–163	158–180
5	11	146–157	154–166	161–184

(continued)

Table 2. *(continued)*

Height Feet	Height Inches	Small frame	Medium frame	Large frame
Men				
6	0	149–160	157–170	164–188
6	1	152–164	160–174	168–192
6	2	155–168	164–178	172–197
6	3	158–172	167–182	176–202
6	4	162–176	171–187	181–207

Height Feet	Height Inches	Small frame	Medium frame	Large frame
Women				
4	10	102–111	109–121	118–131
4	11	103–113	111–123	120–134
5	0	104–115	113–126	122–137
5	1	106–118	115–129	125–140
5	2	108–121	118–132	128–143
5	3	111–124	121–135	131–147
5	4	114–127	124–138	134–151
5	5	117–130	127–141	137–155
5	6	120–133	130–144	140–159
5	7	123–136	133–147	143–163
5	8	126–139	136–150	146–167
5	9	129–142	139–153	149–170
5	10	132–145	142–156	152–173
5	11	135–148	145–159	155–176
6	0	138–151	148–162	158–179

Weights at ages 25–29 based on lowest mortality. Weight in pounds according to frame (in indoor clothing: weight, 5 lbs. for men and 3 lbs. for women); shoes with 1-in heels.

Reprinted with permission from *Statistical Bulletin* (1983; 62:2), Copyright © 1983 Metropolitan Life Insurance Co. Courtesy of Metropolitan Life Insurance Co.

Table 3. Average height-weight tables for people age 65 years and older

Height (inches)	Ages 65–69	Ages 70–74	Ages 75–79	Ages 80–84	Ages 85–89	Ages 90–94
Men						
61	128–156	125–153	123–151			
62	130–158	127–155	125–153	122–148		
63	131–161	129–157	127–155	122–150	120–146	
64	134–164	131–161	129–157	124–152	122–148	
65	136–166	134–164	130–160	127–155	125–153	117–143
66	139–169	137–167	133–163	130–158	128–156	120–146
67	140–172	140–170	136–166	132–162	130–160	122–150
68	143–175	142–174	139–169	135–165	133–163	126–154

(continued)

Table 3. *(continued)*

Height (inches)	Ages 65–69	Ages 70–74	Ages 75–79	Ages 80–84	Ages 85–89	Ages 90–94
			Men			
69	147–179	146–178	142–174	139–169	137–167	130–158
70	150–184	148–182	146–178	143–175	140–172	134–164
71	155–189	152–186	149–183	148–180	144–176	139–169
72	159–195	156–190	154–188	153–187	148–182	
73	164–200	160–196	158–192			
			Women			
58	120–146	112–138	111–135			
59	121–147	114–140	112–136	100–122	99–121	
60	122–148	116–142	113–139	106–130	102–124	
61	123–151	118–144	115–144	112–136	104–128	
62	125–153	121–147	118–144	112–136	108–132	107–131
63	127–155	123–151	121–147	115–141	112–136	107–131
64	130–158	126–154	123–151	119–145	115–141	108–132
65	132–162	130–158	126–154	122–150	120–146	112–136
66	136–166	132–162	128–157	126–154	124–152	116–142
67	140–170	136–166	131–161	130–158	128–156	
68	143–175	140–170				
69	148–180	144–176				

From Master, A.M., Lasser, R.P., & Beckman, G. (1960). *Journal of the American Medical Association, 172,* 658–662; reprinted with permission. Copyright © 1960, American Medical Association.

Table 4. Healthy weight ranges for men and women[a,b]

Height	Weight (in lbs.)
4'10"	91–119
4'11"	94–124
5'0"	97–128
5'1"	101–132
5'2"	104–137
5'3"	107–141
5'4"	111–146
5'5"	114–150
5'6"	118–155
5'7"	121–160
5'8"	125–164
5'9"	129–169
5'10"	132–174
5'11"	136–179
6'0"	140–184
6'1"	144–189
6'2"	148–195

Table 4. *(continued)*

Height	Weight (in lbs.)
6"3"	152–200
6'4"	156–205
6'5"	160–211
6'6"	164–216

[a]USDA (1995).

[b]The chart applies to men and women of all ages. Weight ranges are given to allow for different amounts of muscle and bones in different people of the same height. The higher weights in the healthiest weight range apply to people with more muscle and bone.

Table 5. Step I diet for weight loss

Nutrients	Recommended amount
Total fat	30% or less of total energy
Saturated fat	8% to 10% of total energy
Polyunsaturated fat	Up to 10% of total energy
Monosaturated fat	Up to 15% of total energy
Cholesterol	Less than 300 mg per day
Protein	Approximately 15% of total energy
Carbohydrate	55% or more of total energy
Fiber	20 g to 30 g per day
Sodium	No more than 2,400 mg per day
Other features	
Calorie level	Individualized to achieve weight loss
The diet should be nutritionally balanced.	

Source: DHHS (1993).

Table 6. Major risk factors for the development of osteoporosis

Risk factors	Effect on bone-building nutrients or process
Aging and age-related decline in functions of organ systems	
Skin	Reduced synthesis of previtamin D_3 from 7-dehydrocholecalciferol (provitamin D_3) from the action of sunlight[a,b]
Liver	Reduced ability to convert provitamin D_3 to 25-hydroxycholecalciferol (25-vitamin D or calcidiol), the second step in the activation of vitamin D to its most active form[a,b]
Kidney	Reduced ability to convert calcidiol to 1,25-dihydroxycholecalferol(1,25-vitamin D or calcitriol), the most active form[a,b]
Gastrointestinal system	Reduced absorption of fats, fat-soluble vitamins, and calcium[c]
Endocrine/Menopause	Lack of endogenous estrogen accelerates bone loss immediately after menopause[d]
Genetics	Heredity influences bone mass and strength[d]

(continued)

Table 6.   *(continued)*

Risk factors	Effect on bone-building nutrients or process
Diseases	
Intestinal disorders that cause malabsorption	Chronic liver diseases that cause malabsorption, cystic fibrosis, pancreatic insufficiency, and gluten-sensitive enteropathy impair absorption of fat-soluble vitamins and calcium[c]
Kidney disease	End-stage renal disease causes profound abnormalities in calcium, phosphorus, and vitamin D metabolism leading to osteodystrophy[c]
Medications	Long-term anticonvulsant therapy (phenytoin, phenobarbital, and carbamazipine) interferes with vitamin D metabolism[b,e] Long-term therapy with glucocorticoids interferes with calcium utilization[f]
Hormonal abnormality	
Hypogonadism	Lack of androgen in male and estrogen in female impairs bone acquisition and maintenance[d] Hypogonadism in adults with Down syndrome is significantly associated with reduced bone density[g]
Hyperparathyroidism	Parathyroid hormone stimulates bone calcium release to sustain blood calcium level[c]
Lack of exposure to sunlight	Impaired photosynthesis of vitamin D on the skin[a,b] Dark skin pigmentation, seasonal variation (winter), and use of sunblocks also reduce this photosynthesis[a]
Inadequate calcium and vitamin D intake	Impaired mineralization and maintenance of bone mass and strength[b,d,f]
Lack of physical activity	Lack of mechanical loading to stimulate bone acquisition and maintenance reduces bone mass[d]
Frailty/thinness	Combination of factors reduces bone mass and strength[f]

[a]Hollick (1999).
[b]Ryan, Eleazer, and Egbert (1995).
[c]Heaney (1999).
[d]Marcus (1999).
[e]Tohill (1997).
[f]Krall and Dawson-Hughes (1999).
[g]Center, Beange, and McElduff (1998).

Table 7.   Selected medications and their effects on the gastrointestinal system and nutrients

Drug	Effect
Antipsychotics	
Clozapine (Clozaril)	Constipation, nausea, vomiting, diarrhea, unusual weight gain
Haloperidol (Haldol)	Constipation, weight gain
Thiothixene (Navane)	Constipation, pseudoparkinsonism, persistent tardive dyskinesia
Risperidone (Risperdal)	Constipation, adynamic ileus, gastrointestinal upset, dry mouth, pseudoparkinsonism, tardive dyskinesia, nausea, anorexia, weight gain
Chlorpromazine HCl (Thorazine)	Constipation, tardive dyskinesia, pseudoparkinsonism

(continued)

Table 7. *(continued)*

Drug	Effect
Antimanic	
Lithium carbonate (Eskalith, Lithobid)	Increased thirst, nausea, vomiting, impaired taste
Anticonvulsants	
Valproic acid (Depakene)	May affect appetite and weight, nausea, vomiting, abdominal cramps, diarrhea
Phenytoin (Dilantin)	Interferes with metabolism of vitamins D and K and folic acid (resulting in rickets or osteomalacia)
Clonazepam (Klonopin)	Dry mouth, constipation, diarrhea, increased or decreased appetite
Primidone (Mysoline)	Nausea, vomiting, anorexia, interferes with vitamin D metabolism
Phenobarbital (Barbita, Luminal, Solfoton)	Nausea, vomiting, constipation, interferes with vitamin D metabolism
Carbamazepine (Tegretol)	Nausea, vomiting, mouth ulcers
Antidepressants	
Amitriptyline HCl (Elavil)	Dry mouth, increased appetite, nausea, unpleasant taste, weight gain
Venlafaxine (Effexor)	Nausea, vomiting, dry mouth, constipation
Nortryptyline HCl (Pamelor)	Dry mouth, constipation, increased appetite, nausea, unpleasant taste, weight gain
Paroxetine (Paxil)	Nausea, dry mouth, constipation, diarrhea
Fluoxetine HCl (Proxac)	Dry mouth, nausea, diarrhea
Sertraline HCl (Zoloft)	Dry mouth, diarrhea or loose stools, nausea, constipation
Other	
Laxatives: Mineral oil	Loss of beta-carotene

Sources: Blumberg and Couris (1999) and Lacy, Armstrong, Ingrim, and Lance (1997).

13

Cash and Counseling as a Model to Structure and Finance Community Supports

Lori Simon-Rusinowitz, Kevin J. Mahoney, Dawn M. Shoop,
Sharon M. Desmond, Marie R. Squillace, and Jo-Ann Sowers

As adults with disabilities have sought more dignified and productive personal assistance options that promote choice and autonomy, researchers have sought for these options new financing models that are both cost-effective and responsive to consumer needs (Ansello & Eustis, 1992; Kapp, 1996; Mahoney, Estes, & Heumann, 1991; Simon-Rusinowitz & Hofland, 1993). Furthermore, as long-term care expenditures have risen, policy makers have sought new ways to control costs while maintaining or increasing consumer satisfaction. Concurrently, there is strong interest among the aging and disability communities in consumer-directed care, which was exemplified in the proposed language of the 1994 Health Security Act (H.R. 3600; Kapp, 1996). With this in mind, policy makers and funders have become increasingly interested in a model that

This chapter is adapted from a technical report prepared for the University of Maryland at College Park by Simon-Rusinowitz, Mahoney, Shoop, Desmond, Squillace, Fay, and Sowers (1998), entitled *Determining preferences of adults with developmental disabilities for a cash option: Florida survey results. Background research to support the Cash and Counseling Demonstration and Evaluation*.

The authors acknowledge the support and guidance of the Cash and Counseling Demonstration and Evaluation Team as well as the Florida project staff. In addition, we are grateful to the adults with disabilities and their families in Florida who participated in the survey.

offers people with disabilities a monthly cash allowance, potentially fostering greater autonomy and choice.

Such an approach, known as "cash and counseling," involves disbursing funds through a cash allowance and at the same time providing counseling services (e.g., advice, information, training). This approach enables adults with a developmental disability to purchase the services, assistive devices, or home modifications that best meet their needs. The counseling is intended to help recipients make effective and informed choices from among the community's vendors and at the same time become more adept at managing their own resources (Cameron & Firman, 1995). In principle, cash allowances maximize consumer choice and promote efficiency because consumers who shop for the most cost-effective providers may be able to purchase additional and more personalized services (Kapp, 1996). Generally, adults with a developmental disability are eligible for a traditional care-managed service or some type of cash allowance. To be eligible for the cash allowance, an adult has to demonstrate that he or she can use the cash allowance provided to meet his or her long-term support needs. (If this is not possible, a consumer may have a friend or relative serve as a surrogate decision maker or "representative" to assist with the necessary tasks.) Such a cash and counseling benefit would thus provide financial support for the individual to take charge of meeting his or her long-term care needs.

This chapter discusses lessons from a telephone survey conducted to assess consumers' preliminary interest in a cash and counseling option in Florida, one of three demonstration states in the Cash and Counseling Demonstration and Evaluation (CCDE). The CCDE, which is jointly funded by The Robert Wood Johnson Foundation and U.S. Department of Health and Human Services, Office of the Assistant Secretary for Planning and Evaluation, will test cash and counseling in three state Medicaid programs and compare this model with traditional, case-managed services. This survey has provided background information for the CCDE and has guided several aspects of program development. This discussion focuses on guidance in developing communications and social marketing materials to assist Florida's efforts to inform consumers about the CCDE. It also discusses key policy issues. An actual enrollment of cash option consumers—and the rigorous program evaluation—began in March 2000. We look forward to reporting program evaluation results in the future.

BACKGROUND

Cash and counseling models, whereby local agencies provide home-based services to consumers who have control over the nature and quality of services purchased and provided, have been implemented in mostly small programs serving elders and younger adults with physical disabilities. In these instances, consumers choose to use their cash allowance to pay a friend or relative for personal assistance services, purchase services from a home health agency (or referral services), attend an adult day services program, make needed home modifications, or pay for residence at an assisted living program (Cameron & Firman, 1995). Care management, service coordination, and guardianship services are additional elements of purchased services that can be brokered by consumers who may not have readily available family. The counseling component involves both an assessment of need and consumer information and advice about available services, financing, and available housing options.

Although such financing models have been implemented for several years in small programs for elders and adults with physical disabilities, their application to helping adults with developmental disabilities has only begun to be explored (Herman, 1991; Knoll et al., 1990; Meyers & Marcenco, 1986; Wisconsin Department of Health and Social Services, 1985). Preliminary efforts have been undertaken to develop, implement, and field-test systems through which Medicaid-funded residential and day activity would be directly controlled by individuals with a developmental disability, with the support of their families or caregivers (Cotten & Sowers, 1996; Fenton et al., 1997). In this regard, a major systems change effort, the Self-Determination for Persons with Developmental Disabilities Project, funded by the Robert Wood Johnson Foundation, was implemented in a number of areas across the United States. In these tests, the participating states developed and field tested mechanisms through which "customers" directly control funding for supports. It is interesting that, notwithstanding strong advocacy toward more self-determination among people in the disability community, the movement toward customer-directed support funding has received a great deal of support from those in the academic community who are interested in related policy issues and from those who work for federal and state developmental disabilities agencies.

Most adults with developmental disabilities and their families are just beginning to be introduced to these new concepts and approaches for financing support services (Agosta & Melda, 1996). However, what is generally still unknown is to what extent adults with developmental disabilities and/or their families desire to control such funding and which individual characteristics (e.g., age, sex, ethnicity) define which groups of people prefer to control their own funding. Also unknown are the reasons for their desire to control their own funding and the mechanisms through which they would prefer to do so. The literature regarding application of this model to older adults provides some guidance regarding background characteristics that possibly are related to preferences for consumer direction. For example, Glickman, Brandt, and Caro (1994) found an association between consumer willingness to assume responsibility for directing a home care worker and the following consumer characteristics: previous experience with directing an in-home worker, greater length of time receiving home care services, greater involvement in directing a home care worker, and lower levels of satisfaction with home care services.

Research that indicates differences in long-term care services use and caregiving patterns among some ethnic and cultural minority groups—greater informal care and less reliance on nursing homes among some minority groups compared with their cultural majority counterparts—offers reason to speculate that preferences for consumer direction may differ according to cultural and ethnic group background (Rimer, 1998; Tennestedt & Chang, 1998; Wallace, Levy-Storms, Kington, & Andersen, 1998). The literature that addresses self-determination for adults with developmental disabilities stresses the importance of teaching skills needed to be self-directing—suggesting that it would be important to assess willingness regarding training to learn the skills required of cash option recipients (Abery, 1994; Wolfe, Ofiesh, & Boone, 1996). Yet limited information about participant preferences for self-direction—and specifically the cash option—point to the need to explore further many unanswered questions. Most important among these is which types of adults with developmental disabilities and their representative decision makers or surrogates, and how many, would choose to participate in a cash option program if given the opportunity? In addition, what would their reasons be for this choice? In this chapter, we explore applications of the cash and counseling program to adults with developmental disabilities by drawing upon lessons from a consumer preference survey in Florida (Simon-Rusinowitz et al., 1998).

PERSONAL ASSISTANCE SERVICE PROGRAMS[1]

Personal assistance services (PAS) encompass a range of human and technological assistance provided to people with disabilities who need help with activities of daily living (ADLs), including bathing, dressing, toileting, transferring, and eating, or instrumental activities of daily living (IADLs), such as housekeeping, cooking, shopping, and laundry, as well as managing money and medication or both (Beatty, Richmond, Tepper, & DeJong, 1998; DeJong, Batavia, & McKnew, 1992). Public or private third-party payers use any of three PAS financing methods: cash benefits (payments to qualified consumers or their representative payees), vendor payments (a case manager determines the types and amounts of covered services and arranges for and pays authorized PAS providers to deliver these services), and vouchers (consumers use funds for authorized purchases).

In the United States, most public programs that finance PAS—including such major funders as Medicaid's optional personal care services benefit and home- and community-based long-term care (HCBS) waiver programs—follow a vendor payment model. That is, the program purchases services for consumers from authorized vendors (services providers or equipment suppliers). In some programs, the list of covered services and authorized vendors is restricted. Other programs may cover a broader range of services, including additional adult day services, transportation, home modifications, and assistive devices, and so forth. Participants may sometimes hire independent providers (i.e., workers not employed by home health agencies) to be their in-home aides.

Until recently, the prohibition on direct payments to Medicaid recipients has rarely been questioned. However, many state program officials have come to share the concerns of disability rights advocates who want PAS programs that promote consumer choice and avoid program rules that may foster dependency in the name of consumer protection and/or public accountability (Litvak & Kennedy, 1990, 1991; Litvak, Zukas, & Heumann, 1987). In addition, state officials have a strong interest in achieving program economies. Most Medicaid PAS programs mandate that service coordinators or case managers (usually registered nurses and social workers) assess adults, develop and monitor care plans, and authorize provider payments. Case management thus can be expensive, and researchers and administrators have questioned whether it should be uniformly required (Geron & Chassler, 1994; Jackson, 1994). Hence, there is a growing interest in cash option programs because of potential savings on program administration and enhanced consumer empowerment.

Significant changes have occurred in the field of developmental disabilities since the 1970s—moving from a system in which many individuals with developmental disabilities were institutionalized to one based on community programs and services (Bradley, Ashbaugh, & Blaney, 1994). However, there is a growing recognition for the need to move beyond a system that is still organized around programs and is professionally driven to one that is truly a part of the community and is consumer and family driven (Nisbet, 1992). As in the general disability field, the motivation for these changes comes from a desire to improve the quality of supports available to and the lives achieved by individuals with disabilities, the philosophical belief in consumers' right to direct their own lives, and growing constraints on the availability of federal and state funds (Ashbaugh, Bradley, & Blaney, 1994).

---

[1]Much of this section is drawn from background materials written during the project development phase by Pamela Doty, the Cash and Counseling Demonstration Evaluation project officer at the U.S. Department of Health and Human Services.

Of particular concern are the growing numbers of individuals who are on service waiting lists. One report noted that approximately 200,000 individuals with developmental disabilities are waiting for services in the United States (Hayden & DePaepe, 1994). As it is unlikely that the amount of funding available for services will increase significantly, this number will only grow unless a dramatic change is made in the developmental services and funding system (Smith, 1994). As in the general disability field, there is strong interest in the field of developmental disabilities to promote alternatives to the current vendor payment mechanisms, including support vouchers and cash paid directly to adults with disabilities (or their families), to help adults with disabilities determine what specific supports they need and wish to purchase and to examine how they will manage their financial affairs and oversee the services they obtain (Bradley et al., 1994; Hayden & Abery, 1994).

APPLICATION AND EVALUATION OF THE CASH AND COUNSELING MODEL

Cash allowance programs are very small because they involve "state-only" funds. States cannot use Medicaid to fund cash allowances that permit recipients to purchase their own services because of federal restrictions on direct payments to recipients. Because of these federal regulatory restrictions, large programs with a cash option have not been implemented, and there have not been any large-scale studies of such programs. When the three-state CCDE is completed, this large-scale evaluation will provide information about the costs, benefits, and implementation issues involved in a cash option so that state and federal policy makers can make informed decisions about implementing this long-term care model. However, background research conducted to guide the CCDE design provides information about consumers' and surrogates' level of interest in a consumer-directed cash option and reasons for such interest. In this chapter, we refer to our experiences with one demonstration site—Florida, where we conducted telephone surveys to assess participants' interest in the cash option versus traditional services. Florida's demonstration (called the Consumer Directed Care Program) encompassed several consumer populations, but in this chapter, we focus only on the outcomes derived from the components involving adults with developmental disabilities and their families. We also examine how lessons from the survey can guide Florida's efforts to develop communications and social marketing materials that will inform participants about the cash and counseling program.

Assessing Participant Preferences: Background Research to Support the CCDE

Little research exists to indicate 1) how many potential participants (or their family members or representative—the "surrogate decision makers") would choose a cash option, 2) which participant characteristics might indicate who would choose cash versus agency-based PAS, and 3) which cash option features would be attractive or unattractive to participants and their representatives. Such information is essential in helping a state design various cash option components (including counseling services) and social marketing approaches that would enable adults with disabilities and their representatives to make informed choices between the cash option and their current program.

States' communications and social marketing tasks are critical to heightening interest in a cash and counseling option and are somewhat daunting for several reasons. The cash option is distinct from traditional services, and adults with developmental disabilities often have difficulty understanding such a new and different concept. For adults who have not completed or gone beyond high school, this communication effort is especially challenging. In addition, even for adults who decide that they like the cash option and feel qualified to try it, there is a need to overcome fears and concerns about changing a service that is so important to their daily lives.

Florida Survey

Florida state officials underwrite supports and care provision for dependent populations in a variety of traditional ways. To determine whether a more consumer-responsive method could be viable, they decided to implement a demonstration of the cash option model. As part of the HCBS 1915c Medicaid Waiver and Individual and Family Supports Program demonstration, state officials decided to include children and adults with developmental disabilities and set up the following rules: 1) funds would need to be used for personal assistance services, such as personal care workers, home renovations, and/or assistive devices; 2) each participant had to develop a plan for the use of the cash; and 3) funds could be carried over from month to month for large purchases or emergency needs. States that have tested such efforts typically have predefined a cash payment amount. In doing so, states generally follow current assessment and care planning practices, establish the value of the individual care plan, and offer a cash amount that approximately amounts to what participants would receive in a traditional services program. In Florida, the state's Department of Developmental Services average annual support plan cost is $8,103 for adults with a developmental disability. Counseling services are an integral part of the demonstration. They include services to help potential participants decide whether to select the cash option, and for cash option participants, they include an array of support services, such as support for helping them manage employer responsibilities or locate home modification subcontractors.

At the time of the demonstration, approximately 12,900 adults with developmental disabilities were receiving services from Florida's HCBS Medicaid Waiver and Individual and Family Supports Program. For the telephone survey, we randomly selected approximately 5% of these adults. We adapted a survey instrument that originally was developed for the CCDE to obtain information from elders and adults with physical disabilities (Simon-Rusinowitz et al., 1997). Development of the 154-item survey was guided by three experts in developmental disabilities as well as a variety of self-advocacy and family focus group discussions (see Zacharias, 1997a, 1997b, for a full discussion of focus group findings). The survey comprised four sections: frequency of and satisfaction with current services, perceptions regarding the cash and counseling option, demographic and background variables, and perceptions and demographics of surrogates. In addition, participants were asked questions about functional status; overall physical health; living arrangement; number of informal caregivers; and experience with interviewing, training, hiring, or supervising workers, among others.

The telephone survey, one component of a three-part study, was conducted along with pre- and postsurvey focus groups. This study was designed to

1. Determine preferences for consumer-directed services in general and for a cash option in specific
2. Determine the percentage of consumers and surrogates who would choose the cash option versus traditional services
3. Identify reasons for consumers' and surrogates' preferences
4. Identify demographic and background characteristics of consumers and surrogates who have specific preferences

5. Identify cash option features that are attractive and unattractive to consumers and surrogates
6. Identify what information consumers and surrogates need to decide whether to choose the cash option
7. Identify consumers' or surrogates' needs for counseling and support services
8. Develop strategies to market the cash option
9. Assess the amount and types of services that consumers received under the state's current programs

People Interviewed   A total of 378 adults with a developmental disability participated in the survey interviews; 100 of these adults answered the survey themselves, and the rest chose to have a surrogate or representative decision maker answer for them. (The survey response rate was 53% as 333 people contacted did not participate.) Among the respondents, men and women were almost equally represented and their ages ranged from 19 to 82 years (mean age, 35 years). The respondents represented an ethnically diverse group: approximately two thirds of the respondents were of European heritage, one fifth were African American, and a small number were Hispanic. Approximately two thirds were single; the rest were married, widowed, or divorced. Approximately two thirds lived with their parents, and the same number had informal caregivers. Most rated their overall health as "good," "very good," or "excellent"; only approximately one fifth reported "fair" or "poor" health. Their functional status was measured by asking whether they needed help with five ADLs or ADL skill areas: bathing, dressing, toileting, transferring, and eating. Scores reflected whether and how often a consumer needed help (i.e., consumers could answer yes, no, or sometimes). Based on a scale ranging from 0 to 5, individuals who scored between 0 and 1.5 were considered mildly disabled (they made up approximately three fourths of the group), those who scored between 2 and 3.5 were considered moderately disabled (they made up approximately one fifth), and those who scored between 4 and 5 were considered severely disabled (they made up approximately one tenth). They were asked whether they received any of 18 different services; the majority reported receiving two types: case management and transportation.

Surrogates ($n = 278$) were older (age range, 28–89 years; mean age, 58 years) and mostly female. Approximately one half were mothers, one fifth were sisters, and one tenth were fathers. Close to 60% were married, and most surrogates or representatives lived with a spouse or their children. Most of the surrogates completed high, trade, or vocational school or attended some college; approximately one fifth did not complete high school. Surrogates' racial and ethnic backgrounds were similar to those of the adults with developmental disabilities.

Consumer Interest in Cash and Counseling   When consumers were asked about their interest in the cash option, 44% who answered for themselves expressed interest, as did 38% of surrogates who answered for consumers. Surrogates also were asked about their own interest in the cash option, and 45% were interested. Whether adults with developmental disabilities were interested in participating in a cash and counseling program differed according to their race and ethnicity, level of disability, satisfaction with current services, and personal desire for more say in selecting and scheduling services. Adults who were of Hispanic and African American heritage were more interested in the cash option than were adults of European heritage. Adults with a severe disability were more likely to be interested in the cash option than were adults with a moderate or mild disability. Adults who were most dissatisfied with their current services had the greatest level of interest in the cash option, when compared with those who were satisfied or unsure about their current services. Adults who wanted more say in selecting their services were more interested in the cash option than were those who were unsure and/or did not want more say. The same was true for adults who wanted more control over scheduling services, with more than half interested in the cash option, compared with those who were unsure or who did not want more control.

We were curious about how satisfied adults with developmental disabilities were with their current services and asked them to indicate their agreement or disagreement with the following three statements that began with, "One of the things I don't like about the services I currently receive is that ...": 1) the agencies providing them don't inform me of changes being made, 2) the people providing them are not properly trained, and 3) often the workers and I don't speak the same language. We found that the more they agreed with either of the first two statements, the more interest they expressed in the cash option. Of those adults who believed that agencies did not inform them of changes, slightly more than half were interested in the cash option. In addition, for those who believed that workers were not properly trained, approximately half were interested in the cash option. No such congruence was seen with agreement noted with the third statement.

Adults with developmental disabilities who were interested in the cash option did not differ significantly (compared with those who were not interested) by the following variables: age, gender, education level, marital status, living arrangement, home ownership, presence of informal caregivers or live-in informal caregivers, past or present employment status, experience with supervising or training and hiring or firing workers, self-rating of overall health status, number of different services received, number of different services with which one is dissatisfied, or average cost of services during a 9-month period. The most important considerations that indicated interest in the cash option among adults with developmental disabilities were 1) personal desire, for those who wanted a greater say in the selection of services were more interested in the cash option; 2) race and ethnicity, as adults who were of other than European heritage were more likely to be interested in the cash option; and 3) functional level, for adults with severe impairments were more likely to indicate some interest in the cash option when compared with adults with mild or moderate impairments.

The adults also were asked which of three program characteristics would make them more interested in the cash option: 1) the ability to get services on the days and times you want them; 2) the ability to hire whomever you want to provide personal care services, even a friend or a relative; and 3) the ability to buy different services. Most who were interested in the cash option indicated that any of these items would make them want to become part of the new program. They also were asked about their interest in purchasing various services, including more hours of personal care services; someone to keep them company; grab bars or equipment to help them in the shower; wheelchair, motorized scooter, hospital bed, or chair lift; home remodeling services; exercise equipment; transportation services; laundry services; and housekeeping services. Again, those who were interested in the cash option were significantly more likely to want to purchase the various services when compared with those who were not interested or those who were not sure of their interest level.

Surrogate Interest in Cash and Counseling   As with the adults with developmental disabilities, surrogate interest in the cash option differed significantly by race and ethnic background. More surrogates of Hispanic and African American background were interested than were surrogates of European heritage. Surrogate interest also differed significantly by age of the consumer. As the consumer age increased, surrogate interest waned. Their interest also waned as surrogates themselves got older. However, surrogate interest did not differ by sex, education level, marital status, relationship to the adult with a disability, or living arrangement. Surrogates who were interested in the cash option were also more likely to be interested in controlling the nature of the services received. For example, they liked the idea of being able to interview and hire the worker and believed that receiving cash would offer more flexibility to them and to their relative or friend. Surrogates were asked whether they thought the cash option would make it easier or harder on them. Approximately one third believed that the option would make their job easier, whereas approximately one fifth believed that it would be harder and approximately one half were not sure. Surrogates who were interested in the cash option were significantly more likely to believe that the option would make things easier for them when compared with those who were not interested. Furthermore, surrogates who were interested in the cash option were more likely than those who were not sure or not interested in performing such tasks as hiring, training, scheduling, supervising, paying, and firing one's own worker. Here, age of surrogate was not a factor, for no age-related differences were found in the surrogates' willingness to perform duties associated with the cash option.

Training and Support Needs   Most adults with lifelong disabilities wanted assistance or training in each of the seven tasks associated with the cash option. However, those who were interested in the cash option were significantly more likely to want help or training on each task when compared with unsure or uninterested consumers. They were more likely to want help, compared with uninterested consumers, with doing a quality check on a worker, deciding how much to pay a worker, payroll taxes, finding a worker, knowing what to do when a worker does not show, interviewing a worker, and firing a worker. Likewise, surrogates who were interested in participating in the cash option were more likely to indicate a need for help or training in the oversight tasks. Overall, before deciding to be involved in the cash option, most adults with a disability (regardless of their interest level) wanted more information. They were found to be even more likely to want information if they stated that they were interested in the option or not certain.

COMMENTARY

Information from the Florida survey helps us better understand how cash and counseling programs can be helpful in maintaining older adults with developmental disabilities in their community. We learned that adults who have the most severe disabilities are the ones who are most likely to be interested in the cash option; however, it is important to include adults with different levels of disability in social marketing efforts. Thus, publicity efforts need to focus on reaching the small, more severely disabled group and learning more about factors that would help adults with mild disabilities feel comfortable with choosing the cash option.

Generally, there is a high level of interest in the cash option among surrogates when they are expressing their own views, yet there is a somewhat lower interest when they are speaking as surrogate decision makers for the adults with a disability. Surrogates who express an interest in the cash option generally think that their adult relative or friend with a disability would want to participate, which indicates that this belief would be important to surrogates' support for the new option. As a majority of adults with developmental disabilities generally are represented by a surrogate decision maker, whether parents or another close relative (e.g., sister, brother, aunt), it is reasonable to assume that one of these people would be influential in helping a consumer make decisions about his or her personal care. It is possible that one surrogate decision-maker role may be as an emergency backup worker if the paid worker does not come to work—an important concern expressed by the adults. Another role may be as a paid worker (obtaining payment for additional help or for some of the services now performed gratis).

Surrogates' interest in the cash option generally decreases as their adult relative's age increases and as their own age increases. One reason for this may be that parents of aging adults, who are themselves older, may be worn out from many years of caregiving. Parents may be uninterested in an option that requires more of their time and energy. However, it is interesting that surrogates' willingness to perform cash option tasks did not differ significantly when their age was considered. More plausible may be that aging parents or other surrogates may be increasingly aware (and fearful) that they will not always be around to care for their adult son or daughter.

Surrogates' interest in the cash option generally is related to three variables (in descending order of importance): 1) surrogates' belief that the cash option would offer more flexibility and independence for them, 2) surrogates' willingness to assume responsibility for employer tasks involved in the cash option, and 3) surrogates' belief that the cash option would make it easier on them. For the surrogates who thought that the cash option would be harder, interest in cash was related to a belief that the extra effort would be worthwhile. Thus, cash option characteristics that are deemed attractive to interested adults can provide ideas about social marketing messages (and, more important, direction for designing the cash option). For example, effective materials should address the ability to get services on the days and at the times when they are wanted, and participants should be able to hire whomever they want to provide personal care services, even a friend or a relative, because these program characteristics are especially appealing. Generally, adults find the ability to "buy different services"—especially transportation services, someone to keep them company, exercise equipment, more hours of service, and housekeeping services—an attractive program feature.

Materials directed toward surrogates should highlight the ability to interview and hire workers and to hire a friend or a relative and should promote the attractiveness of increased flexibility for adults with disabilities and their surrogates. Consumers and surrogates who are interested in a cash option should also be informed that there can be peer support from other cash option recipients and that they can back out of the option if they want to return to a traditional funding of services program. Another attractive feature of the cash option that can be used in promoting its availability is that the recipient is not barred from hiring his or her current worker. Social marketing materials should inform potential participants that they can have help or training with the most requested tasks: doing a background check, help with deciding how much to pay a worker, filing payroll taxes, finding a worker, knowing what to do when a worker does not show, and interviewing and firing a worker.

In making the cash and counseling option available in any community, the following should be considered: First, should social marketing efforts use some well-regarded community organizations? Second, at what level should written materials be directed? Will they be equally effective for people with or without a high school education? Third, what about the timing of presenting various issues? For example, what messages are critical "door openers" to be included in general introductory materials? What information should be included in follow-up communication? Fourth, how do you know when potential participants want hands-on assistance as opposed to training that would allow them to function independently? Fifth, should separate materials be developed for specific segments of the population (e.g., according to gender, race, age, surrogate, consumer viewpoint)?

The premise for the cash and counseling approach is that the cash option is a choice that is available to consumers who want to exercise consumer direction. It is not intended to replace traditional services, as the cash option is unlikely to be appropriate for or desirable to all consumers. The Florida survey supports this perspective; although a sizable number of people expressed a preliminary interest in the cash option, many others were uncertain or not interested. Fraud and abuse concerns, related to the possibility that consumers and/or their families might misuse the cash benefit or be exploited by others, must also be considered (Doty, 1997). Thus, procedures to minimize fraud and abuse need to be designed to maintain consumer empowerment principles. However, caution must be used because overly restrictive measures would negate the effect of the consumer-directed intervention. Misuse of the cash benefit includes the possibility that consumers might not pay taxes or their workers. The Florida survey has shown that these possibilities are limited, as a majority of consumers and surrogates who are interested in the cash option said they would want help or training with payroll and taxes. That is, most recipients are likely to elect to have the payrolling and tax withholding for their workers done for them by accounting professionals. This service would limit the amount of cash that consumers need to manage. Consumers who elect not to use accounting professionals may need to participate in a training program and demonstrate competency in payrolling tasks or enter into cooperatives, such as could be provided by independent living centers at little or no cost.

To prevent consumer exploitation by others (and subsequent experiencing of ill effects), the cash option allows and encourages the use of a surrogate or decision maker to assist consumers who are unable to make all decisions independently. Representatives are not paid for their assistance in this function. Although there are many questions to consider regarding surrogate decision makers, we know from the Florida survey that most adults with a developmental disability use representatives. When asked about their own views (versus representing an adult with a disability), almost half of these representatives were interested in the cash option. In the event of possible exploitation by a surrogate under the cash option, counselors will have a role in monitoring all consumers—even those with representatives. For adults who function independently—that is, without representatives—the cash option's training and support services offer further protection against consumer exploitation. We know that the vast majority of consumers who were interested in the cash option wanted these support services and that some states require all consumers and surrogates to participate in some training. The counselors who offer such support services have had specific training in consumer-direction principles as applied in the cash and counseling option to supplement their experience with traditional personal care programs.

Because many adults with a developmental disability prefer to hire whomever they want to provide personal care services, even a friend or a relative, this is an attractive feature of the cash option financing model. However, policy makers often raise concerns about the quality of the care provided by friends or relatives because they may lack formal training. Two studies of California's In-Home Support Services Program found that consumers rated family members and friends as more reliable than workers who were strangers (Barnes & Sutherland, 1995; Benjamin, Matthias, & Franke, 1998). In addition, a study of older Medicaid personal care recipients in Michigan found that consumer satisfaction was related to several indicators of greater consumer control, specifically to that state's policy of encouraging clients to hire family, friends, and neighbors as attendants (Doty, Kasper, & Litvak, 1996). The Florida survey tells us that the cash and counseling demonstration will further our understanding about the quality of services when friends and relatives become paid providers.

In summary, the Florida survey provides evidence that many adults with developmental disabilities and their surrogate decision makers will be interested in the cash and counseling option—a policy that encourages adults with disabilities to make their own decisions and have control over their services. This option has the potential to address the public policy concerns of containing costs and promoting self-determination. We look forward to learning even more about consumers' interest in and satisfaction with a cash option (versus traditional services) as the demonstration and evaluation proceeds and as the choice becomes real, not theoretical.

REFERENCES

Abery, B.H. (1994). A conceptual framework for enhancing self-determination. In M.F. Hayden & B.H. Abery (Eds.), *Challenges for a service system in transition: Ensuring quality community experiences for persons with developmental disabilities* (pp. 345–380). Baltimore: Paul H. Brookes Publishing Co.

Agosta, J., & Melda, K. (1996). Supporting families who provide care at home for children with disabilities. *Exceptional Children, 62,* 271–282.

Ansello, E.F., & Eustis, N.N. (1992). A common stake? Investigating the emerging intersection of aging and disabilities. *Generations, 16,* 5–8.

Ashbaugh, J.W., Bradley, V.J., & Blaney, B.C. (1994). Implications for future practice and systems design. In V.J. Bradley, J.W. Ashbaugh, & B.C. Blaney (Eds.), *Creating individual supports for people with developmental disabilities: A mandate for change at many levels* (pp. 491–508). Baltimore: Paul H. Brookes Publishing Co.

Barnes, C., & Sutherland, S. (1995). *Context of care, provider characteristics, and quality of care in the IHSS program: Implications for provider standards. Interim report to the California Department of Social Services.* Sacramento: California State University, Institute for Social Research.

Beatty, P.W., Richmond, G.W., Tepper, S., & DeJong, G. (1998). Personal assistance for people with physical disabilities: Consumer-direction and satisfaction with services. *Archives of Physical Medicine and Rehabilitation, 79,* 674–677.

Benjamin, A.E., Matthias, R.E., & Franke, T. (1998). *Comparing client-directed and agency models for providing disability-related supportive services at home.* (Report prepared for the Assistant Secretary for Planning and Evaluation, U.S. Department of Health and Human Services, Award No. HHS-100-94-0022.) Los Angeles: University of California, Los Angeles, Center for Child and Policy Studies.

Bradley, V., Ashbaugh, B., & Blaney, B. (Eds.). (1994). *Creating individual supports for people with developmental disabilities: A mandate for change at many levels.* Baltimore: Paul H. Brookes Publishing Co.

Cameron, K., & Firman, B. (1995). *International and domestic programs using "cash and counseling" strategies to pay for long-term care.* Washington, DC: National Council on the Aging.

Cotten, P., & Sowers, B. (1996). *Choice through knowledge: Knowledge = power.* Durham: University of New Hampshire, Institute on Disability.

DeJong, G., Batavia, A., & McKnew, L. (1992). The independent living model of personal assistance in national long-term care policy. *Generations, 16,* 89–95.

Doty, P. (1997). *Internal briefing paper addressing possible fraud and abuse issues in the cash option.* Unpublished manuscript, U.S. Department of Health and Human Services, Office of the Assistant Secretary for Planning and Evaluation, Washington, DC.

Doty, P., Kasper, B., & Litvak, S. (1996). Consumer-directed models of personal care: Lesson from Medicaid. *Milbank Memorial Fund, 74,* 377–409.

Fenton, M., Entrikin, T., Morril, S., Marburg, G., Shumway, D., & Nerney, T. (1997). *Beyond managed care: Volume II.* Durham: University of New Hampshire, Institute on Disability.

Geron, S., & Chassler, D. (1994). *Guidelines for case management practice across the long-term care continuum* (Technical Report). Bristol, CT: Connecticut Community Care.

Glickman, L.L., Brandt, K.B., & Caro, F.G. (1994). *Self-direction in home care for older people.* Boston: University of Massachusetts–Boston, Gerontology Institute and Center.

Hayden, M., & Abery, B.H. (Eds.). (1994). *Challenges for a service system in transition.* Baltimore: Paul H. Brookes Publishing Co.

Hayden, M.F., & DePaepe, P. (1994). Waiting for community services: The impact on persons with mental retardation and other developmental disabilities. In M.F. Hayden & B.H. Abery (Eds.), *Challenges for a service system in transition: Ensuring quality community experiences for persons with developmental disabilities* (pp. 173–206). Baltimore: Paul H. Brookes Publishing Co.

Herman, S. (1991). Use and impact of a cash subsidy program. *Mental Retardation, 29,* 253–258.

Jackson, M.E. (1994). *Rationing case management: Six case studies.* Unpublished report prepared for the U.S. Department of Health and Human Services, Office of the Assistant Secretary for Planning and Evaluation, Washington, DC.

Kapp, M. (1996). Enhancing autonomy and choice in selecting and directing long-term care services. *Elder Law Journal, 4*(1), 55–97.

Knoll, J., Covert, S., Osuch, R., O'Connor, S., Agosta, J., & Blaney, B. (1990). *Family support service in the United States: An end of the decade status report.* Boston: Human Services Research Institute.

Litvak, S., & Kennedy, J. (1990). *New models for the provision of personnel assistance services. Appendix B: Chartbook of tables from FY 1988 personal assistance program survey data* (NIDRR Grant No. G008720134). Berkeley, CA: World Institute on Disability.

Litvak, S., & Kennedy, J. (1991). *Policy issues and questions affecting the Medicaid personal care services optional benefit* (Contract No. HHS-100-89-0025). Oakland, CA: World Institute on Disability.

Litvak, S., Zukas, H., & Heumann, J.E. (1987). *Attending to America: Personal assistance for independent living. A survey of attendant service programs in the United States for people of all ages with disabilities.* Berkeley, CA: World Institute on Disability.

Mahoney, C.W., Estes, C.L., & Heumann, J.E. (Eds.). (1986). *Toward a unified agenda: Proceedings of a national conference on disability and aging.* San Francisco: University of California/World Institute on Disability.

Meyers, B., & Marcenco, M. (1986). *An evaluation of Michigan's family support subsidy program: Coping with the cost.* Detroit: Wayne State University, Developmental Disabilities Institute.

Nisbet, J. (Ed.). (1992). *Natural supports in school, at work, and in the community for people with severe disabilities.* Baltimore: Paul H. Brookes Publishing Co.

Rimer, S. (1998, March 15). Blacks carry load of care for their elderly. *The New York Times,* p. 1.

Simon-Rusinowitz, L., & Hofland, B.F. (1993). Adopting a disability approach to home care services for older adults. *Gerontologist, 33,* 159–167.

Simon-Rusinowitz, L., Mahoney, K.J., Desmond, S.M., Shoop, D., Squillace, M.A., & Fay, R. (1997). Determining consumer preferences for a cash option: Arkansas survey results. *Health Care Financing Review, 19*(2), 73–96.

Simon-Rusinowitz, L., Mahoney, K.J., Shoop, D., Desmond, S.M., Squillace, M.A., Fay, R., & Sowers, J.A. (1998). *Determining preferences of adults with developmental disabilities for a cash option: Florida survey results. Background research to support the Cash and Counseling Demonstration and Evaluation.* Unpublished technical report, University of Maryland, College Park.

Smith, G. (1994). Paying for supports: Dollars, payments, and the new paradigm. In V.J. Bradley, J.W. Ashbaugh, & B.C. Blaney (Eds.), *Creating individual supports for people with developmental disabilities: A mandate for change at many levels* (pp. 481–490). Baltimore: Paul H. Brookes Publishing Co.

Tennestedt, S., & Chang, B.-H. (1998). The relative contribution of ethnicity versus socioeconomic status in explaining differences in disability and receipt of informal care. *Journal of Gerontology, 53B,* S61–S70.

Wallace, S.P., Levy-Storms, L., Kington, R.S., & Andersen, R.M. (1998). The persistence of race and ethnicity in the use of long-term care. *Journal of Gerontology, 53B,* S104–S112.

Wisconsin Department of Health and Social Services. (1985). *Family support guidelines and procedures.* Madison: Author.

Wolfe, P.S., Ofiesh, N.S., & Boone, R.B. (1996). Self-advocacy preparation of consumers with disabilities: A national perspective of ADA training efforts. *Journal of The Association for Persons with Severe Handicaps, 21*(2), 81–87.

Zacharias, B.L. (1997a). *Cash and counseling demonstration and evaluation: A study to determine the preferences of consumers and surrogates for a cash option. Report on Florida focus groups.* Unpublished technical report University of Maryland Center on Aging, College Park.

Zacharias, B.L. (1997b). *Cash and counseling demonstration and evaluation. A study to determine the preferences of consumers and surrogates for a cash option. Report on New York State Focus Groups.* Unpublished technical report, University of Maryland Center on Aging, College Park.

14

Modifying Home Environments

B. Lynn Hutchings, Richard V. Olsen, and Ezra D. Ehrenkrantz

As the quality and availability of health care advances, people with developmental disabilities are increasingly likely to live to old age. Current goals of deinstitutionalization and normalization mean that this population is, for the first time in recent history, living in integrated, community-based environments. Research has shown the benefits of aging in place rather than moving frail individuals to nursing homes or other institutional environments (Heller, 1985). This has prompted research into the advantages of modifying the home for people who are experiencing the physical effects of aging. The need for a physically supportive home is particularly pronounced for older people with developmental disabilities, who face the prospect of having age-related disabilities overlaid onto existing limitations, and particularly for those who are experiencing the resurrection of old limitations, such as people with postpolio syndrome.

Although a fair amount of research probes the environmental needs of people with specific disabilities, such as Alzheimer's disease or other cognitively and/or physically debilitating conditions, very little research has considered the role of the physical environment as it affects people who are aging with developmental disabilities. Furthermore, research needs to confirm that nursing home placement or other forms of institutionalization can be avoided or delayed if these individuals have the appropriate physical and social supports in their homes.

Like the larger population, the population of older people with developmental disabilities is a heterogeneous population with respect to age, health, functional impairments, cognitive abilities, and informal support systems (Adlin, 1993; Krauss & Seltzer, 1986). It includes not only people with intellectual disabilities but also those with cerebral palsy and other neuromuscular disorders, spina bifida, and a host of less-publicized disabilities. This variation means that people with disabilities place a correspondingly wide range of demands on their physical environment. Providers of services and housing to people with developmental disabilities need to ensure that the built environment maintains its ability to meet the needs of higher functioning individuals while simultaneously providing the flexibility to adapt to the worst-case scenario without assuming the trappings of an institution. For example, a group home may include both individuals who are relatively spry and others who use wheelchairs and have severe mobility impairments. Older people, in particular, can move from the high to the low end of the functional abilities spectrum in a relatively short period of time (American Institute of Architects [AIA], 1985). Consequently, environments for older people with and without preexisting disabilities should be designed with maximum flexibility to adapt to these changing needs. It is a good tactic to develop designs and retrofits that are dementia friendly. It is now estimated that 50% of the population older than 85 years (and this is the fastest growing segment of the population) has some form of cognitive or memory impairment. It is important for those who design new homes for people with disabilities to consider people's needs across their entire adult life spans.

Although flexible home designs may be more expensive at the outset, the potential savings over time can mitigate the initial expense by avoiding the many costs associated with a nonsupportive environment. These unwelcome expenditures can include home care and increased staffing at group homes to meet individual needs, nursing home costs, moving expenses, and the total replacement of housing that cannot be modified to meet changing needs. In addition, the supportive environment provided by flexible home design will result in a higher quality of life for people with developmental disabilities. For example, if people are able to prepare their own meals or to continue to use the bathroom without assistance, then their personal dignity and self-esteem are upheld while the cost of care is minimized. People who have led independent lives, such as many of those with postpolio syndrome and spina bifida, are more likely to remain in their homes with minimal personal assistance if their homes are physically accessible and adaptable to their needs as they age. Although some home designs are inherently more flexible than others, there are many ways in which existing housing can be modified to meet the needs of people with the ever-increasing limitations that are likely to occur with advancing age. Although this chapter focuses mainly on modifications that can be made to existing homes, it also discusses considerations for new home design.

MODIFYING ENVIRONMENTS FOR PEOPLE WITH PHYSICAL DISABILITIES

A number of authors have provided information that specifically addresses the needs of people with physical disabilities (Ferguson, 1988; Goldsmith, 1976; Lifchez & Winslow, 1979). For example, Ferguson (1988) provided a conceptual overview of the relationship among environment, behavior, and personal autonomy and choice. For a more pragmatic and architectural approach, *Designing for the Disabled* by Goldsmith (1976) remains a comprehensive design resource. Although written primarily for practicing architects, this third edition of a book first published in 1963 also is oriented toward providers of housing for people with physical disabilities. It includes practical information that is pertinent to the design and retrofit of both public buildings and private dwellings.

Dementia and Aging

Because of the challenges presented by Alzheimer's disease and related dementias and the potential of the physical environment to have an impact both positively and negatively on this population, several excellent resources exist on this subject (e.g., Cohen & Wiesman, 1991; Warner, 1998). *Homes that Help: Advice from Caregivers for Creating a Supportive Home* (Olsen, Hutchings, & Ehrenkrantz, 1993) details recommendations made by 90 long-term caregivers of family members with Alzheimer's disease. This publication focuses on creating an environment that is calm, reassuring, physically safe, and supportive and that provides opportunities for things to do. It includes detailed recommendations for home modifications that support these goals and includes a home safety audit checklist, as well as delineating features that are desirable if the family decides to move.

Calkins and Namazi (1991) also researched home modifications for Alzheimer's care. Fifty-nine in-home caregivers reported on the nature and effectiveness of environmental modifications they had made to address issues that are common to dementia, such as wandering and incontinence. Warner (1998) discussed strategies for providing a safe and secure home for people with dementia and included information on mobility, wandering, activities of daily living, and behavior problems.

Consumer-Based Developmental Disabilities Research

Since 1992, the authors have completed four consumer-based studies on the needs and preferences of adults with developmental disabilities (Olsen, Hutchings, & Ehrenkrantz, 1992, 1995, 1996, 1997). Although all of these studies included older adults, the second two specifically included a smaller subsample of people aging with developmental disabilities and the fourth was concerned solely with this population. A primary goal of the research was to explore the relationship between the home environments of people with both physical and intellectual disabilities and their physical and social functioning and well-being. Consequently, the degree to which their physical environments made it easier or harder to do things on their own was of particular interest. The vast majority of responses indicated the critical nature of accessible design. Findings underscored that accessibility is the pathway to mobility and independence. This was particularly true for people with physical disabilities but also true for people with intellectual disabilities, as their stamina and agility decreased with age. Findings also underscored the importance of people's having a high degree of control over their environments and independence in their actions.

Although information on home design and modifications for both people with physical disabilities and people who are aging are widely available and publications that link this area to specific conditions such as Alzheimer's disease also can be found in the literature, there remains a need for information on home modifications specific to the needs of people aging with developmental disabilities. The Center for Architecture and Building Science Research's (CABSR's) report (Olsen et al., 1997) provided the "first glimpse" of the impact of the physical environment on people with developmental disabilities who are aging. Additional research to gain a better understanding of the complexities of this relationship is needed. Even books on group homes rarely address the actual home design and ways that the physical environment can be modified as the needs of older residents change and increase with advancing age. CABSR's research has addressed this issue, although much work still needs to be done. This chapter integrates the findings from the literature with CABSR's research to provide preliminary guidelines for the wide range of home modification options that may be undertaken to better serve this population.

GENERAL LAYOUT AND FURNISHING CONSIDERATIONS

In designing for older people with developmental disabilities, a simple layout is far preferable to one that includes complex corners and multiple levels. In the wide range of aging and disability studies conducted by CABSR, one-level homes were highly recommended by both people with disabilities and their caregivers. When people have dementia or are experiencing some degree of confusion, open layouts that allow the impaired person to see his or her caregiver contribute to his or her sense of security and decrease feelings of isolation and loneliness. Conversely, the caregiver, who may be a group home manager responsible for other individuals, is able to keep an eye on the person for whom he or she is caring while completing personal and household tasks. Open layouts also enable a confused person to see the bathroom, bedroom, and other areas of the home that he or she may need to enter. An open floor plan also is more conducive to social interaction and casual conversation. In existing homes, the layout can be opened up somewhat by widening doorways and putting window spaces or pass-throughs into preexisting walls between rooms. Unnecessary walls can be replaced with columns. Non–load-bearing walls can be removed. Doors between shared spaces also can be removed to create wider openings and increased visibility. It is important, however, to keep in mind that there is a trade-off between an open plan that is conducive to safety and security and smaller spaces that provide privacy and intimacy. The ideal home will provide space for both.

Although we often think of grab bars and handrails as bathroom modifications, they also can improve safety in other areas, particularly in hallways. Handrails can increase independence by making it possible for people to walk on their own for a longer period of time. They can also help define a path to specific areas of the home (e.g., to the bathroom or the kitchen).

Because older people often lack visual acuity and may not remember to look where they are walking, uncluttered rooms pose fewer safety hazards than crowded spaces. Throw rugs should be avoided, because they are likely to be unnoticed and cause falls. If residents use walkers, canes, wheelchairs, or crutches or shuffle when they walk, then low-pile carpeting or no carpeting are preferable to area rugs. It also will be helpful to remove doorsills, which could trip a shuffler and provide an impediment for people who use assistive mobility devices, such as wheelchairs or scooters. Single steps are considered dangerous for people of all ages, because they are likely to go unnoticed and cause minor accidents. Single steps may be replaced with ramps to accommodate the change in level.

Glass-top cocktail tables, small nesting tables, ottomans, magazine racks, and other low furniture should be kept to a minimum. Small tables and other low furniture, in particular, should not be placed in the center of rooms. Furniture placed against walls is less likely to be tripped over and bumped into. Sharp corners and edges should be avoided whenever possible.

There are certain areas in which it may be helpful to add furniture. Shelves on which to deposit bags and packages temporarily are useful on both sides of exterior doorways. If hallways or stair landings provide sufficient width, then a chair or a bench might provide a much-welcomed resting place. Particularly if residents have trouble hearing, it may be helpful to create seating alcoves, or spaces set off from the general flow of traffic, that eliminate confusing background noise and can be used for conversation (Pynoos & Regnier, 1991).

Multiple-Level Homes

When a person who lives in a multilevel home can no longer safely traverse up and down stairs, there are two options to solve the problem. The first is to modify the house to create one-level living. This can be done by adding rooms to the first level of the house (e.g., a master bedroom and bath suite) and by using existing space in a different way. Several families in CABSR's studies have made dens, dining rooms, or family rooms into bedrooms. This is a viable option, but it generally requires a full bath on the same floor to make it work most efficiently.

The second option is to make stairs more user-friendly. Many people as they become more frail pull themselves up the stairs, one step at a time. A railing on both sides of the stairs, securely anchored into the wall studs or the steps, will support the weight of the person. Vertical hand grips, also anchored into the studs at strategic locations, can serve the same purpose when it is impossible to install a continuous railing. As people's comprehension and vision deteriorate with increasing age, they may have trouble seeing steps or perceiving a step as a change in level. It is important to make sure stairs are well lit. Major changes in illumination between stairways and surrounding areas should also be avoided, because difficulty in adapting to varying light conditions increases the risk of falls (Pynoos, Cohen, Davis, & Bernhardt, 1987). It may be advantageous to highlight the edge of a step by firmly gluing textured strips or reflector tape to the outer edge of the step or by painting the edge of the step a contrasting color. This allows a person to see the edge of the step more easily and know where to place his or her feet. This technique may be undesirable, if not impossible, on carpeted stairways. Interior stairways should have a stable, nonslip surface that prevents slipping. Wylde, Baron-Robbins, and Clark (1994) pointed out that stairs that have no landings and begin at the door threshold are particularly dangerous. Several caregivers in CABSR's studies placed handgrips at the top of such stairways, allowing the user to pull him- or herself up into the room or hall at the top of the stairs.

When people are no longer able to navigate stairs and yet need to live on more than one level, other options include ramps, stair lifts, and elevators. Building codes require that ramps have at least a 1:12 slope (or rise no more than 1 foot for every 12 feet) and recommend a 1:20 slope as easier for people to climb, whether walking or in wheelchairs (Wylde et al., 1994). As previously mentioned, short interior ramps that alleviate the need for one or two steps are often useful modifications to private homes. Longer interior ramps, such as those that would be needed in a split-level home, are rarely feasible because the space required for them would consume a good percentage of the living area of the house.

Stair lifts that feature a seat that moves up and down one side of a stair on a track are often added to single-family homes when residents have trouble navigating stairs. Although lifts that curve and bend around landings are available, straight lifts are less expensive and more commonplace (Wylde et al., 1994). In our research, we have seen these installed to great advantage even in small Cape Cod–style homes. However, lifts with chairs have several disadvantages. First, they lift the person only—not the person's wheelchair. If a person is dependent on a mobility device, he or she must either have an extra device waiting at the top or bottom of the staircase or have someone assist him or her by carrying the device up or down the stairs on an as-needed basis. Second, chair lifts require that a person be able to complete several sequential tasks to operate them safely. The chair must be folded down and locked into position; the person must be able to get on and off the chair, fasten the seatbelt or harness, and operate the lift. Many lifts require that constant pressure be applied to the controls by the rider for the lift to move, although lifts with remote controls are available. People who are confused, have intellectual disabilities, lack good hand dexterity, and/or lack good balance are likely to require assistance with these tasks.

Platform lifts are a more viable option for people who depend on wheelchairs. These mechanisms lift both the person and the wheelchair from one story to another and eliminate the need for transfers. Platform lifts come in two varieties: inclined lifts, which ascend and descend along an existing stairway, and vertical lifts, which rise vertically from one floor to the next but do not operate in a shaft the way an elevator does. Both are useful but costly additions to existing multistory homes. Elevators with fully enclosed cabs can also be added to existing homes, but at even greater expense. Some residential models run on tracks installed vertically along a wall surface, thus freeing the downstairs floor space when the elevator is on an upper floor. People in CABSR's studies who have gone to the trouble and expense of installing these residential elevators all have reported a high level of satisfaction with them. It is important also to install a phone in the elevator in case the elevator malfunctions or the person needs unexpected help.

Kitchens

In many homes, the kitchen serves not only as a place to prepare and eat food but also as a social and activity center. The traditional kitchen is often designed with a "one-size-fits-all" approach. However, this type of design rarely works for people with disabilities who are aging. Wylde et al. (1994) recommended that kitchens provide counters and work surfaces at varying heights ranging between 32 and 36 inches to accommodate people of varying heights or in wheelchairs. Ideally, work surfaces should be located on both sides of the cooktop, sink, and refrigerator, providing a place to put things that are heavy and/or hot. Countertops should have rounded edges and bull-nose corners to avoid injury in case of falls. Wylde et al. (1994) recommended heat-safe surfaces on countertops that have a dull or matte finish so as not to cause excessive glare. If residents use wheelchairs or do not have the strength or balance necessary to stand while preparing food, providing legroom underneath sinks, cooktops, microwaves, and other work surfaces will allow better proximity for someone who is seated in a chair or a wheelchair. When adequate counter space is not available, drawers at appropriate heights can be retrofitted with sliding panels above the interior space, providing a cantilevered work surface to which residents can easily pull up in a wheelchair. If heat-resistant countertops adjacent to the cooktop also are flush in height, people with limited strength can slide pots off the stove without having to lift them. Trash and recycling bins on castors that can be wheeled out from under counters provide a convenient disposal method. Sinks that are relatively shallow will be easier for people to use from a seated position. Lever-type faucets provide an advantage to people with limited hand and wrist mobility, because they do not have to grasp, turn, or twist them. Spray hoses and detachable faucets allow the user to pull a hose out from the faucet's spout to direct the stream of water more easily and efficiently.

Kitchens will have added versatility if they include a desk area that is accessible to wheelchair users. This provides a convenient spot to write recipes and shopping lists and to take notes while on the telephone. This area can double as a safe kitchen work space for people who no longer have the competency necessary to cope with appliances that can be dangerous to them. It should be located some distance away from the cooking area to avoid spills and splashing.

Multiple sources of direct lighting in the kitchen are critical to avoiding accidents and facilitating efficient use of space. Fluorescent lights can be hung underneath cabinets and on walls focusing on sinks and counter workspaces. CABSR's studies have shown that kitchen cabinets have numerous deficiencies for older users. Upper cabinets are rarely within reach of wheelchair users and often require stepstools for anyone below average height. Wylde et al. (1994) recommended lowering kitchen cabinets to a height from 12 to 15 inches above the counter. Below-counter cabinets, which are usually deep, dark, and hard to reach, may be replaced with drawers or pullout shelving. It is possible to purchase vertical units of shelving, which slide out from underneath the countertop, providing easy shelf access from two sides. "Lazy Susans" in corner cabinets improve the use of this space. It also is possible to purchase electronic revolving closet and cabinet systems that greatly facilitate access.

Appliances

Ovens and dishwashers normally have pull-down doors that make them difficult to approach in wheelchairs. This difficulty can be minimized by having adequate counter space and wheelchair space underneath counters on either side of appliances with pull-down doors. Wylde et al. (1994) recommended that ovens be mounted so that the base is 30–34 inches above the floor and easily reachable from both a standing and a wheelchair position. A side-hinged oven door and a pullout shelf located directly beneath the oven are also recommended, because they allow someone to pull a hot container out of the oven and rest it on a shelf, instead of having to pull and lift simultaneously. Refrigerators with side-by-side cold storage and freezer space facilitate use from a variety of positions. For residents with limited dexterity, refrigerators that are equipped with exterior water and ice dispensers may be worth the extra expense. It also is possible to purchase refrigerators that have a small pull-down door within the larger door at wheelchair height. This may be particularly advantageous if it is necessary to make some food easily accessible and other items off limits to people with intellectual and/or memory deficits who might otherwise eat inappropriate foods. Refrigerators with pullout shelves also are available.

Controls on all appliances should be located within easy reach and have clearly visible indicators. It also is possible to install fixtures with controls that are designed to be manipulated by people with limited hand dexterity (Pynoos & Regnier, 1991). Knobs placed at the back of stoves should be avoided because people have to reach across burners to operate them. All controls should be at the front of the cooktop.

It may become necessary to make the stove off-limits to someone who is confused or has memory or other cognitive limitations. There are a variety of ways to accomplish this. Knobs can be removed from the stove, although persistent individuals may still be able to turn the stems. Stove knob covers are available for purchase, as are aluminum covers that completely hide both the burners and the knobs. On electric ranges, the circuit breaker for the stove can be turned off or the fuses that control the stove can be removed. More convenient, a separate circuit breaker or gas switch-off can be installed near the stove but in a concealed place. Be sure to consult with an electrician or your gas company when you explore this option (Olsen et al., 1993).

Bathrooms

Bathrooms can be a source of multiple problems for older people with limited strength and coordination. As discussed, older people may have decreased balance and agility and compromised vision, all of which can make using a bathroom a treacherous necessity. Fortunately, there are many products that can be purchased and modifications that can be made to improve their safety and accessibility for anyone with compromised capabilities. Although larger bathrooms are easier to modify for accessibility, even small bathrooms can be greatly improved by the addition of nonslip flooring, grab bars, raised toilet seats, bath chairs, handheld shower hoses, and faucets with lever controls. Other assistive technology, such as bathtubs with side-hinged doors and molded seats, hydraulic bath seats, sinks, and shower chairs that can be electronically raised and lowered, are available at additional, often considerable, expense. The latter can make it easier for a person with limited use of the lower body, such as someone with spina bifida or postpolio syndrome, to groom him- or herself independently.

People who use assistive devices such as walkers and wheelchairs will often find traditional bathrooms too small to navigate in. Open areas in front of and underneath the sink and around the toilet are particularly essential to people who use wheelchairs. Larger bathrooms also become necessary when people require assistance with grooming, bathing, and toileting and an extra person is needed in the room to help with these activities. In CABSR's study (Olsen et al., 1997), one resourceful woman who lacked sufficient turning radius space in the bathroom adjacent to her master bedroom solved the problem by creating a "roll-through" bathroom. By installing a second bathroom door at the opposite end of the bathroom and opening onto the kitchen, she was able to get to the bathroom easily from these two different areas of the house that were otherwise separated by the living room and a long hall. Doors opening into bathrooms can present a dual problem. First, they may waste valuable navigation space. Second, if a resident falls in the bathroom, he or she may block the door, making it difficult for someone to get in to help him or her. Pocket doors, which slide horizontally into the adjacent wall cavity to open, can alleviate both of these concerns. However, pocket doors may present other problems. People with dementia or some degree of confusion may not remember that the door needs to be slid to the side rather than pushed or pulled. The hardware used to open and close pocket doors may be difficult or impossible for a person with limited hand dexterity to manipulate. If not properly designed and installed, they will not glide open and shut easily.

Grab Bars

All bathrooms should have grab bars bolted into the wall studs and located wherever a person may need support. This includes standing at a sink or vanity table or in the bathtub or shower, climbing into a bathtub, stooping, or going from a standing to a seated position. Although it may necessitate rebuilding walls to include extra wall studs, this is well worth the extra expense and inconvenience. Grab bars that are not firmly mounted are dangerous because they can pull out without warning when too much force is applied. People who participated in CABSR's studies installed grab bars in the bathtub and shower and at the entrance to the shower and tub, near the toilet, and in the front of vanity-type sinks and grooming tables. Pull-down sidebars are available for toilets. Vertically mounted, multilevel handgrips are particularly useful in bathtubs, where people of varying heights pull themselves up from a seated to a standing position. Grab bars not only help people with cerebral palsy and other developmental disabilities that are primarily physical but also steady people with intellectual disabilities who are experiencing the increasing frailty of old age. Pynoos and Regnier (1991) recommended installing towel racks that are heavier than normal and securely bolted into wall studs so that residents who use the racks to steady themselves will have a safe and secure handhold.

Sinks

Height-adjustable sinks allow a person who uses a wheelchair to raise the sink electronically while he or she pulls his or her chair underneath it, then lower it to a height that is more convenient for actual use. Wall-mounted or vanity-type sinks that are not height adjustable can be installed at a height that is convenient for both standard and wheelchair users—generally approximately 32 inches off the ground. Pullout hoses and detachable faucets, although usually designed for use in the kitchen, may also prove helpful at bathroom sinks. If people have limited arm movement and/or hand dexterity, it may be worth investing in a sensor-type faucet that turns on automatically when there is movement under the spout. If a vanity top or sink is particularly deep and faucets are difficult for residents to reach, it is possible to install faucets on the side rather than at the back of the sink. Spouts that pivot are useful in that they can reach well into the center of the sink but also can be turned out of the way. If a person has dementia, however, pivoting faucets can pose a flooding problem if the confused person turns the water on when the spout is not over the sink's basin. Mirrors over the sink and other grooming areas can be tilted slightly away from the wall at the top to give people who are seated a better view of themselves.

Toilets

Older people frequently have trouble lowering themselves from a standing to a seated position and raising themselves back up. For this reason, grab bars near the toilet or special grab bar units that fit around the toilet are highly recommended. Grab bars that can be lowered when needed and raised to a position flush with wall when they are not add a measure of versatility when people of varying degrees of agility are using the same toilet. Although "handicap" toilets have an 18-inch seat height that may make it easier to transfer from a wheelchair, this height will not allow many people's feet to touch the ground and may lead to a feeling of instability and insecurity. Both hydraulic and electronic toilets that lower and raise the user to and from a sitting position are available, but at considerable additional expense.

Bathtubs and Showers

Although many people prefer to have the options of both a bath and a shower as individuals lose dexterity and agility, they often find themselves relegated to one or the other. Wylde et al. (1994) found that people who used walkers, canes, or crutches had greater difficulty using a shower, whereas those who used wheelchairs had greater freedom in a shower. Because bathtubs require that a person lift his or her legs and step over the side onto a wet surface, they may pose safety hazards for people with limited dexterity or fragile balance. Bath mats, bath chairs, and grab bars are the least costly ways to address this problem.

Faucets should be easy to understand, with controls that are easy to grasp and turn. Older people may find faucets with separate hot and cold water controls easier to understand than the premixed (one spout for both hot and cold water) control system, because many of them grew up using the former. Handheld showerheads come highly recommended by subjects in both CABSR's study on aging with developmental disabilities and our Alzheimer's disease research. When people require assistance with bathing, handheld hoses put the control of the water into the hands of the caregiver and prevents him or her from having to move the person around the jet stream. Handheld units that slide up and down along a vertical rod and that can double as an adjustable-height, standard showerhead offer the most versatility. The showerhead should attach and detach easily and offer a variety of sprays and water-stream pressure. The controls should be easily reached from both inside and outside the shower stall. Anti-scald water control systems are widely available and easy to install. They make it possible to preset the water temperature and thereby ensure that residents do not inadvertently burn themselves.

Bath and shower chairs come in a variety of styles and at a range of prices. The term *bath chair* is often a misnomer, because most of them are far too high to give the seated person the opportunity to sit in a bath; many are really shower chairs, and some are designed to fit in bathtubs. CABSR's research has shown that this is an area in which the adage, "You get what you pay for," holds true. Bath chairs that are equipped with a backrest and extend over the side of the tub are usually easier and safer for people who have difficulty stepping over the bathtub's side wall. The disadvantage of these chairs is that a shower curtain cannot be placed inside the tub at the point where the chair extends over the side of the tub. Some bath chairs come with a cut-out area in the seat, making it easier to wash private parts with a handheld shower nozzle. There are bath chairs that have plastic tube frames and mesh seats that are height adjustable when they are not in use. Bathtubs designed with a wide shelf at the back of the tub may help a person to enter and exit the tub if he or she is able to sit on the shelf, swing his or her legs over the side of the tub, and then lower him- or herself into the tub. Options for people who have less dexterity and who want to take a bath but who have difficulty lowering themselves to a seated position in a bathtub are generally more expensive. These types of devices include chairs that can be raised and lowered hydraulically or electronically and side-opening bathtubs with raised, molded seats.

For people who prefer showers and are able to walk, the traditional walk-in shower stall often is a viable option. Grab bars and shower chairs can be used to help a person who does not have the strength or balance to stand unaided. Wylde et al. (1994) warned that some prefabricated shower stalls with molded seats are not particularly functional. They recommended that a shower seat be at least 15 inches deep to provide stability for the user. Seats that fold out of the way offer greater versatility but should be easy to raise and lower.

Roll-in showers are an attractive option for people who use wheelchairs regularly. The entrance to roll-in showers should be flush with the bathroom floor. The shower floor should have a slight slope so that water flows toward the floor drain. The entire shower area should have a waterproof surface, and the floor should have nonslip properties. The shower area should be a minimum of 30 by 60 inches, with a 60-inch opening toward the bathroom; larger areas will, of course, allow easier access. Shower curtains are the easiest way to contain the water spray. Some shower manufacturers provide prefabricated roll-in units. Roll-in shower chairs are widely available; some are made with a cutout seat and rolled directly over the toilet and thus can double as a toilet seat. Wylde et al. (1994) is a particularly good source for anyone modifying or building a bathroom. They not only suggest bathroom plans in a variety of sizes but also provide more detailed analyses of tubs, showers, sinks, and toilets and manufacturer information for many specialized products and fixtures.

Lighting and Heating

Good lighting should be installed in grooming, sink, and bathing areas. It should, of course, be diffused enough not to shine directly into the eyes of the bathroom user. For older people who may take longer to towel off and dress after a bath or a shower, heat lamps can provide an efficient source of well-timed and localized heat.

Outdoor Access

As people with developmental disabilities age and their world is in danger of shrinking as a result of increasing physical, cognitive, and sensory limitations, opportunities to expand their world become paramount. Awareness of the changing seasons, weather, and natural light can help to orient a person who is confused or confined indoors. Even placing a bed or a chair near a window with a view of outdoor life can provide orientation cues and a feeling of connection to a larger world. Lever handles on windows make it easier for people with limited hand dexterity to open and close them independently. Providing safe outdoor access is one of the easiest and healthiest ways to enrich an older person's life. Greenhouses, sunrooms, or lanai and enclosed porches provide varying degrees of protection from the elements and a feeling of safety and security while providing an outdoor feeling. Decks and paved patios or terraces provide stable footing for wheelchairs or people whose balance is shaky. When building decks or patios, it is important to have a smooth surface across which people who use wheelchairs, walkers, and canes can move easily. Paved patios are the easiest way to ensure a smooth surface. When bricks or flagstones are used to create terraces or patios, gaps should be no more than ½-inch wide and boards used for decking should be spaced no more than ¼-inch apart (Wylde et al., 1994). Thresholds between the deck or patio and the house should be kept to a minimum. Even a slightly raised threshold should have beveled edges to avoid a tripping hazard and provide a smooth transition for wheelchair users.

Planters that are hung from deck railings serve a dual purpose. First, they provide an area where people who use wheelchairs can create small herb or flower gardens. Second, they will discourage confused residents from attempting to climb over deck railings. If the yard is uneven or not accessible to residents with mobility impairments, building a deck that encircles all or part of the house can provide freedom of movement and room for exercise that is often impossible indoors. Windscreens can extend the use of decks and porches through three seasons. They can easily be made of thick Plexiglas bolted to deck or porch railings or by hanging heavy plastic or Mylar shades from porch walls or ceilings. Balconies with high, sturdy railings are a good way to provide access to the outdoors while curtailing exit opportunities for people who are likely to wander inappropriately. There are several publications that provide detailed descriptions and plans for building decks and patios (Baldwin, 1990; Beckstrom & Smith, 1995; Ireton, 1997; Mills, 1996; Shakery & Moore, 1991).

PROVIDING A HOMELIKE ENVIRONMENT WITH OPPORTUNITIES FOR ENJOYMENT AND GROWTH

It is important to balance home modifications, some of which may seem institutional, with changes that increase the homelike feeling of the environment. This can be accomplished in several ways (Pynoos & Regnier, 1991). First, modifications can be attractive and residential. Wooden handrails finished to match the home's interior trim and interior ramps that blend with the surrounding floors are examples of this approach.

Second, opportunities can be created for residents to personalize both private and shared spaces. Tables and walls on which people can display framed photographs of themselves and their loved ones and other objects and memorabilia will provide a homelike feeling and give residents a sense of belonging and connection to their environment. Hang framed artwork, pictures, and photographs on walls. Allow residents to select and care for both indoor and outdoor plants. Jenkins (1988) suggested giving group home residents each a small plot of land to plant and tend.

Third, provide opportunities and spaces for meaningful activities. Pynoos and Regnier (1991) suggested areas for crafts and artwork, aquariums, bird feeders and birdbaths, and outdoor herb and sensory gardens. The work of Egli, Roper, Feurer, and Thompson (1999), Robinson (1988), Thompson, Robinson, Dietrich, Farris, and Sinclair (1996a, 1996b), and Thompson, Robinson, Graff, and Ingenmey (1990) provided additional insights into physical and architectural features that are associated with a homelike feeling in group homes for people with intellectual disabilities.

CONCLUSIONS

It has been pointed out that when there is a poor fit between the capabilities of older people and their home environments, they may give up activities unnecessarily or have falls or other accidents (Pynoos & Regnier, 1991). Either of these outcomes can precipitate isolation and/or premature or unnecessary institutionalization. Unsafe environments also can promote dependency and increase feelings of alienation and dissatisfaction, which have the potential to undermine feelings of competency and independence (Langer & Rodin, 1976). People who require constant assistance with activities of daily living are severely limited in their opportunities to be alone. The intrusion on their privacy has the potential to undermine the individual's sense of self and feelings of self-worth. Conversely, when older people are able to continue to do things for themselves and feel that they have a degree of mastery and control over their environment, their sense of self is enhanced (Pynoos & Regnier, 1991).

Home modifications can alleviate some of the costs associated with home care, nursing homes, and housing replacement. More important, providing a home that is safe, supportive, and homelike and that includes opportunities for growth and stimulation can enhance an individual's feelings of competency and independence and sense of self-worth. The individuals in CABSR's study on aging with developmental disabilities who felt good about themselves were people who accepted their disabilities but did not equate them with dependence (Olsen et al., 1997). The challenge faced by their families, friends, service providers, and environmental planners was to provide the environmental supports necessary for maintaining independence and self-esteem.

This chapter focused on the wide range of adaptations that can be made to meet the physical environmental needs of people who are aging with a disability and experiencing increasing impairments. This could lead one to the mistaken conclusion that all or most people with developmental disabilities are frail and have impaired mobility. Nothing could be further from the truth. In our research, we have found an abundance of vibrant, healthy individuals who are eager to continue to live life to the fullest. People who had been recently deinstitutionalized were, for the first time in their lives, reveling in their autonomy, freedom, and self-determination. However, these people will grow older and eventually experience the physical, cognitive, and sensory declines that characterize aging. When that time comes, a supportive home will permit them to age in place. In the meantime, sensitive design and modifications to the physical environment will help them to continue to grow and realize their goals.

REFERENCES

Adlin, M. (1993). Health care issues. In E. Sutton, A.R. Factor, B.A. Hawkins, T. Heller, & G.B. Seltzer (Eds.), *Older adults with developmental disabilities: Optimizing choice and change* (pp. 49–60). Baltimore: Paul H. Brookes Publishing Co.

American Institute of Architects (AIA). (1985). *Design for aging: An architect's guide.* Washington, DC: AIA Press.

Baldwin, E.A. (1990). *Decks and patios: Designing and building outdoor living spaces.* Blue Ridge Summit, PA: Tab Books.

Beckstrom, R.J., & Smith, S.W. (Eds.). (1995). *How to design and build decks.* San Ramon, CA: Ortho Books.

Calkins, M.P., & Namazi, K.H. (1991). Caregivers' perceptions of the effectiveness of home modifications for community living adults with dementia. *American Journal of Alzheimer's Care and Related Disorders and Research, 6*(1), 25–29.

Cohen, U., & Wiesman, G.D. (1991). *Holding on to home: Designing environments for people with dementia.* Baltimore: The Johns Hopkins University Press.

Egli, M., Roper, T., Feurer, I., & Thompson, T. (1999). Architectural acoustics in residences for adults with mental retardation and its relation to perceived homelikeness. *American Journal on Mental Retardation, 104,* 53–66.

Ferguson, R.V. (1988). Environmental design for disabled persons. In R.I. Brown (Ed.), *Quality of life for handicapped people* (pp. 164–183). London: Croom Helm.

Goldsmith, S. (1976). *Designing for the disabled* (3rd ed.). London: RIBA Publications Ltd.

Heller, T. (1985). Residential relocation and reactions of elderly mentally retarded persons. In M.P. Janicki & H.M. Wisniewski (Eds.), *Aging and developmental disabilities: Issues and approaches* (pp. 379–389). Baltimore: Paul H. Brookes Publishing Co.

Ireton, K. (Ed.). (1997). *Porches, decks and outbuildings: The best of* Fine Homebuilding. Newtown, CT: Taunton Press.

Jenkins, D.B. (1988). Design features and exterior spaces. In M.P. Janicki, M.W. Krauss, & M.M. Seltzer (Eds.), *Community residences for persons with developmental disabilities: Here to stay* (pp. 347–364). Baltimore: Paul H. Brookes Publishing Co.

Krauss, M.W., & Seltzer, M.M. (1986). Comparison of elderly and adult mentally retarded persons living in community and institutional settings. *American Journal of Mental Deficiency, 91,* 237–243.

Langer, E., & Rodin, J. (1976). The effects of choice and enhanced personal responsibility for the aged: A field experiment in an institutional setting. *Journal of Personality and Social Psychology, 34,* 191–198.

Lifchez, R., & Winslow, B. (1979). *Design for independent living: The environment and physically disabled people.* London: Architectural Press.

Mills, H. (Ed.). (1996). *Complete deck book.* Menlo Park, CA: Sunset Publishing.

Olsen, R.V., Hutchings, B.L., & Ehrenkrantz, E. (1992). *The group home environment: The residents' perspective* (Unpublished report). Trenton: New Jersey Developmental Disabilities Council.

Olsen, R.V., Hutchings, B.L., & Ehrenkrantz, E. (1993). *Homes that help: Advice from caregivers for creating a supportive home.* Newark, NJ: NJIT Press.

Olsen, R.V., Hutchings, B.L., & Ehrenkrantz, E. (1995). *Along the continuum: Consumers reactions to supported and supervised apartments* (Unpublished report). Trenton: New Jersey Developmental Disabilities Council.

Olsen, R.V., Hutchings, B.L., & Ehrenkrantz, E. (1996). *Deinstitutionalization: The consumers' perspective* (Unpublished report).Trenton: New Jersey Developmental Disabilities Council.

Olsen, R.V., Hutchings, B.L., & Ehrenkrantz, E. (1997). *Issues and concerns of consumers aging with a developmental disability* (Unpublished report). Trenton: New Jersey Developmental Disabilities Council.

Pynoos, J., Cohen, E., Davis, L., & Bernhardt, S. (1987). Home modifications: Improvements that extend independence. In V. Regnier & J. Pynoos (Eds.), *Housing the aged: Design directives and policy considerations* (pp. 277–303). New York: Elsevier Science.

Pynoos, J., & Regnier, V. (1991). Improving residential environments for the frail elderly: Bridging the gap between theory and application. In J.E. Birren, J.E. Lubben, J.C. Rowe, & D.E. Deutchman (Eds.), *The concept and measurement of quality of life in the frail elderly* (pp. 91–119). San Diego: Academic Press.

Robinson, J. (1988). Design features and architectural considerations. In M.P. Janicki, M.W. Krauss, & M.M. Seltzer (Eds.), *Community residences for persons with developmental disabilities: Here to stay* (pp. 327–346). Baltimore: Paul H. Brookes Publishing Co.

Shakery, K., & Moore, R. (1991). *Deck and patio upgrades.* San Ramon, CA: Ortho Books.

Thompson, T., Robinson, R., Dietrich, M., Farris, M., & Sinclair, V. (1996a). Architectural features and perceptions of community residences for people with mental retardation. *American Journal on Mental Retardation, 101,* 292–313.

Thompson, T., Robinson, R., Dietrich, M., Farris, M., & Sinclair, V. (1996b). Interdependence of architectural features and program variables in community residences for people with mental retardation. *American Journal on Mental Retardation, 101,* 315–327.

Thompson, T., Robinson, R., Graff, M., & Ingenmey, R. (1990). Home-like architectural features of residential environments. *American Journal on Mental Retardation, 95,* 328–341.

Warner, M.L. (1998). *The complete guide to Alzheimer's proofing your home.* West Lafayette, IN: Purdue University Press.

Wylde, M., Baron-Robbins, A., & Clark, S. (1994). *Building for a lifetime: The design and construction of fully accessible homes.* Newtown, CT: Taunton Press.

15

Housing and Living Supports

An Asset Management Challenge

DiAnn L. Davies, Robert J. Davies, and Peter Sheridan

This chapter focuses on a concept known as asset management. Although it is not a new concept to the business world, the use of it for meeting housing and living supports needs for people with developmental disabilities is new. The World Bank has estimated that two thirds (or approximately 160–200 million) of all people with severe to moderate disabilities live in poverty. "They belong to the poorest of the poor of the world's population and are acutely affected by shortages in water, food and housing, bad or nonexistent public transportation and health care, and the lack of employment or other income opportunities" (United Nations, 1996). Factor into the equation the reality that people with disabilities are living longer today, and the result is the need for comprehensive, long-term planning when assisting these people with planning for the future.

A comprehensive planning process assures the person a more stable future. Planning should include financial backing, housing, service provision, recreation, employment, transportation, and the development of appropriate and flexible supports as the person ages and should give the person maximum control of life decisions and choices. This process is best approached through the concept of asset management, which includes full participation of the person, the family, the disability agency, other government agencies, and the community at large. Ideally, asset management begins when the individual is very young and continues throughout the aging process. Today, government sources of funding and services, outside of entitlements (Supplemental

257

Security Income [SSI] and Medicaid), are not guaranteed. Therefore, a blending of multiple funding sources is required. Families and provider agencies need to assist people with disabilities to create wealth. The creation of wealth gives a person choice, control, and options well into to his or her senior years.

ASSET MANAGEMENT: A MODEL

When developing housing and services for people with disabilities, one must look at all of options available, not just at what is available from the disabilities services system (see Table 1). Sherraden defined asset building "as accumulated savings that are invested for social and economic development. The investments can be in human, social or tangible assets, most often in education, home ownership, and small business development" (1991, p. 1). In many states, long waiting lists exist for people with disabilities and their families (Hayden & DePaepe, 1994). State-funded services and supports provide only part of the needed resources to ensure a stable future. Exploring solutions that give the family and the person with the disability more control over where they live, with whom they live (if anybody), how long they live in a location, who comes to visit, and the hiring and firing of support staff complete the picture. As Sherraden (1991) also noted, the ultimate standard of success in asset building is intergenerational well-being and asset accumulation and development across generations.

Exploring all options involves a process. The asset management model presented here is designed to help people with disabilities, their families, and support staff explore many new opportunities available to them. This resource-gathering technique applies to all age groups.

The asset management model examines five points of support: 1) the person with the disability, 2) the person's family, 3) the state disability services agency and its providers, 4) other government agencies, and 5) local community and natural supports. Figure 1 portrays a balance of all five components—each part having equal significance. Together these five components create for the person with a disability a scope of available resources that far exceed any one part. Furthermore, if each person involved in the planning process for the individual brings his or her contributions from each of the five component areas, then the options become even greater.

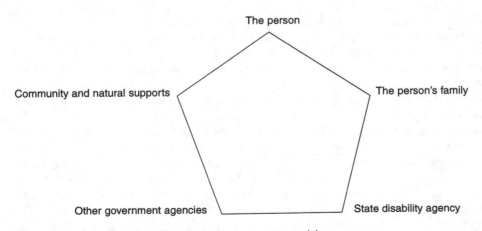

Figure 1.   Asset management: The five asset management model components.

Table 1. Housing and service options for older families

Community senior housing	Run by municipal government or contract agencies; call county or town aging office for information on availability, waiting lists, and rules
Assisted living programs	Often run by local nursing facilities, religious groups, or social agencies; call local religious organizations, churches, and/or the county aging office for availability and other information
In-home supports	Provided through county aging office; can provide in-home supports, transportation, respite, help with medical appointments, shopping, household chores, and other services for older adults
Homeownership	Parents can add support or financial assistance to homeownership and/or can arrange for a reverse mortgage. These steps can ease the transfer when parents move away or die. Call a local advocacy agency or "home of your own" group.
Home environmental modifications	Ramping, internal adaptations, use of assistive technology to help older parents stay in the home; call not-for-profit organizations that may assist with adaptations as well as the county aging office and independent living centers
Housing supports	Help parents of and individuals with disabilities with home maintenance, rental subsidies, weatherization, utility service discounts and payments, and so forth; call the local county aging office for information
Service system assistance	Help with securing financial aid or entitlements, such as Social Security, Medicaid, homeowner's tax benefits, veteran's benefits, and so forth for parents and their children with disabilities
Family assistance and planning	Help for families in organizing and planning for the future; establish goals and time frames for transitions, financial transfers, picking up of caregiving responsibilities by others; setting up guardianships and trusts

Person

All people with disabilities have assets and skills, though varying in degree, to add to the picture. A person's assets are not limited to the dollar amount coming in each year. The person must be involved with daily activities in all aspects of his or her life, including many of the household activities that are part of everyone's normal day. Even the individual with a severe or profound disability is able to contribute to some degree. Examples include mowing the lawn, taking out the garbage, basic housecleaning, and other household maintenance projects. As the individual participates in these daily activities, operating costs may be offset and he or she is engaged directly in life and does not have to have things done for him or her, as is the common practice. If the individual is lacking in basic skills, then supports must focus on the skill acquisition and maintenance. Training and habilitation activities need to target practical areas of daily living that allow the person greater control and independence. For example, John lives in a community residence that has a nice sized yard, which, naturally, needs cutting. Typically, the yard is cut by someone other than those individuals who live in the house. John is not able to cut the yard on his own but with one-to-one staff assistance could be directed to steer a self-propelled mower around the yard. John receives day habilitation (a service that allows him training in the community), which may, for example, include going shopping at the mall once a week. If cutting his own yard is added to his day habilitation training, then the habilitation directly correlates to John's daily living.

People with disabilities may have government financial supports, trust income, employment income, or some combination of these. The individual, the family, and support staff must explore all benefits and entitlements for which the person with disabilities is eligible when developing a plan of support. These benefits and entitlements can include housing subsidies, Social Security Disability, Supplemental Security Income, food stamps, energy assistance, telephone lifeline, food banks, property tax reductions, moderate rehabilitation and environmental modification programs, housing counseling, Medicare, state plan Medicaid services, and services and supports from state developmental disabilities agencies.

People with disabilities need to work if possible. Work gives a dimension and meaning to one's life, but more important, it generates income. People with severe disabilities are now working in supportive and competitive employment situations, and this income assists the person to seek economic independence. Work is the goal of adulthood until retirement. Upon retirement, some people choose to continue to work, become volunteers, travel, or relax. Work and savings help one prepare for retirement by accumulating resources.

Special or supplemental needs trust funds further assist a person with a disability to achieve more financial stability and independence. Trust funds can be set up by third parties (e.g., family members, friends) or by first parties (the individual) if he or she has excess resources. An individual should use money earned from work and not from limited SSI for a first-party trust. These trusts allow the person to continue to receive SSI and Medicaid while having additional funds available for housing and services. A trust is for the benefit of the person with the disability and may be used to purchase items above and beyond what SSI or Medicaid benefits do not cover. A cautionary note: The Social Security Administration (SSA) has precise regulations as to what a trust can purchase for the individual without affecting eligibility. The publication *Provisions: Sample Language for Supplemental Needs Trusts* (Froemming, 1997) is a useful reference tool for writing trusts. Individuals and families should consult a lawyer who is well versed in first- and third-party trusts and SSA regulations before establishing a trust fund. A trustee, who is authorized by the trust to make payments on behalf of the person with the disability, controls the funds. The establishment of a supplemental needs trust should be in the support plan for all people with a disability. Relying only on SSI for income ensures that the individual will remain in poverty for the rest of his or her life.

As the person ages, looking at all angles of his or her life and maximizing and maintaining his or her skills, assets, and activities gives him or her not only financial security but also more control and satisfaction with his or her life. It is as important to prepare for the financial retirement of the person with a disability as it is to prepare for our own retirement. Multiple sources of financial assets mean greater choice and opportunities for housing and services for the individual with a disability.

Family

The family of a person with a disability plays an extensive role in the person's life. Every member of the family has skills and assets. The larger the family, the greater the collective skills and assets. Families add numerous options in the life of a person with a disability. Options may include daily assistance, emotional and financial support, vacations, a trust fund, painting a room or a porch, gifts, holiday gatherings, family picnics and reunions, teaching skills, or just a walk at the end of the day. A new look at the role of the family in future care planning is needed to build housing and living supports for an aging son or daughter with a disability.

Early in one's life, the family provides all life supports. Parents help daughters and sons prepare for their ultimate independence from them. Typically, families with a member with a disability are very close, and their support and care of their son or daughter with a disability is a lifelong activity. Most families want their children to have successful lives and assist them to prepare for adulthood with financial and educational support. Parents may help with a first car, down payment on a house, a loan during hard times, help on a home maintenance project, and many other forms of lifelong support of their children. This also should apply to children who have a disability.

The family of a person with a disability needs to plan for that person's future in greater detail because of the long-term needs of the person. The earlier the family begins planning, the better. Planning should be a dynamic, changing, and flexible process. A plan is something that changes over time as a person grows, graduates, works, and retires. In the field of disabilities, future care planning is a process that families implement to ensure that their child has a secure, stable, and safe future. Such a plan, as Castellani, Bird, and Manning (1995) noted, is intended to be "holistic" by considering the widest range of a person's desires and plans for life rather than specific developmental deficits. The plan may include the appointment of a guardian; financing a trust; the willing of property; directions for the future care of the son or daughter; information concerning legal, medical, religious, and financial directives; and special instructions concerning care, burial, likes and dislikes, and other information only a parent would know. The planning of future services provision and housing needs is as crucial as securing the child's financial future.

When a family begins the planning process, it is important that all family members be involved. Siblings, grandparents, aunts, uncles, cousins, nieces, nephews, and grandchildren should be part of the planning and support for the son or daughter. Close family friends and neighbors, social and religious organizations, and financial and legal advisors should also be involved. Collaboration such as this contributes a significant amount of skills and assets to start formulating the plan. Another benefit of families planning together is that they can share the responsibility to assist the person with the disability in all areas of his or her life. Consequently, as parents, grandparents, aunts, and uncles die, siblings, nephews, nieces, and cousins can pick up some responsibilities, thus giving continuity of support to the individual. The outcome of a future care plan is a financially secure future in which the person with the disability has choices and control over his or her life.

As the person with a disability ages, the significance of a well-prepared plan will become evident. Family members know where and how their daughter or son will live and how he or she will be supported. This gives the family great comfort and ensures quality and security to the daughter or son. The person with a disability also feels more secure knowing that his or her housing, clothing, medical care, and advocate or guardian is a stable part of his or her life. "If you plan, you can provide an environment that best nurtures the independence and dignity of your daughter/son. If you plan, you may provide your daughter/son with what she or he most desires—a life lived to its fullest" (Smith, 1997, p. 2). Change and uncertainty are difficult for all of us, but good future care planning takes much of the guesswork out of the future of a person's life.

Accumulating financial resources for the individual with a disability should begin as early as possible. Just as parents begin saving for college funds for children, so too should the parents of a child with a disability begin saving for future housing and services. The greater the number of people involved in the financial plan, the better. For example, if 10 family members purchase an insurance policy or investments amounting to $10,000 with the beneficiary being a trust fund set up on behalf of the individual with the disability, then the individual with the disability would potentially have a $100,000 trust fund that could be used for housing and services and he or she ages. Because of SSI savings restrictions of $2,000, a supplemental needs trust fund (discussed previously) is advised. Failure to use this form of trust could make the individual with the disability ineligible for SSI and Medicaid benefits. However, through careful planning, a supplemental needs trust can receive gifts, property, and proceeds from estates without affecting the individual's eligibility for benefits. Families can learn more about supplemental needs trusts from provider agencies, trusts and estates sections of their state bar association, and documents listed in the "Additional Reading" section at the end of this chapter.

Depending on the severity of the individual's disability, a guardian or advocate and designated backups may need to be appointed at the age of 18. An advocate is someone who is appointed in an unofficial manner. A guardian is appointed through the court system. As Smith noted, "Guardianship should be viewed as an invaluable tool, but to be so, it must be understood" (1997, p. 37). These people must fully understand and advocate for the individual. A well-educated guardian can make the difference between someone's continuing to live in the community or having to move to a facility (Smith, 1997). The guardian or advocate should be aware of the parents' wishes as well as of the wishes and needs of the person with the disability. The guardian or advocate must also be knowledgeable about the services and supports available for the individual. The role of the guardian or advocate is heightened after the death of the parents. His or her job is to add a voice of support in negotiating the housing and services/support system. Families should contact local service provider to explore the steps necessary to appoint a guardian or an advocate. If the parent wants to be the initial guardian, then the guardianship must be set up before the individual turns 18.

Housing is a major consideration for families that are thinking about the future of their son or daughter with a disability. In some cases, families keep their daughters and sons at home and make arrangements for assistance from other relatives in the event of their death. One possibility is for the individual with the disability to remain in the family home, cooperative, condominium, or apartment and for the residence to be left to the individual with the disability, left in a trust, or given to another relative with a tenancy-for-life clause in the parents' will. This option allows the individual stability in the neighborhood where he or she is known and supported. This decision must be fully discussed with all family members to ensure harmony. This option is not for everyone but should be seriously considered by families that own property. Sometimes selling the parents' property makes more sense so that the proceeds can be used to purchase a townhouse, cooperative, or condominium. A benefit in housing of this type is that the exterior maintenance (e.g., yard care, snow removal) is the responsibility of the owners' association or board. Another benefit is that quite often it is less expensive than single-family housing.

Another scenario is that the house is shared with other people. Home sharing (LePore, Sheridan, & Aloyo, 1993) gives the individual companionship, support, and possible income. Shared housing has had a rich and significant role in U.S. housing and, if trends of the 1990s continue, will be an increasingly popular housing option for older adults well into the future (Shared Housing Resource Center, 1988). For people with a disability, a roommate may be a friend, relative, college student, older person, couple, or single person of the same age. This other person may or may not have a disability. Generally, roommates share the expenses of living together and help one another with chores. Roommates also share recreational interests and provide emotional support. In some situations, one of the roommates helps the other in exchange for housing.

In developing home-sharing opportunities, it is sometimes helpful to have a person initiate the roommate match. That person may be a friend, support staff, or an agency that provides home-sharing matching services. A home-sharing agency may be a services provider agency serving people with disabilities, an agency that serves older people, or a housing agency. Home sharing provides a solution for two basic needs—companionship and independence—and is a cost-effective way to help people share housing expenses, particularly when rents are high and incomes are low. If there is income, it may be more appropriate to pay rent to a trust rather than to the individual. Income to the individual may effect his or her SSI and Medicaid eligibility. In 1988, there were almost 400 home-sharing programs in 42 states (Shared Housing Resource Center, 1988), and the number has grown since then. In New York, for example, there is the Co-op City shared apartment program in the East Bronx and the home-sharing project initiated by the New York State Developmental Disabilities Planning Council and the New York State Research Foundation for Mental Hygiene, in which more than 400 individuals with disabilities were successfully matched. These programs have been and continue to be a key component in meeting the housing needs of older people. Families should check with their local and state government for shared housing programs in their area.

Families may want to collaborate with other families that have sons or daughters with a disability and plan with their children for a mutually benefiting goal. For example, groups of families in Ohio have successfully operated a family consortia program for a number of years. In other states, such groups have either accomplished this type of housing or are in the process of developing this type of future support for their adult children. However, compatibility among families does not guarantee compatibility among their children who may have to live together. In shared housing, there is always the possibility of changing roommates, but this may not always be easy when a group of families join to organize a living situation. Thus, it is very important that the person with the disability be part of any of these discussions. Following the principle "nothing about me without me" is good practice, particularly when matching roommates.

Some families leave their property to a nonprofit services provider in return for life tenancy and services for their son or daughter. This may offer the family or estate some beneficial tax incentives, but the family then looses control of the property. In this situation, ongoing oversight by a guardian or advocate is recommended to ensure the interests of the individual with the disability. This also may be an option for negotiating shared services with others who are receiving services but need housing.

Regardless of which options are pursued, it is essential that families begin the planning process early and update the plan throughout their lives. Families should not wait for governmental programs to solve the services and housing needs of their children but should work collaboratively with government programs to ensure the best future for their son or daughter.

State Developmental Disabilities Agencies

State developmental disability agencies and their staff have a variety of skills and resources. Properly using existing resources by blending them with other resources serves a greater number of people. Thus, there should be discussions with state decision makers, legislators, and advocates on ways to stretch resources in new ways to give people with disabilities and their families more control and flexibility in funding. Support services funds should be portable so that a person with a disability can move from services and housing provider to other providers if dissatisfied with his or her current provider. The investment and reinvestment of funds need careful consideration to ensure that the resources available serve the most people.

State developmental disabilities services funds can and should be used to leverage additional funds from foundations, banks, and other governmental agencies. This leveraging of present services and housing funds with those of municipal and nonprofit housing agencies results in greater housing resources for the person. Services and housing support funds can be used as matching funds in collaborative housing projects with local, affordable housing developers to ensure set-asides for people with disabilities. New developmental disabilities housing funds could be used to leverage lower finance rates with banks under the Community Reinvestment Act of 1977 (PL 95-128) if state developmental disabilities agencies negotiate wisely with financial institutions. State housing finance agencies, community development agencies, and developmental disabilities agencies need to develop collaborative development activities to ensure that adequate housing stock and funding sources for environmental modifications are available for people with disabilities and people who are aging.

Fragmented systems of identifying and funding environmental modifications need streamlining. Collaborative efforts for leveraging funding sources between the private and public sectors need to be developed to address modification issues for aging in place and accessible housing for aging people with lifelong disabilities. In Minnesota, a collaboration among the state vocational rehabilitation system, the building codes division, the private sector, and volunteers resulted in a huge number of low-cost, modular, portable ramps being constructed for people with ambulation difficulties. This type of initiative is an example of what can be done in other parts of the country.

State developmental disabilities agencies need to develop new policy initiatives that focus on adopting universal design in state and national building codes, funding shared housing programs, and encouraging public–private partnerships to services and housing waiting lists. They also need to assist in efforts that ensure that appropriate housing is being developed for people with disabilities as they are aging. Replicating programs from states that have broadened the menu of services and options available for people with disabilities and their families is an important role for the developmental disabilities agency. Support of self-advocacy, person-controlled environments, self-determination, portable funding, and down payment programs for home ownership is another role for the agency. Building the capacity of people with disabilities and their families to gain access to locally funded and state-funded housing and services needs further support from the agency. Families and their children need knowledge of all of the options, not just of the options funded by the developmental disabilities agency. With knowledge comes more control, flexibility, and options. Families can help by opening dialogue with their local state agency about their concerns and needs for their family member with a disability.

Disability agencies have the responsibility to coordinate and facilitate the array of resources available to the person with the disability. This is accomplished through the funding of service coordination, training activities, and interagency collaboration. This coordination and facilitation needs to evolve constantly into more options for people with disabilities as they age. Outcomes should be oriented toward achieving an individual's overall quality of life rather than toward treatment for specific problems (Castellani et al., 1995). Budget initiatives to encourage the evaluation and reinvestment of existing resources are essential in serving more people with existing funds. Evaluation is also necessary to ensure that some people are not overserved while others are underserved. Restructuring funding streams can give individuals and families more control and effectiveness in services provision. Parents have been cost-effective in the spending of family support services funds in family reimbursement programs across the country. Most important, agencies have to be agents of change. As times, philosophy, needs, market demand, personal preferences, and services evolve, disability agencies must be the engines of service system change. Creating new funding streams, regulations, service models, and administrative structures supports the evolution of services to people with disabilities.

Nonprofit and for-profit provider agencies that are under contract with state developmental disabilities agencies have a large role in the development and implementation of many of the topics listed previously. In fact, they may be the catalyst for many of the systems changes needed to secure an appropriate future for aging individuals with disabilities. In other cases, the provider agencies may need training, financial incentives or disincentives, and regulatory requirements to develop a full menu of options for their customers. Developmental disabilities systems need to look outside the traditional box of housing and services to integrate their customers into the mainstream of housing and services.

Other Government Agencies

In developing lifelong plans, one must be aware not only of the developmental disability service system but also of the variety of other agencies that can offer support to people with disabilities. Certainly, the aging services network of area offices and nonprofit agencies must be a large part of planning for the later years of a person's life in an integrated and inclusive environment. One must also use generic, affordable housing agencies, senior housing opportunities, rental subsidies, government-funded environmental modifications, durable medical equipment, and assistive technology.

Government benefits that may be used include SSI, Social Security Disability Income (SSDI), food stamps, property tax exemptions for older adults and people with disabilities, Home Energy Assistance Program, prescription drug programs, rent subsidies, affordable housing, and a diverse array of disability and senior support programs. In planning, one must explore all entitlements and benefits to develop the correct mix of finances and supports necessary at any given time in the life of the person with a disability. Support staff need to examine the restrictions of certain benefits and entitlements to ensure that financial assets from one arena do not jeopardize eligibility in another area.

Other government agencies supply affordable housing, rental subsidies, home ownership assistance, personal care, crisis intervention, and other supportive services. People with disabilities are eligible for a variety of housing funds to help meet their needs. Many people with disabilities have limited incomes, which makes them eligible for all of the low- and moderate-income programs funded by state and federal agencies. Learning about these resources can help in developing options for people with disabilities.

Housing resources sponsored by the U.S. Department of Housing and Urban Development (HUD) include homeless housing and support services, senior housing complexes, moderate rehabilitation of owner-occupied housing (owner must be under 80% of median income), moderate rehabilitation of rental housing if landlord rents to people under 80% of median income, home ownership assistance, housing counseling, environmental modifications, and rental subsidies. There are HUD regional offices throughout the United States or you can access HUD's web site (see Table 2). All applications, notifications of fund availability, lists of foreclosed properties, housing counseling agencies, grants recipients, and other information is available on their web site. Links to web sites for other housing information in cities and states are listed. These funds and programs can be accessed through local nonprofit housing agencies, municipal governments, and counties. In some cases, there are waiting lists; therefore, a first-come-first-serve process or lotteries are used for these funds. Early and frequent contact with the funding entities is important.

In rural areas, the Rural Housing Service (formerly Farmers Home Administration) provides many similar housing programs. The Rural Housing Service is part of the U.S. Department of Agriculture. Funding is provided for moderate rehabilitation, first-time home ownership, and rental subsidies. Some of the loans are at a very low interest rate (as little as 1% depending on income).

At the state level, there may be one or more housing entities that develop affordable housing for people with low and moderate income; state Housing Finance Agencies (HFAs) are the most common. In many states, state developmental disabilities and aging agencies have successfully used HFAs to develop senior housing, home ownership programs for people with disabilities, and affordable and accessible rental housing. HFAs have in some instances set aside a certain percentage of their housing for special needs populations, such as older adults or people with disabilities, in mixed-use or intergenerational housing. The HFAs finance for-profit and nonprofit developers.

In some states, the affordable housing agencies collaborate with nonprofit housing agencies to target low-income housing development. Many of these agencies have set-asides for special needs populations and are interested in working with developmental disabilities and aging services agencies to develop new housing. Many agencies have made vacancies in existing affordable housing available to people with developmental disabilities and older adults. Collaboration with these agencies is essential in developing comprehensive, publicly assisted housing for people with disabilities. Most states have web sites with links to their housing agencies.

Other state agencies may have housing and services supports for older people with disabilities. State social services agencies have emergency services, food, and housing assistance. State offices for the aging have a variety of budget, policy, services, and funding initiatives for the aging populations. Many offices have collaborative activities with developmental disabilities agencies. Comprehensive lists of housing options for older adults exist in some of these state offices. State departments of transportation, parks and recreation, and conservation may have programs and subsidies for older adults, such as reduced fishing license fees, bus pass reductions, and other programs that assist older adults.

Table 2. Web sites for information on housing or related topics

Organization	Web site address
Ability Network	http://www.ability-network.com.au/
The Arc of the United States	http://TheArc.org/
Center for Social Development	http://www.gwbweb.wustl.edu/Users/csd/
The Center for Universal Design	http://www2.ncsu.edu/ncsu/design/cud/index.html
Consortium for Citizens with Disabilities	http://www.c-c-d.org/
disABILTY Information and Resources	http://www.eskimo.com/~jlubin/disabled/index.html
The Foundation Center	http://fdncenter.org/
Housing Assistance Council	http://www.ruralhome.org/
National Low Income Housing Coalition	http://www.nlihc.org/
National Home of Your Own Alliance	http://alliance.unh.edu/
NeighborWorks	http://www.nw.org/
UCPnet: United Cerebral Palsy	http://www.ucp.org/index.htm
United Nations	http://www.un.org/
U.S. Department of Housing and Urban Development (HUD)	http://www.hud.gov/

At the county and municipal levels, many of these same programs and services exist. County and municipal older adult, housing, community development, and planning offices can assist older adults and people with disabilities and their families and support staff in the planning and development of appropriate housing and services. Collaboration and planning with these agencies are essential to the development of a comprehensive array of housing and services options at the local level. Provider agencies and the disability community need to work closely with local government to plan and use community development block grants and HOME funds (a program of the U.S. Department of Housing and Urban Development [HUD]) to develop appropriate local services and housing programs allowed by the sources. This is accomplished through a Consolidated Plan required by HUD. Provider agencies and people with disabilities and their families need to work with local government to ensure that a portion of local HUD funds are allocated for services and housing for people with disabilities and seniors.

Many of the housing and service programs provided at the local level are funded by federal, state, or local government or through nonprofit corporations. If one is seeking services, any of these offices would be a good place to start. Senior housing agencies for people with disabilities are listed in the yellow pages of a local telephone book under "disability." However, if an agency is seeking to develop or expand services, it should be working with municipal, county, and statewide agencies to secure funding.

Community and Natural Supports

Community and natural supports provide numerous opportunities to develop housing and services options. Banks provide grants, volunteers, and lending products. Social services and the religious community are involved in volunteer projects to help with specific situations. Motorcycle clubs build ramps and provide recreation equipment. Habitat for Humanity builds houses. Businesses and corporations give donations of funds, materials, and time to people in need. Families, friends, and neighbors help each other. Building suppliers donate materials to nonprofit corporations for tax benefits or sell products at wholesale costs. Many health clubs have workout buddy programs for people who live in group homes. Telephone company Pioneer Club members build modular and portable ramps for home accessibility. A retired person volunteers to spend a day with a person with a disability. Friends and neighbors paint the house of a friend with a disability. A wealthy citizen of the community makes a donation to make a van accessible to a person with a disability. A radio station, church, volunteer fire company, or social organization holds a fund-raising event for a family in need. All of these are actual examples of how a person with a disability and his or her family have gained access to community and natural supports.

Another source of community supports is the business sector in the form of charitable grants and contributions. Klein noted that there are two basic premises of fundraising: 1) "If you want money, you have to ask for it," and 2) "If you ask enough people, you will get your money" (1996, p. 7). Philanthropic foundations and their corporate equivalents are increasingly contributing more money to nonprofit organizations toward housing and services. It is therefore important that agencies begin now to form collaborations with corporations that make contributions to programs that serve people with disabilities. State and local libraries carry guides in their reference sections on philanthropic foundations and corporations. The Foundation Center (see Table 2), with branches in New York City, Washington, D.C., San Francisco, Cleveland, and Atlanta, also has resource rooms where individuals can conduct research. Although most foundations and corporations do not give to individuals, families should not be discouraged from seeking them out with assistance from a nonprofit organization. Collaborating with a nonprofit organization can be beneficial for all parties concerned. Families could also form their own nonprofit organization. This is not a new concept; in fact, many of the nonprofit organizations that exist today were begun by families who had children with disabilities and who were in need of services. Other business contributions can come from banks, which are required to contribute money to community projects through the Community Reinvestment Act, or local neighborhood corporations. Agencies and individuals can approach these businesses to help with a housing project or a service need.

CONCLUSIONS

The combination of the person, the family, the disability agency, other government agencies, and community and natural supports provides the disability community a whole that is greater than the sum of its parts. It is a reinvention of community and uses private–public partnership to solve today's problems. This approach is a dynamic and successful tool to help solve housing and services needs for people with disabilities and their families. The process, ideally started while the person with the disability is young, can start at any age. What is important is to begin the process. As the process unfolds and the information surrounding the person with a disability grows, the benefits of the asset management model become apparent. The resulting product is a detailed plan for the individual that ensures a stable and financially secure life as he or she grows older— a life filled with choice, safe and affordable housing, and multiple services that provide for a rewarding and fulfilling old age.

REFERENCES

Castellani, P.J., Bird, W., & Manning, B.L. (1995). *Supporting individuals with developmental disabilities in the community.* Albany: New York State Office of Mental Retardation and Developmental Disabilities.

Community Reinvestment Act of 1977, PL 95-128, 12 U.S.C. §§ 2901 *et seq.*

Froemming, R. (1997). *Provisions: Sample language for supplemental needs trusts.* Madison: Wisconsin Council on Developmental Disabilities.

Hayden, M.F., & DePaepe, P. (1994). Waiting for community services: The impact on persons with mental retardation and other developmental disabilities. In M.F. Hayden & B.H. Abery (Eds.), *Challenges for a service system in transition: Ensuring quality community experiences for persons with developmental disabilities* (pp. 173–206). Baltimore: Paul H. Brookes Publishing Co.

Klein, K. (1996). *Fundraising for social change.* Berkeley, CA: Chardon Press.

LePore, P., Sheridan, P., & Aloyo, V. (1993). *It's time for change: Homesharing, a guide to match-up homesharing as a residential option for persons with mental retardation & developmental disabilities.* Albany: New York State Developmental Disabilities Planning Council.

Shared Housing Resource Center. (1988). *National trends and state initiatives in shared housing.* Philadelphia: Author.

Sherraden, M. (1991). *Strategic plan for the program in asset building and community development, 1997–2003.* St. Louis, MO: Washington University, Center for Social Development.

Smith, M.R. (1997). *Planning for the future: A guide for families and friends of people with developmental disabilities.* Albany: New York State Developmental Disabilities Planning Council.

United Nations. (1996). *3 December 1996: International Day of Disabled Persons, Focus on Poverty and Disability (DPI/1865).* New York: United Nations Department of Public Information.

ADDITIONAL READING

Beverly, S. (1997). *How can the poor save? Theory and evidence on saving and asset accumulation in low-income households* [Working paper]. St. Louis, MO: Washington University, Center for Social Development.

Klein, J., & Black, M. (1994). *Extending the American dream: Home ownership for people with disabilities.* Durham: University of New Hampshire, Institute on Disability/A University Affiliated Program.

Pollak, P.B. (1991). *Key issues for shared residences for older persons.* Washington, DC: American Association of Retired Persons.

Resource Center for the Elderly. (1989). *Shared housing manual: How to develop and implement home-sharing programs.* Arlington Heights, IL: Resource Center for the Elderly.

Sherraden, M. (1991). Toward a theory of welfare based on assets. In M. Sherraden, *Assets and the poor: A new American welfare policy* (pp. 145–188). Armonk, NY: M.E. Sharpe.

16

Value-Based Human Resources Management

David B. Henry, Christopher B. Keys, and Alan R. Factor

"They keep asking me who the president of the United States is," Mr. D stated as we were visiting him in his room in a nursing home, "and I keep telling them, 'Donald Duck.' They think I'm senile or have old timer's disease or something." Mr. D is a 78-year-old with a wry sense of humor. He and his sister were born with the physical anomalies and cognitive limitations associated with fetal alcohol syndrome. They lived in Chicago in the house built by their father. After his sister's death, Mr. D lived there alone.

During an extensive heat wave that hung over the city of Chicago in the summer of 1995, more than 400 mostly older Chicagoans died of heat-related causes (Centers for Disease Control and Prevention [CDC], 1995). This tragedy precipitated a local public health panic the week after the hottest day. Teams of police, public health nurses, and social workers were sent into neighborhoods to locate older people who might be at risk from the heat. At the same time, teams of lawyers went to court to suspend their civil rights. Mr. D was one of many older people who were forcibly hospitalized in the week that followed, although he had taken his own precautions to cope with the heat. During that week, representatives of the city's Department of Human Services petitioned the probate court for temporary

We are grateful to the Department of Psychology and the Department of Disability and Human Development at the University of Illinois at Chicago for their assistance with and support of this chapter.

guardianship of Mr. D, who was not informed of the hearing in time to respond. The petition was granted; soon afterward representatives of the department, along with several ambulance attendants, arrived at Mr. D's home and strapped him to a gurney. Mr. D protested, "It's a free country!" to which a social worker responded, "It's not that free." After an examination at the hospital revealed mild dehydration and anemia but no serious medical problems, Mr. D was transferred to a nursing home to regain his strength before returning to his home.

During Mr. D's brief experience with the human services system, he encountered ignorance of and indifference to his cognitive disability in contacts with nurses, physicians, psychologists, and social workers. On numerous occasions, Mr. D's pastor and neighbors informed social services personnel of his intellectual disability to prevent the application of unnecessary restrictions. Each time, the information was ignored. At one point, Mr. D was physically restrained in bed because a physician mistook his cognitive limitation for disorientation.

The situation in which Mr. D found himself has been repeated across the United States. Even though many older adults with intellectual disabilities are seen as part of their communities, their life conditions are easily misunderstood and they are too often viewed as vulnerable and dependent. It is estimated that as many as 60% of people with developmental disabilities in the United States may be unknown to the developmental disabilities services delivery system (Krauss, 1988). As these people age, they, like Mr. D, will become involved with human services systems that provide services to aging adults. Often, their first contact is with the network of programs and services established by the Older Americans Act of 1965 (PL 89-73). The growing emphasis on individual choice and community membership is increasing referrals of older people already served by the developmental disabilities services system. One survey found that approximately half of senior centers reported serving people with developmental disabilities on a regular basis (Rinck, Naragon, & Shollenberger, 1996). These agencies also reported significant problems with serving this population because of a lack of funding, inadequate staffing, lack of staff training, and negative attitudes of other older adults toward people with developmental disabilities.

More generally, many aging-related and developmental disabilities agencies find themselves at the intersection of aging and developmental disabilities without necessarily intending to be there. Both service systems are trying to address the needs of increasing numbers of older people without a parallel growth in resources and while undergoing a change in caregiving philosophy. This trend will continue into the 21st century.

The developmental disabilities services system must redesign a system that initially was established for children and young adults to address a growing population with later-life concerns. This redesign is occurring at a time when services based on the developmental model are giving way to individualized services that are consumer driven and use natural community supports. In this high-demand context, agency leaders confront a set of interrelated management challenges, namely 1) how constructive change can be implemented when staff already face substantial work responsibilities and pressures, 2) how existing staff can be trained and supported to adapt to changing conditions, and 3) how staff energies can be more focused on common goals and values.

Human services organizations that serve the general population, including medical facilities and programs specifically for older adults, espouse positive values for their services similar to those that provide the foundation for most developmental disabilities services today. Values, variously called empowerment, independence, choice, and autonomy, regularly appear in the literature on aging (e.g., Simon-Rusinowitz & Hofland, 1993) and developmental disabilities (Bruininks, 1991; Miller & Keys, 1996). Accrediting organizations such as the Commission for Accreditation of Rehabilitation Facilities (CARF) are using these values in developing standards for services for older adults with developmental disabilities and their families. However, for organizations outside the developmental disabilities services system, the danger is that staff will not provide services that are consistent with these values. Most organizations continue to deliver services that are managed by professionals with little input from consumers. Staff have had little exposure to consumer direction, which can result in questions, confrontations, and challenges to practices and their underlying assumptions. Staff in these environments need to understand and adopt these values and know how to operationalize them with an unfamiliar population. Staff in the aging services network need to recognize that people with developmental disabilities have personalities and personal preferences and are capable of self-direction. Their impairments may require hands-on support to make and implement choices.

Staff in organizations whose policies are perceived to be consistent with their values have higher job satisfaction than do staff in organizations whose practices are perceived to be inconsistent with their values (Balcazar, Mckay, Keys, Henry, & Bryant, 1998). Values are a key motivator for staff. Askvig and Vassiliou (1991) found that 43% of the direct care workers in their sample cited the meaningfulness of their work as a motivator for staying on the job. How can service delivery systems that are devoted to aging people or people with developmental disabilities become more sensitive and responsive to the needs and rights of aging people with developmental disabilities? Training that acclimates staff to the characteristics of aging and developmental disabilities and central values such as empowerment can be enhanced by making core values part of the culture of the organization. However, organizational socialization and reward systems must support implementing these values and changing disempowering attitudes. Otherwise, training is more likely to be perceived as adding more burdens to already overburdened staff and thus may engender resistance to change.

Such values can be incorporated into the culture and be institutionalized in the day-to-day functioning of agencies that encounter people with developmental disabilities in the usual course of service delivery to older people. This chapter presents a method for gathering basic data on the ways in which staff behavior embodies core values. These data can then be used as a foundation for recruiting, training, and evaluating staff, as well as for evaluation of services.

MANAGEMENT BY VALUES

Values provide an anchor in times of change—a basis that directs action when coping with the new demands faced by aging people with developmental disabilities. For example, attention to the organizational values of independence and choice can motivate a staff member to support individuals with developmental disabilities in trying new activities and in establishing new friendships. In all organizations, good work is work that is consistent with organizational values. As Schein (1990) noted, values in organizations are as often implicit as they are explicit. Management by values is the process of explicating and institutionalizing an organization's values through the process of job analysis and the development of selection and evaluation methods (Henry & Keys, 1990a, 1990b; Henry, Keys, & Balcazar, 1991; Keys, Henry, & Schaumann, 1997).

Making attention to values an explicit part of the process of job analysis enables agencies to develop methods for recruitment, selection, training, and performance appraisal that correspond to current values in the field. This enables them to attract employees whose personal values are congruent with those of the agency, train employees in core agency values and their implications for work, and evaluate employees on the basis of the extent to which their work is consistent with the values of the agency.

This method is referred to as value-based job analysis. Job analysis is a collection of methods for defining jobs in terms of the behaviors necessary to perform them (Cascio, 1998). The results of a job analysis usually include job descriptions that cover the physical and environmental characteristics of the work to be done and job specifications that cite the types of knowledge, skill, and ability necessary to do the job. Job analysis is widely used in the for-profit sector for developing selection devices such as tests and structured interviews, for designing jobs, and for developing tools for performance appraisals. The Supreme Court has ruled that job analysis must be a part of validation studies on employee selection devices (*Albemarle Paper Company v. Moody,* 1975). Partly because of the costs involved in having job analysis done by industrial psychologists, it is used less in the nonprofit sector.

As can be seen in Figure 1, value-based job analysis has three basic phases: articulation, data gathering, and instrument development. The first phase is the assessment and articulation of organizational values within the agency, building on the organization's existing mission. This phase involves research, assessment, discussion, and writing and produces a values statement that details the core values of the organization, such as choice, appropriate interpersonal relationships, and an emphasis on personhood over disability or age.

The data collection phase is the process of learning about the ways in which employees' job behaviors express the core values articulated in the first phase. Information on the personal values and attitudes of existing staff and the behaviors, requirements, knowledge, skills, and abilities that are relevant to the jobs in question must be collected from supervisors, job incumbents, and consumers of services. Because information on quality as defined by values is desired, this information is most usefully collected in the form of descriptions of incidents of job behaviors that are relevant to the organizational values in question. The information collected is processed to yield lists of job behaviors and attitudes. These job behaviors and attitudes are then scaled on value dimensions through ratings by job incumbents, managers, and consumers of services.

The third phase is the creation of desired instruments based on the personal and organizational values and the job information collected. These methods are designed to focus human resource and staff development efforts on the core values of the organization. In short, value-based job analysis uses personal and organizational values as a basis for creating an organizational culture in which the goals and paths to good performance are clearly linked to the values of the organization.

In the sections that follow, we consider the basic phases of value articulation and data gathering as they might be applied to an organization that serves aging people with developmental disabilities, using examples from an application of the method in Oakdale Center, a developmental disabilities services environment that provides residential and recreational services, and in St. Margaret's,[1] a facility that provides inter-

---

[1]The names of these agencies have been altered.

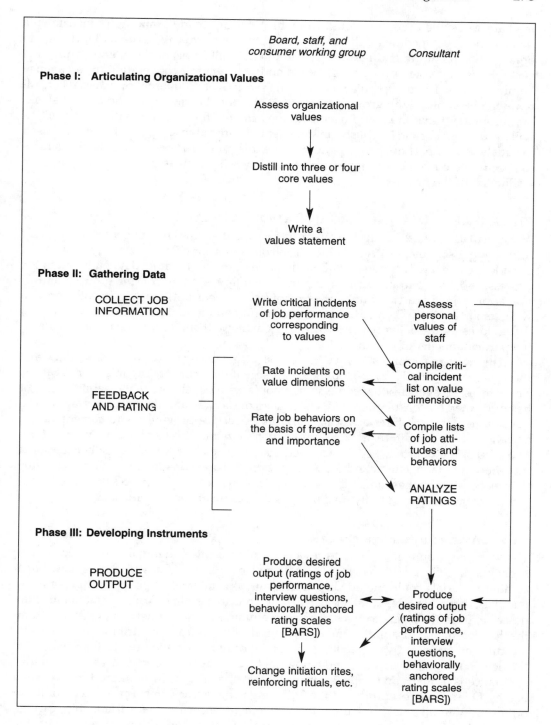

Figure 1.   Value-based job analysis: A three-phase model. Phases and steps in management by values.

mediate and skilled care for retired women. We also provide examples of instruments that can be developed using this method. This process aims at fundamental change in organizational culture and requires commitment at all levels of the agency. Thus, it is best initiated by vote of the agency board and with the full cooperation of top agency administrators. The process also requires the services of an internal or external consultant who is familiar with group process, organizational assessment, and data analysis. We recommend that the board decide, at the time the process is initiated, what action will need to be taken to establish the statement of core values generated by value-based job analysis as a part of agency policy. Before this process is begun, it is also desirable to specify the outcomes of interest and how they will be measured. This will facilitate evaluation of the process.

PHASE I: ARTICULATING ORGANIZATIONAL VALUES

The articulation phase begins by appointing a consultant and forming a working group to develop a statement of core values. The consultant may be a person from inside or outside the agency. This person will facilitate the process, compile data gathered in the process, and draft outputs. Appointing the consultant and the working group is a function appropriately carried out by the organization's board of directors in collaboration with senior executive staff. However, successful completion also requires input from those closest to the delivery of services, namely the staff and consumers who are essential participants in daily agency life.

This working group's first tasks consist of gathering information and data that form the raw material for developing a concise statement of core organizational values. This process in agencies that serve aging people with developmental disabilities might be augmented by consultation with consumers of services and their families, aging and developmental disabilities advocates, and other service provider as to current values and how they might relate to organizational values in services delivery. At St. Margaret's, the board issued a proposed statement of core values and then initiated interviews of management and focus groups of staff and consumers of services for further elaboration, suggestions, and comments. At Oakdale, the process included consumers of services and family members, as well as management and staff.

Step 1: Assess Organizational Values

The working group first needs to review existing printed materials produced by the agency and collect text that may reveal the underlying values of the agency. Such printed materials could include brochures, mission statements, policy and procedures manuals, and other related material. Staff and consumers can contribute statements that describe, from their perspectives, what is really important to this agency. Others from the developmental disabilities and aging communities can also contribute statements in a similar manner, and value statements can be drawn from the literature on values in the developmental disabilities and aging fields (e.g., Heal, 1988, p. 61). The goal of this step is to have many (perhaps 20 or more) statements of values before the next step begins. One such effort produced the following list of values: freedom, choice, comfort, opportunity to take risks, community involvement, security, safety, friendship, caring, support, health, learning, appropriate interpersonal relationships, growth, spiritual development, recognition of sexuality, accessibility, respect of differences, and respect of boundaries.

Step 2: Distill into Three or Four Core Values

Values are choices. Often these are difficult choices between two desirable ends that conflict in particular cases (e.g., choice versus safety). In this phase, members of the working group choose which organizational values statements are closest to expressing the desired core values of the agency. For this group session on values and for all research and intervention activities in this process, minimally intrusive supports should be provided so that all can participate as fully as possible, regardless of physical, sensory, or cognitive limitations. For example, at Oakdale, one person with a disability worked in a team of two with another participant speaking quietly to have a more complete understanding of the values put forth.

One method for completing this in a group in which all participants are sighted is to draw a large bull's eye on a piece of newsprint or butcher paper and post it in a location that can be reached by all participants in the working group. Then, spread on a table the organizational values statements, written on sticky notes, so that all participants can see each statement. The next half hour is carried out in silence as members of the working group take the values statements and place them on the bull's eye as near or far from the center as they desire. Each member may also move statements posted by others. If members decide that two statements express the same core value, then they may be attached to each other.

After this period of individual input, group discussion of the core values ensues. On the basis of early decisions about how the values statement is to be adopted as agency policy (e.g., changes in bylaws, articles of incorporation), the kind of product desired from the process and the next steps in adoption should be discussed. The process of distilling agency values begins with discussion of each value placed at the core of the bull's eye. In discussing each value, there are some key questions that should be addressed:

1. Why is this important? Are there implicit values underlying this stated value? Is the source of a value's importance financial, legal, regulatory, moral, or utilitarian?
2. Are there times when this value needs to be set aside in favor of a more important end? If so, what are they? What other values form the boundaries of the stated value?
3. What perspective can consumers and staff contribute to understanding this value and its operation? How does this value work in day-to-day delivery of services? To what extent does the agency's work currently proclaim this value?
4. In light of the preceding, should this value become more important to the agency's philosophy?

As the discussion continues, three or four core values are likely to emerge. At Oakdale, participants agreed on the importance of choice as a core value and moved it closer to the bull's eye. They saw greater risk to health and safety as a likely consequence of choice and finally affirmed choice and reasonable risk as a core value, limited only when there were substantial risks to health and safety.

Step 3: Write a Values Statement of Organizational Values

The final part of the work of articulation is writing a statement of organizational values in an appropriate form that can be submitted to the board for ratification. For example,

Table 1 illustrates the statement of core values. Note that these values are equally applicable to services for people with developmental disabilities and for aging people. Statements 2 and 3 reflect consideration given by the working group to the boundaries and relative priorities of core values. The values statement provides a framework for the next step in the process, data gathering.

PHASE II: GATHERING DATA

Step 1: Personal Values and Attitudes Assessment: Profile of the "Typical" Staff Member

People tend to be attracted to work that expresses their personal values and attitudes (Katz & Kahn, 1978). For example, Williams (1986) found that people who are attracted to work in the field of developmental disabilities have different values from those of the general population. Williams's (1986) sample valued helpfulness more and achievement less than did the general population. It is likely that a similar principle holds for people who work in the field of aging. Recruiting staff with values that fit those of the hiring agency and those of others in the fields of aging and developmental disabilities can increase the extent to which prospective staff come to work prepared to implement organizational values. For this reason, an important ingredient for developing recruitment and selection materials is a knowledge of the personal values and attitudes of existing staff members.

A personal values assessment may be carried out with a random sample of agency employees. The sample should be random to avoid biases as a result of self-selection, which would misrepresent the attitudes and values of staff as a whole. In an agency with a small number of staff, say, fewer than 100, an attempt might be made to assess all staff members. It is particularly helpful to encourage participation from part-time staff; staff who work evenings, nights, and weekends; and staff who work in environments away from the main office. Often, these staff identify less strongly with agency initiatives.

One of the most frequently used assessments of personal values is the Rokeach Value Inventory (Rokeach, 1973). This inventory asks respondents to rank several statements of values that are desirable end-states ("terminal values") and desirable means to an end ("instrumental values"). Although other measures are available, there are better normative data available for the Rokeach measure than for any other measure of values. Responses to the Rokeach Value Inventory (Rokeach, 1973) can be compared with other samples, such as Williams's (1986) sample of volunteers in developmental disabilities and Rokeach's (1974) normative sample, providing knowledge concerning the extent to

Table 1.   Illustrative statement of core values

1. Participants' assurance of health and safety is a core value as well as a legal mandate.
2. Participants should have an enjoyable experience in this setting. Fun takes precedence over treatment, except where treatment is necessary for health or safety.
3. Participants should be allowed and encouraged to think and act independently, to make choices about their activities, and to take risks except where there is a clear threat to health and safety.
4. Participants should experience positive, age-appropriate interpersonal relationships with staff and with each other.

which staff are high or low on certain values. For example, Williams' (1986) sample of volunteers who worked with people with developmental disabilities placed more emphasis on the value of friendship and were less concerned with a comfortable life than were the members of Rokeach's (1974) normative sample. Williams's (1986) sample also valued helpfulness more and cleanliness less than did the normative sample.

The Community Living Attitudes Scale (CLAS; Henry, Keys, Jopp, & Balcazar, 1996) is an instrument that is suitable for assessing the attitudes of staff toward people with developmental disabilities. This scale measures four aspects of inclusion attitudes: empowerment (freedom to make decisions), exclusion (desire to exclude people with developmental disabilities from community life), sheltering (desire to protect people with developmental disabilities), and similarity (perceived similarity of people with developmental disabilities to themselves and others in society). Henry et al. (Henry, Keys, Balcazar, & Jopp, 1996; Henry, Keys, Jopp, et al., 1996) published means and standard deviations of community and staff samples on the CLAS subscales. These can be used to produce a profile of current agency staff on inclusion-related attitudes.

Step 2: Critical Incident Collection

The attitudes and values assessment provides a profile of the personal values and attitudes of the staff. The next step is to gather data on the ways in which individuals act on their values and the organization's values in their day-to-day work. The critical incident technique (Flanagan, 1954) provided a method for gathering information about jobs that is well suited to value-based job analysis. This method asks individuals who are familiar with the job role to write accounts of events that exemplify positive and negative staff performance. Each account includes the background of the incident, what the individual did that was effective or ineffective, the consequences of the staff person's behavior, and whether the consequences were under the control of the staff person.

For use in the data gathering process for value-based job analysis, the critical incident method can be modified to define good and poor job performance using the organization's values. Supervisors, consumers, and others who are familiar with direct-services jobs in an agency can be instructed to write critical incidents of job behaviors. They also specify which of the organization's values was demonstrated (positively or negatively) in the incident and rate the behavior from excellent to poor according to the value involved. (See Figure 2 for a sample critical incident report form.) This method allows respondents to report any incident they believe to be noteworthy and gives them a value framework within which to evaluate the quality of job performance. This procedure yields incidents of positive and negative job performance that the writers link directly to the core values of the agency. For example, the following incident was written by an Oakdale staff member:

A participant that had problems controlling his anger was encouraged to behave more appropriately by a staff member. The staff member refused to have an adversarial relationship with the participant, and as a result was able to establish better communication with the participant.

This incident was linked to the value of "age-appropriate interpersonal relationships."

Step 3: Feedback and Rating

The goals of feedback and rating are to organize the critical incidents systematically on the value dimensions and to use these incidents to identify the most frequent and important job behaviors and attitudes. The consultant(s) and/or selected working

CRITICAL INCIDENT REPORT

We are interested in collecting descriptions of important actions of our staff in the normal course of doing their jobs. Please write a description of an incident that you believe is representative of particularly good or poor performance. Do not use the staff member's name or the name of any consumers of services in your description. Refer to the parties only as *staff member* and *consumer*. Each description should include the following sections:

1. Background: What led up to the incident?
2. What did the staff member do that was effective or ineffective?
3. Describe the consequences of the staff member's behavior.
4. Describe whether the consequences were under the staff member's control. Why? How?

_____

_____

_____

_____

_____

_____

_____

_____

_____

_____

_____

_____

_____

_____

_____

_____

This incident is related to which important value of our agency? _____

_____

Based on this value, please rate the staff member's performance from 1 (poor) to 6 (excellent) [*circle*]:

Poor   1   2   3   4   5   6   **Excellent**

Figure 2.   Sample critical incident report form.

group members first sort the critical incidents into categories that correspond to the core organizational values. Part of this sorting can be done based on the core organizational values indicated by the writers of the incidents. In cases in which the writer had specified no organizational value as relevant to the incident or had specified more than one value, working group members can independently attempt to classify the incident and place it in the modal class.

The consultant(s) can then review the incidents and extract the job-related behaviors or attitudes described in each one. Table 2 gives examples of job attitudes and behaviors that are associated with the organizational value "positive age-appropriate interpersonal relationships." When these lists of attitudes and behaviors are completed, working group members and job incumbents can rate each job attitude and behavior on two dimensions: 1) the frequency with which it was required in the job specified and 2) its importance to successful job performance. In addition, the working group members rate the original critical incidents, listed under core value headings, on the extent to which each incident represents an example of good or poor work according to the core value to which it was assigned.

Starting with value-based incidents of job behavior, the feedback and rating step produces lists of job attitudes and behaviors and their importance and frequency for each core organizational value. These ratings, along with the lists themselves and the rated critical incidents on value dimensions, can provide rich source material for developing specific instruments that can be used in recruitment, selection, training, and evaluation of staff.

PHASE III: INSTRUMENT DEVELOPMENT

At the end of phase II of value-based job analysis, the raw materials for human resource management by values are in place. In phase III, the organizational values, job behaviors, personal values, and attitudes elicited thus far are used to produce instruments and training materials that are tailored to the agency's needs. More specific, the goal of phase III is for the working group and the consultant(s) to convert the information gathered in the preceding steps into desired materials for staff recruitment, selection, train-

Table 2. Organizational value, personal values, and related incidents of job behaviors

ORGANIZATIONAL VALUE

Participants should experience positive, age-appropriate interpersonal relationships with staff and with each other.

RELATED PERSONAL VALUES
ON WHICH STAFF DIFFERED FROM THE GENERAL POPULATION
Loving others, friendship

CRITICAL INCIDENTS RELATED TO
POSITIVE INTERPERSONAL RELATIONSHIPS

Even though a staff member was not experienced with communicating with a participant who was difficult to understand, the staff member maintained a conversation with the participant until he was absolutely sure what he needed.

When a participant utilized an offensive (and often-expressed) racial epithet, the staff member took the time to clearly and respectfully explain the inappropriateness and consequences of the use of the epithet on others. The participant appeared to be sorry for using the word and didn't say the word again for three days.

ing, or evaluation of staff or services. The following are examples of ways in which source material produced by a value-based job analysis can be used.

For recruitment, the critical incident descriptions can be combined with the value and attitude profiles of the "typical" staff member into realistic job previews (McEvoy & Cascio, 1985; Wanous, 1989). Realistic job previews are printed descriptions of the job that both allow potential employees to self-select in or out of the organization and begin the new employees' socialization into the organization. Oakdale Center found that although greater initial recruitment efforts were necessary, final job candidates were better suited to the jobs than were previous candidates. Table 3 gives an example of a realistic job preview segment.

For selection, the consultant(s) or working group members can prepare a set of interview questions from the value-based critical incidents. Each open-ended question poses a situation taken from a critical incident and asks the interviewee how she or he would respond. A scoring key can be developed to rate responses as good, marginal, or poor in terms of the extent to which the response positively reflected the relevant organizational value (see Table 4 for an example).

The critical incidents and lists of job behaviors and attitudes can be useful in training. They provide specific information on job attitudes and behaviors that are viewed by the organization as exemplary of good performance, which, according to path-goal theories of leadership, enhance performance (Evans, 1970; House, 1971). Using the materials in this way can help employees understand the larger aims of their organizations and how their day-to-day work achieves those aims.

For performance reviews, the critical incidents and ratings on value dimensions can be used to prepare behaviorally anchored rating scales (BARS; Campbell, Dunnette, Arvey, & Hellervik, 1973) for each value dimension, anchored by positive and negative behaviors on the relevant dimension from the critical incident (see Figure 3). These scales assist both supervisors and job incumbents to have a more complete understanding of performance ratings. The scales are anchored in specific behaviors, which are themselves anchored in core organizational values. Information from a value-based job analysis also can be used to construct materials to evaluate services that are outsourced, such as meal programs and home care. As the information gathered is of a specific, behavioral nature, it can be easily converted into questionnaires for use by consumers of agency services or into interviews with consumers for the purpose of evaluating services.

Table 3.   Realistic job preview segments related to positive interpersonal relationships

"Staff must learn to understand participants' forms of communication, whether it be speech, or the use of a computer or a word board, and to be patient in understanding when the participant communicates. Frequently, a staff member's failure to understand properly is the root cause of problems participants have."

"We expect that staff members will interact with participants in a positive, age-appropriate manner. Most important, staff are expected to remember that participants have the same needs for dignity and respect that we all do."

"Being a staff member requires the ability to be patient with participants and to relate well to them even in times of stress. Staff at this agency tend to highly value human relationships, and many develop strong friendships with each other and with the participants they get to know. Staff also place a high value on being helpful and loving. They find it rewarding to help another person overcome communication barriers, have fun, and become more independent."

IMPLEMENTING AND EVALUATING VALUE-BASED CHANGE

Value-based recruitment and selection require agencies to become proactive in the search for suitable staff. The purpose of the realistic job preview is to encourage people who are likely to turn over early or to perform poorly to self-select out of the job before applying. Given this self-selection, without wider recruitment efforts than usual, there may be too small an applicant pool to provide the necessary numbers of staff. Overall, the goal is to find numerous suitable applicants from which to make a selection. Active dissemination of information about job opportunities, coupled with distribution of the realistic job preview, should result in a strong group of suitable applicants. Applicants can then be screened with the interview questions and selected on the basis of their answers.

Value-based methods may be evaluated according to several criteria for success. High staff turnover is a significant problem in human services, including developmental disabilities and aging services (Bergson, 1988; Braddock & Mitchell, 1992; Lakin, 1981; Lakin, Hill, Hauber, & Bruininks, 1983; Wolfensberger, 1988), and is potentially remediated through use of this method. Staff performance changes can be assessed by aggregating information from performance reviews before and after the implementation of the methods. Alternatively, if ratings on the quality of services were collected before the intervention, these can be compared with the quality of service ratings collected after the intervention.

In a test of this method by Henry, Keys, and Schaumann (1993), the primary objective was to reduce staff turnover. They had the agency director collect data on the number of individuals hired, the number leaving voluntarily, and the number terminated. They also reviewed available comparable figures from the previous year, which were typical of other years. In the year in which value-based job analysis was used, only approximately 3% of the new hires either did not arrive to begin their jobs or left during orientation. This represented a statistically significant improvement over the baseline year, which had a 28% early turnover rate. In both years, the termination rate was stable, between 8% and 9%. The director noted in a letter to the consultants, "Although the number of people terminated was almost the same for the two years, many people who were not doing a good job were kept on in the year previous to the baseline year to avoid being shorthanded. That was not the case in the year of the intervention. In the current year, the staff who are with us are all eligible to be retained." In terms of other, less quantifiable indicators of change, the director noted in the same letter that the staff in the intervention year were "extremely dedicated and caring."

Table 4.   Interview question related to positive interpersonal relationships

Participants often spend considerable time in wheelchairs and are unable to move themselves enough to get comfortable. Imagine that a participant lets you know that he or she is uncomfortable in a wheelchair. What would you do?

GOOD RESPONSE: Talk patiently with the participant until I understand exactly what is making him or her uncomfortable, then shift his or her position to a more comfortable one.

MARGINAL RESPONSE: Try to see what is bothering the participant and adjust his or her position until it seems more comfortable. (Here no mention is made of dialogue with the participant.)

POOR RESPONSE: Shift the participant's position so it is more comfortable. (Here there is no mention of analyzing the situation.)

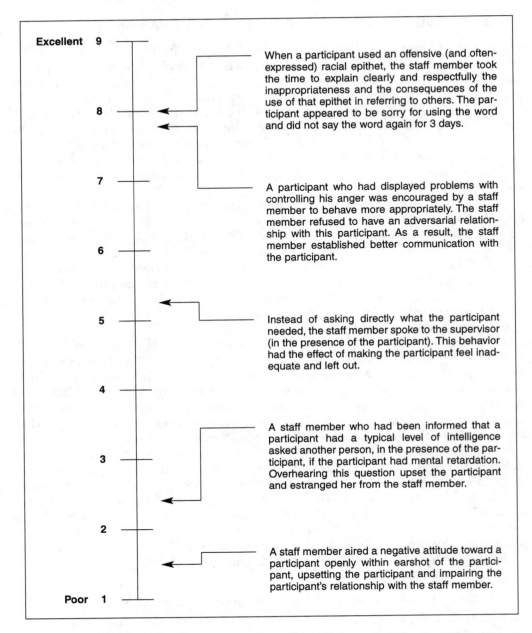

Excellent 9

When a participant used an offensive (and often-expressed) racial epithet, the staff member took the time to explain clearly and respectfully the inappropriateness and the consequences of the use of that epithet in referring to others. The participant appeared to be sorry for using the word and did not say the word again for 3 days.

A participant who had displayed problems with controlling his anger was encouraged by a staff member to behave more appropriately. The staff member refused to have an adversarial relationship with this participant. As a result, the staff member established better communication with the participant.

Instead of asking directly what the participant needed, the staff member spoke to the supervisor (in the presence of the participant). This behavior had the effect of making the participant feel inadequate and left out.

A staff member who had been informed that a participant had a typical level of intelligence asked another person, in the presence of the participant, if the participant had mental retardation. Overhearing this question upset the participant and estranged her from the staff member.

A staff member aired a negative attitude toward a participant openly within earshot of the participant, upsetting the participant and impairing the participant's relationship with the staff member.

Poor   1

Figure 3. Behaviorally anchored rating scale related to positive interpersonal relationships with participants.

CONCLUSIONS

As people with developmental disabilities age, they may move into environments that serve and support other older people or continue in environments that serve people with developmental disabilities. Staff in both aging and developmental disabilities environments will be called on to meet the needs of these people with sensitivity to their abilities and limitations. Training that teaches staff about the nature of developmental disabilities and aging can be augmented by management that articulates agency values and institutionalizes them in the selection, training, and evaluation of staff. This chapter reviewed a method for value-based job analysis that consisted of three basic phases: articulation of values, data gathering, and instrument development. This method can incorporate the input of agency staff, consumers, board members, advocates, and service provider in framing core organizational values. We believe that use of this method can foster team spirit and a sense of mission in work, as staff at all levels see themselves as working to implement common values, such as choice, that are important to all. Such a sense of mission can prevent staff burnout, especially among human services workers (Cherniss, 1980), and provide for constructive change an avenue that does not create additional pressure on staff. A sense of mission in work can relate to decreased turnover and better staff performance.

What is most important is that experience with this method suggests that managers, staff, and consumers of services can work together to strengthen the organizations that are important to them. Using a management-by-values approach to link positive ideals to daily reality, agency leaders may improve their human resource management and increase their capacity to provide older adults with developmental disabilities such as Mr. D with appropriate, sensitive supports and services from human services agencies.

> *Postscript: Later in the summer of 1995, a contingent of church friends and neighbors, led by Mr. D's pastor, accompanied Mr. D to a competency hearing in probate court. With Mr. D's agreement and the consent of the public guardian's office, a longtime neighbor was appointed to be Mr. D's guardian. Accompanied by friends from his church, Mr. D. celebrated his 80th birthday in 1999. He once again lives in his own home and still has his sense of humor.*

REFERENCES

Albermarle Paper Co. v. Moody, 422 U.S. 405 (1975).

Askvig, B.A., & Vassiliou, D. (1991). *Factors related to staff longevity and turnover in a facility serving persons with developmental disabilities: A final report.* Minot: Minot State University, North Dakota Center for Disabilities.

Balcazar, F., Mckay, M., Keys, C., Henry, D., & Bryant, F. (1998). Agency commitment to the values of community inclusion: Effects on staff satisfaction. *American Journal on Mental Retardation, 102,* 451–463.

Bergson, G. (1988). All people have personal assets. *Mental Retardation, 26,* 71–73.

Braddock, D., & Mitchell, D. (1992). *Residential services and developmental disabilities in the United States: A national survey of staff compensation, turnover, and related issues.* Washington, DC: American Association on Mental Retardation.

Bruininks, R.H. (1991). Presidential address 1991. Mental retardation: New realities, new challenges. *Mental Retardation, 29,* 239–251.

Campbell, J., Dunnette, M., Arvey, R., & Hellervik, L. (1973). The development and evaluation of behaviorally-based rating scales. *Journal of Applied Psychology, 57,* 15–22.

Cascio, W.F. (1998). *Applied psychology in human resource management* (5th ed.). Upper Saddle River, NJ: Prentice-Hall.

Centers for Disease Control and Prevention (CDC). (1995). Heat-related mortality: Chicago, July 1995. *Morbidity and Mortality Weekly Report, 44*(31), 577–579.

Cherniss, C. (1980). *Professional burnout in human service organizations.* Westport, CT: Praeger.

Evans, M.G. (1970). Leadership and motivation: A core concept. *Academy of Management Journal, 13,* 91–102.

Flanagan, J. (1954). The critical incident technique. *Psychological Bulletin, 51,* 327–358.

Heal, L.W. (1988). The ideological responses of society to its handicapped members. In L.W. Heal, J.I. Haney, & A.N. Amado (Eds.), *Integration of developmentally disabled individuals into the community* (2nd ed., pp. 49–67). Baltimore: Paul H. Brookes Publishing Co.

Henry D., & Keys, C. (1990a, May). *Management by values: Conceptual issues.* Paper presented at the annual meeting of the American Association on Mental Retardation, Atlanta, GA.

Henry, D., & Keys, C. (1990b, January). *Values and management in the developmental disabilities field.* Paper presented at a meeting of the Agency Executives of the Association of Retarded Citizens of Illinois, Matteson, IL.

Henry, D., Keys C., Balcazar, F., & Jopp, D. (1996). The attitudes of community living staff toward persons with mental retardation, mental illness and dual diagnosis. *Mental Retardation, 34,* 367–379.

Henry, D., Keys C., Jopp, D., & Balcazar, F. (1996). The Community Living Attitudes Scale: Development and psychometric properties. *Mental Retardation, 34,* 149–158.

Henry, D., Keys, C., & Balcazar, F. (1991, October). *Implementing values in services for persons with severe mental illness and developmental disabilities.* Symposium presented at the Midwest Ecological Psychology Conference, Dowagiac, MI.

Henry, D., Keys, C., & Balcazar, F. (1992, May). *Community integration values of community integration workers.* Poster presented at the annual meeting of the American Association on Mental Retardation, New Orleans, LA.

Henry, D., Keys, C.B., & Schaumann, L. (1993, May). *Value-based job analysis: First field trial.* Paper presented at the annual meeting of the American Association on Mental Retardation, Washington, DC.

House, R.J. (1971). A path-goal theory of leadership effectiveness. *Administrative Science Quarterly, 16,* 321–338.

Katz, D., & Kahn, R.L. (1978). *The social psychology of organizations* (2nd ed.). New York: John Wiley & Sons.

Keys, C., Henry, D., & Schaumann, L. (1997). Using value-based job analysis to reduce staff turnover: An organizational culture case study. In M. Montero (Ed.), *Psychology and community: Proceedings of the 25th Inter-American Psychology Conference* (pp. 235–253). Caracas, Venezuela: Sociedad Interamericana de Psicologia.

Krauss, M.W. (1988). Long-term care issues in mental retardation. In J.F. Kavanagh (Ed.), *Understanding mental retardation: Research accomplishments and new frontiers* (pp. 331–339). Baltimore: Paul H. Brookes Publishing Co.

Lakin, K. (1981). Occupational stability of direct-care staff of residential facilities for mentally retarded people. *Dissertation Abstracts International, 42*(1-A), 171.

Lakin, K., Hill, B., Hauber, F., & Bruininks, R. (1983). A response to the GAO report "Disparities still exist in who gets special education." *Exceptional Children, 50,* 30–34.

McEvoy, G.M., & Cascio, W.F. (1985). Strategies for reducing employee turnover: A meta-analysis. *Journal of Applied Psychology, 70,* 342–353.

Miller, A.B., & Keys, C.B. (1996). Awareness, action, and collaboration: How the self-advocacy movement is empowering for persons with developmental disabilities. *Mental Retardation, 34,* 312–319.

Older Americans Act of 1965, PL 89-73, 42 U.S.C. §§ 3058 *et seq.*

Rinck, C., Naragon, P., & Shollenberger, D. (1996). *Senior center perceptions: Interface between aging and disabilities* (NCOA Rep. No. 1). Kansas City, MO: University of Missouri–Kansas City, Institute for Human Development.

Rokeach, M. (1974). Change and stability in American value systems, 1968–1971. *Public Opinion Quarterly, 38,* 222–238.

Schein, E. (1990). Organizational culture. *American Psychologist, 45,* 109–119.

Simon-Rusinowitz, L., & Hofland, B.F. (1993). Adopting a disability approach to home care services for older adults. *Gerontologist, 33,* 159–167.

Smull, M.F. (1997). Helping staff support choice. *AAMR News and Notes, 10,* 8.

Wanous, J.P. (1989). Installing a realistic job preview: Ten tough choices. *Personnel Psychology, 42,* 117–134.

Williams, R. (1986). The values of volunteer benefactors. *Mental Retardation, 24,* 163–168.

Wolfensberger, W. (1988). Common assets of mentally retarded people that are not commonly acknowledged. *Mental Retardation 26,* 63–70.

III Essay

Disability Policy in Taiwan

On the Right Track?

Kuo-yu Wang

Taiwan's government policy for people with disabilities is different from its social policy for other groups of people with special needs. It is a system that has incorporated various policies from different parts of the world. For instance, it uses a registration system that is similar to the Japanese system, and it follows a mandatory employment quota policy that resembles Germany's system. People with intellectual disabilities are generically defined as "disabled" and receive the same services as other people with disabilities under this system.

In 1980, the Welfare Law for People with Disabilities became the first legislation to address specifically provision of social services for people with disabilities. It required that the government establish a system to identify individuals with disabilities and stipulated that an individual's disabilities and degree of self-care skills must fit into one of several categories of disability to get a government-issued identification card ("ID card") as a person with a disability. Since its inception, this identification system has also served as a census of the population with disabilities in Taiwan. This system emphasized the different characteristics of people with disabilities and unfortunately sent a message to society at-large (and to people with disabilities) that unless their disabilities fit the system's definitions, they are not considered "disabled." Currently, the number of people with intellectual disabilities in Taiwan is approximately 61,200, or 0.3% of the total population of 21 million people. Because this number is used to guide the government's budget allocations and service provision, unfortunately, people who lack a disability ID card are not included in the census and therefore are not eligible for services.

This system has its good and bad points. For example, it does identify a class of people who receive special attention. However, it is a static, rather than a dynamic, system of demographic data, meaning that people who enter this system will continue to exist in our statistics, without accounting for deaths. For another example, the ID card never needs to be reissued or renewed. However, this card serves as an entry to applying for services but does not necessarily mean that the government will actually provide the services. Therefore, for many people, having this card has meant receiving only the minimum services. In another example, because this system restricts the definition of disabilities to various categories, individuals whose disabilities occur later in life still need to go through the process of getting this card before receiving services or benefits. Thus, the card functions purely as an accounting system, rather than as a method of planning for services or policy.

REFORMS OF THE DISABILITY POLICY

In 1990, the government, under pressure from disability advocacy groups, revised the law by expanding the provisions of services and, most important, the definition of disability. The categories of disability were expanded to 12, from the previous 6, and restrictions were loosened on defining the degree of severity of disability. The law also imposed on employers a mandatory employment quota system that required the public and private sectors to reserve a certain proportion of job openings for people with disabilities. If they violate the rule, employers must pay a fine.

These 1990 amendments expanded the scope of government intervention in employment, health, and cash assistance programs to people with disabilities, and the amendments created a linkage between cash benefits and the severity of a person's disability. The impact of these new policies has been to give people with disabilities more incentives to apply for the ID cards and enable them to gain access to in-cash aid programs. Since 1990, the number of people with disabilities in the system has continued to increase.

In 1997, the government enacted a second change to the legislation. The name of the legislation was changed from "Welfare Law for People with Disabilities" to "A Bill of Rights Protection for People with Disabilities," and the new legislation adopted a different approach to policy implementation. This second change established rights as the central framework of its policy and clearly stated that the rights of people with disabilities consist of health, education, employment, social services, and access to a social environment. The new law also specified which government officials are obligated to take major roles in satisfying the needs of people with disabilities. For instance, the minister for education was now obligated to provide special education, whereas the minister for labor was to take responsibility for employment policy. The minister for health was to take responsibility for the delivery and design of early intervention programs, and the head of the Bureau of Social Service was to be responsible for providing care for people with disabilities.

The 1997 revisions also created more cash incentives to aid families that have members with disabilities. For instance, the government now exempts low-income people with disabilities from paying their share of national health insurance and provides families with certain cash assistance that is more generous than other social aid programs. In addition, the government provides a tax reduction either to the family with a member with a disability or directly to the individual with a disability. These revisions also provided explicit guidelines for community care, including rehabilitation, day care, meal services, transportation, recreational services, parental education, and various referral services.

Since fiscal year 1990, the various programs that provide cash and services to people with disabilities have accounted for more than 50% of the central government's welfare services budget for various populations in Taiwan. Therefore, the system of providing services and aid to people with disabilities is much more generous than for other groups of people who are in need. How this budget allocation will actually change their lives has not yet been determined; however, from the perspective of the other groups of people who are in need, the people with disabilities seem to be receiving more resources. From the perspective of people with disabilities, the allocation of resources is insufficient to meet their needs.

DISCONNECTED POLICIES

The underlying assumption of Taiwan's disability policy is that people with disabilities are dependent on others to support them. This needs-based distribution system has both strengths and weaknesses. It treats people with disabilities as one category of citizens, as if all people with disabilities have the same needs and can benefit from the same forms of aid. Thus, adults with intellectual disabilities must adjust to fit this general disability system. The system treats them equally within the disability system but treats them unequally outside the disability system. In addition, disability policy in Taiwan has thus created a separate, nonintegrated system that cannot satisfy the needs of an aging population, unless the aging person has an ID card to identify him- or herself as having a disability.

Furthermore, fiscal resources all go to cash assistance programs rather than to the creation of new programs to meet the needs of families located in different areas of Taiwan. The direction of disability policy has focused on compensating people with disabilities by using cash that is shared substantially among budgetary resources. This kind of resource allocation has reduced the flexibility to initiate new programs. Although Taiwanese law specifically pays attention to community-based care systems and services, with this skewed allocation of budgetary resources, it is unclear from where the funds for these programs will actually come. It may be that this unwise allocation of resources may prevent people who need services from receiving them and prevent those who might need more support from receiving it.

In 1980, the first legislation regulating services for older adults was enacted. Under this law, only people age 70 and older were deemed eligible to apply for aging-related services. But because retirement programs in Taiwan began at age 65, there was a gap between the retirement age and eligibility for welfare benefits. In 1997, the government revised the Welfare Law for the Elderly, and the two ages were reconciled. Since then, the age requirement has been consistent—age 65—and the nation's programs and services use this age for eligibility determination. Taiwan's welfare services for older adults have focused mostly on recreational and educational services, and a number of community-based senior centers have been established throughout the island. However, what is still needed is a well-planned home care or community care system.

Currently, approximately 8% of the Taiwanese population is age 65 or older. In the next 20 years or so, the percentage of older adults will increase to between 15% and 20%. It is not known how many of these will be older adults with lifelong disabilities.

Living arrangements for the older population in Taiwan clearly show that a family's ability to provide care or support for their aging parent will be reduced, because the birth rate has already dropped to the replacement rate. In the future, if the government does not adopt a comprehensive policy to target issues related to the aging population, the burden will become even worse for those families. Furthermore, along with increased longevity within the population of people with disabilities, the decrease in family size also implies that there will be fewer available resources within the family to provide supports for older adults with lifelong disabilities, as well as to their older parents. This disconnected system will weaken our ability to allocate resources for long-term care because each of these systems will have its own program and services. People who need such services will not be able to move between the "aging" and "disability" categories, even though the other system may provide better services for them. Sadly, because the Taiwanese welfare system is divided according to characteristics, a solution to the problem of integrating these two systems has not yet been found.

The Taiwanese disability system functions independently, rather than being integrated into other welfare systems. This fragmented approach has created problems for the families of adults with intellectual disabilities, particularly those who are older. This system pays attention to early childhood and school-age children with intellectual disabilities, but not to adult care or services. After the adult child with a disability reaches a certain age, the family must take care of him or her. The research I have done in rural areas clearly shows that those families live one day at a time, with only limited supports from their local government. I can only imagine what will happen to those adults with intellectual disabilities when they get old. Unfortunately, over the years, I have observed a trend toward institutional care for adults with intellectual disabilities. The few institutions that exist in Taiwan have raised their limit of age 30 for admissions to older than age 50. As long as there is not a good alternative to present to families of adults with intellectual disabilities, there is no easy way to stop this trend toward institutional care for older adults with an intellectual disability.

CONCLUSIONS

Inclusion of people with disabilities in various aspects of social life has become a major focus of change in Western countries. Taiwan also has tried to adopt this ideology, but, as evidenced by its legislative reforms and current services system, it has actually created an even more separate disability system than the law intended. This unintended policy consequence is related to two factors: a lack of substantial research data and the perception of disability. The first needs to be addressed in a much more detailed way. The Taiwan government does not have enough data collected about the population with disabilities to be able to gain an overall picture of the size and structure of this population, as well as basic information on education, employment, and living arrangements. Thus, although Taiwan's disability policy has been drawn from Western models, the underlying foundations and operational aspects of these models and their impact cannot be stated explicitly, even by advocates for these policies.

The second is that Taiwan's system has always extrapolated the needs of people with disabilities from their difficulties, rather than see them as human beings. That is, Taiwan's policy pays too much attention to the disability itself, and this attitude transfers into contract policy and programs. Being identified as a person with a disability and having an ID card are essential to Taiwan's system; ironically, this has made people with disabilities a special class of citizens. Their special status eventually separates those with disabilities from others in society; thus, "inclusion" becomes "exclusion."

In the end, disability policy in Taiwan can be categorized as a special system for a special population. The current system perceives people with disabilities as needing to have their rights preserved on the basis of their special characteristics, rather than of their status as general citizens. In the 1990s, through protests, public hearings, and the parents' movement, the public began to recognize the needs of people with disabilities. We have accomplished the tasks of reforming legislation and expanding public funds for both in-kind and in-cash programs. But these changes have not penetrated into the rural areas of Taiwan. One reason is that the financial arrangement between central and local governments has created a "winner take all" situation, leaving the less-developed areas in worse condition.

The care system for people with intellectual disabilities has followed the same path as the rest of Taiwan's disability system. Thus, what happens in the disability system affects people with intellectual disabilities as well. Unless we integrate our disabilities system into other welfare programs, this transformation of inclusion into exclusion will continue to have an adverse impact on older people with intellectual disabilities.

IV

SUPPORTING HEALTH
AND WELLNESS

In Section IV, the assembled chapters address both contributors and impediments to well-being when growing older with lifelong disabilities. Recognizing that one of the key indicators of "wellness" is good health through nutrition, Mughal and Bruckner, in Chapter 17, delineate common nutrition principles and provide guidelines for maintaining the health of older adults with intellectual disabilities in the community. Included in their discussions are an explanation of the nutritional needs of older adults, suggestions for dietary planning, and the application of common guidelines for meal planning and preparation. Their extensive tables and figures are a significant contribution for supporting the health of adults who are living on their own or in family or group environments.

Oral health, a subject long overlooked with regard to healthy aging, is the focus of Chapter 18, by Santos-Teachout, Malmström, Moss, and Handelman. Current epidemiological data indicate that people with developmental disabilities are at high risk for developing a variety of oral diseases and disorders. They note that this increased risk arises from factors such as cognitive or behavioral disabilities and residential and lifestyle issues that can interfere with oral hygiene and dietary habits. Given their risk for poor hygiene, people with intellectual and developmental disabilities need to be involved with primary dental care, and when appropriate, dentistry needs to be part of a coordinated multidisciplinary team approach.

Promoting mental health is the subject of Chapter 19. Cooper reviews how mental health and psychopathology affect people with intellectual disabilities in later life and discusses the more prevalent challenges for people who live in the community. She notes that dementia, depressive episodes, and anxiety disorders are prevalent conditions that warrant particular care and specialist interventions. Psychiatric disorders may present differently in older and younger populations, and there are particular causative factors of psychiatric disorders that are associated with older age. Clearly, and most important, there is reason to suspect that older people with intellectual disabilities may also have a differing range of mental health needs and service requirements than their younger counterparts.

Building on this perspective, Chapter 20 describes the need for functional assessment and presents a model for an ambulatory comprehensive geriatric assessment (CGA) that could serve to identify the presentation and possible causes of functional decline in adults with an intellectual disability. Henderson and Davidson point out that adults referred for a CGA generally present with global declines in functional capability—in particular, decreases in multiple self-care skills and social interaction skills. Many have concurrent disabling conditions not previously appreciated. Caregivers may overlook conditions that are amenable to management or treatment, assuming the presence of nonreversible dementia. The impact of undiagnosed or inadequately treated medical disorders, environmental barriers, and psychosocial factors that pertain to older age may not be identified by most health care providers. Henderson and Davidson make the case that further development of assessment clinics may improve identification of potentially reversible aging-related causes of functional impairment in older adults with intellectual disabilities.

The expression of dementia and related conditions is age associated and as such will affect more adults with the "graying" of the nation's population. Given demographic trends, dementia associated with Alzheimer's disease and other causes has become an additional challenge for providers of services to adults with intellectual disabilities. Janicki, McCallion, and Dalton, in Chapter 21, explicate the challenges that dementia presents to continued community living. The authors consider the dimensions of dementing illnesses and their definitions, scope, and means of identification. In addition, they provide an analysis of the factors, policies, and support structures that can help agencies to provide continued dementia-capable care that allows "aging in place," develop "in-place progression" dementia-specific programs, or choose alternative care environments. They also explore some features of dementia-related behaviors that may need to be taken into account in program design and proffer staff training suggestions and considerations for initiating dementia programs.

The final chapter of the section addresses the final stage of life. Botsford examines the dynamics of end-of-life care and concerns. She notes that as increasing numbers of people with lifelong disabilities survive into old age, staff will regularly encounter end-of-life situations among very diverse individuals in equally diverse community settings. Families, friends, and staff of hospices, hospitals, and home care agencies are asking how best to support people who are confronting the death of aging parents, siblings, housemates, friends, and staff, as well as their own terminal illnesses. With the use of vignettes, Chapter 22 identifies the needs of those who are dealing with end-of-life issues, including terminal illness, dying, death, bereavement, and mourning. Among the supportive strategies and resources presented are death education, advance directives, grief counseling, and inclusion. Helpfully, Botsford cites successful programs that promote staff knowledge and skills and include staff development and training, interdisciplinary ethics committees, and end-of-life committees.

Complementing this section's chapters, Zink's essay offers the insights of a person who has grown older with a lifelong disability and who has encountered the health care system firsthand. Her personal reflections convey the immediacy of these interactions, including the frustrations and challenges of dealing with health care providers who are insufficiently prepared to respond appropriately. Her essay is telling testimony of the still-wide gulf between people who need services and those who, ostensibly, provide them.

17

Food, Nutrition, and Wellness

Dawna Torres Mughal and Timothy L. Bruckner

Food has power. It not only nourishes and fuels the body but also comforts, expresses love and hospitality, reflects social status, portrays aspects of tradition and culture, and can represent reward or punishment. Eating behavior is complex, and many theoretical models and conceptual frameworks have been used to explain it. These include anthropological perspectives (Ritenbaugh, 1981), communication theory (Yarbrough, 1981), and a social psychological framework (Coates, 1981). Why do people eat what they eat? It is widely recognized that knowledge generally is not a significant predictor of adherence to health or medical advice. Therefore, it is important not only to educate people about the nutritional value of food but also to pay attention to the other factors that influence their acceptance and enjoyment of food.

A survey of a national sample of 2,967 American adults showed that taste, nutrition, cost, and weight control concerns influence food choices. Taste, however, was the most important and seemed to be the minimal criterion for food consumption (i.e., the other factors are important as long as the food is viewed as good tasting). Stressing the good taste of healthful foods may, therefore, be a more productive strategy in influencing food choices (Glanz, Basil, Maiback, Goldberg, & Snyder, 1998).

Stressing the blend of good taste and nutrition, Hess said, "Encourage clients to take the time for conscious eating rather than mindless fueling. Paying attention to food temperature, plate presentation, color, texture, and aroma slows the eating process and allows for the food we eat to nourish the body as well as the soul" (1996, p. 656). The sensory appeal of foods is important to people of all ages. It becomes more important when the senses of taste and smell become dull and when people have chronic illnesses

297

and functional impairments. To many older adults, eating is the highlight of the day, a pleasurable experience that they look forward to. Nutrients have value in preventing and treating diseases. If the food that supplies them is flavorful, attractive, and safe, eating may remain one of life's greatest pleasures.

This chapter discusses the guidelines for dietary planning, the energy and nutritional needs of older adults, and the application of the dietary guidelines to planning and preparing healthful meals. The nutrients discussed include carbohydrates, proteins, lipids, fat-soluble vitamins, selected water-soluble vitamins and minerals, and fluid. These are translated into a universal language, which is food. It is not our intent to address the complex nutritional needs associated with various specific disabilities but rather to provide general nutrition guidelines for older adults with developmental disabilities who live at home and in community-based homes.

GUIDELINES FOR DIETARY PLANNING

Foods supply the following nutrients that are vital to health and life: macronutrients (carbohydrates, proteins, and lipids), micronutrients (vitamins and minerals), and fluids. Guidelines for dietary planning have been developed to help people get adequate nutrients from foods. Service providers, caregivers, and older adults can use these guidelines to plan their meals.

Guidelines for dietary planning include the 1989 Recommended Dietary Allowances (RDAs; National Academy of Sciences/National Research Council, 1989), the 1995 Dietary Guidelines for Americans (U.S. Department of Agriculture [USDA], 1995), and the Food Guide Pyramid (USDA, 1996). In addition to these guidelines, the new Nutrition Facts labels found on most processed foods that are sold commercially provide educational information to help consumers select foods. The RDAs, which are numbers intended for professionals' use, and the Dietary Guidelines, which are statements of principles, are translated to food selection via the Food Guide Pyramid and the Nutrition Facts label (Owen, Splett, & Owen, 1999). The uses of the Dietary Guidelines, Food Guide Pyramid, and food labels are coordinated as tools for nutrition education of the public. Because references are made to the Dietary Guidelines as "standards" for dietary planning, these guidelines are explained here.

Recommended Dietary Allowances

The RDAs (see Table 1 in the appendix, which shows the values for older adults) are estimates of nutrient intakes that will meet the requirements of nearly all healthy people (97.5%). An individual whose intake is below the RDA is not necessarily at risk (Nandi, 1998). Because the values are for the healthy population, they may be inadequate for people with illnesses or health problems. In addition, the recommendations for older adults are extrapolated from data derived from experiments in younger people. The last age category is 51 years and older, suggesting that the RDAs may not meet the individual needs of all older people when they are lumped into one general age group (Russell, 1997). Despite the limitations, the RDAs can be used to estimate the probable risk of deficiency for an individual when food intakes are averaged over a sufficient length of time (Jacob, 1998).

In the late 1990s, the Food and Nutrition Board of the Institute of Medicine released new nutrient reference values or Dietary Reference Intakes (DRIs) for Americans and Canadians. The first two reports are the DRIs for calcium, phosphorus, magnesium, vitamin D, fluoride, B vitamins, and choline (Yates, Schlicker, & Suitor, 1998). The reference values are intended to help individuals optimize their health, prevent disease, and, where data are available, avoid consuming too much of a nutrient (Public Policy News, 1998). The DRIs, which expand and replace the 1989 RDAs, include four reference values: the RDA, Adequate Intake (AI), Estimated Average Requirement, and Tolerable Upper Intake Level. Each reference value has a specific use. In planning their diets, individuals can use the RDA and the AI as goals for their daily nutrient intake averaged over time (Yates et al., 1998). The application of the current and the pending DRIs as reference tools for dietary planning and assessment will take several years. In the meantime, the 1989 RDAs will continue to serve their purpose. One notable change is that, in contrast to the 1989 RDAs, the 1997–1998 DRIs include two different life stage groups for older adults (ages 51–70 years and older than age 70 years). Table 2 in the appendix displays the currently available DRIs, including the uses of the four reference values.

1995 Dietary Guidelines for Americans

The seven Dietary Guidelines (see Figure 1 in the Appendix at the end of this chapter) translate science into food-based recommendations for healthy Americans age 2 years and older. They provide the basis for nutrition policy and education activities. The guidelines emphasize the overall diet pattern and the link between diet and physical activity (USDA, 1995). They also use positive messages ("balance," "choose," and "eat") that focus on the total diet rather than negative prescriptions ("avoid" and "don't"). However, they do not specify consumer behavior, and consumers want directions regarding what to do and how to do it (Kennedy, Myers, & Layden, 1996).

In February 2000, the Advisory Committee on the Dietary Guidelines for Americans 2000 presented its recommendations to the Secretary of Agriculture to update the 1995 Dietary Guidelines (USDA, 2000). The committee's recommendations are included in the Appendix at the end of this chapter for informational purposes. The recommended revision has three basic messages, which are the "ABCs for health," with 10 guidelines to point the way to good health. The guidelines are intended for healthy children ages 2 years and older and adults of any age (Advisory Committee, 2000).

Food Guide Pyramid

The USDA Food Guide Pyramid (see Figure 2) is the research-based official food guidance system in the United States. It helps consumers put the Dietary Guidelines into practice by suggesting types and amounts of food for people of different ages and sexes. Emphasizing total diet quality, flexibility, and enjoyment of food, it teaches these three major concepts: variety, moderation, and proportion. *Variety* means eating a wide selection of food within each group and among major food groups. Variety is important because no single food can provide all of the nutrients in adequate amount. *Moderation* means eating food, especially those high in fat and added sugar, in recommended portions and eating fats, oils, and sweets sparingly. *Proportionality* means eating relatively more foods from larger groups (grains, fruits, and vegetables) in the Food Guide Pyramid than from smaller groups (Achterberg, McDonnell, & Bagby, 1994). These concepts are applicable to food plans served at home and in other places. Other food guide pyramids, such as the Asian, Pilipino, Latin American, Mediterranean, Puerto Rican, and vegetarian, are available to meet diverse dietary preferences. A Modified Food Guide Pyramid for 70+ Adults (see Figure 3) was published in 1999 (Tufts University Health and Nutrition Letter [TUHNL], 1999).

Food Label

The new food label helps consumers choose more healthful diets and offers an incentive to food companies to improve the nutritional quality of their product (U.S. Food and Drug Administration [FDA], 1995). Healthy People 2000, a national initiative to promote the nation's health and prevent diseases, has 27 nutrition objectives. One of these is to increase to at least 85% the proportion of people age 18 years and older who use food labels to make nutritious food selections (U.S. Department of Health and Human Services [DHHS], 1996).

Table 3 in the appendix displays the mandatory components of the "Nutrition Facts" panel. Producers may list voluntary components such as monounsaturated fat, polyunsaturated fat, and other nutrients (FDA, 1995). One way of conceptualizing the mandatory components is to divide them into two categories: "yellow light" for slow down or caution, and "green light" for go. The yellow light includes total fat, saturated fat, cholesterol, and sodium (components of which people should have less). The green light includes carbohydrate, dietary fiber, protein, vitamins A and C, iron, and calcium (components of which people should have more). Because of the public's preoccupation with fats and cholesterol, consumers may focus only on the yellow light. They should aim low at nutrients in the yellow light, for which the goal is moderation, and high at those in the green light, for which the goal is 100% of the reference or daily value. Figure 4 provides additional information, including the use of the percentage daily values and of the nutrient descriptors ("free," "low," and several others) that can help in deciding how the food fits the overall diet.

NUTRITIONAL NEEDS OF OLDER ADULTS WITH DEVELOPMENTAL DISABILITIES

The nutrient needs of older adults with developmental disabilities are the same as those of the general population. Nutritional problems frequently found in people with developmental disabilities, such as growth deviation (failure to thrive, obesity, and growth retardation), gastrointestinal disturbances (diarrhea and constipation), and feeding or eating problems, require individualization of dietary modifications (Posthauer, Palmer, Kadlec, Cloud, & Devlin, 1993). Treatment of chronic diseases, such as diabetes, hypertension, coronary artery disease, celiac disease, and osteoporosis, also requires dietary adjustments. Medical nutrition therapy of complex nutrition problems should be referred to qualified dietetics professionals in conjunction with medical consultation.

The following sections summarize the nutritional needs of older adults for selected nutrients and also their energy and fluid needs. The nutrients are linked to their food sources in the Food Guide Pyramid, and issues relevant to certain conditions that alter the energy and nutritional needs of older adults with developmental disabilities are discussed.

Macronutrients

The macronutrients (carbohydrates, proteins, and lipids) yield energy, whereas the micronutrients (vitamins and minerals) do not. Many vitamins and minerals, however, assist in energy-producing cellular reactions. Table 4 in the appendix summarizes the recommended intake, selected major functions, and primary food group sources of the macronutrients.

Proteins Various factors affect protein needs. Because the recommendation is based on body weight, the total value will vary with the person's weight. In addition, inadequate energy intake, inferior protein quality and digestibility (Matthews, 1999), hypermetabolic conditions (fever, infection, pressure ulcers, cancer, and AIDS), and growth will increase protein needs. People who have decubiti, or pressure ulcers caused by skin breakdown on bony prominences, need extra protein and calories for healing and prevention of infection (Neidert, 1998). To optimize the use of protein for tissue building, older people with developmental disabilities should consume sufficient calories to spare protein from being used as an alternate fuel source.

Animal protein is superior in quality to plant protein. Proper combination of plant proteins, however, can improve their quality (Whitney, Cataldo, & Rolfes, 1998). Unlike other plant foods, soy beans provide high-quality protein. One-half cup of cooked and one-half cup of roasted soy beans contain 14 grams and 34 grams of protein, respectively (Messina, 1999), or 28% and 68% of the RDA for a 51+-year-old woman. Many recipes and publications are available to help Americans develop their taste for soy. Consuming the recommended portions of lean meats and low-fat dairy products will supply high-quality protein and also vitamins and minerals while controlling fat, cholesterol, and calorie intake.

Carbohydrates   A diet that is liberal in foods containing complex carbohydrates (starches and fiber) provides not only the bulk of the day's total energy needs but also dietary fiber, vitamins, and minerals. Carbohydrate spares protein from being used for energy and promotes complete fat oxidation, thereby preventing the development of ketosis (i.e., an abnormal increase of ketone bodies in the body in conditions of reduced or disturbed carbohydrate metabolism) (Whitney et al., 1998). At least 100 grams of carbohydrates is the minimum desirable amount to prevent ketosis (Carter, 1999). For example, each of these foods in specified servings contains approximately 15 grams of carbohydrate: 1 slice of bread, ½ cup of mashed potatoes, ½ cup of corn, ½ cup of orange juice, and 1 small apple (American Dietetic Association [ADA] and American Diabetes Association, 1995). The normal functioning of the central nervous system requires a constant normal blood glucose level. Sick older adults who do not or cannot eat enough may develop hypoglycemia, which causes fatigue, weakness, dizziness, headache, confused state, and fainting. Increases in plasma glucose have been reported to enhance memory and other cognitive functions in older adults with Alzheimer's disease and young adults with Down syndrome (Gold, 1995). Table 4 shows that plant foods are the major carbohydrate suppliers, although milk contains a substantial amount of lactose, a naturally occurring simple sugar. One cup (8 ounces) of milk, on the average, has 12 grams of carbohydrate (ADA, 1995).

People who have lactose intolerance may better tolerate fermented milk products, such as yogurt and acidophilus milk, and milk divided into smaller portions (Whitney et al., 1998). Most adults who cannot digest lactose can tolerate up to 250 milliliters (approximately 8 ounces) of milk (Levin, 1999). Milk treated with lactase enzyme is another option (Whitney et al., 1998).

Sugar in moderation can be a part of a healthful diet. The Dietary Guidelines recommend that people choose a diet that is moderate in sugar (USDA, 1995). Good oral hygiene helps prevent dental caries, which are associated with sugar consumption (see Chapter 18).

Dietary fiber, found only in plant foods, has several health benefits (see Table 4). The 1995 Dietary Guidelines recommend that, to help meet their carbohydrate needs, people choose a diet with plenty of vegetables, fruits, and whole grains (USDA, 1995). Legumes from the meat and alternatives group provide approximately 5–8 grams of fiber. Table 5 in the appendix lists the fiber content of selected foods.

A study of adults with intellectual disabilities who lived in community group homes reported that the residents' food intake from the fruit, vegetable, and milk groups was most often deficient (Mercer & Ekvall, 1992). Fiber and fluid intake needs special attention because of the prevalence of constipation in the older population and in people with developmental disabilities. A rational approach is to include two to three servings of whole grains as part of the daily six or more servings of grains, five servings of fruits (whole fruits rather than juice) and vegetables daily, and a serving of legumes at least once or twice a week (ADA, 1998). To prevent bloating and gastrointestinal discomfort, dietary fiber intake should be increased gradually.

Lipids   Because excessive fat intake contributes to obesity and obesity is associated with diabetes, hypertension, and heart disease, people are advised to reduce their fat intake. Wells, Turner, Martin, and Roy (1997) pointed out that most of the risk factors for cardiovascular diseases are at least as prevalent among people with intellectual disabilities as in the general population. These risk factors include obesity, hypertension, and high blood cholesterol level. Excessive intake of saturated fat and cholesterol is a risk factor for hypercholesterolemia, atherosclerosis, and heart disease, with saturated fat being more so. The National Cholesterol Education Program (DHHS, 1993), therefore, recommends a diet controlled in total fat, saturated fat, and cholesterol as described in Table 3. This concept is consistent with the 1995 Dietary Guidelines for Americans and the Healthy People 2000 objectives (DHHS, 1996).

Although the public health message advises people to limit their saturated fat intake, it is important to note that individual saturated fats have different effects on blood cholesterol level. Saturated fatty acids that have shorter carbon chains (12, 14, and 16 carbons) raise blood cholesterol; of these, the one with 14 carbons has the greatest effect. These saturated fatty acids are lauric (12 carbons), myristic (14 carbons, predominant in coconut and palm kernel oils), and palmitic (16 carbons, predominant in palm oil, butter, and other animal products). In contrast, stearic acid, a longer-chain saturated fatty acid (18 carbons, found in animal products such as beef, cheese, cream, and certain plant foods and oils) has a neutral effect and may even lower total cholesterol (Kris-Etherton & Yu, 1997).

Many consumers have become concerned about the link of trans-fatty acid intake to heart disease. Partial hydrogenation of vegetable oils to make margarine, vegetable shortening, or frying fats changes the structure of polyunsaturated fatty acids, thereby forming trans-fatty acids. Hydrogenation is a chemical process that changes the liquid vegetable oils to hard and plastic products (Groff & Gropper, 2000). Trans-fatty acids have been reported to raise blood levels of low-density lipoprotein cholesterol (LDL; "bad cholesterol"), lower high-density lipoprotein cholesterol (HDL; "good cholesterol"), and increase the ratio of total cholesterol to HDL cholesterol. These abnormal values are risk factors for heart disease (Ascherio & Willett, 1997). Research findings have contributed to the recent recommendations that information about the amount of trans fats be added to food labels.

The value of dietary cholesterol reduction in treating hypercholesterolemia in people 70 years old and older has been questioned. Aggressive intervention to lower blood cholesterol is not indicated for severely incapacitated people or for those who have life-threatening diseases (Carter, 1999). Because many factors contribute to the development of heart disease, the better approach to prevention and treatment is multiple risk factor intervention. This includes control of hypertension, obesity, and diabetes mellitus; cigarette smoking cessation; and an increase in physical activity (DHHS, 1993). Balancing its bad reputation, cholesterol has several important uses in the body (see Table 4). The liver synthesizes cholesterol, and various factors, in addition to diet, can affect cholesterol balance (Groff & Gropper, 2000). If older adults and people with developmental disabilities find modified diets too restrictive and, consequently, do not enjoy their food and eat less, liberalization of the diet may increase food intake, improve nutritional status, and enhance the quality of life (ADA, 1997).

The overwhelming volume of information about what to eat and what not to eat has confused the public and raises the question, What is a practical dietary guide for older people with developmental disabilities and their caregivers? The USDA Food Guide Pyramid, with its principles of variety, moderation, and proportion, remains a good, simple tool. Implementation of dietary guidelines and diet prescriptions should be tailored to the individual's nutritional or health goals. There are times when extra dietary fats and the life-sustaining calories that they provide are necessary. One diet does not fit all individuals.

Energy   Many factors affect individual calorie needs. In general, with aging, people require less energy as a result of decreased basal metabolic rate and physical activity. The average energy allowances for the reference man and woman, 51 years of age and older, are 2,300 kilocalories and 1,900 kilocalories per day, respectively. A coefficient of variation of ±20% is used for the range of light to moderate activity (National Academy of Sciences/National Research Council, 1989). On the basis of body weight, the average energy allowance is 30 kilocalories per kilogram of body weight. This should be adjusted to the level of physical activity and other factors that could change calorie requirement. For example, people with Down syndrome or Prader-Willi syndrome need fewer calories than people with athetoid cerebral palsy (Cloud, 1997). A common-sense approach is to monitor appetite, food intake, and usual body weight for changes. Unintentional weight change is a good practical sign of the imbalance between energy intake and expenditure, whatever the cause may be. To underscore this, Mercer and Ekvall (1992) noted that the energy intake of adults with intellectual disabilities who lived in intermediate care facilities and in group homes was significantly one third below the RDA. When energy intake is inadequate, the intake of essential nutrients likely is low (Hogan & Evers, 1997; Mercer & Ekvall, 1992). Increasing energy intake from nutritious foods is, therefore, a dietary priority.

Commentary

In general, carbohydrates should provide 50%–60% of the day's total calories, protein 10%–15%, and fat 25%–30%. This calorie distribution translates to selecting primarily plant foods (grains, fruits, and vegetables) in the Food Guide Pyramid and a moderate amount of animal foods (meats and dairy) and using fats, oils, and sweets sparingly. When energy needs are reduced, meals should be planned carefully so that the foods are rich in nutrients but low in calories.

Micronutrient Needs

Fat-Soluble Vitamins   The fat-soluble vitamins include vitamins A, D, E, and K. Because they are fat soluble, their absorption is reduced by conditions that impair fat absorption. Table 6 in the appendix summarizes the RDAs, selected major functions, and primary food group sources of these vitamins.

Vitamin A   Although the mean intake of vitamin A in older people tends to exceed the RDA, many older people have poor intake (Schlenker, 1998). Even if dietary intake is adequate, several factors affect the actual use of the vitamin in the body. These factors include long-term laxative use, such as mineral oil (Blumberg & Couris, 1999), and chronic diseases of the liver, pancreas, and gastrointestinal tract, which cause fat mal-absorption. Chronic alcohol ingestion, by inducing liver disease, and several drugs (phenobarbital and ethanol) can adversely affect vitamin A metabolism and utilization. Excessive vitamin A intake is toxic, and the widespread vitamin A supplement use by older adults is a health concern (Suter, 1999). Because fat-soluble vitamins are stored in the body, vitamins A and D, particularly, have greater toxicity potential than the water-soluble vitamins.

Vitamin A absorption in adults with Down syndrome was studied repeatedly because adults with Down syndrome often exhibited symptoms of vitamin A defi-ciency. These symptoms are hyperkeratotic lesions of the skin, increased incidence of upper respiratory tract infection, and poor visual ability to adapt to darkness. Results of the studies regarding impaired vitamin A absorption are conflicting and inconclusive (Patterson & Ekvall, 1993). Two to three servings of fruits and three to five servings of vegetables supply beta-carotene, which is converted to vitamin A in the intestinal tract, and the meat and the dairy groups provide the preformed vitamin A. Bright or deep yellow fruits and vegetables (also dark green) are generally rich in beta-carotene (Whitney et al., 1998).

Vitamin D   The vitamin D status of older people, especially of those with devel-opmental disabilities, deserves special attention. In fact, it was found that vitamin D intake of adults with intellectual disabilities who live in community group homes was significantly one third less than the RDA (Mercer & Ekvall, 1992). Anticonvulsant ther-apy increases risk for vitamin D and calcium deficiency because the drug interferes with vitamin D metabolism. Other factors that compromise vitamin D status include age-related changes in the skin, liver, and kidney; these organs play an important role in vitamin D synthesis and activation. Many frail older adults, shut-ins, and care-dependent individuals have reduced sun exposure and, consequently, reduced vitamin D production on the skin. Also, aging skin has lost its efficiency in this process (Ryan, Eleazer, & Egbert, 1995). Dark skin pigmentation can partially inhibit the conversion of vitamin D precursor on the skin, as indicated by a study of young African American women and women of European heritage (Harris & Dawson-Hughes, 1998). Decreased renal mass associated with aging can reduce the production of the most active form of the vitamin D hormone, 1,25 dihydroxycholecalciferol, by the kidney. Insufficient con-sumption of vitamin D–fortified milk, because of lactose intolerance, can further increase the risk (Ryan et al., 1995). Vitamin D promotes calcium absorption; vitamin D deficiency therefore causes calcium deficiency (Groff & Gropper, 2000). Because vitamin D deficiency can cause secondary calcium deficiency, it has a role in the development of osteoporosis. The increased prevalence of osteoporosis has been observed in rela-tively younger adults with intellectual disibilities (Center, Beange, & McElduff, 1998).

As Table 6 shows, only a few foods, primarily animal foods (liver, egg yolk, fatty fish, butter, and fortified milk), supply vitamin D (Whitney et al., 1998). One quart (4 cups) of milk is fortified with 400 international units (IU) of vitamin D, sufficient to meet the 1989 RDA and the new AI for 50- to 70-year-olds but is only 66% of the AI for those older than 70 years. A study of 376 older women (65–67 years old) in a multicen-ter osteoporosis trial showed that milk supplied 50% of the dietary vitamin D intake (Kinyamu, Gallagher, Rafferty, & Balbourn, 1998), indicating that milk is a primary source of dietary vitamin D. Because many older adults and people with developmen-tal disabilities may not be able to get sufficient vitamin D from foods alone, they should be exposed to sunlight as a major source of additional vitamin D. A daily supplementation of 10 micrograms (400 IU), alone or combined with calcium supplement, has been suggested for those with low sun exposure (Suter, 1999). Long-term megadoses of vitamin D, however, can be toxic (Whitney et al., 1998).

Vitamin E   Vitamin E is a group of chemically related substances that have the biological activity of alpha-tocopherol. Among the eight forms (stereoisomers) of vitamin E, RRR-alpha-tocopherol is the most biologically active. The different forms have different antioxidant activities and physiological effects (Traber, 1999).

The RDA for vitamin E can be obtained easily from foods. As shown in Table 6, wheat germ, safflower, and sunflower oils are particularly rich in the most biologically active form of vitamin E (RRR-alpha-tocopherol) (Traber, 1999). The public's fat phobia and the medical prescription for low-fat diets for older people can reduce the intake of fat-soluble vitamins. Because of fat malabsorption associated with cystic fibrosis, children with this disease can develop deficiency (Traber, 1999).

The antioxidant action of vitamin E has been studied in relation to heart disease, cancer, cataracts, depression, dementia, and immune function status (Traber, 1999). These emerging issues may have contributed to the widespread use of vitamin E supplementation in this country. As a group, older adults in the United States are the biggest users of vitamin E supplementation. A study indicated that a 4-month daily supplementation with 80–800 IU (55–182 milligrams) all-rac-alpha-tocopherol (7–23 times the RDA for individuals 51 years of age and older) was safe (i.e., it did not have adverse effects on kidney and liver functions, hematological status, bleeding time, and other outcome measures in 88 healthy older adults [ages 65 years and older] who had normal vitamin K status and who were not taking anticoagulants) (Meydani et al., 1998). Vitamin supplement users who are receiving anticoagulant therapy should be aware that pharmacological doses of vitamin E (and A) counteract the blood-clotting function of vitamin K and can increase the blood-thinning effect of anticoagulants, such as aspirin and coumarin (Olson, 1999). They should also note that chemically synthesized vitamin E is less biologically potent than the naturally occurring form. The pills that contain the synthetic vitamin E (all-rac-alpha-tocopherol) are labeled "dl-alpha-tocopherol." Those that contain the natural vitamin E (RRR-alpha-tocopherol) are labeled "d-alpha-tocopherol" (Traber, 1999).

Vitamin K   Vitamin K deficiency is rare in healthy adults. It can be induced, however, by certain medications and diseases. Phenytoin anticonvulsant (Blumberg & Couris, 1999), coumarin anticoagulants, salicylates, broad-spectrum antibiotics, and pharmacological doses of vitamins A and E antagonize vitamin K action. Sulfaquinoxaline, neomycin, and other broad-spectrum antibiotics can sterilize the bowel and impair vitamin synthesis by the gut bacterial flora (Olson, 1999). People who have vitamin K deficiency are at risk for developing bleeding tendencies because the synthesis of certain blood-clotting factors is impaired (Suter, 1999). Table 6 shows that vitamin K is obtained not only from foods but also from intestinal microflora synthesis.

Water-Soluble Vitamins   The water-soluble vitamins include vitamin C (ascorbic acid) and the B vitamins (thiamin, riboflavin, niacin, vitamin B_6 or pyridoxine, folate, vitamin B_{12}, pantothenic acid, and biotin). The 1989 RDAs (see Table 1) have established allowances for all of them except pantothenic acid and biotin. Because they are water soluble, the amount that exceeds the body's needs is excreted in the urine. Like their fat-soluble counterparts, the water-soluble vitamins are needed in small amounts and do not yield usable energy. The vitamins, however, are powerful helpers in energy metabolism and cellular processes. Deficiency diseases can result from primary or secondary deficiencies of certain vitamins. For example, deficiencies of vitamin C, thiamin, and folate (also vitamin B_{12}) cause scurvy, beriberi, and anemia, respectively.

Vitamin C   Vitamin C has many essential functions in the body (see Table 6). In general, fresh fruits and vegetables are rich sources of vitamin C. For example, 1 cup of orange juice, on average, supplies 100 mg of vitamin C, or 166% of the RDA for individuals ages 51 years and older. Vitamin C is easily destroyed by heat, light, air, and alkali. Vegetables should be cooked in small amounts of water for a short time (Whitney et al., 1998). As noted previously, adults with intellectual disabilities living in intermediate care facilities and group homes were found to have deficient intake of fruits and vegetables (Mercer & Ekvall, 1992). Poor dentition and chewing and swallowing difficulties tend to limit a person's fruit and vegetable consumption. Soft fruits and vegetables or their juices can be used instead. Older shoppers, particularly those on fixed incomes, may perceive the relatively high cost of fruits and vegetables as a barrier to eating these foods. Considering their notable nutritional contributions to the diet, fruits and vegetables are "good buys."

Folate   Because of the potential role of folate status in reducing the risk factor (elevated blood homocysteine level) for heart disease, in maintaining cognitive function in older adults, and in the development and management of psychiatric disorder and depression in older adults, folate has received increased attention (Miller, 1999; Suter, 1999). Miller (1999) reviewed studies that related high homocysteine blood level (one indicator of folate deficiency) with dementia of the Alzheimer type. Reports regarding reduced folate absorption in older adults are conflicting (Suter, 1999). From a disease prevention standpoint, folate helps prevent neural tube defect, such as spina bifida (Koehler, Pareo-Tubbeh, Romero, Baumgartner, & Garry, 1997).

Table 6 shows that the new RDA (400 micrograms) for folate is twice the 1989 RDA and is expressed in dietary folate equivalent (DFE) (Food and Nutrition Board, 1998) to correct for the higher bioavailability of synthetic folic acid relative to food folate. DFE converts all forms of dietary folate, including synthetic folic acid in fortified products, to an amount that is equivalent to food folate (Bailey, 1998).

Folate and vitamin B_{12} have complex interrelated biochemical functions in DNA synthesis that promote cellular growth, including red blood cell formation. Deficiencies of either one or both can cause blood abnormalities, such as megaloblastic anemia. Certain medications interfere with folate utilization and may increase folate requirement. These medications include triamterene, a diuretic and antihypertensive agent; the anticonvulsants phenytoin and phenobarbital; barbiturates, both sedative and anticonvulsant; sulfasalazine, an antidiarrheal agent used in treating Crohn's disease; and methotrexate, an antimetabolite used to treat cancer (Blumberg & Couris, 1999; Herbert, 1999) and rheumatoid arthritis. High intake of alcohol, combined with an inadequate diet, is one of the major contributors to clinical folate deficiency (Blumberg & Couris, 1999).

When people with developmental disabilities need folate supplementation, it is important to assess their vitamin B_{12} status also. High folate intake superimposed on vitamin B_{12} deficiency can mask vitamin B_{12} deficiency, which occurs in many older adults and has serious consequences (i.e., folate can correct the megaloblastic anemia but not the neurological damage induced by vitamin B_{12} deficiency). To prevent this "masking effect," it is recommended that total folate intake be limited to less than 1 mg per day (FDA, 1996). In view of folate fortification of certain grain products, screening for vitamin B_{12} deficiency using modern methods and treating the deficiency are, therefore, important health promotion strategies (Koehler et al., 1997).

Folate is widely distributed in foods (see Table 6). Because oxidation during cooking and storage can destroy as much as half of folate in foods (Whitney et al., 1998), vegetables should not be overcooked or held in steam tables for a long time.

Vitamin B_{12}   The 20% increase in the new RDA for vitamin B_{12} (see Table 6) considers the needs of older people who have reduced absorption of the food-bound vitamin as a result of atrophic gastritis. The prevalence of atrophic gastritis increases with age (Suter, 1999). Vitamin B_{12} is found naturally only in animal foods. Older people generally consume limited amounts of these foods and may be able to meet the RDA for vitamin B_{12} mainly by consuming vitamin B_{12}–fortified foods (e.g., breakfast cereals) or a supplement containing vitamin B_{12}. People with atrophic gastritis can absorb the crystalline vitamin B_{12} better than they can food-bound vitamin B_{12} (Koehler et al., 1997).

Lack of intrinsic factor, as a result of genetic defect or stomach injury, impairs vitamin B_{12} absorption and causes pernicious anemia.[1] Intrinsic factor, a protein made and released by the stomach, is essential to vitamin B_{12} absorption (Groff & Gropper, 2000). Intramuscular injection of vitamin B_{12} is necessary to circumvent this abnormality in absorption.

Minerals   People of all ages need calcium, an important mineral that is responsible for bone mineralization and strength. Calcium deficiency, caused by inadequate intake or secondary to vitamin D deficiency, medication use, or diseases that reduce absorption, is a risk factor for the development of osteoporosis. Osteoporosis is a major problem that affects women (McBean, Forgac, & Finn, 1994) and also people with intellectual disabilities (Center et al., 1998) and with celiac disease (Mora et al., 1998). The inappropriate food intake often seen in people with intellectual disabilities reduces calcium intake (Mercer & Ekvall, 1992). In addition, certain factors can affect the amount of calcium actually absorbed from food. The efficiency of digestion, the health of the intestinal tract, and interfering factors (e.g., medications such as antacids and tetracycline) can reduce calcium absorption (Blumberg & Couris, 1999). Long-term therapy with glucocorticoids, by interfering with calcium utilization, can induce osteoporosis (Lukert & Raisz, 1990). The interrelated function of calcium and vitamin D in bone health has already been discussed in the previous section. Because osteoporosis, like many other chronic diseases, has a multifactorial cause, its prevention and treatment should be multifaceted. Bone health maintenance requires other nutrients (protein, vitamins C and K, phosphorus, fluoride, and several others) in addition to calcium and vitamin D (McBean et al., 1994). Prevention should start early because "osteoporosis is a pediatric disease with a geriatric outcome" (McBean et al., 1994, p. 669).

Table 6 shows that the recommended calcium intake ranges from 800 mg/day to 1,500 mg/day. The preferred source of calcium is calcium-rich foods. Two to three cups of milk and other dairy products (e.g., yogurt) in the Food Guide Pyramid can supply approximately 600–900 mg of calcium, or one half to three fourths of the recommended AI for older adults. Results of a multicenter, randomized, controlled trial with 204 healthy older adults between 65 and 85 years of age showed that the addition of three 8-ounce cups of fluid milk to these individuals' usual consumption of dairy products for 12 weeks resulted in positive bone balance as measured by specific outcomes. This means that new bone formation exceeded old bone destruction. Bone

---

[1]Severe hyperchromic anemia (marked by a progressive decrease in number and increase in size and hemoglobin content of the red blood cells and by pallor, weakness, and gastrointestinal and nervous disturbances) is associated with reduced ability to absorb vitamin B_{12} as a result of the absence of intrinsic factor.

formation and bone resorption are natural processes that occur in bone remodeling throughout life. The researchers concluded that it is feasible to increase calcium intake through dietary sources and that these dietary changes affect bone formation favorably (Heaney et al., 1999).

People who do not consume milk products or who are lactose intolerant may use calcium-fortified products and calcium supplements. Although some green leafy vegetables (beet greens, kale, Swiss chard, turnip greens, collard, and Chinese cabbage) provide some calcium, people may not eat them frequently or in sufficient amounts. In addition, spinach contains oxalate, a calcium binder that reduces the absorption of this mineral. Meat alternatives, such as legumes (soy beans, black-eyed peas, and navy beans), can provide significant amounts when consumed frequently (Whitney et al., 1998). Table 7 in the appendix lists the calcium content of selected foods.

In general, older adults with developmental disabilities may not be able to meet the recommended calcium intake from foods alone. Calcium supplementation may be beneficial. A review and evaluation of several clinical trials showed that additional calcium supplement added to standard antiresorptive therapy (estrogen, alendronate, and calcitonin) generally decreased bone loss. The benefits were associated with a calcium intake of 1,200 milligrams (Nieves, Komar, Cosman, & Lindsay, 1998).

Fluids   Dehydration is life threatening. Older adults and their caregivers, therefore, must ensure adequate hydration at all times and recognize signs of dehydration (Lipschitz, 1992). In clinical practice, different formulas are used to calculate fluid needs depending on the medical conditions that cause fluid retention or losses. Under normal conditions, for a reference older man and woman whose average energy allowance is 2,300 kilocalories and 1,900 kilocalories, respectively, the total fluid is 2,300 milliliters (9 c) and 1,900 milliliters (8 c). This is based on 1 milliliter of fluid per kilocalorie intake (Kleiner, 1999). The general recommendation is six to eight glasses of water per day. Alternative fluid sources, such as fruit juices and watery food, are palatable and provide needed nutrients and calories. Although caffeine and alcoholic beverages are fluid, they have a diuretic effect and can increase fluid loss (Kleiner, 1999).

Emerging Issues

Space does not allow the discussion of many other nutrients (thiamin, riboflavin, niacin, pyridoxine, pantothenic acid, biotin, and many important minerals) known to benefit health. The exclusion does not imply that they are less important. All nutrients are equally important, working in concert to produce the desired outcomes. These are exciting times for research in nutrition, as studies continue to expand our knowledge of the nutrients and other substances in foods. Antioxidants, carotenoids, flavonoids, isoflavones, carnitine, creatine, phytoestrogens, and other ingredients sound more like a pharmacy than a food pantry.

Basic research has indicated the potential value of dietary carotenoids and possibly vitamin C in reducing the risk for developing advanced age-related macular degeneration (AMD). AMD is the leading cause of irreversible blindness among people older than 65 years. Increasing the consumption of foods that are rich in certain carotenoids (dark green, leafy vegetables) may have a protective effect (Seddon et al., 1994). West et al. (1994) reported the protective effect of vitamin A, vitamin C (ascorbic acid), vitamin E (alpha-tocopherol), and beta-carotene. The hypothesis regarding antioxidant therapy for AMD is promising but unproved (Seddon & Henekens, 1994). Additional studies are needed to make rational recommendations for the prophylactic or therapeutic use of these substances.

Commentary

Food supplies the energy and nutrients that the body needs in health and disease. People need the same nutrients, but the amounts may vary depending on the individual's physiological and medical condition. Eating proper amounts of diverse foods from each food group and across groups; drinking adequate fluids; and being physically, socially, and mentally active are part of the recipe for healthful living and aging. People can and should get nutrients primarily from foods. If illness cannot make this possible, then nutrition supplements, in consultation with qualified health professionals, may be necessary. Older adults need to be educated regarding spending their money on unproven remedies that are not effective in treating health problems. Because many medications can adversely affect food intake and nutrient utilization, education about medications is an essential health promotion strategy.

MEAL PLANNING

Using the Food Guide Pyramid in Building Healthful Meals

The next section explains the use of the Food Guide Pyramid in meal planning for older adults. The basic principles are intended for healthy Americans ages 2 years and older (USDA, 1996). Dietary modifications can be made to fit individual needs; however, the principle for such changes is the same (i.e., the diet should be nutritionally balanced as much as possible).

The Food Guide Pyramid emphasizes the three groups of plant foods—grains, fruits, and vegetables—as the foundation of a healthful diet and the source of most of the day's energy intake. The foundation consists of six to eleven servings of grain products, three to five servings of vegetables, and two to four servings of fruits. Whole-grain, enriched, or fortified high-fiber products and vitamin A– or vitamin C–rich fruits and vegetables with roughage should be chosen. Moderate amounts of animal foods should be added to this (i.e., two or three servings from the meat group and two or three servings from the dairy group). Not classified as a food group, fats, oils, and sweets in the tip of the pyramid should be used sparingly (USDA, 1996). Because of the importance of normal hydration, at least eight glasses of water should be added to the foundation of the pyramid (Kleiner, 1999; TUHNL, 1999). Alternating legumes (beans) for meat at least twice a week will increase fiber intake (ADA, 1998; TUHNL, 1999). As noted before, a "Modified Food Pyramid for 70+ Adults" (see Figure 3) is available.

Each of the five food groups shows a range of servings to allow for differences in energy needs. A day's meals, planned using the lowest number, will contain approximately 1,600 kilocalories, an appropriate level for many sedentary women and older adults. Using the middle and highest numbers, the meals will provide 2,200 and 2,800 kilocalories, respectively. The amount of fat in the lowest, middle, and highest calorie levels is 53 grams, 73 grams, and 93 grams, respectively (USDA, 1996). Table 8 in the appendix displays the meal plans for the three calorie levels.

Vegetarian Diets

As long as the variety and amounts of food are adequate, vegetarian diets can meet the RDAs for nutrients. Because lacto-ovovegetarians eat dairy products and eggs, they, as a group, consume a nutritionally adequate diet. Iron, zinc, and B vitamins need special attention when diets exclude their major sources, such as meat, fish, and poultry. Because vegans eat only foods of plant origin, they need to supplement their diet with a source of vitamin B$_{12}$. This vitamin is found naturally only in animal products. Calcium and vitamin D sources also need special attention (USDA, 1995).

Fats and Sugars

Naturally occurring or added fats, represented by the symbol ● in the pyramid, are present in foods. This fat symbol is more predominant in the meat and dairy groups and in fats, oils, and sweets. The symbol ▼ in the pyramid represents added sugar (USDA, 1996). The tip of the pyramid has many of the symbols, and the grain and dairy groups have some. Regardless of these symbols, no food group has to be excluded from the diet. The concepts of variety, moderation, and proportion suggest that all foods can fit into a healthful diet.

Defining Serving Sizes

Table 9 in the appendix shows the USDA's (1996) definition of single servings of foods in each of the five food groups. The USDA (1993) has suggested a 1,600-kilocalorie meal plan for older women and a 2,400-kilocalorie meal for older men. Table 10 in the appendix shows the 1,600-kilocalorie meal plan and examples of foods in each group. Foods from each group can be added to the basic plan to increase calories and nutrients.

Other countries have developed methods for teaching meal planning. One example, commonly used in Europe, is the plate model, a visual method for teaching healthful eating through the use of pictures, graphs, charts, and food replicas. A dinner plate, serving as a pie plate, shows the proportion of the plate that should be covered by foods from the food groups. The vegetables cover one half of the plate; the grain products (pasta, potato, or rice), one fourth; meat and meat alternatives, one fourth; and fruits, low-fat milk or yogurt, and grains (bread, rolls, or crisp bread) are on the side. The plate model's effectiveness and application to other populations need to be evaluated (Camelon et al., 1998). Because the method is simple and visual, it has potential utility for teaching many older adults with developmental disabilities.

Controlling Dietary Fat and Cholesterol Intake

Dietary fat and cholesterol intake can be controlled through proper selection and preparation of foods. In general, foods from animals (meat and dairy groups) are higher in fat than foods from plants. Cholesterol is found naturally only in animal products, and saturated fats (with some exceptions) also predominate in these foods. Certain vegetable oils, such as coconut and palm, are predominantly saturated fats. Using unsaturated fats in place of saturated fats, within the total fat limit, is recommended for lowering blood cholesterol. Monounsaturated fats include olive, peanut, and canola oils. Polyunsaturates include safflower, corn, soybean, sunflower, and cottonseed (USDA, 1996). Hydrogenation (a chemical process) of unsaturated vegetable oils to make margarine and shortening changes the unsaturated to saturated fats. Partially hydrogenated vegetable oils (e.g., those used in many margarines and shortenings) contain trans-fatty acids, a form of unsaturated fats that may raise blood cholesterol level (USDA, 1996). Controlling the total fat intake helps control the consumption not only of saturated fats and extra calories but also of trans-fatty acids. Strategies should focus on total diet quality rather than on single nutrients. Choosing moderate amounts of lean cuts of meat and fish and low-fat milk and milk products helps reduce fat and cholesterol intake.

Several preparation techniques, such as low-fat cooking and recipe modification, can also reduce dietary fat and cholesterol. Skimming fat from soups and gravies, baking meat on a rack to drain the fat, trimming visible fat from meat, using more egg whites than yolks in certain recipes, and substituting low-fat ingredients for high-fat ones (e.g., yogurt or buttermilk for sour cream, skim milk for whole milk) are just some of the many ways to reduce fat and calorie intake (USDA, 1993).

A certain amount of fat is needed in the diet, and some older people with developmental disabilities who need to gain weight may need to eat more fat. Fat enhances the flavor of food. A fat-free, "cardboard taste" diet is not very palatable.

Salt and Sodium

The daily value or reference standard for sodium is 2,400 milligrams per day. This limit is based on the link between excess sodium and hypertension (USDA, 1995). Table salt (sodium chloride) is approximately 40% sodium. One teaspoon of salt contains 2,000 milligrams of sodium (USDA, 1996; Whitney et al., 1998). Without counting grams of sodium on the food label, people can control their sodium intake through proper food selection and preparation. The major sources of sodium include the salt added to cooking and at the table, as well as processed foods, with some containing much more sodium than others. Table 11 in the appendix shows the average sodium content of foods by food group. If people find the reduced-sodium meals tasteless and unappetizing, they can use seasonings, such as herbs and spices, which are excellent flavor enhancers. Because of their reduced taste sensitivity, older adults may enjoy more highly seasoned foods.

Alcohol

Alcohol is both a food and a drug. As a food, it provides 7 kilocalories per gram without nutritional value. As a drug, it depresses the central nervous system, irritates the gastrointestinal tract, damages the liver, and causes neurological damage. It can also interfere with certain medications and cause adverse reactions (Whitney et al., 1998).

The best advice is not to drink at all. If people drink, however, they should do so in moderation. *Moderation* means one drink per day for women and no more than two drinks per day for men. A drink is equivalent to 12 ounces of regular beer (150 kilocalories) or 5 ounces of wine (100 kilocalories) or 1.5 ounces of 80-proof distilled spirits (100 kilocalories) (USDA, 1995).

Boosting the Appetite

Results of a survey of older adults showed that food presentation, taste, and temperature (cold foods were cold enough and hot foods were appropriately hot) influenced satisfaction with food service. The type of diet (modified or regular) did not predict dietary satisfaction, indicating that therapeutic or texture-modified diets can be made as appealing as regular diets (O'Hara et al., 1997).

Attention to food preparation and presentation and to the total dining environment can boost appetite, food intake, and satisfaction. With consideration of an individual's chewing and swallowing ability, textures can be added to soft foods. For example, soft vegetables cut into pieces can be added to mashed foods, and crunchy cereal can be mixed with yogurt. Chewing foods thoroughly to release the flavor and eating with other people can enhance the enjoyment of meals ("Promoting elderly appetite," 1993). Table 12 in the appendix lists some quick and easy ways to improve food and nutrient intake in older people with developmental disabilities. Creativity in using available resources, attractive plate presentation, and a pleasant and caring environment contribute to the making of enjoyable and nutritious meals.

Physical Activity

Regular physical activity and a well-balanced diet contribute to good health. It is recommended that people accumulate 30 minutes or more of moderate-intensity physical activity on most (preferably all) days of the week (USDA, 1995). The 30 minutes can be accumulated using shorter bouts of 8–10 minutes each. For older adults, moderate-intensity physical activities, such as gardening, walking, grocery shopping with a grocery cart, pushing a stroller, putting away groceries, and water aerobics, are realistic exercises. They should do what they enjoy. People can adjust the length of their exercise time according to the intensity of their physical activity ("Promoting physical activity and health," 1996). Balancing energy intake with energy expenditure on physical activity can help prevent unwanted weight gain in older adults with developmental disabilities. Regular physical activity helps to maintain muscle. Muscle maintenance helps reduce the risk of falls and fractures (USDA, 1995).

Food Safety

Safe food handling practices should be followed. People with developmental disabilities, especially when older, may have weak immune systems and, therefore, may be at high risk for problems related to food safety. Walter, Cohen, and Swicker (1997) reported that staff and consumers in a variety of community-based homes for people with developmental disabilities need food safety training. The authors suggested that education regarding safe food preparation, including storage and handling procedures, would be beneficial for staff and consumers.

One of the Healthy People 2000 objectives is to reduce infections caused by key food-borne pathogens (DHHS, 1996). The FDA and the USDA have published extensive consumer guidelines for shopping and for food preparation and storage at home. The first cardinal rule of safe food preparation at home is to keep everything clean. This applies to the food preparation area and, most important, to the cook. Food handlers should wash their hands thoroughly before preparing the meal and after handling raw meat or poultry and should cover long hair with a net or a scarf. Cuts or sores on their hands should be completely covered. If the sore or cut is infected, the cooks should not handle foods at all. Raw vegetables should be washed thoroughly. The second cardinal rule is to keep hot foods hot and cold foods cold. Cooking meats thoroughly, refrigerating leftovers promptly, protecting foods promptly from cross-contamination after cooking, and keeping foods below 40° F and above 140° F to prevent the growth of pathogenic bacteria are valuable guidelines to follow (FDA, 1997).

CONCLUSIONS

Food and nutrition are part of good medicine that will help older adults with developmental disabilities live a healthy life. As Berry said, "When a patient leaves the doctor with a drug prescription in one hand, he or she should have a nutritional prescription in the other" (1993, p. 7). The nutritional prescription, unlike bad-tasting medicine, however, should be packaged in good-tasting, safe food that is attractively presented as a feast to the senses. The sensory appeal will make the medicine go down to nourish both the body and the soul.

REFERENCES

Achterberg, C., McDonnell, E., & Bagby, R. (1994). How to put the Food Guide Pyramid into practice. *Journal of the American Dietetic Association, 94,* 1030–1035.

Advisory Committee on Dietary Guidelines. (2000). *Report of the Advisory Committee on Dietary Guidelines, 2000.* Washington, DC: U.S. Department of Agriculture.

American Dietetic Association. (1997). Position of the American Dietetic Association: Health implications of fiber. *Journal of the American Dietetic Association, 97,* 1157–1159.

American Dietetic Association. (1998). Position of the American Dietetic Association: Liberalized diets for older adults in long-term care. *Journal of the American Dietetic Association, 98,* 201–204.

American Dietetic Association and American Diabetes Association. (1995). *Exchange lists for meal planning.* Alexandria, VA/Chicago: Authors.

Ascherio, A., & Willett, W.C. (1997). Health effects of trans-fatty acids. *American Journal of Clinical Nutrition, 66*(4 Suppl.), S1006–S1010.

Bailey, L.B. (1998). Dietary reference intakes for folate: The debut of dietary folate equivalents. *Nutrition Reviews, 56,* 294–299.

Berry, E.M. (1993). Nutrition: Rx for chronic disease. *Worldview, 5,* 7.

Blumberg, J.B., & Couris, R. (1999). Pharmacology, nutrition, and the elderly: Interactions and implications. In R. Chernoff (Ed.), *Geriatric nutrition: The health professional's handbook* (2nd ed., pp. 342–365). Gaithersburg, MD: Aspen Publishers.

Camelon, K.M., Hadell, K., Jamsen, P.T., Ketonen, K.J., Kotamaki, H.M., Makimatilla, S., Tormala, M.L., & Valve, R. (1998). The plate model: A visual method of teaching meal planning. *Journal of the American Dietetic Association, 98,* 1155–1158.

Campbell, W.W. (1996). Dietary requirements of older people. Is the RDA adequate? *Nutrition Today, 31,* 192–197.

Carter, W.J. (1999). Macronutrient requirements for elderly persons. In R. Chernoff (Ed.), *Geriatric nutrition: The health professional's handbook* (2nd ed., pp. 13–26). Gaithersburg, MD: Aspen Publishers.

Center, J., Beange, H., & McElduff, A. (1998). People with mental retardation have an increased risk of osteoporosis: A population study. *American Journal on Mental Retardation, 103,* 19–28.

Cloud, H. (1997). Expanding roles for dietitians' work with persons with developmental disabilities. *Journal of the American Dietetic Association, 97,* 189–190.

Coates, T.J. (1981). Eating: A psychological dilemma. In Proceedings of the Workshop on Nutrition Education Research: Applying Principles from the Behavioral Sciences. *Journal of Nutrition Education, 13*(Suppl. 1), S12–S13.

Food and Nutrition Board, National Academy of Sciences, Institute of Medicine. (1998). Dietary reference intakes: Recommended intakes for individuals. *Nutrition Today, 33,* 257–259.

Glanz, K., Basil, M., Maiback, E., Goldberg, J., & Snyder, D. (1998). Why Americans eat what they do: Taste, nutrition, cost, convenience, and weight concerns as influences on food consumption. *Journal of the American Dietetic Association, 98,* 1118–1126.

Gold, P. (1995). Role of glucose in regulating the brain and cognition. *American Journal of Clinical Nutrition, 61*(Suppl.), 987S–995S.

Groff, J.L., & Gropper, S.S. (2000). *Advanced nutrition and human metabolism* (3rd ed.). Belmont, CA: West/Wadsworth.

Harris, S.S., & Dawson-Hughes, N. (1998). Seasonal changes in plasma 25-hydroxyvitamin D concentrations of young American black and white women. *American Journal of Clinical Nutrition, 67,* 1232–1236.

Heaney, R.P., McCarron, D.A., Dawson-Hughes, B., Oparil, S., Berga, S.L., Stern, J.S., Barr, S.I., & Rosen, C.J. (1999). Dietary changes favorably affect bone remodeling in older adults. *Journal of the American Dietetic Association, 99,* 1228–1233.

Herbert, V. (1999). Folic acid. In M.E. Shils, J.E. Olson, M. Shike, & C.A. Ross (Eds.), *Modern nutrition in health and disease* (9th ed., pp. 433–446). Baltimore: Williams & Wilkins.

Hess, M.A. (1996). Food for the soul as well as the body. *Journal of the American Dietetic Association, 96,* 656.

Hogan, S.E., & Evers, S.E. (1997). A nutritional rehabilitation program for persons with severe physical and developmental disabilities. *Journal of the American Dietetic Association, 97,* 162–166.

Jacob, A. (1998). The Recommended Dietary Allowances: A nutrition practitioner's perspective. *Nutrition Reviews, 56,* S48–S52.

Kennedy, E., Myers, L., & Layden, W. (1996). The 1995 Dietary Guidelines for Americans: An overview. *Journal of the American Dietetic Association, 96,* 234–237.

Kinyamu, H.K., Gallagher, J.C., Rafferty, K.A., & Balbourn, K.E. (1998). Dietary calcium and vitamin D intake in elderly women: Effect on serum parathyroid hormone and vitamin D metabolite. *American Journal of Clinical Nutrition, 67,* 342–348.

Kleiner, S.M. (1999). Water: An essential but overlooked nutrient. *Journal of the American Dietetic Association, 99,* 200–206.

Koehler, K.M., Pareo-Tubbeh, S.L., Romero, L.G., Baumgartner, R.N., & Garry, P.J. (1997). Folate nutrition for older adults: Challenges and opportunities. *Journal of the American Dietetic Association, 97,* 167–173.

Kris-Etherton, P.M., & Yu, S. (1997). Individual fatty acid effects on plasma lipids and lipoproteins: Human studies. *American Journal of Clinical Nutrition, 65*(5 Suppl.), S1628–S1644.

Levin, R.J. (1999). Carbohydrate. In M.E. Shils, J.E. Olson, M. Shike, & C.A. Ross (Eds.), *Modern nutrition in health and disease* (9th ed., pp. 49–65). Baltimore: Williams & Wilkins.

Lipschitz, D.A. (1992). Nutritional needs of the elderly: An approach to rational management. *Long Term Care Forum, 2,* 9–15.

Lukert, B.P., & Raisz, L.G. (1990). Glucocorticoid-induced osteoporosis: Pathogenesis and management. *Annals of Internal Medicine, 112,* 352–364.

Matthews, D.E. (1999). Proteins and amino acids. In M.E. Shils, J.E. Olson, M. Shike, & C.A. Ross (Eds.), *Modern nutrition in health and disease* (9th ed., pp. 11–48). Baltimore: Williams & Wilkins.

McBean, L.D., Forgac, T., & Finn, S.C. (1994). Osteoporosis: Visions for care and prevention—A conference report. *Journal of the American Dietetic Association, 94,* 668–671.

Mercer, K.C., & Ekvall, S.W. (1992). Comparing the diets of adults with mental retardation who live in intermediate care facilities and group homes. *Journal of the American Dietetic Association, 92,* 356–358.

Messina, M. (1999, June). *Soybean and health.* Paper presented at the Soy Connection Dietitian Seminar, Cleveland, OH.

Meydani, S.N., Meydani, M., Blumberg, J.B., Leka, L.S., Pedrosa, M., Diamond, R., & Schafer, E.J. (1998). Assessment of the safety of supplementation with different amounts of vitamin E in healthy older adults. *American Journal of Clinical Nutrition, 68,* 311–318.

Miller, J.W. (1999). Homocysteine and Alzheimer's disease. *Nutrition Reviews, 57,* 126–129.

Mora, S., Barera, G., Ricotti, A., Weber, G., Bianchi, C., & Chiumello, G. (1998). Reversal of low bone density with a gluten-free diet in children and adolescents with celiac disease. *American Journal of Clinical Nutrition, 67,* 477–481.

Nandi, B.K. (1998). Harmonization of Recommended Dietary Allowances: Implications and approach. *Nutrition Reviews, 56,* S53–S56.

National Academy of Sciences (NAS)/National Research Council (NRC). (1989). *Recommended dietary allowances.* Washington, DC: National Academy Press.

National Institutes of Health (NIH). (1994, June 6–8). NIH consensus statement on optimal calcium intake. *NIH Consensus Statement, 12*(4), 1–31.

National Institutes of Health (NIH). (1997). *Eating hints for cancer patients* (NIH Publication No. 97-2079). Washington, DC: Author.

Neidert, K.C. (Ed.). (1998). *Nutrition care of the older adult: A handbook for dietetics professionals working throughout the continuum of care.* Chicago: American Dietetic Association, Consultant Dietitians in Health Care Facilities Practice Group.

Nieves, J.W., Komar, L., Cosman, F., & Lindsay, R. (1998). Calcium potentiates the effect of estrogen and calcitonin on bone mass: Review and analysis. *American Journal of Clinical Nutrition, 67,* 18–24.

Nutrition labeling of food. (1996). 21 C.F.R. pt. 101.9.

O'Hara, P.A., Harper, D.W., Kangas, M., Dubeau, J., Borsutzky, C., & Lemire, C. (1997). Taste, temperature, and presentation predict satisfaction with food services in a Canadian continuing-care hospital. *Journal of the American Dietetic Association, 97,* 401–405.

Olson, R.E. (1999). Vitamin K. In M.E. Shils, J.E. Olson, M. Shike, & C.A. Ross (Eds.), *Modern nutrition in health and disease* (9th ed., pp. 363–380). Baltimore: Williams & Wilkins.

Owen, A.L., Splett, P.L., & Owen, G.M. (1999). *Nutrition in the community: The art and science of delivering services* (4th ed.). New York: WCB/McGraw-Hill.

Patterson, B., & Ekvall, S.W. (1993). Down syndrome. In S.W. Ekvall (Ed.), *Pediatric nutrition in chronic diseases and developmental disorders: Prevention, assessment, and treatment* (pp. 149–156). New York: Oxford University Press.

Pennington, J.A.T. (1998). *Bowes and Church's food values of portions commonly used* (17th ed.). Philadelphia: Lippincott-Raven.

Posthauer, M.E., Palmer, K., Kadlec, S., Cloud, H.H., & Devlin, C. (Eds.). (1993). *Clinical criteria and indicators for nutrition services in developmental disabilities, psychiatric disorders, and substance abuse.* Chicago: American Dietetic Association.

Promoting elderly appetite. (1993). *Worldview, 5,* 5.

Promoting physical activity and health. (1996, Fall). *Food and Nutrition News, 68,* 1.

Public Policy News. (1998). Translating the science behind the dietary reference intakes. *Journal of the American Dietetic Association, 98,* 756.

Ritenbaugh, C. (1981). An anthropological perspective on nutrition. In Proceedings of the Workshop on Nutrition Education Research: Applying Principles from the Behavioral Sciences. *Journal of Nutrition Education, 13*(Suppl. 1), S12–S13.

Rock, C.L., Jacob, R.A., & Bowen, E. (1996). Update on the biological characteristics of the antioxidant micronutrients: Vitamin C, vitamin E, and the carotenoids. *Journal of the American Dietetic Association, 96,* 693–702.

Russell, R.M. (1997). New views on the RDAs for older adults. *Journal of the American Dietetic Association, 97,* 515–518.

Ryan, C., Eleazer, P., & Egbert, J. (1995). Vitamin D in the elderly: An overlooked nutrient. *Nutrition Today, 30,* 228–233.

Schlenker, E.D. (1998). *Nutrition in aging* (3rd ed.). Boston: McGraw-Hill/WCB.

Seddon, J.M., & Henekens, C.H. (1994). Vitamins, minerals, and macular degeneration. *Archives of Ophthalmology, 112,* 176–178.

Seddon, J.M., Ajami, U.A., Sperdotto, R.D., Hiller, R., Blair, N., Burton, T., Farber, M.D., Graqoudos, E.S., Haller, J., Miller, D.T., Yanuzzi, L.A., & Willett, W. (1994). Dietary carotenoids, vitamins A, C, and E, and advanced age-related macular degeneration. *JAMA: Journal of the American Medical Association, 272,* 1413–1420.

Suter, P.M. (1999). Vitamin status and requirements. In R. Chernoff (Ed.), *Geriatric nutrition: The health professional's handbook* (2nd ed., pp. 27–62). Gaithersburg, MD: Aspen Publishers.

Traber, M.G. (1999). Vitamin E. In M.E. Shils, J.E. Olson, M. Shike, & C.A. Ross (Eds.), *Modern nutrition in health and disease* (9th ed., pp. 347–362). Baltimore: Williams & Wilkins.

Tufts University Health and Nutrition Letter (TUHNL). (1999). *New food guide pyramid specifically for people 70 and older.* Medford, MA: Tufts University.

U.S. Department of Agriculture (USDA). (1993). Food facts for older adults: Information on how to use the Dietary Guidelines (Home and Garden Bulletin No. 252). Hyattsville, MD: Human Nutrition Information Service.

U.S. Department of Agriculture (USDA). (1995). *Dietary Guidelines Advisory Committee: Report of the Dietary Guidelines Advisory Committee on the dietary guidelines for Americans to the Secretary of Health and Human Services and the Secretary of Agriculture.* Washington, DC: Dietary Guidelines Advisory Committee.

U.S. Department of Agriculture (USDA). (1996). The food guide pyramid (Home and Garden Bulletin No. 252). Washington, DC: Author.

U.S. Department of Agriculture (USDA). (2000). News release. Available http://www.usda.gov/news/releases/2000/02/003/.

U.S. Department of Health and Human Services (DHHS). (1993). *Cholesterol education program: Second report of the Expert Panel on Detection, Evaluation, and Treatment of High Blood Cholesterol in Adults—Executive summary* (NIH Publication No. 90-3096). Washington, DC: National Cholesterol Education Program Expert Panel.

U.S. Department of Health and Human Services (DHHS). (1996). *Healthy People 2000: National health promotion and disease prevention objectives—Midcourse review and 1995 revisions.* Washington, DC: Author.

U.S. Food and Drug Administration (FDA). (1995, May). *The new food label* (Publication No. BG95-12). Available http://vm. cfsan.fda.gov/~Ird/cons0693.txt.

U.S. Food and Drug Administration (FDA). (1996, February 29). *Folic acid fortification. Office of Public Affairs Fact Sheet.* Available: http://vm.cfsan.fda.gov/dms/wh-folic.html.

U.S. Food and Drug Administration (FDA). (1997). *Food safety musts: The unwelcome dinner guest—Preventing food borne illness.* Available http://vm.cfsan.fda.gov/~dms/fdunwelc.html.

Walter, A., Cohen, N.C., & Swicker, R.C. (1997). Food safety training needs exist for staff and consumers in a variety of community-based homes for people with developmental disabilities. *Journal of the American Dietetic Association, 97*, 619–625.

Wells, M.B., Turner, S., Martin, D.M., & Roy, A. (1997). Health gain through screening—coronary heart disease and stroke: Developing primary health services for people with intellectual disability. *Journal of Intellectual and Developmental Disability, 22*, 251–263.

West, S., Vitale, S., Hallfrisch, J., Munoz, B., Muller, D., Bressler, S., & Bressler, N.M. (1994). Are antioxidants in supplements protective for age-related macular degeneration? [Abstract]. *Archives of Ophthalmology, 112*, 222–227.

Whitney, E.N., Cataldo, C.B., & Rolfes, S.R. (1998). *Understanding normal and clinical nutrition* (5th ed.). Belmont, CA: Wadsworth.

Yarbrough, P. (1981). Communication theory and nutrition research. In Proceedings of the Workshop on Nutrition Education Research: Applying Principles from the Behavioral Sciences. *Journal of Nutrition Education, 13*(Suppl. 1), S16–S27.

Yates, A., Schlicker, S.A., & Suitor, C.W. (1998). Dietary Reference Intakes: The basis for recommendations for calcium and related nutrients, B vitamins, and choline. *Journal of the American Dietetic Association, 98*, 669–706.

Appendix

Tables and Figures

Table 1. Recommended dietary allowances for adults ages 51 years and older[a]

Dietary component	Men[b]	Women
Energy (kcal)	2,300.0	1,900.0
Protein (g)	63.0	50.0
Vitamin A (μg RE)[c]	1,000.0	800.0
Vitamin D (μg)[d]	5.0	5.0
Vitamin E (mg α TE)[e]	10.0	8.0
Vitamin K (μg)	80.0	65.0
Vitamin C (mg)	60.0	60.0
Thiamin (mg)	1.2	1.0
Riboflavin (mg)	1.4	1.2
Niacin (mg NE)[f]	15.0	13.0
Vitamin B_6 (mg)	2.0	2.0
Folate (μg)	200.0	150.0
Vitamin B_{12} (μg)	2.0	2.0
Calcium (mg)	800.0	800.0
Phosphorus (mg)	800.0	800.0
Magnesium (mg)	350.0	280.0
Iron (mg)	10.0	10.0
Zinc (mg)	15.0	12.0
Iodine (μg)	150.0	150.0
Selenium (μg)	70.0	55.0

Reprinted with permission from Recommended Dietary Allowances, 10th edition. Copyright © 1989 by the National Academy of Sciences. Courtesy of the National Academy Press, Washington, DC.

[a]The allowances, expressed as average daily intakes over time, are intended to provide for individual variations among most people as they live in the United States under our usual environmental stresses. Diets should be based on a variety of common foods to provide other nutrients for which human requirements have been less well defined. Weights and heights for reference adults are central medians for the U.S. population of the designated age as reported by NHANES II. The use of these figures does not imply that the height-to-weight ratios are ideal.

[b]Median weight and height for men = 77 kg (170 lb); 173 cm (68 in). Median weight and height for women = 65 kg (143 lb); 160 cm (63 in).

[c]RE = retinol equivalents; 1 RE = 1 μg retinol or 6 μg beta-carotene.

[d]As cholecalciferol; 10 μg cholecalciferol = 400 IU of vitamin D.

[e]α TE = α-tocopherol equivalents, 1 mg d-α = 1 TE.

[f]NE = niacin equivalent; 1 NE = 1 mg of niacin or 60 mg of dietary tryptophan.

317

Table 2. Food and Nutrition Board, Institute of Medicine/National Academy of Sciences dietary reference intakes: Recommended levels for individual intake[a]

Life stage group	Calcium (mg/d)	Phosphorus (mg/d)	Magnesium (mg/d)	Vitamin D[b,c] (μg/d)	Fluoride (mg/d)	Thiamin (mg/d)	Riboflavin (mg/d)	Niacin[d] (mg/d)	Vitamin B6 (mg/d)	Folate[e] (μg/d)	Vitamin B12 (μg/d)	Pantothenic acid (mg/d)	Biotin (mg/d)	Choline[f] (mg/d)
Infants														
0–6 mo	210*	100*	30*	5*	0.01*	0.2*	0.3*	2*	0.1*	65*	0.4*	1.7*	5*	125*
7–12 mo	270*	275*	75*	5*	0.5*	0.3*	0.4*	4*	0.3*	80*	0.5*	1.8*	6*	150*
Children														
1–3 yr	500*	460	80	5*	0.7*	0.5	0.5	6	0.5	150	0.9	2*	8*	200*
4–8 yr	800*	500	130	5*	1*	0.6	0.6	8	0.6	200	1.2	3*	12*	250*
Males														
9–13 yr	1,300*	1,250*	240	5*	2*	0.9	0.9	12	1.0	300	1.8	4*	20*	375*
14–18 yr	1,300*	1,250*	410	5*	3*	1.2	1.3	16	1.3	400	2.4	5*	25*	550*
19–30 yr	1,000*	700	400	5*	4*	1.2	1.3	16	1.3	400	2.4	5*	30*	550*
31–50 yr	1,000*	700	420	5*	4*	1.2	1.3	16	1.3	400	2.4[h]	5*	30*	550*
51–70 yr	1,200*	700	420	10*	4*	1.2	1.3	16	1.7	400	2.4[h]	5*	30*	550*
>70 yr	1,200*	700	420	15*	4*	1.2	1.3	16	1.7	400	2.4[h]	5*	30*	550*
Females														
9–13 yr	1,300*	1,250*	240	5*	2*	0.9	0.9	12	1.0	300	1.8	4*	20*	375*
14–18 yr	1,300*	1,250*	360	5*	3*	1.0	1.0	14	1.2	400[h]	2.4	5*	25*	400*
19–30 yr	1,000*	700	310	5*	3*	1.1	1.1	14	1.3	400[h]	2.4	5*	30*	425*
31–50 yr	1,000*	700	320	5*	3*	1.1	1.1	14	1.3	400[h]	2.4	5*	30*	425*
51–70 yr	1,200*	700	320	10*	3*	1.1	1.1	14	1.5	400	2.4[g]	5*	30*	425*
>70 yr	1,200*	700	320	15*	3*	1.1	1.1	14	1.5	400	2.4[g]	5*	30*	425*

Pregnancy													
≤18 yr	1,300*	400	5*	3*	1.4	1.4	18	1.9	600[i]	2.6	6*	30*	450*
19–30 yr	1,000*	350	5*	3*	1.4	1.4	18	1.9	600[i]	2.6	6*	30*	450*
31–50 yr	1,000*	360	5*	3*	1.4	1.4	18	1.9	600[i]	2.6	7*	30*	450*
Lactation													
≤18 yr	1,300*	360	5*	3*	1.5	1.6	17	2.0	500	2.8	7*	35*	550*
19–30 yr	1,000*	310	5*	3*	1.5	1.6	17	2.0	500	2.8	7*	35*	550*
31–50 yr	1,000*	320	5*	3*	1.5	1.6	17	2.0	500	2.8	7*	35*	550*

Reprinted with permission from Dietary Reference Intakes. Copyright © 1998 by the National Academy of Sciences. Courtesy of the National Academy Press, Washington, DC.

[a]Recommended Dietary Allowances (RDAs) are in bold type and Adequate Intakes (AI) are in ordinary type followed by an asterisk (*). RDAs and AIs both may be used as goals for individual intake. RDAs are set to meet the needs of almost all (97%–98%) individuals in a group. For healthy breastfed infants, the AI is the mean intake. The AI for other life-stage and gender groups is believed to cover needs of all individuals in the group, but lack of data or uncertainty in the data prevents the ability to specify with confidence the percentage of individuals covered by this intake.

[b]As cholecalciferol: 1 μg cholecalciferol = 40 IU vitamin D.

[c]In the absence of adequate exposure to sunlight.

[d]As niacin equivalent (NE): 1 mg of niacin = 60 mg of tryptophan; 0–6 months = preformed niacin (not NE).

[e]As dietary folate equivalents (DFE): 1 DFE = 1 μg food folate = 0.6 μg of folic acid (from fortified food or supplement) consumed with food = 0.5 μg of synthetic (supplemental) folic acid taken on an empty stomach.

[f]Although AIs have been set for choline, there are few data to assess whether a dietary supply of choline is needed at all stages of the life cycle, and it may be that the choline requirement can be met by endogenous synthesis at some of these stages.

[g]In view of evidence linking folate intake with neural tube defects in the fetus, it is recommended that all women capable of becoming pregnant consume 400 μg of synthetic folic acid from fortified foods and/or supplements in addition to intake of food folate from a varied diet.

[h]Because 10%–30% of older people may malabsorb food-bound B_{12}, it is advisable for those older than age 50 years to meet their RDA mainly by consuming foods fortified with B_{12} or a supplement containing B_{12}.

[i]It is assumed that women will continue consuming 400 μg of folic acid until their pregnancy is confirmed and they enter prenatal care, which ordinarily occurs after the end of the periconceptional period—the critical time for formation of the neural tube.

Reference Values of the Dietary Reference Intakes (DRIs) (Table 2)

The DRIs include four reference values for the nutrient intakes by Canadians and Americans. These values are defined as follows.

Recommended Dietary Allowance (RDA) is the average daily dietary intake that is designed to meet the nutrient requirements of nearly all individuals (97%–98%) in the life stage and gender group. This value is intended as a goal for dietary intake by individuals (Yates, Schlicker, & Suitor, 1998). The RDAs have been set for phosphorus, magnesium, thiamin, riboflavin, niacin, vitamin B_6, folate, and vitamin B_{12} for individuals (except infants) in different life stage and gender groups (see Table 2).

Adequate intake (AI) is the daily dietary intake recommended when scientific information is not available to set the RDA, and it can be used to set goals for individuals' nutrient intake. AI is based on observed or experimentally determined approximations of the average nutrient intake by a defined population or subgroup that appear to sustain a defined nutritional state (Food and Nutrition Board, National Academy of Sciences, Institute of Medicine, 1998). AIs have been set for calcium, vitamin D, fluoride, pantothenic acid, biotin, and choline (Table 2).

Estimated average requirement (EAR) is the dietary intake level, averaged over time (1 week for most nutrients), estimated to meet the requirement of 50% of the individuals in a life stage and gender group. EAR is used as the basis for setting the RDA and may be used for assessing the adequacy of groups' intakes and for planning adequate intakes by groups (Food and Nutrition Board, National Academy of Sciences, Institute of Medicine, 1998).

Tolerable upper intake level (UL) is the highest intake level that is unlikely to have harmful health effects for almost all individuals in the group. This maximum level, with high probability, can be tolerated biologically. UL applies to chronic daily nutrient intake. It is not intended as a recommended intake, as intakes above the RDA and AI by healthy individuals have no established benefits (Food and Nutrition Board, National Academy of Sciences, Institute of Medicine, 1998).

Table 3. Mandatory components on "nutrition facts" of the food label and daily values

Components	Unit of measure listed on label	Daily reference value (DRV)[a]
Total calories	Calories	
Calories from fat		
Total fat	Grams (g)	Less than 65 g
Saturated fat	Grams (g)	Less than 20 g
Cholesterol	Milligrams (mg)	Less than 300 mg
Sodium	Milligrams (mg)	Less than 2,400 mg
Total carbohydrate	Grams (g)	300 g
Dietary fiber	Grams (g)	25 g
Protein	Grams (g)	50 g is Reference Daily Intake (RDI) (not shown on label)
Vitamin A	% of RDI	5,000 IU is RDI (not shown)
Vitamin C	% of RDI	60 mg is RDI (not shown)
Calcium	% of RDI	1,000 mg is RDI (not shown)
Iron	% of RDI	18 mg is RDI (not shown)

Source: FDA (1995).

[a]The DRVs for total fat, saturated fat, carbohydrate, dietary fiber, and protein are based on a 2,000-kilocalorie diet.

Table 4. Macronutrients, recommended intake, selected functions, and major food group sources

Nutrients	Recommended intake	Selected functions	Major food group sources
Protein	RDA: 0.8 g/kg of body weight (NRC, 1989) 1.0–1.25 g/kg body weight or average of 1.0 g/kg (Campbell, 1996; Carter, 1999; Lipschitz, 1992) 14%–15% of total calorie intake (Carter, 1999); this assumes adequate calorie intake No Dietary Reference Intake (DRI)	Builds, maintains, and repairs tissues (e.g., growth, wound healing) Synthesis of hormones, which control body processes; enzymes, which aid chemical reactions; antibodies to fight infection Blood clotting factors Part of organic matrix in the bone Regulates fluid balance Alternative source of energy: 4 kcal/g	Meat, fish, poultry, eggs, dried beans, and nuts Milk, yogurt, and cheese Animal foods supply high-quality protein.
Carbohydrates	No RDA or DRI General guideline: 55%–60% of total day's calories (Carter, 1999; Levin, 1999) Greater proportion should be complex (starches and fiber). Sugars should be used in moderation (USDA, 1995).	Major fuel source: 4 kcal/g Spares protein Glucose serves as the fuel for the brain and nervous system.	Bread, cereal, rice, and pasta Vegetables: Starchy kinds Above are good sources of complex carbohydrates. Fruit: Fructose, naturally occurring simple sugar Milk: Lactose, same as above Top of the pyramid: Sweets
Carbohydrate dietary fiber	No RDA or DRI General guidelines: 25 g to 35 g/day, (Carter, 1999) 25 g for 2,000-kcal and 30 g for 3,000-kcal diet (USDA, 1995)	Maintains bowel regularity Reduces risk for colorectal cancer and diverticulosis Soluble fraction (pectin in fruits, beta-glucan in oat bran and kidney beans), along with a healthy diet, may lower high blood cholesterol. Not digested by humans, dietary fiber yields an insignificant number of calories.	Bread, cereal, rice, and pasta Vegetables Fruit: whole and with skin Meat group: legumes (dried beans)

(continued)

Table 4. *(continued)*

Nutrients	Recommended intake	Selected functions	Major food group sources
Lipids	No RDA or DRI Guidelines: Limit total fat to less than 30% of total calories and saturated fatty acids to 8%–10%; monounsaturated fatty acids, up to 15%; and polyunsaturated fatty acids up to 15% of total calories. Limit cholesterol to less than 300 mg per day (DHHS, 1993).	Most concentrated source of energy: 9 kcal/g Carrier of fat-soluble vitamins; improves flavor and texture of foods, e.g., baked products Cholesterol is used to make bile acids, which aid in fat digestion; steroidal sex hormones (androgen, estrogen, and progesterone); adrenocortical hormones; and vitamin D (Groff & Gropper, 2000).	Top of the pyramid: Fats and oils Visible fats (e.g., butter, margarine, salad dressing, oils) Invisible fats: Hidden fats Meat: High-fat meats Milk: High-fat milk and milk products Grain: Certain items (e.g., croissants, muffins, biscuits)

Source: Whitney Cataldo, and Rolfes (1998) unless other references are noted.

Table 5. Dietary fiber content of selected foods

Food groups and foods	Fiber (g)	Calories
Bread, cereal, rice, and pasta		
Cereal		
Oatmeal, instant, 1 packet	5.5	158
Oatmeal, cooked, ½ cup	2.0	73
Ready-to-eat cereal		
All Bran, ½ cup	10.0	81
Bran, 100%, ½ cup	8.3	75
Frosted Miniwheats, 1 cup	6.3	201
Breads		
Branola, 1 slice	3.0	90
Whole wheat, 1 slice	1.9	69
Rye, 1 slice	1.9	83
Wheat, stoneground	2.0	60
Bran, country, 1 slice	5.0	80
Fruit		
Apple, raw, with skin, 1 medium	3.7	81
(Same apple, without skin)	2.4	73
Apricots, raw, 3 medium	2.5	51
Banana, raw, 1 medium	2.7	105
Orange, navel, raw, 1 fruit	3.1	60
Papaya, raw, 1 medium	5.5	119
Peach, raw, 1 medium	1.7	37
Strawberries, raw, 1 cup	3.4	45
Meat alternatives		
Baked beans, homemade, 1 cup	13.9	382
Beans, canned, ½ cup	≅6.0	152
Chickpeas, boiled, ½ cup	6.0	135
(Legumes are generally high in dietary fiber.)		

(continued)

Table 5. *(continued)*

Food groups and foods	Fiber (g)	Calories
Vegetables		
Broccoli, boiled, ½ cup	2.3	22
Brussels sprouts, boiled, ½ cup	2.0	30
Carrots, boiled, ½ cup	2.6	35
Corn, boiled, ½ cup	2.3	89
Green peas, boiled, ½ cup	4.4	62
Potato, baked, with skin, 1	4.8	220
Potato, baked, without skin, 1	2.3	145
Acorn squash, baked, ½ cup cubes	4.5	57

Source: Pennington (1998).

Table 6. Micronutrients, recommended intake, selected functions, and major food group sources

Nutrients	Recommended intake	Selected functions	Major food group sources
Fat-soluble vitamins			
Vitamin A	RDA: 1,000 retinol equivalent (RE) for men 800 RE for women (National Academy of Sciences/National Research Council, 1989) No Dietary Reference Intake (DRI)	Essential for vision, cellular differentiation, growth, reproduction, bone development, and the immune system Beta-carotene has antioxidant properties (Groff & Gropper, 2000).	Vegetable and fruit groups Rich yellow, deep orange, and dark green are rich in beta-carotene, which is converted to vitamin A in the intestinal tract. Vegetables: Broccoli, butternut squash, carrots, spinach, turnip greens Fruits: Apricots, cantaloupes, mangos, peaches Meat and dairy groups supply preformed vitamin A. Meat items: Egg yolk, liver Milk: Whole milk, vitamin A–fortified low-fat milk

(continued)

Table 6.   *(continued)*

Nutrients	Recommended intake	Selected functions	Major food group sources
Vitamin D	RDA: 5 μg (200 IU) (NRC, 1989) Adequate Intake (AI) 10 μg (400 IU) for 51- to 70-year-old, and 15 μg (600 IU) for >70-year-old men and women, in the absence of sunlight Expressed as cholecalciferol 1 μg of cholecalciferol = 40 IU of vitamin D (Food and Nutrition Board, 1998)	Aids in bone mineralization and maintenance Regulates calcium absorption and utilization Acts as a hormone	Meat: Fatty fish, egg yolk Milk: Vitamin D–fortified milk and milk products Top of the pyramid: Fats Butter, vitamin D–fortified margarine
Vitamin E	RDA: 10 mg α-tocopherol equivalent (TE) for men, 8 mg α-TE for women 1 mg α tocopherol = 1 α TE (NRC, 1989) No DRI	Acts as an antioxidant in various biochemical reactions Protects cell membrane from damaging effects of oxidation	Plant oils and their products: Wheat germ, safflower, sunflower, cottonseed, vegetable shortening, margarine Alpha tocopherol Predominate in olive, canola, safflower, and sunflower oils (Rock, Jacob, & Bowens, 1996)
Vitamin K	RDA: 80 μg for men, 65 μg for women (NRC, 1989) No DRI	Helps in the synthesis of blood clotting factors and of bone protein (Groff & Gropper, 2000)	Vegetable: Dark green leafy vegetables, cabbage family Milk: Milk Nonfood sources: Synthesized by bacterial flora in the gut
Water-soluble vitamins			
Vitamin C (or ascorbic acid)	RDA: 60 mg for men and women (NRC, 1989) No DRI	Helps in synthesis of protein (organic matrix for bone formation and tissue repair, e.g., wound healing)	Fruit and vegetable groups (fresh has higher content)

(continued)

Table 6. *(continued)*

Nutrients	Recommended intake	Selected functions	Major food group sources
		Antioxidant activities protect cell membrane from oxidative damage Aids in production of certain hormones Assists in synthesis of neurotransmitters, which affect brain chemistry (Groff & Gropper, 2000)	Vegetables: Broccoli, green pepper, tomatoes Fruits: Citrus, strawberries, kiwi
Folate (or folacin or folic acid)	RDA: 200 μg for men, 180 μg for women (NRC, 1989) DRI RDA: 400 μg for 51- to 70- and >70-year-old men and women Expressed as Dietary Folate Equivalent (DFE) 1 DFE = 1 μg food folate = 0.6 μg of folic acid (Food and Nutrition Board, 1998)	Works closely with Vitamin B_{12} in DNA synthesis and, therefore, new cell formation, including red blood cell production. Helps prevent neural tube defects (spina bifida)	Vegetables: Dark green leafy vegetables Fruit: Orange juice Meat and meat alternatives: Liver, legumes, seeds Other sources: Fortified foods Grains: Cereals
Vitamin B_{12} (or cobalamin)	RDA: 2.0 μg for men and women (NRC, 1989) DRI: AI: 2.4 μg for men and women, 51 to 70 and >70 years old (Food and Nutrition Board, 1998)	Works closely with folate in DNA synthesis and new cell formation as described previously Maintains the sheath of the nerves	Meat: Found naturally only in animal products Other sources: Vitamin B_{12}–fortified products
Minerals Calcium	RDA: 800 mg for men and women (NRC, 1989) DRI: AI: 1,200 mg for 51 to 70 and >70 years old (Food and Nutrition Board, 1998) Men, 25–65 years old: 1,000 mg Men 65 years old: 1,500 mg Postmenopausal women <50 years old, on estrogen: 1,000 mg Same women not on estrogen, and women <65 years old: 1,500 mg (NIH, 1994)	Essential for bone formation and maintenance— mineralization or hardening of bones Aids in blood clotting Assists in muscle contraction	Milk: Milk, cheese, yogurt Vegetables: Dark greens, e.g., beets, turnips, kale, collards, spinach Meat alternatives: Dried beans Other sources: Calcium-fortified orange juice and soy milk

Source: Whitney Cataldo, and Rolfes (1998) unless other references are noted.

Table 7. Calcium content of selected foods

Foods	Calcium (mg)	Calories
Milk and milk products		
Milk, whole, plain, 1 cup	274	139
Milk, 1% fat, 1 cup	300	102
Milk, 2% fat, 1 cup	297	121
Milk, nonfat, 1 cup	302	86
Cheese, American and Swiss, processed, 1 oz	172	101
Cheese, cheddar, 1 oz	204	114
Cottage cheese, 1% fat, 1 cup	138	164
Cottage cheese, 2% fat, 1 cup	155	203
Feta, 1 oz	140	75
Mozzarella, part skim, 1 oz	183	72
Yogurt, many varieties, 1 cup	300 (Average)	90–250
Meat alternatives		
Beans, vegetarian, canned, 1 cup	127	236
Beans, old-fashioned, canned, ½ cup	100	180
(Dried beans generally are high in calcium.)		
Vegetables		
Beet greens, boiled, ½ cup	82	19
Chinese cabbage, boiled, ½ cup	79	10
Collards, frozen, boiled, ½ cup	179	31
Kale, frozen, boiled, ½ cup	90	20
Mustard greens, boiled, ½ cup	76	14
Okra, boiled, ½ cup, slices	77	30
Spinach, frozen, boiled, ½ cup	122	21
Turnip greens, boiled, chopped, ½ cup	125	25

Source: Pennington (1998); product name brands are omitted.

Table 8. Sample 1-day meal plans at three kilocalorie levels

Food groups	Number of servings		
	1,600 kcal	2,200 kcal	2,800 kcal
Grain	6	9	11
Vegetable	3	4	5
Fruit	2	3	4
Milk	2–3[a]	2–3[a]	2–3[a]
Meat and meat alternatives[b] (ounces)	5	6	7
Water (at least six to eight glasses)			
Total fat (grams)	53	73	93
Total added sugars (teaspoons)	6	12	18

Adapted from USDA (1996).
[a]Women who are pregnant or breastfeeding, teenagers, and young adults to age 24 need three servings.
[b]Meat group amounts are in total ounces, not servings. See Table 9 for definitions of serving sizes.

Table 9. Examples of single serving sizes of foods in the food groups

Food group and food	Size of a single serving
Bread, cereal, rice, and pasta	
Bread	1 slice
Ready-to-eat cereal	1 ounce
Cooked cereal, rice, or pasta	$\frac{1}{2}$ cup
Vegetable	
Raw leafy vegetables	1 cup
Other vegetables, cooked or chopped, raw	$\frac{1}{2}$ cup
Vegetable juice	$\frac{3}{4}$ cup
Fruit	
Apple, banana, or orange	1 medium
Chopped, cooked, or canned fruit	$\frac{1}{2}$ cup
Fruit juice	$\frac{3}{4}$ cup
Milk, yogurt, and cheese	
Milk or yogurt	1 cup
Natural cheese	$1\frac{1}{2}$ ounces
Process cheese	2 ounces
Soy-based beverage with added calcium	1 cup
Meat, poultry, fish, dry beans, eggs, and nuts	
Cooked lean meat, poultry, or fish	2–3 ounces
($\frac{1}{2}$ cup of cooked dry beans, or 1 egg, or 2 tablespoons of peanut butter, or $\frac{1}{2}$ cup of tofu, or $2\frac{1}{2}$ ounces of soy burger, or $\frac{1}{3}$ cup of nuts count as 1 ounce of lean meat)	

Table 10. Sample 1,600-calorie meal plan for older women[a,b,c]

Food group	Number of servings	Examples of foods and serving sizes
Bread	6–9	2 slices whole-wheat toast, 2 small corn muffins, 1 small whole-grain roll, 3 squares of graham crackers. (Three servings can be added to the above.)
Vegetable	3–4	$\frac{3}{4}$ cup vegetable juice (no salt added), $1\frac{1}{2}$ cup mixed greens, $\frac{1}{2}$ cup stewed tomatoes (no salt added), $\frac{1}{2}$ cup yellow corn (fresh or frozen) (Choose orange, yellow, or dark green vegetables and those with roughage.) (One serving can be added.)
Fruit	2–3	$\frac{1}{2}$ medium grapefruit, 1 medium fresh peach (Choose rich or deep yellow, whole fruits, and those high in vitamin C.) (One serving can be added.)
Milk	2	1 cup skim milk, $1\frac{1}{2}$ oz Swiss cheese
Meat	2	3 oz sirloin steak (lean, broiled), 1 ounce turkey, 1 ounce ham (2 ounces can be added) Use $\frac{1}{2}$ cup legumes as a meat substitute two to three times per week.

(continued)

Table 10.   *(continued)*

Food group	Number of servings	Examples of foods and serving sizes
Fats, oils, and sweets		2 teaspoons margarine (soft), 1 tablespoon French dressing (low-calorie), 1 cup lime sherbet, 1 cup lemonade (1½ tablespoons of jelly and 1 teaspoon of margarine can be added to this)
Water		At least six to eight glasses

Adapted from USDA (1993).

[a]For the 1,600-kilocalorie meal plan, use the lower number. For the 2,400-kilocalorie level, add more servings from certain food groups, as noted.

[b]According to the USDA (1993), the 1,600-kilocalorie meal plan has 46 g of fat (26% of the total kcal), 18 g of saturated fat (10% of the total kcal), 185 mg of cholesterol, 2,190 mg of sodium, and 18 g of dietary fiber. The amount of fat, saturated fat, cholesterol, and sodium meets the recommendations of the National Cholesterol Education Program (USDA, 1993). The dietary fiber is consistent with the recommendation of 11.5 g/1,000 kcal (FDA, 1995).

[c]Foods can be added to increase the energy level of the meal plan. The older person's preferences and tolerance should be taken into consideration in planning this menu. Foods have been set up this way purposely (rather than in a menu format) to show their placement in the food groups and the total number of servings from each group. If mixed dishes such as casseroles and soups are used, individual ingredients can be identified and categorized in the appropriate food group. Some food items can be classified in more than one group. For example, legumes, which belong to the meat group, are also vegetables. It should be counted as one or the other, not both (USDA, 1996).

Table 11.   Sodium content of selected foods by food group

Food group and foods	Sodium (mg)
Bread, cereal, rice, and pasta	
Cooked cereal, rice, pasta, unsalted, ½ cup	Trace
Ready-to-eat cereal, 1 ounce	100–360
Bread, 1 slice	110–175
Vegetable	
Vegetables, fresh or frozen, cooked without salt, ½ cup	Less than 70
Vegetables, canned or frozen with sauce, ½ cup	140–460
Tomato juice, canned, ¾ cup	660
Vegetable soup, canned, 1 cup	820
Fruit	
Fruit, fresh, frozen, canned, ½ cup	Trace
Milk, yogurt, and cheese	
Milk, 1 cup	120
Yogurt, 8 ounces	160
Natural cheeses, 1½ ounces	110–450
Processed cheeses, 2 ounces	800
Meat, poultry, fish, dry beans, eggs, and nuts	
Fresh meat, poultry, fish, 3 ounces	Less than 90
Tuna, canned, water pack, 3 ounces	300
Bologna, 2 ounces	580
Ham, lean, roasted, 3 ounces	1,020

(continued)

Table 11. *(continued)*

Food group and foods	Sodium (mg)
Other	
Salad dressing, 1 tablespoon	75–220
Catsup, mustard, steak sauce, 1 tablespoon	130–230
Soy sauce, 1 tablespoon	1,030
Salt, 1 teaspoon	2,000
Dill pickle, 1 medium	930
Potato chips, salted, 1 ounce	130
Corn chips, salted, 1 ounce	235
Peanuts, roasted in oil, salted, 1 ounce	120

Source: USDA (1996).

Table 12. Some dietary ways to increase food and nutrient intake

Goal	Diet method to move toward goals
Combating poor appetite	Eat small meals throughout the day; eat whenever you are hungry. Keep nutrient- and calorie-packed snacks handy.
	Add variety to the menu.
	Eat with other people. Socialization can improve appetite.
	Serve an attractive plate. Simple garnishes can add a special touch to the eye appeal of foods.
	Take advantage of your "good" days when your appetite is better. Eat and enjoy as much food as you can then.
Increasing protein intake	
Using milk and milk products	Add grated cheese to soups, sauces, casseroles, vegetable dishes, mashed potatoes, and meatloaf.
	Mix cottage cheese or ricotta cheese with casseroles, scrambled eggs, and gelatin.
	Use milk in beverages or cooking.
	Add powdered milk to regular milk and milk drinks and to casseroles, meatloaf, mashed potatoes, and sauces.
	Add chopped, hard-cooked eggs to salads and salad dressing, vegetables, and cream sauce.
	Add extra eggs or egg whites to scrambled eggs and omelets.
	Use prepared breakfast mixes in milk or milk shakes.

(continued)

Table 12.   *(continued)*

Goal	Diet method to move toward goals
Using meat and meat alternatives	Roll a banana in chopped nuts. Sprinkle nuts or wheat germ on fruit, cereal, ice cream, or yogurt. Spread peanut butter on sandwiches, toast, crackers, muffins, waffles, pancakes, and fruit slices. Blend peanut butter with milk drinks, beverages, soft ice cream, and yogurt. Cook and use dried peas, legumes, beans, and bean curd (tofu) in soups, or add them to casseroles, pasta, and grain dishes that also contain meat. Add chopped, cooked meat or fish to vegetables, salads, casseroles, soups, sauces, and biscuit dough. Use it also in omelets and sandwich filling.
Increasing calories Using fats, oils, and sweets	Add butter or margarine to cream soups and gravies, mashed and baked potatoes, rice, pasta, hot cereal, and cooked vegetables. Use table cream in soups, sauces, egg dishes, puddings, and custard. Mix table cream with pasta and mashed potatoes. Use table cream in making hot chocolate. Add honey, jam, or sugar to bread, cereal, milk drinks, and fruits. Scoop sour cream on fresh fruits and add brown sugar.
Using cereal	Sprinkle granola on vegetables, yogurt, ice cream, custard, pudding, and fruit.
Using dried fruits	Add dried fruits to cereals and baked product recipes. Cook and eat them for breakfast or as snacks. Mix them with cottage cheese, yogurt, or ice cream. Add them to baked product recipes (breads and cookies).

Source: National Institutes of Health (NIH) (1997).
This list is not comprehensive. Tips were chosen for their ease and convenience.

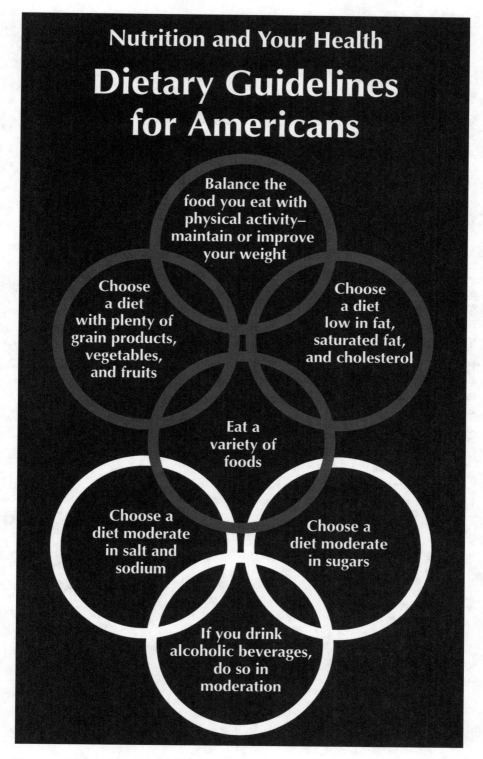

Figure 1. Dietary Guidelines for Americans. (*Source:* U.S. Department of Agriculture [1995].)

Dietary Guidelines for Americans 2000: Aim, Build, Choose for Good Health

A   Aim for fitness.
Aim for a healthy weight.
Be physically active each day.

B   Build a healthy base.
Let the pyramid guide your food choices.
Eat a variety of grains daily, especially whole grains.
Eat a variety of fruits and vegetables daily.
Keep foods safe to eat.

C   Choose sensibly.
Choose a diet that is low in saturated fat and cholesterol and moderate in total fat.
Choose beverages and foods that limit your intake of sugars.
Choose and prepare foods with less salt.
If you drink alcoholic beverages, do so in moderation.

Source: U.S. Department of Agriculture (2000). Available http://www.usda.gov/news/releases/2000/02/003/.

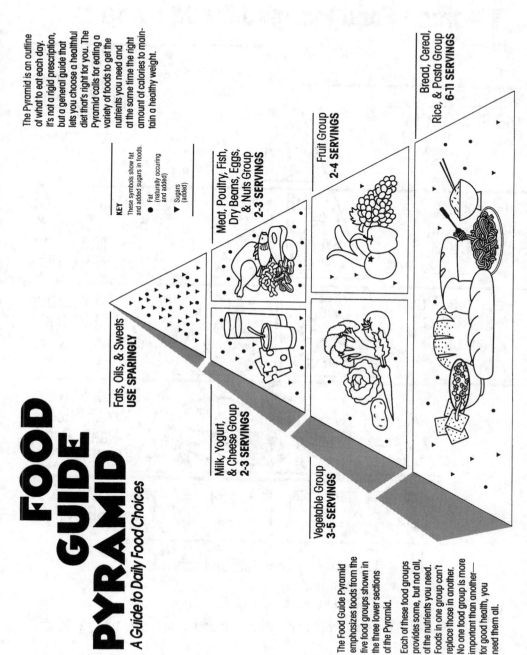

FOOD GUIDE PYRAMID
A Guide to Daily Food Choices

The Food Guide Pyramid emphasizes foods from the five food groups shown in the three lower sections of the Pyramid.

Each of these food groups provides some, but not all, of the nutrients you need. Foods in one group can't replace those in another. No one food group is more important than another— for good health, you need them all.

Fats, Oils, & Sweets
USE SPARINGLY

The Pyramid is an outline of what to eat each day. It's not a rigid prescription, but a general guide that lets you choose a healthful diet that's right for you. The Pyramid calls for eating a variety of foods to get the nutrients you need and at the same time the right amount of calories to maintain a healthy weight.

KEY
These symbols show fat and added sugars in foods.
● Fat (naturally occurring and added)
▼ Sugars (added)

Milk, Yogurt, & Cheese Group
2-3 SERVINGS

Meat, Poultry, Fish, Dry Beans, Eggs, & Nuts Group
2-3 SERVINGS

Vegetable Group
3-5 SERVINGS

Fruit Group
2-4 SERVINGS

Bread, Cereal, Rice, & Pasta Group
6-11 SERVINGS

Figure 2. Food Guide Pyramid. (*Source:* U.S. Department of Agriculture, U.S. Department of Health and Human Services [1996].)

333

Tufts University's
Modified Food Pyramid for 70+ Adults

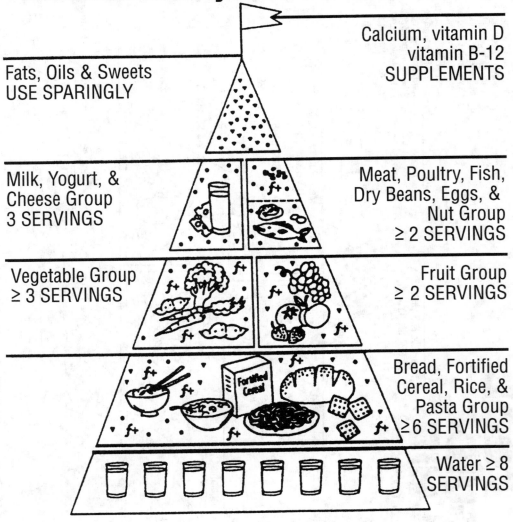

Calcium, vitamin D
vitamin B-12
SUPPLEMENTS

Fats, Oils & Sweets
USE SPARINGLY

Milk, Yogurt, &
Cheese Group
3 SERVINGS

Meat, Poultry, Fish,
Dry Beans, Eggs, &
Nut Group
≥ 2 SERVINGS

Vegetable Group
≥ 3 SERVINGS

Fruit Group
≥ 2 SERVINGS

Bread, Fortified
Cereal, Rice, &
Pasta Group
≥6 SERVINGS

Water ≥ 8
SERVINGS

- Fat (naturally occurring and added)
▼ Sugars (added)
ƒ+ Fiber (should be present)

These symbols show fat, added sugars, and fiber in foods.

Figure 3. New Food Guide Pyramid specifically for people ages 70 years and older. (Reprinted with permission from *Tufts University Health and Nutrition Letter,* Copyright © April 1999 by Tufts University Health and Nutrition Letter, New York.)

Tuft University's New Food Guide Pyramid (NFGP) for 70+ Adults (Figure 3) was devised by researchers at the Human Nutrition Research Center on Aging at Tufts University. The recommendations discussed in the text are consistent with those of the NFGP's. A summary of the NFGP's recommendations follows (Tufts University Health & Nutrition Letter, 1999).

Fluid

Drink plenty of fluid—at least eight glasses of water, juice, or milk daily—to help prevent or correct constipation. The important role of adequate fluid in older adults' health is conveyed by the placement of fluid in the foundation of the pyramid.

Fiber

Emphasize fiber to prevent or correct constipation, and consume at least 20 grams of fiber daily. This can be obtained by choosing whole fruits, high-fiber cereals, and beans for a main dish twice a week.

Enriched and/or Fortified Cereal, Rice, and Pasta

Choose enriched and/or fortified cereals. These will help increase the intake of nutrients, particularly of vitamin B_{12}, of which many older adults, because of atrophic gastritis, may absorb less from food. Older adults with atrophic gastritis can absorb the vitamin B_{12} added to cereal better than they can the food-bound version.

Vegetables

Choose deeply colored vegetables (dark green, orange, and yellow vegetables). These are rich in vitamin C, beta-carotene, and folate. Folate may reduce the risk for heart disease by lowering blood homocysteine level. In addition, eat more cruciferous vegetables, such as kale, cabbage, broccoli, and cauliflower. These vegetables contain phytochemicals that may help prevent cancer.

Milk, Cheese, and Yogurt

"Think milk," and strive to consume at least three servings of calcium-rich foods (milk, yogurt, cheese, and calcium-fortified orange juice).

Meat, Poultry, Fish, Dry Beans, Eggs, and Nuts

Eat a variety of meats (lean cuts), including fish, a good source of omega-3 fatty acids. These fatty acids may help lower the risk for heart disease.

Supplements

The flag at the top of the pyramid indicates that older adults may need supplementation when they cannot obtain enough of the nutrients from foods. The nutrients that may need to be supplemented are vitamins B_{12} and D and calcium.

Nutrition Facts

Serving Size ½ cup (114g)
Servings Per Container 4

Amount Per Serving

Calories 90   Calories from Fat 30

	% Daily Value*
Total Fat 3g	**5%**
Saturated Fat 0g	**0%**
Cholesterol 0mg	**0%**
Sodium 300mg	**13%**
Total Carbohydrate 13g	**4%**
Dietary Fiber 3g	**12%**
Sugars 3g	
Protein 3g	

Vitamin A	80%	•	Vitamin C	60%
Calcium	4%	•	Iron	4%

* Percent Daily Values are based on a 2,000 calorie diet. Your daily values may be higher or lower depending on your calorie needs:

	Calories	2,000	2,500
Total Fat	Less than	65g	80g
Sat Fat	Less than	20g	25g
Cholesterol	Less than	300mg	300mg
Sodium	Less than	2,400mg	2,400mg
Total Carbohydrate		300g	375g
Fiber		25g	30g

Calories per gram:
Fat 9   •   Carbohydrate 4   •   Protein 4

Figure 4.   Sample food label. More nutrients may be listed on some labels.

CONSUMERS' GUIDE FOR USING THE NUTRITION FACTS

The information on the new food label (Figure 4) is required by federal regulations ("Nutrition Labeling of Food," 1996). On the nutrition panel, "Nutrition Facts" replaced "Nutrition Information per Serving." The NLEA regulations cover not only the components on the label but also the type size, style, spacing, and contrast used (FDA, 1995).

Daily Values

Two sets of dietary standards comprise the Daily Values; these are the Daily Reference Values (DRVs) and Reference Dietary Intakes (RDIs).

Daily Reference Values DRVs, based on a 2,000-kilocalorie daily intake, have been set for energy-producing nutrients: fat, carbohydrate (which includes fiber), and protein. The DRVs will vary with the total calorie intake; that is, they will be lower for an intake less than 2,000 kilocalories and higher for an intake greater than 2,000 kilocalories (FDA, 1995).

DRVs have also been set for cholesterol, sodium, and potassium, nutrients that do not yield calories. These do not change with the total daily caloric intake. DRVs for the energy-producing nutrients are calculated based on a 2,000-kilocalorie daily intake. The calculation and the resulting daily value for each nutrient are as follows (FDA, 1995):

- Total fat: 30% of the total energy or 65 grams
- Saturated fat: less than 10% or 20 grams
- Carbohydrate: 60% or 300 grams
- Protein: 10% of the calories or 50 grams (This applies only to adults and to children older than age 4 years.)
- Fiber: 11.5 grams per 1,000 kilocalories or 24 grams per 2,000 kilocalories (The value used is 25 grams.)

The above DRVs for fat and saturated fat represent the uppermost limit, which is considered to be desirable for disease risk reduction. The same limit applies to the following DRVs for cholesterol and sodium, which remain the same for all calorie levels (FDA, 1995):

- Cholesterol: Less than 300 mg
- Sodium: Less than 2,400 mg

Reference Daily Intake RDI is just a name change for the term *U.S. RDA,* a label reference that the FDA introduced in 1973 for vitamins, minerals, and protein in voluntary nutrition labeling. The values are the same. The RDIs for the mandatory vitamins and minerals on the food label are as follows (FDA, 1995):

- Vitamin A: 5,000 IU
- Vitamin C: 60 mg
- Calcium: 1.0 g
- Iron: 18 mg

Calculating an Individual's Daily Value

As stated previously, the Daily Values for energy-producing nutrients are based on a 2,000-kilocalorie diet. What are the Daily Values for total fat, saturated fat, and carbohydrate for an older woman who, for example, has estimated energy needs of 1,600 kilocalories?

Given the daily values for fat (less than 30% of the total calories), saturated fat (less than 10% of the total calories), and carbohydrate (60% of the total calories), and the calorie values fat, 9 kcal/g, and carbohydrate, 4 kcal/g, this person can calculate her personal Daily Values. For example:

$$1,600 \text{ kcal (total calories)} \times .30 \text{ (or } 30\%) = 480 \text{ kcal from fat}$$

$$480 \text{ kcal}/9 \text{ kcal} = 53 \text{ g of fat}$$

$$1,600 \text{ kcal} \times .10 \text{ (or } 10\%) = 160 \text{ kcal from saturated fat}$$

$$160 \text{ kcal}/9 \text{ kcal} = 17 \text{ g of saturated fat}$$

$$1,600 \text{ kcal} \times .60 \text{ (or } 60\%) = 960 \text{ kcal from carbohydrate}$$

$$960 \text{ kcal}/4 \text{ kcal} = 240 \text{ g of carbohydrate}$$

Nutrient Content Descriptors
Federal guidelines specify which terms can be used to describe nutrient levels and how these can be used. Examples of the specifications follow (FDA, 1995):

- Free: The product contains no amount or a very small amount of components, such as fat, saturated fat, cholesterol, sodium, sugars, and calories. Synonyms are "without," "no," and "zero."
- Low: The synonyms are "little," "few," and "low source of."
  - Low fat: 3 g or less per serving
  - Low saturated fat: 1 g or less per serving
  - Low sodium: 140 mg or less per serving
  - Very low sodium: 35 mg or less per serving
  - Low cholesterol: 20 mg or less and 2 g or less of saturated fat per serving
  - Low calorie: 40 calories or less per serving
- Lean and extra lean
  - Lean: Less than 10 g fat, 4.5 g or less saturated fat, and less than 95 mg cholesterol per serving and per 100 g
  - Extra lean: Less than 5 g fat, less than 2 g saturated fat, and less than 95 mg cholesterol per serving and per 100 g
- High: 20% or more of the Daily Value for a particular nutrient in a serving
- Good source: 10% to 90% of the Daily Value for a particular nutrient in a serving
- Reduced: A nutritionally altered product contains at least 25% less of a nutrient or of calories than the regular or reference product.
- Less: The food, whether altered or not, contains 25% or less of a nutrient or of calories than the regular or reference product.

- Light: This can mean two things:
  - The nutritionally altered product contains one third fewer calories or one half the fat of the reference food. If the food derives 50% or more of its calories from fat, the reduction must be 50% fat.
  - The sodium content of a low-calorie, low-fat food has been reduced by 50%. In addition, "light in sodium" may be used if sodium has been reduced by 50%.
- More: A serving of food, whether altered or not, contains a nutrient that is at least 10% of the Daily Value more than the reference food. The 10% of Daily Value guideline also applies to "fortified," "enriched," and "added" claims, but in these cases the food must be altered.

Regulations also cover various health claims regarding nutrient–disease connection, such as calcium and osteoporosis, fat and cancer, and folic acid and neural tube defects (FDA, 1995).

18

Oral Health Care

Rosemeire R. Santos-Teachout, Hans Malmström,
Mark E. Moss, and Stanley L. Handelman

Oral diseases are some of the most prevalent health problems in American society. To a large degree, health behaviors determine the amount of oral disease that an individual experiences, but early intervention can reduce the impact of the disease process. For any adult to enjoy a high quality of life, it is important that the oral cavity be healthy and well functioning. Unfortunately, it is recognized that for many adults with developmental disabilities, dental needs often go unmet (Nowak, 1976).

Although the epidemiology of dental diseases in people with intellectual disabilities has not been studied extensively, some studies have provided an indication of the extent of dental diseases and problems. Furthermore, it is generally acknowledged that the most prevalent oral diseases and disorders among adults with lifelong disabilities are dental caries (Nowak, 1984; Scott, Marsh, & Stokes, 1998), periodontal disease (Johnson & Young, 1963), bruxism (i.e., grinding or clenching of teeth; Tesini & Fenton, 1994), erosion (Tesini & Fenton, 1994), malocclusion (Scott et al., 1998) mucosal pathology, and xerostomia (i.e., salivary gland hypofunction; Scott et al., 1998). Yoder and Schimmele (1997) evaluated the oral health of 393 adults with intellectual disabilities and determined that, compared with the general population, they had higher rates of missing teeth and were more commonly toothless. In addition, periodontal disease was significantly more prevalent, and oral hygiene was poorer. Studies also show that there is an increased rate (and severity) of bruxism in adults with intellectual disabilities compared with the general population (Tesini & Fenton, 1994). In addition, Scott et al. (1998) found that oral mucosal pathology and moderate to severe malocclusion were up to

341

seven times as frequent among adults with intellectual disabilities than among the general population, although dental caries were less prevalent. In an Australian study of adults with intellectual disabilities, Beange, McElduff, and Baker (1995) found that dental disease was the most frequent health problem, occurring in 86% of the adults evaluated. Such studies are telling, for they indicate that dental disease may be underdiagnosed in people with lifelong disabilities. In a comprehensive geriatric assessment study of 24 older adults with intellectual disabilities, Carlsen, Galluzzi, Forman, and Cavalieri (1994) found that adding dental evaluation to the assessment protocol resulted in a marked increase of otherwise undiagnosed oral diseases.

COMMON ORAL DISEASES

Recognizing the importance of oral health and dental disease prevention, as well the general underuse of dental services among adults with intellectual disabilities who live in the community, we offer in this section a brief overview of the prominent dental diseases and oral health problems and suggestions with regard to common practice for their treatment or remediation.

Dental Caries

Dental caries, or tooth decay, is the local destruction of the enamel and underlying dentine (the hard tissue that makes up the bulk of the tooth) of a tooth so that cavities form and infection can gain access to the pulp (Youngson, 1992). Often, such infection can destroy the internal blood vessels and nerves and kill the tooth. Treatment requires root canal therapy or extraction.

Causes   Dental caries is the destruction of the tooth as a result of acid demineralization. Plaque-forming bacteria metabolize sugar components in the diet, creating a local acidic environment that results in dissolution of tooth enamel followed by destruction of dentin and the pulp (tooth nerves, capillaries, and tooth-forming tissue), which can lead to an infection and tooth abscess. The rate of formation of a carious lesion, or cavity, is a function of 1) the frequency of eating sugar or refined carbohydrate snacks, especially between meals, and resultant frequent lowering of the pH, 2) the availability of the fluoride ion to counteract the process through remineralization, 3) the quality and frequency of oral hygiene of the individual, especially related to the use of fluoride toothpaste and mouth rinses; and 4) the flow and the quality of saliva to remove and neutralize acids. Saliva production can be reduced by salivary gland disease or the use of certain medications. Lack of saliva can increase the number of bacteria and the formation of plaque on teeth and can prolong the damaging effect of a low pH (Dodds & Wefel, 1999; Nikiforuk, 1985).

Signs and Symptoms   Cavitation occurs after a significant amount of hard tissue loss and usually is determined by the dentist clinically and with the aid of a dental radiograph. The dental caries mainly occurs in the pits and fissures (grooves) of posterior teeth at the contact between adjacent teeth or around the necks of teeth. Initially, dental caries is white or chalky and then tends to turn brown. Dental caries causes sensitivity to cold and hot, sweets, and, in more advanced stages, causes spontaneous pain.

Treatment   In the very early stages, topical fluoride may reverse the progression of the disease. When the dental decay has progressed to the dentin, restorative procedures are required by a dentist.

Periodontal Disease

Periodontal disease (gum and supporting bone disease) is any disorder of the peri-odontium (the tissues surrounding and supporting the teeth). The most common type of periodontal disease is chronic gingivitis (inflammation of the gums) and periodonti-tis (inflammation of the periodontal membranes around the base of the teeth and loss of bone that holds the teeth) (Youngson, 1992).

Causes Because periodontal disease is bacterial in origin, inflammation and infec-tion are the hallmarks. Dental plaque primarily composed of bacteria that accumulate around the gum line has been demonstrated to be the most important factor in the development of gingivitis and periodontal disease (Lindhe, 1989; Loe, Theilade, & Jensen, 1965). The inflammatory reaction may cause damage to the surrounding con-nective tissue structures, including alveolar bone.

Signs and Symptoms Warning signs of advanced periodontal disease include red, swollen, and/or bleeding gums and persistent bad breath. If left untreated, the gum infection damages the bone and supporting tissues. Alveolar abscess may develop, and if bone loss continues, the tooth may become loose. Early and moderate periodontal disease may exhibit few, if any, symptoms, although bleeding when brushing is a com-mon finding.

Treatment In the early stages of the disease, good oral hygiene habits and fre-quent professional oral prophylaxis (cleaning) can stop progression of the disease and reverse the process. Investigators have demonstrated the efficacy of prophylaxis visits three or four times a year (Axelsson & Lindhe, 1981). In advanced stages, gum surgery may be necessary to remove the calculus, plaque, and bacteria to reestablish a cleans-able environment (Lindhe, 1989).

Bruxism

The American Academy of Orofacial Pain defines *bruxism* as a diurnal or nocturnal parafunctional activity including clenching, gnashing, and grinding of the teeth (Okeson, 1996). Awareness of bruxism, with either grinding or clenching, is reported by 6%–20% of adults.

Causes Occlusal interference historically was considered a major cause of brux-ism by "triggering" parafunctional activity via a proprioceptive feedback mechanism (Krough-Poulsen & Olsson, 1966). However, subsequent research has demonstrated that experimentally placed defective occlusal contacts in people with bruxism tend to reduce masticatory muscle activity during sleep rather that enhance it (Rugh, Barghi, & Drago, 1984). In addition, it has been shown that occlusal adjustments do not stop brux-ism (Bailey & Rugh, 1980). Psychological stress has been implicated as a cause of brux-ism (Lavigne & Montplaisir, 1995; Marbach, Lennon, & Dohrenwend, 1998). People who were exposed to stressful experimental stimulus showed increased masticatory muscle activity. However, it is not clear how such experimentally induced muscle activ-ity relates to bruxism. In addition, altered brain chemistry has been associated with bruxism (Lobbezoo, Soucy, Montplaisir, & Lavigne, 1996).

Signs and Symptoms Dental attrition is discovered by visual observation of the occlusal surface of the teeth and the presence of clenching activity. Patients may report that they clench or grind their teeth at night. Myofacial pain, temporomandibu-lar joint noises (e.g., clicking, crepitus), limitation of jaw movements, and tension-type headaches are symptoms of bruxism (Marbach et al., 1998). However, many patients who seem to be engaging in bruxism nightly may have no masticatory muscle pain at all (Lobbezoo & Lavigne, 1997; Lundh, 1995).

Treatment   An occlusal appliance, made of hard acrylic, that fits over the occlusal and incisal surfaces of the teeth in one arch is commonly used to treat bruxism. The appliance may provide a more stable or functional joint position and protect the teeth and supportive structures from abnormal forces that may create breakdown and tooth wear (Okeson, 1989).

Erosion

Erosion consists of an irreversible loss of tooth structure from the external surface. It is a pathological, chronic, localized, painless loss of dental hard tissue chemically etched away from the tooth surface by acid and/or chelation without bacterial involvement (Impeeld, 1996).

Causes   The acids responsible for erosion are not products of bacteria, as in dental caries; they stem from dietary, occupational, or intrinsic sources, such as recurrent vomiting, regurgitation, or reflux. It is frequently associated with eating disorders of psychosomatic origin, such as nervous vomiting, anorexia nervosa, or bulimia as a result of self-induced regurgitation or vomiting. Somatic causes include pregnancy; alcoholism; disulfiram (Antabuse) therapy for alcohol abuse; and gastrointestinal disorders such as gastric dysfunction, chronic obstruction, hiatus hernia, duodenal and peptic ulcers, and gastroesophageal reflux disease (Scheutzel, 1996).

Signs and Symptoms   The clinical aspect of erosion consists of thin enamel aspect appearance confined to the palatal of the maxillary teeth and occlusal surfaces of the maxillary posterior teeth as result of daily vomiting or regurgitation. Additional buccal erosion can also be present if there is frequent exposure to dietary acids (Scheutzel, 1996). The dissolution of the enamel surface may cause increased tooth sensitivity to cold or hot, or sweets but frequently is painless. However, if this process is slow, an increased sensitivity may be delayed. Depending on the severity and longevity of erosion, the process may lead to total destruction of the dentition.

Treatment   Buffering systems such as calcium or phosphate added to drink could reduce the amount of dental enamel dissolved. Fluoride therapy may improve the acid resistance of enamel against erosion as well, and the use of bicarbonate mouth rinse may neutralize the acid after the consumption of fruit juices. Other suggestions for minimizing erosion potential include modifications of route of intake by use of a straw, which is the least harmful method of imbibing sugar-containing drinks (Grenby, 1996).

Malocclusion

Malocclusion is the misalignment of teeth in the upper and lower jaw. In normal occlusion, the posterior teeth of the upper and lower jaw should be in balanced contact, and the upper anterior teeth should overlap slightly and touch the lower anterior teeth.

Causes   Malocclusion is considered a developmental condition. In most instances, malocclusion and dentofacial deformities are caused not by some pathological process but by moderate distortions of normal development, although early tooth loss related to dental caries and oral habits can cause malocclusions. Often, these problems result from a complex interaction among multiple factors that influence growth and development. These factors include 1) genetic influences; 2) environmental influences; and 3) specific causes of malocclusion such as disturbances in embryological development, skeletal growth disturbances, muscle dysfunction, and trauma to the teeth (Proffit & Fields, 2000).

Signs and Symptoms   Misaligned (crowded) teeth are the most common sign of malocclusion (in approximately 40% of children and 85% of youths). The second most common finding is excessive protrusion of maxillary incisors (Proffit & Fields, 2000). Although unusual, a severe malocclusion may compromise all aspects of oral function. Adults with severe malocclusion routinely report difficulty with chewing; after treatment, patients say that the masticatory problems are largely corrected (Ostler & Kiyakha, 1991). Research indicates that malocclusion does not increase caries or periodontal disease (Helm & Petersen, 1989). The most common concern of adults with malocclusion is psychosocial problems related to impaired dentofacial aesthetics (Jenny, 1975).

Oral Mucosal Lesions

Candidiasis   Also known as *thrush,* candidiasis is an infection caused by the common fungus of the genus *Candida.* This infection affects the warm, moist areas of the body, such as the mouth. The most common oral mucosal lesion is a mycotic infection. Oral manifestation can be acute or chronic with various degrees of severity and forms. Young infants and older adults frequently are affected. Estimates of disease frequency range up to 5% of neonates and 10% of older adults who are debilitated and live in institutions. In individuals with dentures, this condition can be present in those who demonstrate deep folds at the commissures of the lips secondary to overclosure. In addition, it can be present at the hard palatal mucosa predominantly beneath maxillary complete denture (Eyre & Nally, 1971; Pindborg, 1986; Regezi & Sciubba, 1999; Rockoff, 1979).

Causes   Candidiasis is caused by *C. albicans,* a microorganism that is a normal inhabitant of the oral cavity in a majority of healthy people. Infection with this microorganism reflects a local or systemic immunocompromised health status or may be related to local factors.

Signs and Symptoms   Candidiasis is characteristically white, soft to gelatinous plaques or nodules that grow centrifugally and merge. Wiping away the plaques with a gauze sponge or cotton swab leaves an erythematous, eroded, or ulcerated surface that often is tender. Lesions are moderately painful, fissured, eroded, and encrusted.

Treatment   This condition can be treated simply with topical applications of nystatin suspension. In denture-related disease, nystatin cream may be used on the affected tissue and in the denture itself to provide prolonged contact and to eliminate the organisms in the denture material.

Recurrent Aphthous Ulcer   Recurrent aphthous ulcer (i.e., canker sore) is a non-traumatic ulceration that affects mucous membranes. Incidence has been reported to be 20%–60%, depending on the population studied (Janicki, 1971). The ulcers are not followed by vesicles, and they appear on the vestibular, buccal mucosa, tongue, soft palate, fauces, and floor of the mouth.

Causes   Although the causes of aphthous ulcer are unknown, factors such as alterations of the immunologic system, microbiological balance, nutrition, hormonal alterations, stress, trauma, and food allergies have been reported (Regezi & Sciubba, 1999).

Signs and Symptoms   An aphthous ulcer can be a single, painful oval ulcer covered with a yellow fibrinous membrane and surrounded by an erythematous halo. When the lateral or ventral surfaces of the tongue are affected, pain tends to be out of proportion to the size of the lesion. It can last for 7–10 days. Tingling or burning occurs before the appearance of the lesion. When lesions are present, there may be pain, especially when eating and drinking.

Treatment   Corticosteroids offer the best chance for disease containment. In severely affected patients, systemic steroids may be used, but in patients with mild to moderate disease, only topical therapy is justified (Hay & Reade, 1984; Regezi & Sciubba, 1999; Wilson, 1980).

Xerostomia (Salivary Gland Hypofunction)

Salivary gland dysfunction results in xerostomia, a condition often found in older adults. This condition consists of dryness of the mouth as a result of decreased salivary flow.

Causes   Xerostomia can result from medication use (at least 400 prescribed medications can cause xerostomia as a side effect, especially when multiple medications are used). If the xerostomia is medication induced, the older adult's physician should be consulted regarding the possibility of changing the medication or dosage. Other causes include 1) radiation therapy for head or neck tumors, 2) chemotherapeutic agents used for cancer and immunosuppression therapy, 3) physiological disorders (e.g., fibrosis of parotid glands subsequent to mumps, blockage of salivary duct), or 4) primary or secondary Sjögren's syndrome (Rounds & Papas, 1991). Sjögren's syndrome is an autoimmune process that causes xerostomia as a result of lymphocytic replacement of salivary glands (Regezi & Scuibba, 1999).

Signs and Symptoms   The consequences of a reduction in salivary flow are a decrease and possible loss of the lubrication of the mouth with decreased bacteriostatic power of the saliva and increased risk for developing dental caries. Dry mouth, a burning sensation of oral mucosa, changes in taste and swallowing, tongue mobility, and wearing of a removable appliance become affected and more difficult.

Treatment   In cases of burning sensation, lidocaine provides temporary relief from pain (Fox, Busch, & Baum, 1987; Regezi & Sciubba, 1999). In addition to xerostomia fungi and bacterial infections, nutritional deficiencies, hormone imbalances, and mechanical trauma are possible causes of burning mouth syndrome. Empirical treatment is frequently the approach most clinicians use for patients with this problem. Antifungal agents, solutions containing tetracycline, nystatin, and diphenhydramine hydrochloride (i.e., Benadryl), or topical steroids are some of the most commonly used agents.

ORAL HEALTH AND LIFELONG DISABILITIES

Dental problems are commonly observed in people with lifelong disabilities and generally are related to their cognitive and/or physical impairments, which may lead to difficulties in learning and/or practicing preventive dental hygiene (Stiefel, Truelove, Chin, & Mandel, 1992) and may make early intervention more difficult. If a patient does not cooperate during attempts to perform a dental examination, it may have adverse consequences, for failure to do an adequate examination may contribute to neglect and the increasing severity of oral disease. In addition, access to dental services can be a factor in dental health among people with lifelong disabilities. For example, Gabre and Gahnberg (1997) found that residential situation and lifestyle issues may be important factors in examination compliance. They observed that people who had more severe forms of intellectual disabilities and were living in institutions had a lower incidence of dental caries than did individuals who had mild intellectual disabilities and were living in supervised apartments in the community. The authors attributed these differences to the decreased supervision of dental hygiene and nutritional habits in adults who live in the community. Others, such as O'Donnell (1994), have observed that there may be significant barriers to routine dental care as a result of the disappearance of institution-based dental facilities and to the dearth of community practitioners who are experienced with the special dental problems and oral health needs of adults with intellectual and other developmental disabilities.

Syndrome-specific factors are also important in predicting dental problems. Adults with Down syndrome, who have a variety of impaired defense mechanisms for infection, have high rates and increased severity of relatively early-age onset periodontal disease compared with adults with other causes of intellectual disabilities (Barnett, Press, Friedman, & Sonnenberg, 1986; Cohen, Winer, Schwartz, Shklar, 1961; Johnson & Young, 1963; Santos, Shanfeld, & Casamassimo, 1996). Among adults with Down syndrome, other dental concerns include malocclusion, microdontia, aberrant patterns of tooth eruption, cone-shaped teeth, hypoplastic enamel, anodontia, and supernumerary teeth (Modeer, Barr, & Dahllöf, 1990; Reuland-Bosma & van Dijk, 1986). Rubinstein-Taybi, Noonan, and Cockayne syndromes, associated with intellectual disabilities, also pose dental problem issues (Nowak, 1976). Having another type of developmental disability may also contribute to dental problems. For example, gingival hyperplasia can occur as a result of taking medication for seizures (epilepsy), and enamel defects and tooth fractures can result from increased bruxism and falls that may occur among adults with cerebral palsy. Relatively common medical conditions found among people with intellectural disabilities, such as gastroesophageal reflux and rumination, can also impair dental health. Furthermore, adults who may also have psychiatric or behavior problems may have dental disease as a result of aberrant eating habits and other behaviors (i.e., pica, self-injury, pouching) as well as be affected adversely by having to take psychotropic medications (Tesini & Fenton, 1994).

Some adults with cerebral palsy, Down syndrome, or Apert syndrome may have craniofacial anomalies that may further compromise oral health. Nowak (1976) pointed out that approximately 40% of people with congenital maxillofacial anomalies have intellectual disabilities. Furthermore, people with severe intellectual disabilities, who tend to have higher rates of syndrome conditions and associated developmental disabilities such as cerebral palsy, display higher rates of malocclusion than do people with mild intellectual disabilities. Among adults with Down syndrome, class III malocclusion is a common problem (Reuland-Bosma & van Dijk, 1986). Adults with other intellectual disabilities and hypotonic perioral muscles often display a class II malocclusion with anterior open bite. Mouth breathing is also commonly found in adults with associated neuromotor abnormalities.

Reports in the dental and medical literature suggest that poor oral health may also be associated with higher risks of developing coronary artery disease (Beck, Garcia, Heiss, Vokonas, & Offenbacher, 1996; Herzberg & Meyer, 1996) or undergoing premature labor (Offenbacher et al., 1996). It has been suggested that poor oral health may also have a negative impact on diabetic control and increase the risk of aspiration pneumonia; however, these suggestions are still speculative and need research validation. Such comorbidity demonstrates that dentists and other oral health specialists should be an integral part of the health care team for individuals with lifelong disabilities.

PREVENTION AND TREATMENT

Prevention of dental disease should include both educational and behavioral approaches aimed at incorporating basic oral hygiene practices and appropriate dietary habits into the daily routine of adults with lifelong disabilities. It should also include regularly scheduled oral examinations and preventive dental interventions initiated by a dental care team.

Educational and Behavioral Approaches

Dental educational and behavioral programs need to take into account the cognitive and physical capability of older adults with lifelong disabilities and should involve the individual, caregivers, and others who are intimately involved with the adult. Such programs need to be integrated into the daily life activities of the residence or life situation of the individual. Any such programs should also include nutritional counseling, specifically focusing on reducing sugar-containing snacks and substituting with non–sugar-containing snacks (Chapter 12). Nicolaci and Tesini (1982) documented one approach to such a dental education and behavior program. They reported that the introduction of their program resulted in improved oral health of recipients with lifelong disabilities. The oral hygiene training program was designed so that it could be administered by direct care staff. As part of the outcome assessment, oral examinations conducted at 6-month intervals demonstrated significant improvement in the adults' oral hygiene scores and calculus deposit and debris indices.

Adults with cognitive and motor impairments (e.g., those attributed to cerebral palsy) or visual impairments may benefit from diligent staff assistance or assisting devices (Nowak, 1976). Adults may also benefit from modified manual toothbrushes, sonic toothbrushes (Day, Martin, & Chin, 1998), or electric toothbrushes (Carr, Sterling, & Bauchmoyer, 1997) as part of their dental hygiene regimes. Desensitization practices using facial-oral stimulation or music therapy may enhance cooperation (Davila & Menendez, 1986). Evidence seems to point to the conclusion that educational and behavioral oral health intervention directed toward people with intellectual disabilities or their caregivers can help to optimize mechanical plaque removal, the cornerstone of preventive oral health programs.

Oral Examinations and Preventive Therapeutic Interventions

Dental Prophylaxis Practices   In general, maintenance dental examinations and prophylaxis should be performed every 6 months. Yet such intervals may vary without adverse results. Maurer, Boggs, Mourino, and Farrington (1996) conducted a retrospective study of the effect of recall intervals (i.e., frequency of dental visits) on the development of dental caries in 83 people with intellectual disabilities. They found no statistical relationship between recall interval and caries formation, although there was a trend toward increased risk for caries after 12-month recall intervals. However, gingival status was not evaluated in this study, and the authors suggested that shorter recall intervals may be required for people with existing gingivitis and periodontal disease. As poor oral hygiene is a major problem for many people with lifelong disabilities, high-risk groups require closer monitoring for the development of oral disease. In people with active gingivitis or periodontal disease, 3-month recall intervals may be indicated. In people without dental disease or with stabilized dental disease, a 6-month recall interval may be optimal for dental prophylaxis and a yearly recall interval is optimal for oral examinations.

Antimicrobial Agents   The use of chlorhexidine may be a beneficial prophylactic component of a comprehensive oral management program for any adult with intellectual disabilities. Stiefel, Truelove, Chin, Zhu, and Lerrox (1995) evaluated the efficacy of incorporating chlorhexidine swabbing in the oral health care of 44 adults with severe intellectual disabilities. The adults in the study were randomly selected into chlorhexidine treatment and placebo control groups. Those who were treated with chlorhexidine demonstrated significantly improved plaque scores over the control group; however, no significant differences were noted in regard to gingivitis, calculus, or pocket depth. Adverse effects of chlorhexidine, such as stained teeth or calculus build-up, were minimal.

Stabholz and colleagues (1991) evaluated the topical application of a sustained-release polymer containing chlorhexidine in 30 individuals with Down syndrome. They demonstrated that this method of chlorhexidine delivery resulted in a statistically significant improvement in plaque and gingival indices and a reduction in the bacterial flora count, compared with a placebo-control group. Burtner, Low, McNeal, Hawell, and Smith (1991) evaluated the effect of chlorhexidine on a number of adults with intellectual disabilities who were unable to brush their own teeth. One group had 0.12% chlorhexidine spray applied twice daily and was compared with that of a group receiving a placebo spray. The results indicated that the chlorhexidine treatment group had reduced plaque and gingivitis. These studies support the contention that chlorhexidine, when applied via a variety of topical delivery systems, can serve as an adjunctive therapy to mechanical plaque removal in helping to control plaque formation and gingival inflammation in selected individuals with intellectual disabilities.

Topical Fluoride   Systemic and topical fluoride use is considered the main reason for the decline in dental caries experienced in many Western countries. Fluoridation of community water supplies is the most cost-effective preventive mechanism; other fluoride treatment is also effective in prevention of dental caries. Fluoride functions in several ways. When given systemically, fluoride alters the structural composition of the teeth. Some individuals with intellectual and other developmental disabilities may benefit from the prescription of additional topically administered fluoride (Jones & Berg, 1992). When given topically, fluoride alters the composition of the surface layer of enamel. Both processes make the teeth more resistant to acid challenges and carious breakdown. Fluoride also assists in the remineralization process, so enamel that has begun to lose mineral content through caries can be replenished with new minerals. If there is little or no fluoride in the water supply, then fluoride supplementation (in the form of fluoride drops, chewable tablets, vitamins with fluoride, or fluoride gel) should be given daily. Before prescribing supplementation, practitioners should know the exact concentration of fluoride in the locality's drinking water, as levels in bottled, well, and tap water vary greatly. As a caution, parents with young children with disabilities should be aware of the fluoride content of water in the child care environment. Excessive concentration of fluoride in young children can result in fluorosis, a brown discoloration with white specks on the permanent teeth (Stookey & Beiswinger, 1999).

Antibiotic Therapy   Primary treatment of adult periodontitis includes oral hygiene education, scaling and root planing, and periodontal surgery. The adjunctive use of systemic and local antibiotic therapy such as doxycycline for the treatment of periodontitis has been suggested. These antibiotics have been used as an adjunct to scaling and root planing in selective individuals with adult periodontitis. The recommended dosage for doxycycline as an adjunct to periodontal treatment is 100 mg per day. This concentration inhibits microorganisms associated with adult periodontitis. A recently introduced dose of doxycycline (20 mg) twice daily reduces elevated collagenase activity in the gingival tissues and fluid of individuals with adult periodontitis. The plasma and tissue concentration of the dosage is well below the concentration required to inhibit microorganisms associated with adult periodontitis. A significant reduction of the pocket depth when using 20 mg of doxycycline twice daily as an adjunct after scaling and root planing compared with scaling and root planing alone was demonstrated by Golub, Ryan, and Williams (1998). However, clinical trials have not included individuals with developmental disabilities. Although a nonantimicrobial dose of doxycycline may be effective as an adjunct to periodontal therapy in individuals with lifelong disabilities, further research needs to be performed to justify its use.

Orthodontic Treatment   Becker and Shapira (1996) described the difficulty in providing orthodontic treatment to people with lifelong disabilities because of behavioral issues and the limited availability of orthodontists who work with people who have special needs. The primary purpose in the general population of the treatment of malocclusion is aesthetic. For the most part, however, the impact of malocclusion on dental disease and function is minimal.

COORDINATION OF DENTAL CARE WITH OTHER HEALTH CARE SERVICES

Dentists who work with people with intellectual disabilities need to be apprised of their patients' medical and mental health status, medications, and medication allergies. Physicians can often help dentists with patient-specific conscious sedation regimens. Mental health providers can assist in desensitization programs or relaxation programs for people with intellectual disabilities who are fearful of dental procedures. For individuals who require general anesthesia for dental care, careful case management can consolidate dental interventions with other intrusive procedures, such as gynecological or ophthalmologic examination. Optimal oral health practices require a team approach with the inclusion of the adult, caregivers, and other health care providers in the treatment plan.

Identification of Dental Care Resources

Dental delivery systems for people with lifelong disabilities require a significant degree of coordination at the community level. Local dental societies can provide the names of dentists who are capable of providing care for people with special needs. For individuals who are eligible for dental care under Medicaid coverage, private practitioners who accept the Medicaid fee schedule is one option. Public-supported clinic facilities such as dental schools, hospitals, health centers, and state-operated facilities that may have a dental team are another option. Unfortunately, many rural or otherwise small communities may not have easy access to special dental resources. Organizations that work on the behalf of adults with disabilities are a good source of information on referrals.

In the United States, one resource for information is the American Dental Association and Foundation of Dentistry for the Handicapped (1800 15th Street, Suite 100, Denver, CO 80202; 1-800-365-7229; www.nfdh.org). The foundation is a national, charitable organization that is dedicated solely to meeting the oral health needs of citizens with special physical, medical, and mental disabilities.

PREPARING FOR A DENTAL VISIT

Oral Hygiene

Some adults may resist the daily practice of oral hygiene because they may not understand the reason for the procedure, may not be able to perform the procedure, or may place little, if any, value in the health of their mouth. Therefore, depending on the nature of the disability, it may be necessary for a parent, guardian, or other caregiver to provide the care. An initial desensitization program as described in the next section may be applied for individuals who are fearful of or resistant to daily oral care. The use of facial stimulation and music therapy prescribed for daily oral hygiene, as described by Davila and Menendez (1986), can desensitize the individual with a disability to accept dental care at home or in the dental office.

Maintaining good oral hygiene can be a difficult task to accomplish. In most situations, someone else must accept the responsibility for the person's oral hygiene. The individual who is responsible should be given a step-by-step demonstration and then given the opportunity to perform the techniques with the individual. This provides an opportunity to make corrections and gain additional support and reinforcement. Printed materials and videotapes can reinforce the knowledge and skills of the caregiver (Schmidt, Leach, Nicolaci, Sutton, & O'Donnell, 1981). If the individual uses a wheelchair, then the caregiver should stand behind the person and use one arm to support the head while using the other arm to manipulate the toothbrush or floss. For individuals who are able to follow commands, a comprehensive task analysis for teaching tooth brushing can be used (Horner & Keilitz, 1975). Before training, the adult can be brought into a room with a sink, a toothbrush, a tube of toothpaste, a paper cup, and a box of tissues and asked to brush his or her teeth using these materials. The presence or absence of each step in the task analysis is recorded on a data sheet. The adult is assessed a second time, and the level of prompt required for performance of each step is recorded (no help, verbal instruction, demonstration by a clinician with verbal instruction, or graduated guidance with verbal instruction). These data, combined with those from the first assessment, can be used to develop an individualized treatment plan for brushing. Such an approach can offer a framework through which dental care providers can track support staff in their roles in providing oral care for people with lifelong disabilities and may also prepare them to accept dental care.

Desensitization Program for Oral Care

A desensitization program can be used to reduce the fear that an individual experiences when faced with the unknown or an unpleasant past experience in dentistry and to provide relaxation and techniques for cooperative behavior for dental examination and caregiver daily oral care practices (Davila & Menendez, 1986; Horner & Keilitz, 1975; Nowak, 1976). Relaxation music, symbolic experiences, oral motor exercises, and proper handling all are part of the program. The program can be carried out daily for 3 weeks before the scheduled dental screening examination. Table 1 describes the principles that should be adhered to for the desensitization program to be successful for individuals with limited capabilities.

If the individual needs to be held to complete the program or examination, remember to use a soft, calm voice and a firm, gentle touch. Rubbing the arms while holding may be comforting. If the individual requires handling techniques because of abnormal

Table 1. Dental contact desensitization program

Implement the program in a distraction-free environment (preferably in a separate room).

Instruct the person to lie on his or her back (people with reclining wheelchairs may remain in their chairs for proper positioning).

Play relaxation tapes while explaining to the person what is about to happen.

Place your hands on the center of the person's forehead. Slowly move your hands away from each other, progressing smoothly to the jaw line and the chin. Continue until the individual starts to appear relaxed (usually after eight strokes).

Place your hands on the individual's jaw joints and move them in small circles along the jaw line to the chin. Consider using a lotion and perfume as olfactory stimulants for relaxation.

Place your hands on the person's cheeks and press down firmly. Hold for approximately 30 seconds.

Put on rubber (i.e., latex) gloves. (Be sure the person is not allergic to latex.) Tell the person that you will put your fingers in his or her mouth and rub his or her gums. Place one finger on the person's lips and wait for him or her to open his or her mouth. Rub each quadrant of the gums two or three times. Do not rub between the jaws and teeth, because you may be bitten.

End the experience by touching the person's face lightly and telling the person that you are done.

tone and reflexes, then transfer him or her onto the examination table using correct transfer techniques. Do not feel rushed. Try to position the head into flexion using a blanket or towel roll. Flexion of the knees may be maintained by using the same method. If objects get caught in the individual's mouth because of abnormal oral reflexes, then place the individual in a sitting position, with the head bent forward. Promote relaxation by rubbing his or her arms or back. Wait for the individual to release the object. Do not try to pull the object out. Return to the examination position after you remove the object.

Devices and Materials

Adults with intellectual disabilities and motor impairment (e.g., caused by cerebral palsy) or visual impairment may benefit from staff assistance and/or modified manual toothbrushes, sonic toothbrushes (Day et al., 1998), or electric toothbrushes (Carr et al., 1997). Selection of a toothbrush should be dictated by the individual's dental health and manual dexterity. Both manual and power toothbrushes can be modified by altering the angle of the handle, increasing the length of the handle, enlarging the diameter of the handle with the addition of foam rubber or tape, or improving the grip by addition of a Velcro strap (Nowak, 1976).

Commercial mouth props are available to assist in keeping the mouth open during plaque removal. If the person cannot or will not open his or her mouth, then gently stroke the cheeks and the inferior border of the mandible. With the teeth apart, the prop can be moved into position between the two arches. The teeth should be cleaned on one side, both maxillary and mandibular, before transferring the prop to the opposite side. A mouth prop can be made by securing together five or six tongue depressors with adhesive tape.

Table 2. Useful information to have available for the dental visit

Medical	Review of systems, medications, allergies
Dental	Past dental experience, traumatic injuries
Oral habits	Use of toothbrush, toothpaste, and floss
Social	Residential setting, name of agency, family involvement
Dietary factors	Meal contents, textures, sugar intake (in medication and food); fluoride supplementation orally and topically
Levels of communication and perceptual ability and skill	Information on ability to perceive, as this may be greater than the ability to communicate
Level of cognitive functioning	Information on ability to follow commands
Etiologic/Diagnostic	Conditions that may pose special considerations for dental care, such as Down syndrome, congenital rubella, or other syndromes
Behavior management	Suggestions on how to have the person respond to an attempt at intraoral instrumentation

Preparation for the Dental Visit

Table 2 provides a list of things that should be taken care of before the visit. This information should be available to the practitioner and given to the receptionist or practitioner upon arrival.

What to Expect at the Dental Visit

The initial visit to the dentist should be a good experience. At this visit, the dentist performs an initial behavioral assessment and determines methods and techniques to be used in considering the individual's problems and needs. As familiarity grows, the ability to obtain compliant behavior will increase.

To meet the objectives of the first visit, the individual should receive radiographs, oral prophylaxis, and an evaluation. If the person presents for an initial visit with a primary complaint and is not there for routine examination and prophylaxis, he or she should still have an examination. However, instead of an oral prophylaxis, an attempt should be made to address the chief complaint. The desensitization program started at home should play a great role in this visit. The chair should not be reclined all the way during the first visit. Many individuals will become much more fearful, anxious, and agitated when they are placed "belly-up." This is a very vulnerable position and should be avoided until the provider has determined that the adult can tolerate it. When the dentist is ready to attempt contact with the oral region, the use of a lotion can help to desensitize the adult. The dentist may use a disposable oral swab that has been dipped in a NutraSweet solution and blotted to wipe over the adult's lips. After this, the provider may attempt to have the adult open his or her mouth and have his her gingival tissues wiped with the swab. During the first visit, the provider generally attempts to perform a behavioral assessment. As the provider develops an understanding of the challenging behaviors that the individual may exhibit, he or she can become better able to manage them.

Behavior Management in the Dental Office

Dental and oral care should be provided in the least restrictive environment. However, after an individual's behavioral assessment, it may be determined that premedication for sedation is indicated to aid in reaching the treatment objectives of the dental plan. A recommendation for premedication for sedation is formulated on an individual basis and should be coordinated with the individual's primary physician. Many drugs are available for sedative use, but generally for oral administration, drugs such as Valium (diazepam), Halcion (triazolam), and Noctec (chloral hydrate) are used.

Treatment Planning

Once the oral examination and necessary health care consultation have been conducted and the diagnostic information has been obtained, an individualized treatment plan can be developed. The clinician must consider the urgency of the oral problems and limiting factors (e.g., financing) that may influence the level of rehabilitation appropriate to the individual's needs. The primary goal of the dental treatment plan is to eliminate all sources of oral infection and restore teeth to allow the person to be free of discomfort. Rehabilitative procedures for people with intellectual and other developmental disabilities generally address their oral condition and have a predictable outcome, depending on the person's oral health issues, adaptive limitations, behavioral obstacles, and cognitive function. In addition, capability of the individual, supporting staff, and/or family and caregivers to provide daily oral health activities must be considered.

CONCLUSIONS

Although more research is necessary, current epidemiological data indicate that people with intellectual and other developmental disabilities are at relatively high risk for a variety of oral diseases and disorders, such as dental caries, erosion, oral mucosal pathologies, periodontal disease, and malocclusion. This increased risk arises from a variety of factors, including cognitive and behavioral disabilities, residential and lifestyle issues that can interfere with oral hygiene and diet habits, syndrome-specific issues, and associated disabilities. Policy makers and other health care providers need to recognize the importance of good dental care in promoting health and well-being. Oral hygiene practices, which may require special educational and behavioral interventions, are the cornerstone of preventive dental care. The frequency of regularly scheduled dental visits for prophylaxis and examinations needs to be based on the oral health status and risks of each individual. A variety of adjunctive treatments may be helpful in optimizing oral health. People with intellectual disabilities and complicated medical or behavioral needs require a coordinated, multidisciplinary team approach.

The following health care processes are recommended for ensuring sound oral health and dental disease prevention:

- Education and behavioral interventions that ensure that appropriate dietary habits need to be established and that oral hygiene practices should be a part of the daily life of people with lifelong disabilities and should be directed toward individuals with disabilities and their caregivers to the maximum extent possible.
- Schedule dental visits for oral examinations and prophylaxis at 3-month intervals for those with active disease and those at high risk for oral disease (which may be many people with intellectual disabilities) and every 6 months for people judged to

be at low risk by the dental care team. This should be part of the overall health maintenance program for people with lifelong disabilities.

• Preventive therapies, such as fluoride or use of antimicrobial agents, should be implemented when indicated.

• Multidisciplinary team approaches incorporating input from medical and mental health providers as well as dentists and dental hygienists need to be adopted to ensure optimal oral health.

REFERENCES

Axelsson, P., & Lindhe, J. (1981). Effect of controlled oral hygiene procedures on caries and periodontal disease in adults: Results after 6 years. *Journal of Clinical Periodontology, 8,* 239–248.

Bailey J., & Rugh, J. (1980). Effect of occlusal adjustment on bruxism as monitored by nocturnal EMG recordings. *Journal of Dental Research, 59,* 327.

Barnett, M.L., Press, M.L., Friedman, D., & Sonnenberg, E.M. (1986). The prevalence of periodontitis and dental caries in a Down's syndrome population. *Journal of Periodontology, 57,* 288–293.

Beange, H., McElduff, A., & Baker, W. (1995). Medical disorders of adults with mental retardation: A population study. *American Journal on Mental Retardation, 99,* 595–604.

Beck, J., Garcia, R., Heiss, G., Vokonas, P.S., & Offenbacher, S. (1996). Periodontal disease and cardiovascular disease. *Journal of Periodontology, 67*(Suppl. 10), 1123–1137.

Becker, A., & Shapira, J. (1996). Orthodontics for the handicapped child. *European Journal of Orthodontics, 18*(1), 55–67.

Burtner, A.P., Low, D.W., McNeal, D.R., Hawell, T.M., & Smith, R.G. (1991). Effects of chlorhexidine spray on plaque and gingival health in institutionalized persons with mental retardation. *Special Care in Dentistry, 11,* 97–100.

Carlsen, W.R., Galluzzi, K.E., Forman, L.F., & Cavalieri, T.A. (1994). Comprehensive geriatric assessment: Applications for community-residing elderly people with intellectual disability/developmental disabilities. *Mental Retardation, 32,* 334–340.

Carr, M.P., Sterling, E.S., & Bauchmoyer, S.M. (1997). Comparison of the Interplak and manual toothbrushes in a population with mental retardation/developmental disabilities (MR/DD). *Special Care in Dentistry, 17,* 133–136.

Cohen, M.M., Winer, R.A., Schwartz, S., & Shklar, G. (1961). Oral aspects of mongolism: Part I. Periodontal disease in mongolism. *Oral Surgery, Oral Medicine, and Oral Pathology, 14*(1), 92–107.

Davila, J.M., & Menendez, J. (1986). Relaxing effects of music in dentistry for mentally handicapped patients. *Special Care in Dentistry, 6,* 18–21.

Day, J., Martin, M.D., & Chin, M. (1998). Efficacy of a sonic toothbrush for plaque removal by caregivers in a special needs population. *Special Care in Dentistry, 18,* 202–206.

Dodds, M.W.J., & Wefel, J.S. (1999). The developing carious lesion. In N.O. Harris & F. Garcia-Godoy (Eds.), *Primary preventive dentistry* (5th ed., pp. 41–61). Stamford, CT: Appleton & Lange.

Eyre, J., & Nally, F.F. (1971). Oral candidosis and carcinoma. *British Journal of Dermatology, 85,* 73–75.

Fox, P.C., Busch, K.A., & Baum, B.J. (1987). Subjective reports of xerostomia and objective measures of salivary gland performance. *Journal of the American Dental Association, 115,* 581–584.

Gabre, P., & Gahnberg, L. (1997). Inter-relationship among degree of mental retardation, living arrangements, and dental health in adults with mental retardation. *Special Care in Dentistry, 17,* 7–12.

Golub, L.M., Ryan, M.E., & Williams, R.C. (1998). Modulation of the host response in the treatment of periodontitis. *Dentistry Today, 17,* 102–109.

Grenby, T.H. (1996). Lessening dental erosive potential by product modification. *European Journal of Oral Science, 104,* 221–118.

Hay, K.D., & Reade, P.C. (1984). The use of an elimination diet in the treatment of recurrent aphthous ulcerations of the oral cavity. *Oral Surgery, Oral Medicine, and Oral Pathology, 57,* 504–507.

Helm S., & Petersen, P. (1989). Causal relations between malocclusion and caries. *Acta Odontologica Scandinavica, 47,* 217–221.

Herzberg, M.C., & Meyer, M.W. (1996). Effects of oral flora on platelets: Possible consequences in cardiovascular disease. *Journal of Periodontology, 67*(Suppl. 10), 1138–1142.

Horner, R.D., & Keilitz, I. (1975). Training mentally retarded adolescents to brush their teeth. *Journal of Applied Behavior Analysis, 8,* 301–309.

Impeeld, T. (1996). Dental erosion: Definition, classification and links. *European Journal of Oral Science, 104,* 151–155.

Janicki, M.P. (1971). Recurrent herpes labialis and recurrent aphthous ulcerations: Psychological components. *Psychotherapy and Psychosomatics, 19,* 288–294.

Jenny, S. (1975). A social perspective on need and demand for orthodontic treatment. *International Dental Journal, 25,* 248–256.

Johnson, N.P., & Young, M.A. (1963). Periodontal disease in mongols. *Journal of Periodontology, 34,* 41–47.

Jones, K., & Berg, J.H. (1992). Fluoride supplementation. *American Journal of Diseases of Childhood, 146,* 1488–1491.

Krough-Poulsen, W.G., & Olsson, A. (1966). Occlusal disharmonies and dysfunction of the stomatognathic system. *Dental Clinics of North America, 10,* 627–635.

Lavigne, G.J., & Montplaisir, J.Y. (1995). Bruxism: Epidemiology, diagnosis, pathophysiology and pharmacology. In J.R. Fricton & R. Dubner (Eds.), *Orofacial pain and temporomandibular disorders: Advances in pain research and therapy* (Vol. 21, pp. 387–404). Philadelphia: Lippincott-Raven.

Lindhe, J. (1989). *Textbook of clinical periodontology* (2nd ed.). Copenhagen: Munksgaard.

Lobbezoo, F., Soucy, J.P., Montplaisir, J.Y., & Lavigne, G.J. (1996). Striatal D2 receptor binding in sleep bruxism: A controlled study with iodine-123-iodobenzamide and single photon emission computed tomography. *Journal of Dental Research, 75,* 1804–1810.

Lobbezoo, F.S., & Lavigne, G.J. (1997). Do bruxism and temporomandibular disorders have a cause-and-effect relationship? *Journal of Orofacial Pain, 11,* 15–23.

Loe, H., Theilade, E., & Jensen, S.B. (1965). Experimental gingivitis in man. *Journal of Periodontology, 36,* 177–187.

Lundh, J.P. (1995). Pain and the control of muscles. In J.R. Fricton & R. Dubner (Eds.), *Orofacial pain and temporomandibular disorders: Advances in pain research and therapy* (Vol. 21, pp. 103–115). Philadelphia: Lippincott-Raven.

Marbach, J.J., Lennon, M.C., & Dohrenwend, B.P. (1998). Candidate risk factors for temporomandibular pain and dysfunction syndrome: Psychological health behavior, physical illness and injury. *Pain, 34,* 139–151.

Maurer, S.M., Boggs, A.M., Mourino, A.P., & Farrington, F.H. (1996). Recall intervals: Effect on treatment needs of the handicapped patient—A retrospective study. *Journal of Clinical Pediatric Dentistry, 20,* 123–126.

Modeer, T., Barr, M., & Dahllöf, G. (1990). Periodontal disease in children with Down's syndrome. *Scandinavian Journal of Dental Research, 98,* 228–234.

Nicolaci, A.B., & Tesini, D.A. (1982). Improvement in the oral hygiene of institutionalized mentally retarded individuals through training of direct care staff: A longitudinal study. *Special Care in Dentistry, 2,* 217–221.

Nikiforuk, G. (1985). *Understanding dental caries: 2. Prevention: Basic and clinical aspects.* Basel, Switzerland: S. Karger.

Nowak, A.J. (1984). Dental disease in handicapped persons. *Special Care in Dentistry, 4,* 66–69.

Nowak, A.J. (Ed.). (1976). *Dentistry for the handicapped patient.* St. Louis: C.V. Mosby.

O'Donnell, J.P. (1994). Dental care for special needs individuals: A new barrier to access [Editorial]. *Special Care in Dentistry, 14,* 178–179.

Offenbacher, S., Katz, V., Fertik, G., Collins, J., Boyd, D., Maynor, G., McKalg, R., & Beck, J. (1996). Periodontal infection as a possible risk factor for preterm low birth weight. *Journal of Periodontology, 67*(Suppl. 10), 1103–1113.

Okeson, J.P. (1989). *Management of temporomandibular disorders and occlusion* (2nd ed.). St. Louis: Mosby.

Okeson, J.P. (1996). *Orofacial pain: Guidelines for assessment, diagnosis, and management.* Chicago: Quintessence Publishing Co.

Ostler, S., & Kiyakha, H.A. (1991). Treatment exceptions vs. outcomes in orthognathic surgery patients. *International Journal of Adult Orthodontics and Orthognathic Surgery, 6,* 247–256.

Pindborg, J.J. (1986). *Atlas of diseases of the oral mucosa* (4th ed.). Philadelphia: W.B. Saunders Co.

Proffit, W.R., & Fields, H.W. (2000). *Contemporary orthodontics* (3rd ed.). St. Louis: Mosby.

Regezi, J.S., & Sciubba, J. (1999). *Oral pathology: Clinical pathologic correlation* (5th ed.). Philadelphia: W.B. Saunders Co.

Reuland-Bosma, W., & van Dijk, J. (1986). Periodontal disease in Down's syndrome: A review. *Journal of Clinical Periodontology, 13,* 64–73.

Rockoff, A.S. (1979). Chronic mucocutaneous candidiasis: Successful treatment with intermittent oral doses of clotrimazole. *Archives of Dermatology, 115,* 322–323.

Rounds, M.C., & Papas, A.S. (1991). Preventive dentistry for the older adult. In A.S. Papas, L.C. Niessen, & H.H. Chauncey (Eds.), *Geriatric dentistry: Aging and oral health* (pp. 323–325). St. Louis: Mosby–Year Book.

Rugh, J.D., Barghi, N., & Drago, C.J. (1984). Experimental occlusal discrepancies and nocturnal bruxism. *Journal of Prosthetic Dentistry, 51,* 548–553.

Santos, R., Shanfeld, J., Casamassimo, P. (1996). Serum antibody response to Actinobacillus actinomycetemcomitans in Down's syndrome. *Special Care in Dentistry, 16,* 80–83.

Scheutzel, P. (1996). Etiology of erosion: Intrinsic factors. *European Journal of Oral Science, 104,* 178–190.

Schmidt, S.M., Leach, M., Nicolaci, A.B., Sutton, R.D., & O'Donnell, J.P. (1981). The dental health educator and programs for institutions with persons who are mentally retarded. *Special Care in Dentistry, 1,* 174–178.

Scott, A., Marsh, L., & Stokes, M.L. (1998). A survey of oral health in a population of adults with developmental disabilities: Comparison with a national oral health survey of the general population. *Australian Dental Journal, 43,* 257–261.

Stabholz, A., Shapira, J., Shur, D., Friedman, M., Guberman, R., & Sela, M.W. (1991). Local application of sustained-release delivery system of chlorhexidine in Down's syndrome population. *Clinical Preventive Dentistry, 13,* 9–14.

Stiefel, D.J., Truelove, E.L., Chin, M.W., & Mandel, L.S. (1992). Efficacy of chlorhexidine swabbing in oral health care for people with severe disabilities. *Special Care in Dentistry, 12,* 57–62.

Stiefel, D.J., Truelove, E.L., Chin, M.W., Zhu, Z.C., & Lerrox, B.G. (1995). Chlorhexidine swabbing applications under various conditions of use in preventive oral care for persons with disabilities. *Special Care in Dentistry, 15,* 159–165.

Stookey, G.K., & Beiswinger, B.B. (1999). Topical fluoride therapy. In N.O. Harris & F. Garcia-Godoy (Eds.), *Primary preventive dentistry* (5th ed., pp. 199–241). Stamford, CT: Appleton & Lange.

Tesini, D.A., & Fenton, S.J. (1994). Oral health needs of persons with physical or mental disabilities. *Dental Clinics of North America, 38,* 483–498.

Wilson, C.W. (1980). Food sensitivities, taste changes, aphthous ulcers and atopic symptoms in allergic disease. *Annals of Allergy, 44,* 302–307.

Yoder, K.M., & Schimmele, R.G. (1997). The oral health of Indiana's independent, disabled adults. *Journal of the Indiana Dental Association, 76*(3), 7–11.

Youngson, R.M. (1992). *Dictionary of medicine.* Glasgow: HarperCollins.

19

Community-Oriented Assessment of and Interventions for Mental Health Needs

Sally-Ann Cooper

As people with intellectual disabilities age, their needs may change. It is important for families, caregivers, professionals, and caregiving organizations to understand how needs change, and it is important that each individual with intellectual disabilities has his or her needs met as fully as possible at each stage of his or her life. Administrators of services also must understand how health and social care needs change with age so that individuals receive appropriate, quality services. There has been a considerable increase in the life expectancy of people with intellectual disabilities; the average age at death has increased from 18 years in the 1930s to over 65 years in the 1990s (Carter & Jancar, 1983; Janicki, Dalton, Henderson, & Davidson, 1999; Puri, Lekh, Langa, Zaman, & Singh, 1995). More individuals are living into old age, and so it can be anticipated that a larger number of people with intellectual disabilities will experience changing needs associated with aging, including social care, physical health, and mental health. This chapter focuses on their mental health needs.

SPECIAL CONSIDERATIONS REGARDING CARE NEEDS
Dementia, depressive episodes, and anxiety disorders are prevalent conditions associated with aging among the general population and warrant particular care and specialist interventions. In addition, the presentation of psychiatric disorders in older

adults can be different from that of the younger population. Particular causes of psychiatric disorders are associated with older age, and prognosis of psychiatric disorders in older people may differ from that of younger people. Older people with intellectual disabilities may also have a differing range of mental health needs and service requirements when compared with younger adults with intellectual disabilities (Cooper, 1997a, 1997b). This suggests that special consideration should be given to the needs of older adults.

The life spans of people with certain different causes of intellectual disabilities (that relate to associated physical disorders) vary, as do the behavior phenotypes (psychiatric and behavioral associations) of specific causes of intellectual disabilities. Psychiatric associations may occur as a result of genetic factors, cerebral dysfunction, or epilepsy: These factors cause both intellectual disabilities and psychiatric disorders (e.g., Prader-Willi syndrome is associated with intellectual disabilities and with psychosis; Down syndrome is associated with intellectual disabilities and with dementia). People with some causes of intellectual disabilities do not live as long as people with other causes of intellectual disabilities. The main reason for shortened life span of some groups is the multiple physical disorders that are also associated with some causes of intellectual disabilities (due to common causation—chiefly genetic factors—of both the intellectual disabilities and the physical disorders). For example, obesity (as well as intellectual disabilities) is a feature of Prader-Willi syndrome, and extreme obesity causes a range of health-related disorders (e.g., diabetes and atheroma) that reduce life span; Down syndrome is associated with congenital heart disease and predisposition to chest infections, which may reduce life span. People with mild intellectual disabilities of unknown cause are less likely to have physical disorders than those with certain syndromes and so enjoy a longer life. Consequently, there are population differences between older and younger adults in terms of cause of intellectual disability. This also may contribute to population differences with regard to associated psychiatric and behavior disorders and also the level of intellectual disabilities (as these differ for different causes of intellectual disabilities).

Some specialized care services may provide care specifically for older people with intellectual disabilities; but when people with intellectual disabilities age, they are often a minority in their social care environment. Many will have moved into residential care homes or other supported living arrangements when they lose their parents or when parents are no longer able to provide daily care. There is a diversity of care arrangements for older people with intellectual disabilities. Some use services developed for the general population of older people, others use services developed for adults with intellectual disabilities; in both environments, the older person with intellectual disabilities is likely to be in the minority. One potential consequence of this is that mental health needs might be overlooked or wrongly ascribed to being "normal" for that person; hence, assessment and intervention might not be sought for the individual. In environments that are designed for the general population of older people, mental health needs of the person with intellectual disabilities may be inadvertently thought to be a typical aspect of intellectual disabilities. In environments that are designed for adults with intellectual disabilities, mental health needs may in error be thought to be a typical part of aging (Cooper, 1997a).

Families and caregivers need access to accurate knowledge of the types of health needs experienced by older people with intellectual disabilities and of the availability of treatments, interventions, and supports. Professionals also must have an accurate knowledge base, and there is a need for flexibility and experience within the health services.

CAUSES OF MENTAL HEALTH NEEDS

There are two stages to psychiatric assessment: 1) determining the range of psychiatric symptoms and signs that the person has (i.e., the descriptive psychopathology), which can be classified into a number of possible descriptive diagnoses, and 2) determining the cause of the disorder (i.e., the causes of the person's mental health needs). Psychiatric disorders are often multifactorial in origin. The treatment care plan is devised, in an individualized way, taking into account both the descriptive diagnosis and the presumed causes. Psychiatrists commonly use two frameworks to conceptualize the causes of psychiatric disorders. These are the division into biological (physical), psychological, social, and developmental risk factors and the division into predisposing, precipitating, and maintaining factors. Using these two frameworks can be helpful when considering the vulnerability of older people with intellectual disabilities to psychiatric disorders. Within each of the categories, one can consider the risk factors for psychiatric disorders that are relevant to the whole population, the risk factors that are of particular relevance to older people, and the risk factors that are of particular relevance to adults with intellectual disabilities.

Each individual is different, so assessments must be individualized. Whereas a particular risk factor may cause a particular psychiatric disorder in one person, it may not in another person. Because the cause of a psychiatric disorder in any one person often is multifactorial, assessment should always be conducted in a structured way and cover all areas: biological, psychological, social, and developmental. If a relevant risk factor is identified, the assessment should still be completed to cover all other possible relevant areas. Examples of risk factors are listed next. This is not a comprehensive list of all possible risk factors, but it illustrates examples within a commonly used framework.

Biological/Physical

- *General population:* Genetic predisposition to psychiatric illness/family history of psychiatric illness; relationship between epilepsy and psychiatric illness (e.g., schizophrenia); physical disorders associated with psychiatric illness (e.g., disseminated sclerosis, carcinoma of the breast, hepatitis, mononucleosis, thyroid disorder, parathyroid disorders, pain); head injury; drugs (e.g., antihypertensives, steroids, beta-agonists, antiepileptics, anticholinergics)
- *Older people:* Neurodegenerative disorders (e.g., Parkinson's disease); cardiovascular disorders and other physical disorders associated with psychiatric illness (e.g., hearing impairment); increased sensitivity to drugs; physical frailty with loss of independence and confidence
- *People with intellectual disabilities:* Behavior phenotypes (e.g., dementia and depression are associated with Down syndrome; anxiety is associated with fragile X syndrome; anxiety and depression are associated with phenylketonuria; self-injury is associated with Lesch Nyhan syndrome, Smith Magenis syndrome, and Prader-Willi syndrome); epilepsy; cerebral dysfunction; sensory impairments; other physical disorders related to the cause of intellectual disabilities that are associated with psychiatric illness (e.g., hypothyroidism is associated with Down syndrome and can cause psychiatric illness)

Psychological

- *General population:* Adverse events in infancy and childhood that affect personality development, predisposing people to psychiatric disorders in adult life, low self-esteem, poor self-image and low self-confidence, and restricted coping strategies (e.g., childhood sexual abuse, neglect or physical abuse, loss of parent in childhood)
- *Older people:* Adjustment to loss of youth and physical health; bereavement of friends, family, and spouse; and retirement
- *People with intellectual disabilities:* Adverse events that affect personality development (e.g., rejection in infancy and childhood, difficulties with parent–child bonding, moves between foster homes, institutional wards, residential schools, placement breakdown, lack of consistent parental figure to internalize); bullying, neglect, exploitation, and abuse; and problems between the balance of protection versus autonomy/choices

Social

- *General population:* Life events, unemployment, poor housing, poverty, social isolation, lack of confidants, and level of expressed emotion within families
- *Older people:* Social isolation, poverty, loss of social role, and lack of transportation
- *People with intellectual disabilities:* Lack of opportunities for occupation, recreation, and education; lack of transportation; lack of confidants; restricted social networks; lack of choice; poverty of environment; stigma; and frequent changes in residential and senior center staff with lack of consistency and frequent loss

Developmental

- *People with intellectual disabilities:* Limited communication skills and behavior patterns reflecting developmental age

PREVALENCE OF MENTAL HEALTH NEEDS

There is limited information from which one can draw conclusions on the prevalence of mental health needs in older people with intellectual disabilities. Although there have been several studies, few have taken a population-based approach and individually assessed all study participants. When this has been undertaken, other differences between study methodology limit comparisons, such as the age range of the participants and the diagnostic criteria used for psychiatric disorder. Corbett (1979) studied 110 adults with intellectual disabilities age 60 years and older using criteria of the *International Classification of Diseases, Eighth Revision* (World Health Organization, 1974). Lund (1985) studied 94 Danish adults with intellectual disabilities age 45 years and older and used modified criteria from the *Diagnostic and Statistical Manual of Mental Disorders, Third Edition* (American Psychiatric Association, 1980). Moss and Patel (1993) studied 105 adults with intellectual disabilities age 50 years and older using criteria from the *Diagnostic and Statistical Manual of Mental Disorders, Third Edition, Revised* (American Psychiatric Association, 1987). Cooper (1997b) studied 134 people with intellectual disabilities age 65 years and older using criteria from the Diagnostic Criteria for Research version of the *International Classification of Diseases, Tenth Revision* (World Health Organization, 1993). Their findings suggest that mental health needs are prevalent among older adults with intellectual disabilities and include the full range of disorders. Dementia and anxiety disorders are common, and depression is frequent. Schizophrenia, mania, and obsessive-compulsive disorder, although less common disorders, also occur in older adults. The studies varied in terms of the findings for the prevalence of behavior disorders, possibly because of the use of differing definitions and measurement instruments. However, behavior disorders have been found to be as prevalent in older as in younger adults, when the same methods of assessment are used (Cooper, 1997b; Corbett, 1979). Similarly, autism is found in similar numbers of older as younger adults.

Consequently, it seems that older adults with intellectual disabilities require access to health care for disorders that are similar to those that occur in younger adults with intellectual disabilities, but they also have additional health needs related to aging. Of particular note are dementia and anxiety disorders. Dementia is associated with Down syndrome (Holland, 1999; Holland & Oliver, 1995; Oliver & Holland, 1985) and occurs in a larger proportion of people with Down syndrome when they reach middle and older age. However, it seems that people with intellectual disabilities of other causes are also at increased risk for dementia when compared with the age-matched general population. This is a replicated finding when comparisons are drawn across the population-based studies that have included individual assessments of study participants, with rates for dementia being approximately 12% for people age 50 years and older (Cooper, 1997b; Lund, 1985; Moss & Patel, 1993) and approximately 22% for those age 65 years and older (Cooper 1997b; Lund, 1985). These rates remain high even after excluding people with Down syndrome, as the older cohorts included few people with Down syndrome. Although the present population structure means that few people with intellectual disabilities require services for dementia, for reasons discussed previously, the numbers are increasing.

ASSESSMENT OF MENTAL HEALTH NEEDS

Assessment is the first necessary step when an older person acquires mental health needs. The assessment is undertaken to describe and understand the cause of the person's needs and to be able to devise the most effective treatment care plans. Assessments should, therefore, be undertaken when a person acquires new problems or when management plans for existing problems are not proving to be effective.

A change in the behavior of an older person with intellectual disabilities almost always indicates a health need. Consequently, changed behavior (of any type) should be assumed to indicate ill health, unless a full assessment has demonstrated otherwise. Change in behavior includes the onset of new symptoms and behaviors, the exacerbation of preexisting symptoms or behaviors, or sometimes a reduction in behaviors that are typical for that person. Hence, the onset of physical aggression in a person who is not usually aggressive, an increase in severity and frequency of a person's usual aggression, and a reduction in the severity and frequency of physical aggression all may be indicative of ill health (physical or psychiatric). Similarly, repeated early-morning waking by a person who usually sleeps well, repeated waking even earlier in the morning by a person who always wakes early, and repeated sleeping late in the morning in a person who usually wakes early all may indicate physical or psychiatric ill health. Relatives or caregivers are advised to seek advice from a health professional should the person with intellectual disabilities change his or her behavior.

Psychiatric assessment includes determining the presenting psychopathology to make the descriptive diagnosis and then establishing the cause. Delineating psychopathology requires reference to the person's usual state for each symptom to establish whether it (e.g., waking early in the morning) is indeed a "symptom" or a longstanding trait that is usual for the person. Although some symptoms may always be considered atypical (e.g., hearing voices talking together about you when there is no one there, referred to as *third-person auditory hallucinations*), this is not the case for the majority of symptoms. This is one of the main differences between psychiatric assessments that are undertaken with a person of average ability, whereby symptom checklists may be used by untrained staff, and psychiatric assessments that are undertaken with a person with intellectual disabilities, whereby symptoms checklists used by untrained staff have limitations. Dementia is an easily understood example: A low score on an ability test (e.g., the Mini-Mental State Examination [Folstein, Folstein, & McHugh, 1975]) may suggest the presence of dementia or acute confusion in a member of the general population but could not be used in the same way to evaluate a person with intellectual disabilities, who may always have had the same low score on the test. This is true not just for dementia but for almost all psychiatric disorders in people with intellectual disabilities.

In view of the detail involved in accurately measuring psychopathology, it is essential that information be available from an informant with background knowledge of the person with an intellectual disability (i.e., someone who knows the person's usual personality). In addition, when the cause of a person's descriptive diagnosis is being established, information is required not just on current factors (e.g., any other health needs they have, use of drugs, social circumstances and life events, developmental factors) but also about his or her past (e.g., past health needs, illnesses, and treatments; past and present health among family members; details of the individual's personal history from conception through childhood and adult life). Family members, particularly parents, usually have this detailed level of knowledge about their relative with intellectual disabilities. However, many older adults with intellectual disabilities will have lost their parents and may no longer be in contact with living relatives. In such a situation, the person best qualified to contribute to the individual's assessment is the one who knows her or him best now and has known her or him the longest. Sometimes, this means that information has to be collected from several informants to complete an assessment. Such a psychiatric approach clearly differs from the well-established psychological approach of functional analysis of behavior. These two different assessment approaches can often be used in a complementary way, particularly for people whose presentation seems to be complex.

The assessment of mental health needs, or change in behavior, necessarily will include some assessments of physical health (to establish the cause of the descriptive diagnosis). A good example of this is the need to distinguish psychiatric disorders from certain types of epilepsy (e.g., complex partial seizures) and from possible side effects of antiepileptic drugs. In view of the known interactions between antiepileptic drugs and psychotropic drugs, knowledge of both is also required when assessments are undertaken and during prescribing, in addition to awareness that psychotropic drugs affect seizure threshold and so can affect epilepsy control. During assessment, physical health is usually assessed during the history taking (by inquiring about sets of symptoms associated with physical disorders, health problems in the present and past, and drug treatments in the present and past), sometimes by undertaking a full or limited (i.e., only certain bodily systems) physical examination and by the use of special investigations. Which special investigations are required depends on the information gathered in the history and physical examination. When an older person presents with mental health needs, the minimal level of special investigations undertaken should include tests to check a full blood count (e.g., to detect anemia), urea and electrolytes (e.g., to detect renal failure), liver function, calcium level, and thyroid function. In some circumstances, other tests may be required (e.g., other blood tests, electrocardiogram, computed tomography head scan, magnetic resonance imaging head scan, electroencephalogram). The purpose of such tests is to determine whether there are any physical causes for the descriptive diagnosis that warrant treatment.

MANAGEMENT OF MENTAL HEALTH NEEDS

The treatments, interventions, and supports that are required to manage the mental health needs of an older person with intellectual disabilities depend on the findings of the assessment. Some elements are always important. These include offering full information to caregivers or family members and the person with intellectual disabilities as far as she or he is able to understand the cause of the problem and discussing the likely benefits and possible side effects of treatments. When possible, information about how the problem may progress in the future and the services and supports that are available can also be useful. Caregivers may have concerns and questions, which need to be fully explored and answered as completely as is possible. Discussions of diagnosis can sometimes have a high emotional impact and so take time and must be undertaken in a sensitive way. Almost all treatment approaches require the support of the person's caregiver(s), whether this is simply helping the person to take the right dose of medication at the right time or implementing specific behavioral care plans. Similarly, evaluating the effectiveness of treatment plans is reliant on information and observations of caregiver(s), so, again, their support and agreement to any proposed treatment plan is essential if it is to succeed. Implementation of treatment plans often involves working across several environments or agencies, as well as with families or residential caregivers and directly with the person with intellectual disabilities. Recognizing caregivers' needs is also important and may include time spent discussing concerns, worries, and stresses and practical support, such as setting up regular respite care.

Whatever the type and cause of the person's mental health need, correcting any other additional problems is likely to be of benefit in terms of maximizing functional ability (e.g., correcting anemia, providing eye glasses and hearing aids, providing properly fitting footwear, cutting toenails).

Providing appropriate opportunities for occupation, education, and recreation is essential for an individual to achieve a good quality of life, regardless of her or his mental health state. These areas of social care, however, assume even greater importance for individuals with certain types of mental health needs. For example, a person with dementia requires the opportunities to have an enjoyable, meaningful, and quality life and also benefits from the opportunities to practice individual skills in social environments; a person who is recovering from a depressive episode may gain confidence from relearning skills lost during the episode and may benefit from reintegration into leisure activities.

In addition to the general approaches described previously, the older person with mental health needs is likely to require specific treatments or interventions. The treatment plan will often be multifaceted, and it is unusual for only one treatment to be implemented. Delivery of treatment plans often requires more than one health care professional, together with the person with intellectual disabilities and her or his family or caregiver(s), and staff working for other agencies, charities, or advocacy groups. The following sections detail examples of specific treatment approaches.

Pharmacotherapy

Drugs can be effective in the treatment of certain disorders. The correct choice of drug will depend on the person's type of psychiatric disorder, the cause of a person's intellectual disabilities, and any other physical disorders they may have; additional consideration should be given to the likely efficacy of the drug balanced against possible side effects. Possible drug treatments include antipsychotic drugs, antidepressant drugs, mood-stabilizing drugs, antimanic drugs, anxiolytic drugs, cognitively enhancing drugs, and drugs from other groups that can have an effect on mental state (e.g., certain antihypertensive drugs, antiepileptic drugs, antiarrhythmic drugs). In the United Kingdom, antipsychotic drugs are often used for their anxiolytic properties because of their efficacy and because of the tolerance that is developed and the addiction associated with other anxiolytic drugs, which are, therefore, prescribed only infrequently and in special circumstances (e.g., benzodiazepines). Within each group of drugs are several different classes (drugs that are thought to have similar properties), so the exact choice of drug will depend on the person's individual circumstances. Often the choice is guided by the drug's side effect profile (i.e., selecting the drug with the lowest risk of side effects for a given level of efficacy). Sometimes it is determined through knowledge of a person's cause of intellectual disability (e.g., the first-line antidepressant to be used for a person with Down syndrome who becomes depressed is a selective serotonin reuptake inhibitor, in view of the person's relative serotonin deficiency; other classes of antidepressants and augmentations with lithium or use of other mood-stabilizing drugs are second-line approaches). Sometimes choice is determined through a consideration of a person's other health needs (e.g., a beta-blocker would not be prescribed for anxiety if a person had asthma; certain antipsychotic drugs would be avoided if the person just had a myocardial infarction).

Mental health disorders that may respond to pharmacotherapy include depression, mania, anxiety, obsessive-compulsive disorder, schizophrenia or other delusional disorders, possibly dementia (although the outcome of results from treatment trials with people with intellectual disabilities are still awaited), tic disorders, behavior disorders in some individuals, and certain aspects of autism. In most of these cases, however, it would be usual for pharmacotherapy to be combined with other types of treatment to maximize treatment outcome.

All drugs, including those that can be purchased over the counter, carry the risk that the person may develop side effects. The majority of people do not develop side effects to drugs prescribed to treat mental health needs, but a small but significant proportion of people do. It is difficult to predict which individuals will develop drug side effects unless they have been treated with the same drug or class of drug previously. Therefore, it is important that the prescribing doctor must alert relatives or caregivers to the possible side effects and ask them to check whether any such problems occur. It is essential that medical follow-up be routinely provided when a person with intellectual disabilities is prescribed drugs for mental health needs. This is required in the long as well as short term. Such follow-up is required to assess whether the drugs are effective (if not, they should be changed or discontinued) to assess whether side effects are occurring and, if so, to reduce or eliminate side effects by changes to the drug, either by using additional drugs or discontinuing the drug (depending on the individual's circumstances). When drugs are prescribed on a "repeat prescription" over a period of years, without specialist follow-up, there is the potential for problems. Ultimately, however, this is dependent on local health care resources. In the United Kingdom and

Ireland, such a role would be provided by a psychiatrist specializing in intellectual disabilities, but in other countries, general psychiatrists or neurologists may provide this specialist role.

After assessment, the management of mental health needs should review other drug treatments that the person is receiving and whether these are effective and still required. It may be possible to reduce or withdraw some drug treatments. Some drugs prescribed for physical disorders can mimic or precipitate mental health needs, so a review of drugs is always required as part of the assessment process.

Electroconvulsive Treatment

Electroconvulsive treatment (ECT) is rapid and highly effective and usually is used for the treatment of people with very severe depression. It is used when there is a need for rapid recovery (e.g., the person is not drinking fluids because of the severity of his or her depression, and so it would not be safe to wait for antidepressant drugs to work) or when other treatments for depression have failed. ECT is given as a course of treatments, usually two per week, evaluated at weekly intervals to judge how long the course should be (6–10 treatments is average, but sometimes fewer or more are required). ECT is given under brief general anesthetic and with the use of muscle relaxant drugs to avoid problems associated with seizure activity, such as those witnessed when ECT was first introduced decades ago. There are risks associated with ECT, should the person react adversely to the anesthetic.

Psychological Treatments

There is a diverse range of psychological treatments. At a simple level, this may include supportive psychotherapy—listening to and empathizing with a person's problems and trying to educate and support. More specific interventions include psychodynamic psychotherapies and behavioral psychotherapies. Behavioral psychotherapies include many different types of interventions, depending on a person's need, and are beyond the scope of this chapter. Specific behavioral treatments may include anxiety management training or for those at a lower developmental level, the use of semihypnotic forms of relaxation, Snoezelen rooms, soft music, aromatherapy, foot spas, and so forth. For individuals whose anxiety disorder includes a phobic component, desensitization programs using a hierarchical approach can be helpful. Modified response-prevention programs may be helpful for individuals with obsessive-compulsive disorder. Sleep hygiene programs can be of benefit for some people. Behavioral programs may be devised after conducting a functional analysis of behavior. Reward programs can be meaningful and helpful for some people.

Social Treatments

Changes in a person's social milieu can be of benefit in the care of mental health needs. Poverty of environment may need to be addressed, but overstimulating environments also can be disadvantageous for some people. Provision of occupational, educational, and recreational opportunities can be highly beneficial as previously discussed. Social work with the person within the family or care environment can also be beneficial for some people.

Developmental Treatments

Developmental approaches can be beneficial for some people with mental health needs. This may include developmental approaches to skill acquisition and retention and specific treatments for maladaptive behaviors associated with a person's developmental level (e.g., head banging). The development of verbal or alternative communication skills and approaches can be of particular importance for some people. Through skill development, confidence may be enhanced. The original focus on specific goals may lead in a subtle way to the gradual development of a therapeutic, trusting relationship with the health care worker, which may bring benefits for other psychological work.

MANAGEMENT OF DEMENTIA

The management of dementia warrants special comment because of its prevalence among older people with intellectual disabilities and middle-age people with Down syndrome and also because of the public misconception that dementia is untreatable. Dementia is a progressive disorder associated with loss of cognitive functioning and skills and onset of noncognitive symptoms, such as change in sleep pattern, anxiety, loss of concentration, apathy, psychotic symptoms, agitation, and aggression. However, individuals with intellectual disabilities and dementia can still enjoy a rewarding and high quality of life, bring love and pleasure to their families, and contribute as valuable members of society. The likelihood of this is enhanced when the appropriate care is made available. It is essential that social care needs be addressed and regularly reviewed because the person's needs change as the dementia progresses. The general elements of care introduced in the "Management of Mental Health Needs" section of this chapter are equally relevant in treating a person with dementia as for treating individuals with other mental health needs. These include the following:

- Maximizing functional ability through treating all other possible problems
- Discussing the person's problem; providing information and education
- Providing emotional and practical support for families and caregivers
- Providing educational, recreational, and occupational opportunities to enhance quality of life and skill retention

In addition, the treatment care plan for a person with intellectual disabilities and dementia should minimize the cognitive features of dementia. This includes using reality orientation techniques, putting identifying pictures on doors, using daily pictorial planners and timetables with regular verbal reinforcement, using reminiscence groups, using pictorial life history books, practicing skills, and possibly using cognition-enhancing drugs.

The treatment care plan should also focus on minimizing noncognitive symptoms of dementia. This presence of noncognitive symptoms of dementia can cause significant distress for people with an intellectual disability and their family or caregiver but is also the area within dementia management in which health care professionals can make a significant difference to symptoms. The exact treatment plans that are required depend on the problem and symptoms and the cause of the symptoms (i.e., a full assessment is always required before a treatment care plan can be devised). For example, a person is experiencing the onset of physical aggression toward her or his caregiver, in the context of a dementing illness, whereas previously she or he was never aggressive. The aggression may be due to a number of reasons:

- A response to hallucinations or delusions (this symptom might be alleviated by prescribing antipsychotic drugs, provided they do not affect the person's cognitive functioning)

- Aggression as a motor component or agitation associated with extreme anxiety (this symptom might be alleviated by prescribing antipsychotic drugs, anxiolytic drugs, and behavioral approaches to relaxation)
- A change in sleep habit (e.g., the aggression may occur only during the night when the person gets up and is insistent on leaving for the day center, thinking it is morning, and her or his caregiver tries to encourage her or him back into bed; this may benefit from sleep hygiene programs, other behavioral care plans for the caregiver to follow, and, in some situations pharmacotherapy)
- Catastrophic reactions, whereby the demands being placed on the individual with intellectual disabilities and dementia now outstrip his or her capacity to deal with them, resulting in seemingly "unprovoked" episodes of aggression (this symptom may be handled by offering educational and behavioral advice to the caregiver and may also require practical support such as respite care and day care away from the person's home)
- A superimposed depressive episode (this would require standard treatment for depression in its own right)

Management is best provided within the person's own home, using a multiprofessional, multiagency approach (see also Chapter 21). Moving the person to other caregiving environments can increase disorientation and always requires careful planning when such moves are unavoidable. The full agreement of relatives and caregivers regarding which treatment care plans are implemented is essential. It is important to recognize the needs of relatives and caregivers as well as those of the person with intellectual disabilities and dementia and for the appropriate support to be made available.

In the future, strategies for the prevention of dementia may become as important, or more important, than the management of dementia itself. Many factors influence the risk that a person has for developing dementia. Examples include family history (genetics), cause of intellectual disabilities, head injury earlier in life, the number of additional physical disorders as well as specific physical disorders (e.g., Parkinson's disease, cardiovascular disease), smoking history (tobacco use), hormonal factors and drug history, use of anti-inflammatory drugs and antioxidant drugs, age, and possibly gender. Some of these factors may be modifiable and provide an avenue in the future to identify ways to reduce an individual's risk for acquiring dementia.

MENTAL HEALTH SERVICES FOR OLDER PEOPLE WITH INTELLECTUAL DISABILITIES

Health services vary in different countries and within countries. However, the structure of local services is less important than the function of the services. If older people with intellectual disabilities are to obtain quality specialist health care, then it is essential that there be an identified local provider who is responsible for meeting these needs or for making special arrangements to meet the needs. The needs of this older population differ from the younger cohort of adults with intellectual disabilities because of different prevalences of psychiatric disorders (e.g., dementia), different prevalences of underlying causes of intellectual disabilities and levels of intellectual disabilities, differences in associated physical disorders, gender distribution, and social care provision. Their needs also differ from those of older people of average ability in terms of the types and distribution of mental health needs and needs associated with intellectual disabilities. Consequently, current health services for younger people with intellectual disabilities and for older people of average ability are unlikely in isolation to be able to meet the needs of older people with intellectual disabilities. The small population size presents difficulties in the development of specialized services. Solutions may lie in health services being flexible and working collaboratively with other health care providers and other agencies that work with people with intellectual disabilities. Some guidelines have been produced by the Royal College of Psychiatrists (1997) of the United Kingdom.

Often, when relatives or caregivers note that a person's needs have changed, the first contact point is either a general practitioner or a community intellectual disabilities team (see also Chapter 20). It is essential that these professionals have either the skills to undertake the required work or the knowledge to refer to the specialist services where the necessary assessments can be undertaken so that the appropriate treatment care plans can be devised and implemented.

CONCLUSIONS

Because of the changing life span of people with intellectual disabilities, more older people will require support, assessment, and treatment as a result of mental health needs. At present, the trends in life span can be noted and the mental health needs of the current cohort of older people with intellectual disabilities can be described, but anticipation of the exact level of need in the future is speculative. However, one can state that there is a need for greater awareness of the mental health needs of older adults with intellectual disabilities; there is a need to educate caregivers about possible mental health needs and to encourage them to seek input from health professionals when individuals with intellectual disabilities change behavior. Specialized intellectual disabilities health services need to be able to respond to such requests and deliver effective health care. The development of effective prevention strategies and enhancement of protective factors to reduce mental health needs also require greater emphasis.

REFERENCES

American Psychiatric Association. (1980). Diagnostic and statistical manual of mental disorders (3rd ed.). Washington, DC: Author.
Carter, G., & Jancar, J. (1983). Mortality in the mentally handicapped: A fifty year survey at the Stoke Park group of hospitals (1930–1980). Journal of Mental Deficiency Research, 27, 143–156.
Cooper, S.-A. (1997a). Deficient health and social services for elderly people with learning disabilities. Journal of Intellectual Disabilities Research, 41, 331–338.
Cooper, S.-A. (1997b). Epidemiology of psychiatric disorders in elderly compared with younger adults with learning disabilities. British Journal of Psychiatry, 170, 375–380.
Corbett, J.A. (1979). Psychiatric morbidity and mental retardation. In F.E. James & R.P. Snaith (Eds.), Psychiatric illness and mental handicap (pp. 11–25). London: Gaskell.
Folstein, M.F., Folstein, S.E., & McHugh, P.R. (1975). "Mini-mental state": A practical method for grading the cognitive state of patients for the clinician. Journal of Psychiatric Research, 12, 189–198.
Holland, A.J. (1999). Down's syndrome. In M.P. Janicki & A.J. Dalton (Eds.), Dementia, aging, and intellectual disabilities: A handbook (pp. 183–197). Philadelphia: Brunner/Mazel.
Holland, A.J., & Oliver, C. (1995). Down's syndrome and the links with Alzheimer's disease. Journal of Neurology, Neurosurgery, and Psychiatry, 59, 111–115.
Janicki, M.P., Dalton, A.J., Henderson, C.M., & Davidson, P.W. (1999). Mortality and morbidity among older adults with intellectual disability: Health services considerations. Disability and Rehabilitation, 21, 284–294.
Lund, J. (1985). The prevalence of psychiatric morbidity in mentally retarded adults. Acta Psychiatrica Scandinavica, 72, 563–570.

Moss, S., & Patel, P.C. (1993). The prevalence of mental illness in people with intellectual disability over 50 years of age, and the diagnostic importance of information from carers. *Irish Journal of Psychology, 14,* 110–129.

Oliver, C., & Holland, A.J. (1985). Down's syndrome and Alzheimer's disease: A review. *Psychological Medicine, 16,* 307–322.

Puri, B.K., Lekh, S.K., Langa, A., Zaman, R., & Singh, I. (1995). Mortality in a hospitalised mentally handicapped population: A 10-year survey. *Journal of Intellectual Disability Research, 39,* 442–446.

Royal College of Psychiatrists. (1997). *Meeting the mental health needs of people with learning disability. Part 2. Elderly people with learning disability* (Council Report CR56). London: Gaskell.

World Health Organization. (1974). *Mental disorders: Glossary and guide to their classification in accordance with the eighth revision of the International Classification of Diseases (ICD-8).* Geneva: Author.

World Health Organization. (1993). *ICD-10 classification of mental and behavioral disorders: Diagnostic criteria for research.* Geneva: Author.

20

Comprehensive Adult
and Geriatric Assessment

C. Michael Henderson and Philip W. Davidson

Neither *old age* nor *intellectual disability* is a medical diagnosis. The tremendous medical and functional heterogeneity seen in people who are older or who have intellectual disabilities makes it difficult to generalize about the specific health care and social supports needs of these populations. Most older people and most people with intellectual disabilities can obtain satisfactory health care from primary care providers without special training in geriatrics or developmental disabilities. However, additional health care expertise may be needed by specific older people, for example, those who experience functional decline secondary to age-related conditions. Likewise, children and adults with intellectual disabilities may need specialty evaluation for conditions that cause functional decline and that are associated with the underlying cause of the intellectual disabilities (hence termed *syndrome-specific*) or that result from associated developmental disabilities.

Significant reforms have resulted in changes in the residential and habilitative supports of people with intellectual disabilities (see Trent, 1994, for a description of these changes in the United States). These reforms have led to a near convergence of the life expectancy of most people with intellectual disability with that of the general population (Janicki, Dalton, Henderson, & Davidson, 1999). Increasing numbers of older people with intellectual disabilities have resulted in increased risks for acquiring age-related conditions that can cause functional decline. Sweeny and Wilson (1979) recognized the potential combinations of impairing conditions caused by intellectual disabilities, syndrome-specific conditions, and concurrent noncognitive developmental disabilities, along with that caused by age-related conditions. The term *double jeopardy* was used to describe this overlap. As neither aging nor intellectual disability is an inherently jeopardizing situation but rather a manifestation of the continuum of the universal human need for societal supports, this term has not been widely used. However, Walz, Harper, and Wilson (1986) acknowledged that new clinical and social services would need to be developed to address the needs of many aging people with intellectual disabilities. It is the argument of this chapter that certain older adults (and some younger adults) with intellectual disabilities (e.g., those who exhibit functional decline) may need expert and comprehensive evaluation that focuses on both general age-related and developmental disability–related issues.

Because developmental disabilities by definition occur during infancy, childhood, and adolescence, medical issues associated with intellectual disability are well recognized within pediatric medicine. The comprehensive and interdisciplinary assessment of children with intellectual disabilities and other developmental disabilities has been well developed since the 1960s (see Farrell & Pimental, 1996). The development of University Affiliated Programs in the 1960s (Magrab & Schmidt, 1980) and the enactment of federally mandated educational supports for children with special needs in the 1970s (Tucker & Goldstein, 1991) provided major prompts for the development of this intervention. Pediatricians-in-training acquire a familiarity with physical developmental disabilities or syndrome-specific issues, seen in many younger people with intellectual disabilities, through patient-based clinical training provided by developmental pediatricians as well as in texts (i.e., Batshaw, 1997; Capute & Accardo, 1996; and Pueschel & Pueschel, 1992). In addition, pediatrics has always acknowledged the importance of the biopsychosocial development of children. One of the unfortunate legacies of institutionalization is that academic internists who teach trainees may lack familiarity with medical issues associated with intellectual disabilities. Also, an emphasis on organ system–based subspecialties may not be conducive to the teaching of broader issues of normal and atypical adult development. Family medicine has avoided some of these pitfalls. Having numerous interactions between medical providers who treat adults with and without intellectual disabilities is a new phenomenon for both internists and family physicians who are based in the community. Finally, medical providers who are trained to see adults may have difficulty obtaining medical histories or conducting physical examinations on people who are nonverbal or not cooperative.

FUNCTIONAL CAPABILITY AND MEDICAL CONDITIONS

Functional capability is an integral concept in understanding intellectual disabilities. The new conceptual paradigm of intellectual disability presented by the American Association on Mental Retardation (Luckasson et al., 1992) is based on the determination of adaptive behavior limitations and needs for supports, as well as on IQ score criteria. Down syndrome is an example of a condition in which relatively high rates of syndrome-specific medical problems can worsen the adaptive limitations posed by the intellectual disability (Ziring et al., 1988). Primary care internists and family physicians who see adults with Down syndrome may not know that conditions such as hearing and visual impairments, hypothyroidism, and cervical spinal myelopathy are relatively common and, therefore, may erroneously attribute functional impairments to behavioral and cognitive issues associated with the intellectual disability. Chicoine, McGuire, and Rubin (1999) described a comprehensive assessment program for adults with

Down syndrome. An interdisciplinary team, including a family physician, social worker, audiologist, and nutritionist, evaluated 148 adults with Down syndrome who presented with functional decline. In addition to behavior disorders, high rates of psychiatric conditions such as affective disorders or adjustment reactions were identified, as well as relatively high rates of probable Alzheimer's dementia, vitamin B_{12} deficiency, endocrinologic problems (especially hypothyroidism and menopause), and sensory impairments. In many cases, individuals required treatment of multiple concurrent conditions to return to functional baseline (Chicoine et al., 1999).

Functional capability is also an important issue in geriatric medicine. Functional capability has been defined as older people's "ability to participate in the arena of daily living" (Solomon, 1988, p. 342). More specific, conceptualizations posited by Kane and Kane (1981), Katz, Ford, Moskowitz, Jackson, and Jaffee (1963), and Lawton and Brody (1969) have led to an overarching concept of functional capability, incorporating discrete skills such as physical and mental abilities, skill areas such as activities of daily living (ADLs) and instrumental activities of daily living (IADLs), and more global capabilities such as engaging in social activities and using community resources and opportunities. The importance of function in geriatrics derives from the fact that although there is wide individual variability, declines in function are associated with older age. Pope and Tarlov (1991) described pronounced declines in basic life activity measures from ages 55 and older, with a 50% risk for developing a significant age-related disability by age 85. Geriatric medicine also acknowledges older age as a dynamic life stage. The maintenance of optimal functional capability is crucial for the developmental tasks of older people. The geriatric medicine perspective recognizes the interaction among age-related disease, the effects of normal aging, and the capability to act in the "arena of daily living" (for a text-length review, see Abeles, Gift, & Ory, 1994).

COMPREHENSIVE GERIATRIC ASSESSMENT

Comprehensive geriatric assessment (CGA) is an intervention that addresses, among other issues, problems that can cause functional impairment in older adults (American Geriatrics Society [AGS], 1999). CGA is typically a three-step process that begins with defining who is to be assessed, proceeds to carrying out the assessment and developing recommendations, and ends with disseminating or sometimes implementing the treatment recommendations. Gaitz and Baer (1970), Kane and Kane (1981), and Solomon (1988) emphasized the need for multifunctional diagnostic models to be used in the assessment of the biopsychosocial status of aging people. These models call for a comprehensive, time-intensive, and interdisciplinary approach, with assessment occurring across various functional domains. Team members, each with different skills in assessing physical and mental health and social and environmental issues, individually and collectively make findings and recommend treatment and services (Satin, 1994; for text-length reviews of geriatric assessment principles, see Gallo, Reichel, & Anderson, 2000; Rubenstein, Wieland, & Bernabei, 1995).

CGA outcomes have been described as diagnosing and prioritizing problems and developing prevention, treatment, and rehabilitation strategies that improve or maintain function, reduce unnecessary use of services, and prolong survival (Rubenstein, 1995). CGA models have been developed in a number of environments, including inpatient and hospital-based acute care and rehabilitation units, day hospital and nursing home programs, outpatient office-based programs, academic centers, and home health teams. Staffing of CGA teams differs according to model goals and environments; however, such teams minimally contain a physician, nurse, and medical social worker with geriatric population experience (Williams, 1987). Extended teams may include a mental health specialist, physical therapist, occupational therapist, dentist, nutritionist, podiatrist, audiologist, optometrist, and others. Individual model staffing is generally based on resources and personnel availability rather than on programmatic needs (AGS, 1999).

CGA efficacy is becoming increasingly better understood. A meta-analysis of the effectiveness of four office-based "ambulatory" CGA models was described by Stuck, Wieland, Rubenstein, Siu, and Adams (1995). A beneficial effect on the number or length of acute hospitalizations was noted in all four programs. Only one program measured physical and cognitive functional status on follow-up, with favorable results reported. In a large-scale examination of the need for CGA patient selection to improve functional outcomes, Cho et al. (1998) examined the role of specific chronic medical illnesses and conditions on the functional status of older people enrolled in an in-home CGA and preventive care program. Thirteen common and age-related chronic illnesses and conditions (hypertension, osteoarthritis, coronary artery disease, obesity, undernutrition, urinary incontinence, sleep disorders, falls, gait/balance disorders, hearing and visual impairments, depression, and unsafe home environment) were assessed annually by geriatric nurse practitioners in consultation with study geriatricians. Findings indicated that although functional status was equivalent in the participants at baseline, the presence of certain target conditions was associated with significant functional decline during the 3-year study period. Four conditions (coronary artery disease, gait/balance disorders, depression, and unsafe home environment) were linked with declines in IADLs, and four conditions (hypertension, urinary incontinence, gait/balance disorders, and depression) were associated with declines in ADLs. In addition to "patient targeting," the impact of CGA on the functional status of older patients is generally directly linked to the degree of patient care responsibility that is assumed by the CGA team after assessment (Rubenstein, 1995).

It has been observed that older adults with intellectual disability may have a variety of conditions that have the potential to cause functional decline. Generally, this information is derived either from smaller-group longitudinal studies, which have targeted specific age-related diagnoses, or from large-scale studies of the general health status of older people with intellectual disabilities within a geographical region. Examples of the former include the documentation, among older adults with intellectual disabilities, of relatively high rates of falls and fractures (Tannenbaum, Lipworth, & Baker, 1989), psychiatric disorders (Day, 1985), sensory impairments (Evenhuis, 1995), conditions that cause mobility impairments (Evenhuis, 1997), and dementia (Zigman, Schupf, Haveman, & Silverman, 1997). Janicki and Jacobson (1986) conducted a large-scale health survey of older adults with intellectual disabilities in New York state and found that potentially disabling medical and neuropsychiatric conditions were commonly reported. These findings have been confirmed in other large-scale studies (Ashman & Suttie, 1996; Hand, 1994; Van Schrojenstein Lantman-de Valk et al., 1997). Kapell, Nightengale, Lee, Zigman, and Schupf (1998) conducted a study of the prevalence of chronic medical conditions in 278 older people (age range, 45–72 years) with intellectual disabilities based on medical record reviews and caregiver interviews. In comparison with the general population, there was a comparable prevalence of several common age-related disorders (diabetes, ischemic heart disease, stroke, and ulcers) and an increased prevalence of thyroid disease, nonischemic heart disease, and sensory impairments. This study found significant differences in types of age-related disorders in people with intellectual disabilities with and without Down syndrome.

CGA models for people with intellectual disabilities have been described. Gambert, Crimmins, Cameron, Bacon-Prue, and Gupta (1988) reported on such a program and found that CGA provided more detailed clinical information than medical chart reviews. Carlsen, Galluzzi, Forman, and Cavalieri (1994) reported on CGA for 24 older adults with intellectual disabilities. In this model, CGA team members included a geriatrician, dentist, geriatric nurse practitioner, and psychiatric nurse practitioner. Compared with medical record review, CGA led to a statistically significant increase in a variety of medical and dental diagnoses. Psychiatric diagnoses were also increased but did not reach statistical significance. The importance of these studies lies in the finding that the in-depth clinical assessment provided by CGA yields more accurate patient profiles than can be obtained through health surveys or medical record review. The implication, drawn from these two studies, was that primary care providers lacking in time or expertise were missing age-related and other clinical diagnoses.

ROCHESTER CAGA MODEL METHOD

The ID/DD Comprehensive Adult and Geriatric Assessment Clinic (henceforth referred to as CAGA), affiliated with the University of Rochester School of Medicine and Dentistry and Monroe Community Hospital, was established in 1995. This outpatient, office-based model combines expertise from university-based programs in geriatrics and developmental disabilities. Personnel include a pediatrician, internist, or geriatrician with training in developmental disabilities, a medical social worker, and a geriatric nurse. The clinic operates one half day a week. Grants, Monroe Community Hospital resources, and fees for service (for the medical evaluation only) fund the clinic. The referral region encompasses a large area in western New York state. Caregivers from local state and nonprofit agencies that provide services to adults with intellectual disabilities refer adults to the clinic. Referral criteria include adult age, the presence of an intellectual disability, and functional decline from a previous baseline as defined by caregivers.

The first author of this chapter, along with collaborators from the University of Rochester Strong Center for Developmental Disabilities, conducted a study of the first 50 adults seen at the CAGA.[1] The investigators posed a number of questions. The first question involved selection by referring caregivers. The investigators suspected that a functional decline referral criterion would result in people presenting with specific losses in self-care skills (e.g., ambulation, continence) caused by well-defined diseases or disorders (e.g., arthritis, detrusor hyperreflexia, dementia). Another question, in a sample defined by functional decline and not chronological age, was that of differential aging trajectories arising from syndromes or associated developmental disabilities. Posited examples included relatively early-onset conditions in specific groups, such as dementia in people with Down syndrome or musculoskeletal problems in people with cerebral palsy. The last question arose from uncertainty about the role that the model would play in treatment and management of conditions. It was thought that this comprehensive model would, like that documented by Carlsen and colleagues (1994), play a robust role in uncovering diagnoses missed by community-based health providers.

The study was conducted during a 2-year period. All of the 50 participants had identifiable primary care physicians, and all had received hearing and visual assessment within 18 months of the CAGA. Twenty-nine adults were receiving psychiatric

[1]This research was supported by Grant No. P-30AG08665 from the National Institute on Aging to the University of Rochester Alzheimer Disease Center.

care, and neurologists followed 16 (for epilepsy) at the time of presentation to CAGA. The participants enrolled in the study were not restricted to older adults because of the presumption that individuals with intellectual disabilities and specific syndromes or associated developmental disabilities might exhibit differences in the age of onset of various age-related conditions. The average age of the adults at presentation was 51 years (the range was ages 29–75 years). There were 25 men and 25 women. Residences included community-based group homes (43 people), supervised apartments (2 people), foster-family homes (2 people), and kin-based homes (3 people). Fifty-six percent (28) of the adults had mild or moderate intellectual disabilities, and 44% (22) had severe or profound intellectual disabilities. Twenty-eight percent (14) had Down syndrome, and 20% (10) had cerebral palsy–associated physical disability.

Initial evaluations took approximately 3 hours per individual. The medical assessment included a thorough medical records review (to obtain information about previously identified medical or neuropsychiatric problems), medication history, visual and auditory status, and medical histories relevant to the period of decline as provided either by caregivers or by the adults. Complete physical examinations were performed, and most participants had clinically indicated laboratory or x-ray studies. Social evaluations included a review of residential and vocational histories as well as information obtained from staff or the adults regarding stressful life situations including bereavement, problems with caregivers or peers, personal trauma, and changes in the social environment (e.g., staff turnover, moves). The nursing assessment emphasized functional capability, hygiene, nutrition, and safety issues. Caregivers and primary care physicians received written CAGA reports. In addition, as-needed consultations were obtained from neurologists, psychiatrists, sleep physicians, and other medical subspecialists. Follow-up and case closure occurred on-site or via telephone and was open-ended and aggressive in an attempt to maximize the diagnostic yield and ensure compliance with treatment recommendations.

ROCHESTER CAGA MODEL FINDINGS

Presentation of Functional Decline

Caregivers identified two types of functional decline. The first was a decline in self-care skills (ADLs) and other skill areas based on physical and/or cognitive performance. The second and more common type was deterioration in the quality of social interactions. Only one adult showed decline in self-care skills alone. Nine adults (average age, 47 years) had declines in social interactions alone. Forty adults (average age, 53 years) showed decline in both self-care skills and social interactions. The majority of the participants who exhibited declines in self-care skills had decrements in three or more ADLs. The participants who exhibited declines in social interaction skills manifested these changes in a variety of ways—apathy and lack of motivation, aggressiveness or irritability, social withdrawal, or lack of compliance with caregiver instructions.

Clinical Conditions Implicated in Functional Decline

The CAGA model focused on conditions that had the potential to cause or contribute to the identified functional decline. CAGA led to the endorsement (or, in some cases, refutation) of previously diagnosed conditions. The participants' pre-CAGA conditions with the potential to cause or contribute to present or future functional decline and for which treatment or management was already received or recommended at the time of assessment were multiple and are delineated in Table 1. These findings indicate fairly

Table 1. Comparative diagnosed conditions pre- and post-CAGA

Condition	Presenting conditions (pre-CAGA) ($N = 50$)	Diagnosed conditions (post-CAGA) ($N = 50$)
Sensory impairments		
Visual (total)	39	
Corrective lenses	(33)	
Blindness	(6)	
Hearing (hearing aid)	14	
Mental health (total)	29	
Affective disorder	(12)	6
Behavior disorder	(11)	
Psychotic disorder	(6)	
Gastrointestinal	29	14
Endocrinological	18	0
Musculoskeletal (pain)	9	14
Cardiovascular	7	0
Respiratory (total)	7	7
Obstructive sleep apnea	(2)	(4)
Urinary tract	4	4
Neurologic (total)	17	5
Epilepsy	16	3
Dementia	1	
Delirium (total)	(0)	8
Adverse drug effect		(6)
Metabolic		(2)
Other medical disorders		6
Hypothyroidism		(2)

CAGA, Comprehensive Adult and Geriatric Assessment.

robust diagnostic efforts by existing community-based primary care and subspecialty medical providers.

Many individuals' pre-CAGA diagnosed conditions were believed to have been inadequately treated or managed. In addition, CAGA identified many conditions that had the potential to cause or contribute to present functional impairment, and new treatment or management regimens were recommended. Post-CAGA recommended changes in the treatment or management of medical conditions that had the potential to affect functional status at the time of assessment are also outlined in Table 1 (and do not include the teaching of environmental interventions to address sensory impairments—these interventions were recommended for all subjects with identified sensory impairments).

Psychosocial Issues

In addition to the medical conditions identified among the participants, CAGA led to the identification or endorsement of psychosocial issues that were believed to have a negative impact on functional capability. CAGA identified six cases of bereavement, only one of which had been explicitly addressed by caregivers. CAGA recognized 11 cases of inappropriate residential or day program situations, 6 of which were in the process of being addressed by caregivers.

Case Examples

The majority of the participants had multiple and concurrent medical conditions and psychosocial issues that had the potential to contribute to functional impairment. The following case studies convey that, in most cases, functional decline was multifactorial in origin.

> N.R., a 70-year-old man with mild intellectual disability, was seen in the CAGA clinic for a 2-year course of functional decline in both self-care and social interaction skills secondary to noncompliance, apathy, and irritability. Clinical conditions noted before CAGA included visual impairment secondary to refractive error and cataracts, mixed-cause hearing loss, gait impairment secondary to cerebral palsy and osteoarthritis, continence issues related to colostomy placement (for an episode of fecal impaction that resulted in bowel obstruction), medically treated esophageal reflux, and psychosocial issues including the near-coincident deaths of his mother and siblings (for which he was receiving bereavement counseling). CAGA revealed esophageal pain secondary to inadequately treated esophagitis, previously unidentified and multiple sites of musculoskeletal pain, and the suspected worsening of the hearing impairment. CAGA recommendations included changing his anti-reflux medications, starting regular doses of acetaminophen, and repeat audiologic testing (which led to a new recommendation for a hearing aid).

> B.J., a 64-year-old woman with mild mental impairment, presented with a 6-month course of functional decline associated with cognitive changes, irritability and sadness, and daytime somnolence. Conditions diagnosed before CAGA included well-controlled epilepsy, visual impairment secondary to astigmatism and cataracts, medically treated recurrent constipation, nonambulatory status secondary to cerebral palsy and flexion contractures, and obesity. CAGA revealed inadequately treated constipation, bereavement issues (B.J.'s mother had died 2 years before assessment), and suspected obstructive sleep apnea. CAGA recommendations included changes in her bowel regimen, bereavement counseling, and referral to a sleep laboratory (which led to a diagnosis of severe obstructive sleep apnea and a subsequent prescription for BiPAP).

Summary of Findings

The first and most striking finding identified during repeated assessments was how functional decline was defined by caregivers. The investigators had expected that loss of specific self-care skills would be emphasized. However, most adults presented with negative changes in the quality or types of their social interactions. Matson and Hammer (1996) emphasized the crucial role that social skills play in enabling social activity. As even basic self-care skills such as ADLs require that subjects be able to work with caregivers and get along with peers, in many cases the deterioration of social skills was the preeminent criterion for the caregiver's definition of functional decline.

The second important finding was that the participants tended to have global decrements in self-care and social skills areas. It is possible that those who were referring the adults to CAGA believed that health service provider could adequately address individuals with isolated or clearly delineated functional losses. Given this bias, it is not surprising that the adults had multiple potentially disabling conditions and that many of these conditions (e.g., delirium, dementia, affective disorders, sleep disorders, painful conditions) had the potential to cause changes in state, affect, and cognition.

Another important finding was the presence of concurrent and even interrelated potentially disabling conditions. This finding replicated that of Chicoine et al. (1999) in their work with adults with Down syndrome who exhibited functional decline. It was not unusual for the adults to have multiple physical (special sensory, pain-causing, motoric) and mental health conditions with the potential to impair function. Although the CAGA model identified a number of "missed diagnoses," many of the impairing conditions (epilepsy, mental health disorders, visual and hearing impairments) had been identified before CAGA. Determining the association and relative impact of these concurrent diagnoses on the functional decline of individual adults was difficult. One of the important services provided by CAGA was the synthesis of functional status as well as multiple preexisting and new diagnoses into coherent, holistic personal profiles that could be understood by caregivers. Comprehensive assessment led to caregiver education, and informal feedback from those who referred the adults indicated that this was a major benefit of CAGA.

An additional observation, based in part on the decision to receive referrals prompted by functional decline and not chronological age, was the varying relationship between specific age-related conditions and adults' ages. Although some geriatric diagnoses were clearly associated with chronological age (e.g., prostate disease), others were not (e.g., probable dementia, in which half of the diagnoses were made in individuals older than age 70 years and half were identified in a cluster of younger adults—all but one had Down syndrome—with an average age of 50 years). Another (incidentally found) example was a cluster of younger ambulatory adults with x-ray–documented osteopenia (i.e., reduction in bone volume to below normal levels) who were receiving ongoing anticonvulsant therapy. These individuals, who represented approximately one third of the adults with epilepsy, had an average age of 39 years. Subsequent work-up revealed no obvious metabolic causes for the bone demineralization other than a possible interplay between nutritional factors and anticonvulsant drugs.

Several specific diagnoses and conditions were surprisingly common. High visual and hearing impairments rates were expected; however, in many cases identification had not led to clearly communicated or implemented treatment or management strategies. Obstructive sleep apnea, although previously described in case series of people with intellectual disability and specific syndromes (Hultcrantz & Svanholm, 1991; Kotugal, Gibbons, & Stith, 1994; Richards et al., 1994; Telakivi, Partinen, Salmi, Leinonen, & Harkonen, 1987; Tirosh & Borochowitz, 1992) was identified in more than 10% of the adults. In addition, a significant number of adults exhibited adverse drug effects. These were almost always caused by central nervous system medications. Anderson and Polister (1993) pointed out relatively high rates of psychotropic medications in a survey of adults with intellectual disability. In this study, approximately 20% of adults were taking three or more medications with primary central nervous system effects. The potential for additive drug effects or other drug interactions was clearly present. The diagnosis of functionally impairing adverse drug effect was made only in adults in whom alterations of the medication regimen were possible and resulted in functional improvement. The amount of drug-induced impairment was probably an underestimation.

Another important finding was the common presence of possible pain or discomfort. Conditions with the potential to impair function by causing pain-related agitation included degenerative musculoskeletal conditions, constipation, reflux esophagitis, and allergic rhinitis. In many cases, these conditions had been recognized before CAGA but were determined by CAGA to be inadequately treated. Delineating the presence, importance, and adequate treatment of pain in participants with functional decline and limited language capabilities was difficult. However, this determination was addressed to the extent possible through participant reports or by the careful solicitation of caregiver observations (see McGrath, Rosmus, Canfield, Campbell, & Hennigar, 1998). In some cases, physical examination maneuvers duplicated caregiver observations by eliciting facial expressions that were consistent with acute pain. Finally, the psychosocial diagnosis of bereavement was an important cause of functional impairment in approximately 10% of these participants. Given the postulated cognitive vulnerability of some people with intellectual disability to work through the bereavement process, our experience suggests that vigilance is required to identify and treat this potentially reversible psychological cause of functional decline (see Deutsch, 1985; Harper & Wadsworth, 1993; Kloeppel & Hollins, 1989; Wadsworth & Harper, 1991).

CONCLUSIONS

The application of a CAGA model for people with intellectual disability like the one described here can serve a number of goals. The first is to obtain clinical experience based on the in-depth assessments of a (necessarily small) number of older adults who are exhibiting functional decline. Patterns and associations may thereby be established between possibly underdiagnosed conditions and the functional capability and quality of life of larger segments of the population of people with intellectual disability. Some examples from the Rochester model include (possible) pain, sleep disorders, adverse drug effects, and bereavement. A second goal is to serve as education and training centers for prompting learning in aging and intellectual disability, both for direct caregivers and clinical trainees in a variety of disciplines. A third and highly specific potential goal is to bring a different perspective to adults with intellectual disability who are using mental health services. Approximately 60% of the adults in the project described in this chapter were receiving psychiatric services before CAGA. In the Rochester referral area, it seems that targeting complex individuals who are already using mental health services and who are not doing well could lead to more comprehensive medical and even psychosocial diagnostic assessment. A fourth goal, specifically for older patients, is to serve as a point of intersection between the intellectual disability and the general aging services system. The geriatric experience of the CAGA physician, nurse, and social worker served as the basis for referrals to services that were not readily accessible or known to caregivers who were providing case management, habilitation, or residential services to older adults with lifelong disabilities.

Team composition can vary according to model goals and available resources. Teams with mandatory representation by multiple subspecialists can lose focus, flexibility, and cost-effectiveness. The effectiveness of the team will likely reflect appropriate assessment time and the aggregate expertise of a relatively small group. However, given the complexity of assessing the problems of older people presenting for CGA (Wollstadt, Glasser, & Nutter, 1997), much less those of complex adults and older adults with intellectual disability, the team should be able to gain access to a wide array of disciplines for consultation. A core team of geriatrician, geriatric nurse clinician, and medical social worker, as described in the Rochester model, should have referral lines to mental health, drug information, neurology, rehabilitation, dentistry, dietary, audiology, optometry, and ophthalmology services.

A major question involves the measurement of efficacy of a complex intervention like CAGA. The efficacy of CAGA compared with existing services can be determined only when the goal of the model is clear cut. Is CAGA being implemented to increase diagnoses or to have a demonstrated positive impact on functional capability? The experience of the Rochester CAGA model confirms the findings of previous investigators that comprehensive assessment increases diagnostic yield. However, the use of functional decline, not chronological age, as the entry criterion in the Rochester CAGA model gives some clues as to how the issue of function can be approached in future studies. Changes in measurements of self-care skills may not be sufficient. Tools that address social skills, either directly (see Matson, 1994, and Matson, Helsel, Bellack, & Senatore, 1983) or indirectly, by documenting aberrant behaviors (see Aman, Singh, Stewart, & Field, 1985) should be considered as outcomes measures. The next step, if study participants act as their own controls, is to implement longitudinal and standardized CAGA protocols, preferably with preassessment and follow-up data collection.

More accurate outcome data (and, probably, greater model efficacy) will be attained if the model sidesteps the issue of varying capabilities of primary care providers and caregivers by assuming the clinical management of CAGA-identified conditions. In addition, the likelihood of encountering high levels of mobility and sensory impairments raises the concern of environmentally induced handicap (World Health Organization, 1980). Adults and older adults with intellectual disabilities and functional decline cannot be adequately assessed in isolation from their social and physical residential and day program environments.

If a comprehensive assessment model for adults and older adults with intellectual disability is set up, it is proposed that the following be considered. The ongoing biopsychosocial development of people with (or without) lifelong disability does not end after childhood and restart in older age. A life span approach may be necessary to address subpopulations with disabilities who have differing aging trajectories. As geriatricians, at least in the United States, are either family physicians or internists, this leads to a concept of specially trained developmental physicians who can cover the adult age spectrum (in which the deficiency or lack of expertise in developmental disabilities is most acutely felt). This concept can be characterized as a life-span developmental assessment model as opposed to an exclusive older age assessment model. The provision of this type of comprehensive, interdisciplinary, and developmental model should be made available to all adults with intellectual disability who are experiencing functional decline. A strong case for periodic assessment can also be made for young adults who have complex biopsychosocial needs and who are graduating from pediatric developmental disabilities centers and services. In addition, the Rochester CAGA model suggests that targeting adults of all ages with intellectual disability who are receiving mental health services and who are not doing well may provide useful clinical information. Finally, an assessment model that is based on adult development and function could serve as an intersection point between disability services and services systems that are directed toward people who have other types of cognitive, behavioral, or physical disabilities. In the United States, this will entail a broader focus on the "disabling process" rather than on the arbitrary distinctions imposed by medical subspecialties that focus on specific diseases.

Older people with developmental disabilities need to be introduced to the expertise and services that are available to other older people. The wonderful, documented increase in the life expectancy of people with intellectual disabilities indicates that increasing numbers of older adults with such disabilities will acquire age-related conditions and, therefore, a need for geriatric expertise (Pope & Tarlov, 1991). For reasons of cost-effectiveness, complex interventions such as CGA should be targeted toward older adults who are experiencing functional decline or who have or who are at risk for developing geriatric conditions. New methodologies, such as dementia screens already developed for people with intellectual disability (see Evenhuis, Kengen, & Eurlings, 1990; Geyde, 1995), will be needed to accommodate the special needs of this population. An intersection between developmental disabilities and aging services should naturally result; teaching, training, and, perhaps, the useful sharing of methodologies across disciplines could take place. The end result might be a step toward the enhanced preservation of function and quality of life of older people with and without lifelong disabilities.

REFERENCES

Abeles, R.P., Gift, H.C., & Ory, M.G. (Eds.). (1994). *Aging and quality of life*. New York: Springer Publishing Co.

Aman, M.G., Singh, N.N., Stewart, A.W., & Field, C.J. (1985). The Aberrant Behavior Checklist: A behavior rating scale for the assessment of treatment effects. *American Journal of Mental Deficiency 89*, 485–491.

American Geriatrics Society (AGS). (1999). *Geriatrics review syllabus: A core curriculum in geriatric medicine* (4th ed.). Dubuque, IA: Kendall/Hunt Publishing Co.

Anderson, D.J., & Polister, B. (1993). Psychotropic medication use among older adults with mental retardation. In E. Sutton, A.R. Factor, B.A. Hawkins, T. Heller, & G.B. Seltzer (Eds.), *Older adults with developmental disabilities: Optimizing choice and change* (pp. 61–75). Baltimore: Paul H. Brookes Publishing Co.

Ashman, A.F., & Suttie, J. (1996). The medical and health status of older people with mental retardation in Australia. *Journal of Applied Gerontology, 15*, 57–72.

Batshaw, M.L. (Ed.). (1997). *Children with disabilities* (4th ed.). Baltimore: Paul H. Brookes Publishing Co.

Capute, A.J., & Accardo, P.J. (Eds.). (1996). *Developmental disabilities in infancy and childhood* (2nd ed.; 2 vols.). Baltimore: Paul H. Brookes Publishing Co.

Carlsen, W.R., Galluzzi, K.E., Forman, L.F., & Cavalieri, T. (1994). Comprehensive geriatric assessment: Applications for community-residing elderly people with mental retardation/developmental disabilities. *Mental Retardation, 32*, 334–340.

Chicoine, B., McGuire, D., & Rubin, S. (1999). Specialty clinic perspectives. In M.P. Janicki & A.J. Dalton (Eds.), *Dementia, aging, and intellectual disabilities: A handbook* (pp. 278–293). Philadelphia: Brunner/Mazel.

Cho, C.Y., Alessi, C.A., Cho, M., Aronow, H.U., Stuck, A.E., Rubenstein, L.Z., & Beck, J.C. (1998). The association between chronic illness and functional change among participants in a comprehensive geriatric assessment program. *Journal of the American Geriatrics Society, 46*, 677–682.

Day, K. (1985). Psychiatric disorder in the middle-aged and elderly mentally handicapped. *British Journal of Psychiatry, 147*, 660–667.

Deutsch, H. (1985). Grief counseling in mentally retarded clients. *Psychiatric Aspects of Mental Retardation Reviews, 4*, 17–20.

Evenhuis, H.M. (1995). Medical aspects of ageing in a population with intellectual disability: I. Visual impairment. II. Hearing impairment. *Journal of Intellectual Disability Research, 39*(pt. 1), 19–33.

Evenhuis, H.M. (1997). Medical aspects of ageing in a population with intellectual disability: III. Mobility, internal conditions, and cancer. *Journal of Intellectual Disability Research, 41*, 8–18.

Evenhuis, H.M., Kengen, M.M.F., & Eurlings, H.A.L. (1990). *Dementia Questionnaire for Mentally Retarded Persons*. Zwammerdam, The Netherlands: Hooge Burch, Institute for Mentally Retarded People.

Farrell, S.E., & Pimental, A.E. (1996). Interdisciplinary team process in developmental disabilities. In A.J. Capute & P.J. Accardo (Eds.), *Developmental disabilities in infancy and childhood: Vol. I. Neurodevelopmental diagnosis and treatment* (2nd ed., pp. 431–441). Baltimore: Paul H. Brookes Publishing Co.

Gaitz, C.M., & Baer, P.E. (1970). Diagnostic assessment of the elderly: A multifunctional approach. *Gerontologist, 10,* 47–52.

Gallo, J.J., Reichel, W., & Anderson, L.M. (2000). *Handbook of geriatric assessment* (3rd ed.). Gaithersburg, MD: Aspen Publishers.

Gambert, S.R., Crimmins, D., Cameron, D., Bacon-Prue, A., & Gupta, K. (1988). A geriatric assessment program for the mentally retarded elderly. *New York Medical Quarterly, 8,* 144–147.

Geyde, A. (1995). *Dementia scale for Down syndrome: Manual.* Vancouver, British Columbia, Canada: Geyde Research and Consulting.

Hand, J.E. (1994). Report of a national survey of older people with lifelong intellectual handicap. *Journal of Intellectual Disability Research, 38,* 275–287.

Harper, D.C., & Wadsworth, J.S. (1993). Grief in adults with mental retardation: Preliminary findings. *Research in Developmental Disabilities, 14,* 313–330.

Hultcrantz, E., & Svanholm, H. (1991). Down syndrome and sleep apnea: A therapeutic challenge. *International Journal of Pediatric Rhinolaryngology, 21,* 263–268.

Janicki, M.P., & Jacobson, J.W. (1986). Generational trends in sensory, physical, and behavioral abilities among older mentally retarded persons. *American Journal of Mental Deficiency, 90,* 490–500.

Janicki, M.P., Dalton, A.J., Henderson, C.M., & Davidson, P.W. (1999). Mortality and morbidity among older adults with intellectual disability: Health services considerations. *Disability and Rehabilitation, 21,* 284–294.

Kane, R.A., & Kane, R.L. (1981). *Assessing the elderly: A practical guide to measurement.* Lanham, MD: Lexington Books.

Kapell, D., Nightengale, A.R., Lee, J.H., Zigman, W.B., & Schupf, N. (1998). Prevalence of chronic medical conditions in adults with mental retardation: Comparison with the general population. *Mental Retardation, 36,* 269–279.

Katz, S., Ford, A.B., Moskowitz, R.W., Jackson, B.A., & Jaffee, N.W. (1963). Studies of illness in the aged. The index of ADL: A standardized measure of biological and psychosocial function. *JAMA: Journal of the American Medical Association, 185,* 914–919.

Kloeppel, D.A., & Hollins, S. (1989). Double handicap: Mental retardation and death in the family. *Death Studies, 13,* 31–38.

Kotugal, S., Gibbons, V.P., & Stith, J.A. (1994). Sleep abnormalities in patients with severe cerebral palsy. *Developmental Medicine and Child Neurology, 36,* 304–311.

Lawton, M.P., & Brody, E.M. (1969). Assessment of older people: Self-maintaining and instrumental activities of daily living. *Gerontologist, 9,* 179–186.

Luckasson, R., Coulter, D.L., Polloway, E.A., Reiss, S., Schalock, R.L., Snell, M.E., Spitalnik, D.M., & Stark, J.A. (1992). *Mental retardation: Definition, classification, and systems of supports* (Special 9th ed.). Washington, DC: American Association on Mental Retardation.

Magrab, P.R., & Schmidt, L.M. (1980). Interdisciplinary collaboration: A prelude to coordinated service delivery. In J.O. Elder & P.R. Magrab (Eds.), *Coordinating services to handicapped children: A handbook for interagency collaboration* (pp. 13–23). Baltimore: Paul H. Brookes Publishing Co.

Matson, J.L. (1994). *Matson evaluation of social skills for individuals with severe retardation: MESSIER.* Baton Rouge, LA: Scientific International Publications.

Matson, J.L., & Hammer, D. (1996). Assessment of social functioning. In J.W. Jacobson & J.A. Mulick (Eds.), *Manual of diagnosis and professional practice in mental retardation* (pp. 157–163). Washington, DC: American Psychological Association.

Matson, J.L., Helsel, W.J., Bellack, A.S., & Senatore, V.C. (1983). Development of a rating scale to assess social skills deficits in mentally retarded adults. *Applied Research in Mental Retardation, 5,* 81–89.

McGrath, P.J., Rosmus, C., Canfield, C., Campbell, M.A., & Hennigar, A. (1998). Behaviors carers use to determine pain in non-verbal, cognitively impaired individuals. *Developmental Medicine and Child Neurology, 40,* 340–343.

Pope, A.M., & Tarlov, A.R. (Eds.). (1991). *Disability in America: Toward a national agenda for prevention.* Washington, DC: National Academy Press.

Pueschel, S.M., & Pueschel, J.K. (Eds.). (1992). *Biomedical concerns in persons with Down syndrome.* Baltimore: Paul H. Brookes Publishing Co.

Richards, A., Quaghebeur, G., Clift, S., Holland, A., Dahiltz, M., & Parkes, D. (1994). The upper airway and sleep apnea in the Prader-Willi syndrome. *Clinical Otolaryngology, 19,* 193–197.

Rubenstein, L.Z. (1995). An overview of comprehensive geriatric assessment: Rationale, history, program models, basic components. In L.Z. Rubenstein, D. Wieland, & R. Bernabei (Eds.), *Geriatric assessment technology: The state of the art* (pp. 1–9). Milan, Italy: Editrice Kutrice.

Rubenstein, L.Z., Wieland, D., & Bernabei, R. (Eds.). (1995). *Geriatric assessment technology: The state of the art*. Milan, Italy: Editrice Kutrice.

Satin, D.G. (1994). The interdisciplinary, integrated approach to professional practice with the aged. In D.G. Satin (Ed.), *The clinical care of the aged person: An interdisciplinary perspective* (pp. 391–403). Oxford, UK: Oxford University Press.

Solomon, D.M. (1988). National Institutes of Health Development Consensus Statement. Geriatric assessment: Methods for clinical decision making. *Journal of the American Geriatrics Society, 36,* 342–347.

Stuck, A., Wieland, D., Rubenstein, L., Siu, A., & Adams, J. (1995). Comprehensive geriatric assessment: Meta-analysis of main effects and elements enhancing effectiveness. In L.Z. Rubenstein, D. Wieland, & R. Bernabei (Eds.), *Comprehensive geriatric assessment technology: The state of the art* (pp. 11–25). Milan, Italy: Editrice Kutrice.

Sweeney, D.P., & Wilson, T.V. (Eds.). (1979). *Double jeopardy: The plight of aging in mid-America.* Ann Arbor: University of Michigan, Institute for the Study of Mental Retardation and Related Disabilities.

Tannenbaum, T., Lipworth, L., & Baker, S. (1989). Risk of fractures in an intermediate care facility for persons with mental retardation. *American Journal on Mental Retardation, 93,* 444–451.

Telakivi, T., Partinen, M., Salmi, T., Leinonen, L., & Harkonen, M. (1987). Nocturnal periodic breathing in adults with Down's syndrome. *Journal of Mental Deficiency Research, 31,* 31–39.

Tirosh, E., & Borochowitz, Z. (1992). Sleep apnea in fragile X syndrome. *American Journal of Medical Genetics, 43,* 124–127.

Trent, J.W., Jr. (1994). The remaking of mental retardation: Of war, angels, parents, and politicians. In J.W. Trent, Jr., *Inventing the feeble mind: A history of mental retardation in the United States* (pp. 225–268). Berkeley: University of California Press.

Tucker, B.P., & Goldstein, B.A. (1991). *Legal rights of persons with disabilities: An analysis of federal law.* Horsham, PA: LRP Publications.

Van Schrojenstein Lantman-de Valk, H.M., van den Akker, M., Maaskant, M.A., Haveman, M.J., Urlings, H.F., Kessels, A.G., & Crebolder, H.F. (1997). Prevalence and incidence of health problems in people with intellectual disability. *Journal of Intellectual Disability Research, 41,* 42–51.

Wadsworth, J.S., & Harper, D.C. (1991). Grief and bereavement in mental retardation: A need for a new understanding. *Death Studies, 15,* 281–292.

Walz, T., Harper, D., & Wilson, J. (1986). The aging developmentally disabled person: A review. *Gerontologist, 26,* 622–629.

Williams, M. (1987). Outpatient geriatric assessment. *Clinics in Geriatric Medicine, 3,* 175–183.

Wollstadt, L.J., Glasser, M., & Nutter, T. (1997). Variations in functional status among different groups of elderly people. *Family Medicine, 29,* 394–399.

World Health Organization. (1980). *International classification of impairments, disabilities, and handicaps: A manual of classification relating to the consequences of disease.* Geneva: Author.

Zigman, W., Schupf, N., Haveman, M., & Silverman, W. (1997). The epidemiology of Alzheimer disease in intellectual disability: Results and recommendations from an international conference. *Journal of Intellectual Disabilities Research, 41,* 76–80.

Ziring, P.R., Kastner, T.A., Friedman, D.L., Pond, W.S., Barnett, M.L., Sonnenberg, E.M., & Strassburger, K. (1988). Provision of health care for persons with developmental disabilities living in the community: The Morristown model. *JAMA: Journal of the American Medical Association, 260,* 1439–1444.

21

Supporting People with
Dementia in Community Settings

Matthew P. Janicki, Philip McCallion, and Arthur J. Dalton

Harriet, a woman with Down syndrome, was 59 years old when she died. She had lived most of her life with her parents. That is, until the past 15 years, when they had become too old to continue to provide for her and arranged for Harriet to move to a small group home. They also arranged for their other daughter to visit Harriet and take her home on holidays. Harriet had enjoyed a full life. Her parents had taken her with them everywhere they went. Her father had been an attorney and had a sizable practice. His income had helped his family live well, and Harriet benefited from his largess. As Harriet's parents grew older, they realized that Harriet most likely would outlive them as they were some 40 years older than Harriet. The group home was their answer for her continued comfortable life in her own old age. Harriet was quite capable—she knew her way around housework and could shop and use the local buses to visit her sister and her friends. About 5 years ago, her sister had begun to notice that she was becoming forgetful and was having more difficulty with her language. She commented about this to the staff director, and he arranged for the agency physician to examine Harriet. The assessment was uncertain, but the physician asked the couple who staffed the home to keep a log about

This chapter was supported in part by Grant No. H133B980046 from the National Institute on Disability and Rehabilitation Research, U.S. Department of Education, to the Rehabilitation Research and Training Center on Aging with Mental Retardation at the University of Illinois at Chicago.

Harriet and jot down what she could and could not do. During the year, the log revealed an increasing number of losses in Harriet's capabilities. Whereas previously she had enjoyed shopping and traveling by herself, she had now become fearful and uncertain. Her coordination was beginning to deteriorate, and there was suspicion that she may have had several seizures. Upon reassessment, the examination revealed what some at the agency were already suspecting: Harriet was experiencing the onset of Alzheimer's disease. Unfortunately, the disease progressed quickly so that within 3 years, Harriet had become a person who was unfamiliar to those who previously knew her. It was at this point that Harriet's sister and the staff at the agency wrestled with what to do next.

As more people with intellectual disabilities survive to old age, the same problems that affect other people in old age will affect them (Janicki, Dalton, Henderson, & Davidson, 1999). One major impairment that occurs in old age (but not a normal expectation of aging) is dementia—primarily the result of Alzheimer's disease but also from other causes. Dementia is a term applied to adults who experience progressive mental deterioration linked to neuropathological changes in the brain. It affects between 2% and 10% of older adults in North America and Europe (Evans et al., 1990; Folstein, Bassett, Anthony, Romanoski, & Nestadt, 1991), and the prevalence seems to double at 5-year intervals after age 65. There are several causes of dementia, each with a somewhat different course and prevalence. Alzheimer's disease is the most common cause, accounting for between 50% and 75% of all dementias in the general population, and represents a significant risk factor for people with Down syndrome (Holland, 1999). It has been estimated that between 3 million and 5 million people in the United States are affected by Alzheimer's disease. The causes, treatment, and prevention of this disease are not known, but risk factors include family history, the presence of the apolipoprotein E gene-E4, head injury, and Down syndrome.

Alzheimer's disease is a degenerative disease of the brain that slowly kills brain cells and affects memory and cognition. Simply put, the disease affects the brain such that brain cells no longer function in the way they did. Cells that store memories and order how to perform daily tasks are lost, and learning cannot be retrieved. People with dementia lose not only their memory but also orientation skills and their ability to perform everyday activities that they usually could do in the past (see Table 1). Dementia may present as "functional retardation" in adults with previously normal levels of functioning. However, there are important differences between dementia and intellectual disability. Dementia occurs in later age, adversely affects already known or learned behaviors, and progressively leads to total debilitation and eventual death. Conversely, intellectual disabilities are present from birth or originate in early childhood and affect a person's potential to learn or the manner in which new things are learned but generally do not impair life functions (unless in severe forms) and are not typically associated with pathological cognitive decline in old age.

CHARACTERISTICS OF DEMENTIA

Dementia is a loss of intellectual functions of sufficient severity to interfere with daily functioning of the individual affected (Alzheimer's Disease and Related Disorders Association, 1992). It is sometimes progressive, as with Alzheimer's disease, and sometimes precipitous, as with vascular dementia. Vascular, or multi-infarct, dementia is caused by small ruptures of the blood vessels in the brain (or strokes). Here the dementia is the result of trauma to the brain, whereas dementia associated with Alzheimer's

Table 1.   Clinical characteristics of dementia

Early stage	*Behavior:* Onset features (short-term memory, language disruption, vocational dysfunction) *Diagnosis:* Initial diagnosis *Care management:* Support compensations *Time frame:* 1–5 years (less in people with Down syndrome)
Middle stage	*Behavior:* Pronounced losses and decline (distinct losses in language, comprehension, disorientation, confusion, short-term memory loss, activities of daily living losses, personality changes) *Diagnosis:* Confirmatory diagnosis *Care management:* Close supervision, controls for wandering, day activities *Time frame:* 5–15 years (less in people with Down syndrome)
Late stage	*Behavior:* Significant decline and complete loss of function and basic skills, long- and short-term memory losses, loss of balance and ambulation *Diagnosis:* Upon autopsy *Care management:* Complete oversight and total care, infirmity, danger of infection and pneumonia, death *Time frame:* 3–5 years (less in people with Down syndrome)

From Dalton, A.J., & Janicki, M.P. (1999). Aging and dementia. In M.P. Janicki & A.J. Dalton (Eds.), *Dementia, aging, and intellectual disabilities: A handbook* (p. 26). Philadelphia: Brunner/ Mazel; adapted by permission from Taylor & Francis, Philadelphia, PA. All rights reserved.

disease is the result of a disease of the brain. Dementia affects each person differently because the cause and course of brain damage underlying the dementia vary by individual; because each person's brain is organized differently, people have different lifelong styles of thinking or processing information, and each person's history, medical status, personality, and lifestyle are unique (Weaverdyck, 1997). With regard to observable changes, Sloane (1997) noted the "four A's" of Alzheimer's disease and their behavioral complications: amnesia (loss of memory), apraxia (loss of ability to coordinate learned movements), aphasia (inability to speak or understand), and agnosia (inability to recognize what is seen). These, in aggregate, reflect the losses experienced as part of the disease course (Lovestone, 1998).

Dementia is age-associated because it happens mostly to people in old age. It occurs less frequently among the young-old and more frequently among the old-old. Approximately 5% of the older population (people ages 60 years and older) is affected by some form of dementia; among people who are older than age 85, approximately 25% to 45% are affected (Evans et al., 1990). Generally, the interval from estimated onset to initial diagnosis is between 2 and 3 years, and the interval between confirmatory diagnosis and death can range from between 3 and 15 years (Alloul et al., 1998; Brawley, 1997). Among people with Down syndrome, these intervals are compressed; the time from estimated onset to death generally ranges from between 1 and 9 years. Among people with intellectual disabilities, it has been reported that prevalence of dementia can range from high (Cooper, 1997) to normative (Janicki & Dalton, 1997a, 2000). At the high end, Cooper (1997; see also Chapter 19) reported a British study that showed that overall, approximately 22% of older people with intellectual disabilities may be affected by dementia (with 16% for people age 65–74, 24% for people age 75–84, and 70% for people ages 86–94 years). At the low end, Janicki and Dalton (1997a) reported a U.S. study that showed a prevalence of dementia of 3% for people ages 40 years and older, 6% for people ages 60 years and older, and 12% for people ages 80 and older. Comparative rates for adults with Down syndrome were approximately 22% for adults ages 40 years and older and 56% for adults ages 60 years and older.

In addition to dementia, people with intellectual disabilities may present with a variety of co-morbid conditions. Studies of adults with Down syndrome have shown that late-onset seizures and sensory problems are common among adults who are affected by dementia (Alvarez, 1996; Brodtkorp, 1994; Evenhuis, 1997; McVicker, Shanks, & McClelland, 1994; Prasher & Corbett, 1993). There are indications that certain psychiatric symptoms and behavior disturbances are also coincident in later stages of dementia (Prasher & Filer, 1995). Among a group of adults with varying etiologies, Cooper (1997) found psychotic symptoms co-occurring in approximately one quarter; the most common symptoms were persecutory delusions and visual hallucinations. Behavior disturbances that are symptomatic of dementia are also prevalent, in particular, changes in sleep patterns, impaired concentration, restlessness, wandering, reduced quantity of speech, changes in appetite, and onset of or increase in aggression. Depression has also been noted to co-occur (Burt & Aylward, 1999; Meyers, 1999). These changes are often associated with various types of dementia. Little is known about the prevalence of the different types of dementia in adults with intellectual disabilities; however, among adults with Down syndrome, dementia of the Alzheimer's type seems to be the most prevalent. Furthermore, among adults with Down syndrome, the onset and course of the disease are atypical and may be more problematic because adults with Down syndrome are younger when affected (Visser et al., 1997) and in some instances experience a more precipitous disease-related decline (Janicki & Dalton, 1999). Death usually occurs from a variety of acute causes, including pneumonia and heart failure (Moss, Lambe, & Hogg, 1998).

DETERMINING THE PRESENCE OF DEMENTIA

Diagnosis of dementia is done by exclusion; that is, assessments are performed in an attempt to determine whether any other causes may be underlying the behavioral presentation. When no other causes can be determined, then a possible or probable determination of dementia is made.[1] Definite diagnosis of Alzheimer's disease or another underlying cause of dementia can only be made postmortem. In general, preliminary impressions are usually obtained by a screening instrument, such as the Mini-Mental State Examination (MMSE; Folstein, Folstein, & McHugh, 1975), but formal diagnoses are obtained after use of more comprehensive measures (American Psychological Association, 1998). In contrast to screening methods that are available to the general population (such as the MMSE), there is no singular standard screening instrument that is readily applicable to all people with intellectual disabilities (because of their variability of intellectual abilities). Burt and Aylward (1999) noted that a standard clinical

---

[1] Generally, a *possible* diagnosis is ascribed if there are classic symptoms present indicating dementia (absent other neurological, psychiatric, or systems disorders) and there are variations in the onset, presentation, or clinical course of deterioration. A *probable* diagnosis is ascribed when the clinical course is established by clinical examination and confirmed by neurological tests, there are deficits in at least two areas of cognition, there is a progressive worsening of memory and other cognitive functions, and there is an absence of other brain diseases or disturbances of consciousness. A *definite diagnosis* is made by clinical criteria for probable Alzheimer's disease and histopathological evidence obtained from a biopsy or autopsy (adapted from Williams, 1995).

history; laboratory tests; and medical, neurological, and radiological studies are generally used to arrive at a diagnosis. These are supplemented by behavioral observations and rating scales standardized specifically for this population. There are several such scales that may be applicable for screening adults with intellectual disabilities for dementia (see Aylward, Burt, Thorpe, Lai, & Dalton, 1995, 1997, for a full discussion). The American Association on Mental Retardation (AAMR) and the International Association for the Scientific Study of Intellectual Disabilities (IASSID) have issued guidelines that recommend that the initial evaluations be done for all adults with Down syndrome beginning at the age of 40 years and for all others at the age of 50 years to help identify sensory, motor, and other age-associated changes that could precede the appearance of any cognitive changes associated with dementia (Janicki, Heller, Seltzer, & Hogg, 1996). Most standardized measures of adaptive behavior are useful in capturing baseline and follow-up data in the event that signs or symptoms of dementia occur at a later date. Furthermore, having such data available is useful upon referral to a specialist for a formal diagnosis (see Janicki & Dalton, 1999).

CARE CHALLENGES

Immediate family members and other caregivers often find that agencies are poorly equipped to provide practical guidance for the care of adults with dementia and intellectual disabilities (see Fray, 2000). Many people with intellectual disabilities are unable to provide verbal self-reports and often cannot follow verbal or spoken instructions readily. These problems hamper the introduction of effective care management strategies. Also, physicians with experience in the diagnosis and treatment of older individuals with intellectual disabilities are hard to find. Family practitioners, geriatricians, and many other health professionals who are accessible may not be aware of the special needs of individuals with intellectual disabilities who are affected by dementia and its impact on care providers.

The occurrence of dementia among individuals with intellectual disabilities has a profound impact on the quality of life of affected individuals and on their families, friends, and caregivers (Antonangeli, 1995; Koenig, 1995; Marler & Cunningham, 1994; May, Fletcher, Alvarez, Zuis, & Cavallari, 1996; Newroth & Newroth, 1981; The Arc of the United States, 1995). People with intellectual disabilities are more likely to have difficulties with communication (McCallion, 1999), experience problems with everyday activities (Moss & Patel, 1997), and be in jeopardy of losing their housing (Cohen, 1999). Also, because most people with intellectual disabilities experience lifelong limitations in verbal and communication skills, there is a greater likelihood that dementia will be well advanced before a diagnosis is made. Dementia-related behavior changes may include a greater number of ongoing health problems and diminished capacity of self-directed activities, as well as significant changes in personality and behavior control (Moss & Patel, 1997). These changes will have a significant impact on a person's personal situation and overall quality of life.

When presented with progressive decline, care providers are often faced with the problem of how to handle constructively the diminishing abilities of people who had been relatively independent and capable of extensive self-direction for most of their lives. When the adult has lived at home or been part of the intellectual disabilities care system, caregivers and staff have come to expect progressive increases in skills and independence. Thus, the presentation of a disease course that undermines these expectations can be disconcerting. Such presentation may pose difficulties for staff, and the contradiction between the reality that the disease presents and the ideology that has been the basis for the delivery of care in the field of intellectual disabilities will have to be addressed. For example, as described by Davis (1999), Duggan, Lewis, and Morgan (1996), Hammond and Benedetti (1999), Prasher (1999), Service, Lavoie, and Herlihy (1999), Udell (1999b), and Visser et al. (1997), adults with Down syndrome can experience a precipitous decline in function; as a result, care management practices can take a substantial emotional toll on family and staff resources. Adults with etiologies other than Down syndrome may have a later onset and even longer duration of decline, stretching responsible care agency resources in different ways.

As noted, the AAMR and the IASSID have issued a set of practice guidelines for the care of individuals with intellectual disabilities and dementia (Janicki et al., 1996). These practice guidelines provide specific suggestions for assessment and service provision as well as a rational basis for making clinical decisions and developing programs that are specifically responsive to the needs of individuals who are affected by dementia. The guidelines were developed on the basis of the following assumptions: 1) Each person's needs must determine how care is provided, 2) age-associated changes are a normal part of life, 3) people with Down syndrome are at greater risk for developing Alzheimer's disease, 4) some behavior changes may look like dementia but may be due to other causes and be reversible, and 5) the individual's own abilities and levels of function should be the basis for evaluating subsequent changes (Janicki et al., 1996).

The AAMR and IASSID practice guidelines call for an initial screening for dementia followed by periodic reviews combined with the implementation of care management practices that are tightly coupled to the expected sequence of functional changes as the individual progresses through the stages of dementia. For example, a program for managing incontinence could be prepared and kept "on the shelf" to be available when the individual shows signs so that it can be immediately implemented at the time when it may be most effective and least embarrassing for the affected individual. The practice guidelines distinguish situations that require only a screening procedure from those that require a more comprehensive assessment. Recommended is a three-step course of action that involves recognizing changes, conducting assessments and evaluations, and instituting medical and care management. These are detailed in the AAMR and IASSID documents.

CARE MODELS AND PRACTICES

In the general population, most out-of-home models of care focus primarily on long-term care in nursing facilities. Nearly one fifth of all nursing facilities in the United States offer care for residents with Alzheimer's disease or other residents with special needs in special units. A survey conducted by the federal Agency for Health Care Policy and Research showed that approximately 3,240, or close to one fifth, of the 17,000 nursing facilities in the United States have one or more special nursing units, and approximately 2,130 facilities have a unit (average unit size of 34) that is dedicated to the care of adults with Alzheimer's disease ("Nearly One Fifth of Nursing Homes," 1998). When care at home becomes untenable, most families or local health authorities will seek institutional placement in a long-term care facility for an affected relative or adult. Alternative models exist but generally are not mainstream options because of a lack of viable funding. These include small board and care homes dedicated to the community care of adults affected by dementia (Monmaney, 1997; "One Facility's Approach," 1993). In addition, voluntary associations, such as the Alzheimer's Association, have evolved to help provide supports to caregivers and to assist with training, education, and advo-

Table 2. Dementia care development considerations

Will you need to alter or modify the physical space or building features? Is there a source of funds to do this? Can the building be modified easily? How will the modifications affect the other people in the home? Will "risk minimization" improvements hinder the ability of others to get in and out of the home?

Will you need to increase, augment, or alter your staff? Will you need staff who are more experienced with nursing care? Will you need more staff on duty at certain times? What additional training will staff need to receive?

How long will the person reside in the home? What are the expectations for the course of the disease (if Alzheimer's disease is involved) or the impairment (if a condition other than Alzheimer's disease is involved)?

Will others in the home be affected similarly? Are there others in the home who may be at risk for developing dementia? Are there others who may be at risk for developing other age-related conditions that will necessitate that they receive more extensive physical care?

Will there be additional costs associated with providing continued care? Will additional staff be needed? Will nursing assistance need to be purchased? Will building or yard modifications need to be paid for? Will altered staffing patterns require additional costs (e.g., more nursing personnel)?

Is a source of funds readily available to cover additional expenses? Does the annual budget allow for incremental increases in expenses? Is the funding agency attuned to budgeting for additional costs of care on an annual basis? Does the license of the home permit more intense levels of care and compensate for them accordingly?

What will be the character of the home in 2 years? in 5 years? in 10 years? Will the person affected have a short-term or long-term progression of impairment associated with dementia? Will others be affected similarly, and thus, in aggregate, will they change the character of the home over time? Is the expectation that the home may become a nursing care home over time?

Which supports will be available as the character of the home changes over the years? Will you be able to add staff or purchase outside help? Will the agency endorse these efforts? Will it be possible to modify programs and supports as the needs of residents change?

To what extent is the agency receptive to dementia-related care at the home? Does the agency's housing policy permit nonambulatory care? Does the agency's housing policy support aging in place? Is it possible to have access to staff from other divisions to help with day activities, trips, and other specialty program endeavors?

Which outside resources can be called on to help in latter-stage dementia care? Can the local Alzheimer's Association chapter provide aid? Do visiting nurse services provide in-home visits to group homes? Is a hospice program available to help? Can staff receive counseling or other supports for end-of-life challenges? What assistance can the local agency on aging provide?

cacy. There has not been a similar level of Alzheimer support development among agencies that offer out-of-home services to people with intellectual disabilities.

Among agencies within the intellectual disabilities system, development considerations are complex and the responses to the presence of dementia are varied. Table 2 illustrates a number of programmatic questions that affect decision making. Managers of such agencies, when confronted with dementia-related decline among the people they serve, often choose one of three approaches (or some mingling of the three). The first option is to follow "aging-in-place" precepts and arrange supports for the person in the home or living environment and ensure that supports are dementia capable. *Dementia capable* is defined as being skilled in working with people with dementia and their caregivers, knowledgeable about the kinds of services that may help them, and aware of which agencies and individuals provide such services. Furthermore, it means being able to serve people with dementia, even when services are being provided to other people as well. In contrast, *dementia specific* means that services are being provided specifically for people with dementia (Alzheimer's Disease and Related Disorders Association, 1997). This approach is consistent with the three critical components of adaptive dementia care: program development, staff development, and environmental design (Grant & Sommers, 1998). The response to onset and diagnosis is to rearrange care to accommodate the effects of stage-related decline and eventual greater personal care needs. The second option is to follow an "in-place progression" model and by developing a dementia specialty program in which a number of people with similar needs are provided with a range of residential accommodations and care in a specialized care setting. Such programs generally provide for people in mid- to late-stage dementia and provide on-site services as the adult progresses to end-stage dementia. The third option, not model based, involves referring the person to a generic extended care or nursing facility.

Aging-in-Place Support Model

Table 3 illustrates the aging-in-place, or readaptation, model, which begins with an equilibrium-of-function phase, proceeds through two change and adjustment phases, and ends with a reestablished equilibrium-of-function phase (Janicki, 1998). Five dimensions (programmatic aspects, care situation, staff capabilities, physical structure, and prognosis) define the changing conditions of the home. In the first phase, the care situation is static, and residents function within generally defined expectations of skill levels and behaviors (as defined upon entry). Only when the onset of dementia becomes remarkable does the dynamic tension in the home become evident, and then dissonance emerges between preestablished and redefined expectations. Staff capabilities may become challenged; because change in one or more of the residents may still be in an early phase, the physical structure dimension may remain unaffected. The prognosis is for emerging difficulties.

At this point, an agency may choose to address the dissonance in one of two ways: introduce supports to address the source of the change, or remove the source of change (i.e., it may support staff and housemates affected by a resident with dementia, or it may remove the resident from the home). If the latter is chosen, it means that the agency has opted for the second or third option. If the former is chosen, the agency has conducted an assessment and has noted that within the care situation, a significant disruption has occurred, usually defined by the changing behaviors of one or more individuals, increased stress levels among the staff, disruptions of routines, and an uncertainty of how to proceed. This stage in agency response can be brief, if the new behaviors are marked and acute, or prolonged, if the new behaviors are more subtle and episodic. However, if the onset of dementia is marked, confirmed by assessment, and administratively defined as part of the care management intent of the residence, then resources can be provided to address the changing nature of the home and emphasis is given to staff redeployment or training. Prognosis is linked to the assumed life course of the dementia and the nature of the disease presentation and duration that is expected. In reality, the home will experience prolonged care management challenges and difficulties. The problem situation and recognition phase is one that requires the most attention, for in many instances, if left unattended, the problem can lead to significant management problems in the home. These may be manifested by staff dissatisfaction and turnover, adverse behavioral impact on housemates, and a

Table 3. Model for redefining services decision making in group or family homes affected by dementia

Circumstances	Typical situation	Emerging problem	Adaptation	Typical situation
Care situation	Static condition	Care and behavior challenges to static care management	Significant disruption	Redefined static condition
Staff capabilities	Established expectations	Dissonance between established and new expectations	Realization of change and staff retention or redeployment and training	Redefined expectations
Physical structure	Predefined environment	Predefined environment	Select environmental modifications	Redefined environment
Prognosis	Continued homeostasis	Emerging difficulties	Prolonged difficulties	Redefined continued homeostasis

fluctuation in the treatment approach for the affected individual. Given adequate intervention by the agency (staff support, training and possible redeployment, alterations to the physical environment, and changes in care management of the person affected by dementia), the expected prognosis is a redefined base or equilibrium of function. This means a return to a static condition, albeit redefined but appropriate to the needs of the person with dementia, the expectations of staff, and the environment.

Structuring Agencies to Support Aging in Place

An agency mission statement or the agency culture should reflect an adherence to a philosophical belief that aging in place is the chosen course. Furthermore, the agency has to back this up with an investment in sound management of the home, close scrutiny of staff capabilities and emotional strength, commitment to additional training and clinical supports, and a fiscal investment in making environmental modifications to the home. It also means that the agency and staff must make a commitment to becoming dementia capable. Yet the most important ingredient in this approach is the staff. Weaverdyck, Wittle, and Delaski-Smith (1998), in studying an analogous care situation to a group home that experienced change over a 5-year period, noted that the emotional challenge to residents and staff as the program's residents progressed through stages of dementia was profound and needed constant attention from management. They noted that capable and dedicated staff are the factor that "makes or breaks" this type of endeavor and that staff burnout is a significant problem, particularly when insufficient support is offered. Weaverdyck et al. also noted that in such situations there is an expectation of staff–resident bonding and that although such bonding can be advantageous in terms of quality of care, progressive decline in residents places emotional demands on staff who then require a great deal of support from management.

Structural Dynamics that Affect Commitment

Two additional considerations apply in this approach: quantity and repetition. Assuming that a small number of individuals are residents in a home, one occurrence of dementia can be manageable and, if not recurring, generally will not disrupt the organization and culture of the home. However, if all of the residents of the home are at the age of being at risk for developing dementia, then the probability is that others will manifest the condition (particularly if they have Down syndrome). When this is the case, a question arises: What is the tipping point at which the aggregate of individuals who are affected means that the residence is no longer the home it was but has become a specialty care residence (as per the second approach). "Tipping point" is the ecological demarcation of the difference between two particular conditions. When dementia is present, the milieu of a home will change as a result of the nature of the care needed. In most settings, this can come about as the result of one individual (demand severity) or several individuals (massed demand). It is also affected by time, as outlined in the previous model. Also at issue is how many people are affected at any particular time (quantity) and, if only one at a time is affected, how often this occurrence repeats itself (repetition). Agencies should take note of the tipping-point notion in identifying decision points at which they may need to reassess staff assignments and deployment, as well as the cost for operating the home.

Another notion to consider is what Janicki and Dalton (1999) termed the *threshold effect*. In contrast to tipping point, which is an ecological concern, the threshold effect is a managerial aspect and defines when the care demand situation shifts so notably that staff can no longer provide the expected level of care. This notion is less concerned with defining the change in character of the care setting but more with its demand characteristics. Such a shift may occur when one or more instances of dementia are evident in residents and no readaptation has taken place. Staff function according to the tenets of the original static condition state, because the emerging problem state is perceived as overwhelming to them. The threshold effect has two facets: tolerance and capability. Tolerance considers which level of demand the staff are willing to endure before they balk, and capability considers staff skills and resources to deliver needed care or their ability to adapt these skills to deliver needed care. The threshold effect can be used to explain why referrals to long-term care facilities often occur. It can also lead agencies to consider specialty programs.

In-Place Progression Model

The second option is to set up a dementia-specific environment (see Weaverdyck et al., 1998). The premise is that specialized staff and a specialized environment are best to provide long-term care for individuals in the later stages of Alzheimer's disease or related dementias. Design issues include case mix, length of stay, admission and retention criteria, staffing and staff training, and design features. With regard to case mix, Weaverdyck et al. (1998) noted that such in-place progression programs are applicable to individuals with dementia progressing from mid- through terminal stage. Thus, case mix and length of stay (or duration) are factors when considering the composition of individuals in such a home. For example, with the known shorter duration of Alzheimer's disease among adults with Down syndrome, the interval from midstage to death can be from 1 to 5 years. For adults with other causes, the interval is usually much longer and the midstage less defined. Thus, determining how long people will live within the program and the setting of admission criteria can be very important. Weaverdyck (personal communication, June 1, 1999) noted that in the general population, admission can be based on the following inclusionary criteria: confirmed diagnosis of mid- to late-stage dementia, intact ambulation/mobility and eating capabilities, and the onset of problems associated with continence and behavior. However, in the few examples we have encountered, admission into a specialized intellectual disabilities program has been based more on the presence of diagnosed dementia and agency-perceived (but not articulated operationally) need for a specialized residence.

If diagnosis of dementia will be the primary factor in admission for most agencies, then consideration needs to be given to the degree to which the person is affected by dementia. If the functional limitations noted by Weaverdyck are to be applicable, then it should be established that the person to be admitted is functioning at a level that is discordant from their "personal best" or norm (i.e., the criteria reflect losses and not typical functioning). The criteria also need to reflect a need for specialized services or oversight by staff as a result of behaviors that are different from those generally found in dependent adults with intellectual disabilities. Such criteria may include losses in activities of daily living (ADLs) from previously competent levels, behavior disturbances that are difficult to manage or adjust in a typical housing situation (e.g., excessive verbal or physical aggression, rummaging and hoarding, shadowing, extreme emotional volatility), and disorientation and wandering.

Consideration should also be given to the expected rate of decline among residents. The nature of a specialized care program can change precipitously as the nature of the residents changes. Hepburn, Petrie, Peterson, and VanLoy (1995) noted that even in special dementia care units, case mix is a factor, with supports in the home shifting from ambulatory care to nursing care as the residents become more infirm and eventually spend most, if not all, of their time in bed. Dementia in people with intellectual disabilities may be a lingering condition or progress quickly. Hammond and Benedetti (1999) and Udell (1999b) reported instances of duration from recognized onset to death of less than 2 years. Janicki and Dalton (2000) noted that duration differences emerge between people with Down syndrome and those with other causes. They noted that long-duration dementia (i.e., more than 10 years) was found in only 7% of adults with Down syndrome, whereas it was found in 29% of adults with other causes of intellectual disabilities. Thus, consideration should be given to how the home will be staffed when the character of the residents changes from ambulatory to nonambulatory as well as when the case mix varies because of new admissions as a result of the early deaths of some residents and because others remain ambulatory but incapacitated for longer periods of time.

Staffing   The care agency must consider whether to staff the home with people who are more adept at dementia care or more familiar with caring for individuals with intellectual disabilities. Given the overlap of intellectual disabilities and the main effects of a dementing process, this consideration requires careful thought. With an emphasis on primary dementia care, it may be more fruitful to assign staff who are more adept with caring for people with declining abilities than who are more adept at promoting new learning or training. Hurley and Kennedy (1997) noted that a key staff characteristic is the ability to commit to the unique demands of caring for someone with dementia. Being successful in other care settings may not mean that the potential staff person is appropriate for a dementia care program. Experience has shown that working in a care setting for people with intellectual disabilities is a useful background (Udell, 1999a). However, staff have to accept that the progressive decline they will witness is organically based and not a function of behavior manipulation. They also have to be willing to adapt their thinking from functioning within the tenets of a developmental model (which stresses progressive growth) to a dementia care model (which stresses maintenance and compensation for progressive deterioration). Thus, a reorientation of staff practices is necessary, as is training to create a working dementia care environment. Specialized staff training on dementia and dementia care practices can be the decisive factor in preventing burnout, retaining staff, and providing a quality dementia-capable program environment (Alfredson & Annerstedt, 1994; Grant, Kane, Potthoff, & Ryden, 1996).

Home Design   Most workers agree that a single-level design that avoids stairs and other access barriers is optimum (Hutchings, 1999). Included in the design are typical home-like features, except that greater emphasis is placed on the therapeutic use of public and private spaces and on designs that provide a secure, safe setting while encouraging and permitting movement and connectedness to the outside. Specific physical design recommendations are available from a number of resources (see, e.g., Brawley, 1997; Cohen & Weisman, 1991; Olsen, Ehrenkrantz, & Hutchings, 1993; Warner, 1998) and organizations (Alzheimer's Disease and Related Disorders Association, 1997). Table 4 illustrates some situations and offers administrative and clinical recommendations for addressing them.

Implementation of an in-place progression model program requires planning data (determining the numbers of people currently affected and projections of numbers potentially similarly affected over the next 5, 10, or more years); the availability of funds

Table 4. Design objectives and situational management in community group homes providing dementia care

Objective	Situational management
Ensure safety and security	Eliminate situations that may pose danger because of pica, wandering, disorientation, and behavior
Support functional abilities	Emphasize activities that support self-image and mastery, involvement with group activities, maintenance of skills
Assist with wayfinding and orientation	Design physical space to help with orientation, consider choice of colors, texture, patterns, placement of rooms and pathways, and cues and guides for movement
Prompt memory	Provide cues for long-term memory recall and orientation: pictures, familiar objects, color schemes, keepsakes, and personal artifacts
Establish links with a familiar, positive past	Combine productive activities with simulation of previous life involvement; use pictures, photographs, and familiar objects to link to favorable past
Convey expectations and elicit and reinforce appropriate behavior	Establish criteria for acceptance of behavior; adapt responses to stages and daily functioning situation; respond to the person within a framework of how the person views his or her present life and situation
Reduce agitation	Provide environmental situations that minimize disorientation and worry; institute controls over behavioral or environmental situations that act as stimuli to behavioral outbursts or difficulties
Facilitate privacy	Maintain balance between public and private spaces; respect need for privacy in personal space and places for visiting with family or friends; install screens or privacy partitions in areas of bathing or toileting
Facilitate social interactions	Provide for both passive (observing) and active (interacting) socialization experiences; provide activities that engage memories and productive functioning
Stimulate interests and curiosity	Maintain a familiar environment but also provide opportunities for exploration and new experiences
Support independence, autonomy, and control	Provide for choice making, particularly with regard to personal space and personal matters; involve the person in decision making but under selected conditions
Facilitate involvement of family and friends	Encourage visits and involvement of family, friends, and others with whom the person is familiar

Adapted from Brawley (1997).

to underwrite, develop, and cover operations expenses; and training and education capacities for ensuring a continued source of personnel. Interagency agreements for the development and management of small community group homes for people affected by dementia, regardless of premorbid diagnosis, should be explored as they could also help agencies that serve people with intellectual disabilities share costs with other providers (e.g., area agencies on aging, home health agencies, hospitals, nursing facilities, Alzheimer's providers) over the long term.

Referral Out

The third option, referral out, asks the question, "Why do adults with dementia end up in long-term care settings?" Outside of major postoperative or specialized nursing care, most older adults in the general population do so because they can no longer care for themselves and their informal support structures have broken down (Mittelman, Ferris, Shulman, Steinberg, & Levin, 1996) or their behavior has become more problematic (Reisburg, Ferris, & DeLeon, 1989). In the former, the situation of a surviving spouse with diminishing stamina and spirit who can no longer cook or provide for self-care and who has no proximate family is typical as is the person with dementia being without a day-to-day caregiver because of death, illness, other commitments, and geographical distance. In such situations, a nursing facility becomes a board and care option that, along with medication, health management, and socialization, provides for the individual's primary care needs. Criteria for admission to such facilities generally are set in state regulations or policies and involve a preadmission screening, generally using a standard instrument. Such instruments look for loss of abilities in ADLs and instrumental activities of daily living (IADLs) and note the need for basic personal care assistance and the presence or absence of direct support from family members (e.g., the Care Needs Assessment Pack for Dementia [McWalter et al., 1998]). In most states, adults with intellectual disabilities easily pass through these nursing facility screens, as their ADLs, IADLs, and personal care levels generally are already below or at the threshold for admission (Governor's Commission on Mental Retardation, 1996).

Not all housing and care options for people with dementia entail direct admission to nursing facilities (Alzheimer's Disease and Related Disorders Association, 1998). Alternative options for what could be termed generic Alzheimer's care include retirement housing, senior apartments or senior living settings, assisted living settings, and continuing care retirement communities (Grant & Sommers, 1998). The first serves people who are considered to be the most independent, and, if staff are present, they rarely have training in dementia and provide no assistance with medication or personal care. However, visiting nurses or other in-home services can be arranged, and these settings might be appropriate for people who are minimally impaired by dementia (i.e., during early stages) and capable of living on their own. The second option, assisted living, board and care or group homes, and related housing, generally provides a private room, meals, access to cooking facilities, on-site staff, and a protected environment (Assisted Living Quality Coalition, 1998). Some will be able to provide for people with dementia; others will not. Many assisted living facilities, particularly ones that are operated by proprietary organizations, offer special memory or dementia care programs and are appropriate for people who may no longer be able to care for themselves. Continuing care retirement communities (CCRC) are usually multifaceted housing programs that offer a range of levels of care and generally are private pay. People with early-stage dementia can secure housing with the assurance that as they decline, the CCRC program will adapt to their needs and provide varying levels of care (Sloan,

Shayne, & Conover, 1995). Finally, some nursing facilities offer special dementia care units and programs that are designed to provide specialized care for people with mid- to late-stage needs.

Agencies may resort to referral out because of a number of factors, including the threshold effect noted previously, lack of congruence with agency mission (i.e., not pre- pared to provide health care or long-term care for people with diminishing capacities), costs (lack of adequate reimbursement for actual costs for care from government agen- cies), and inadequate staff capabilities or training capacities (Cohen, 1999). To justify referral out, we have observed that some intellectual disabilities agencies argue that nursing care facilities are better qualified to provide care for people with intellectual dis- abilities and dementia because of their focus on "nursing care," or having specialized nursing care staff, and because their size would permit provision of such care at a less expensive daily rate. Some even propose to develop special units within existing nurs- ing facilities that are dedicated to people with intellectual disabilities. These proposals generally suggest augmenting nursing facility staff with staff from the disability agency so that such units may be jointly operated. The main thrust of these proposals is to pro- vide housing and dementia care as it is provided to other older people who are affected by dementia and to provide for an economy of scale relative to costs (noting "bigger is cheaper"). Yet for those agencies that are reluctant to refer out, particularly those that are parent based and that may have no other option because of low reimbursement levels from state funding agencies, there are additional concerns over the seeming lack of qual- ity control in nursing facilities ("Toward Nursing Home Reform," 1999), the reported higher quality of life among adults who have moved out of nursing facilities (Heller, Factor, Hsieh, & Hahn, 1998) and, more important, the inadequacy of specialized atten- tion for people with lifelong cognitive deficits (Cohen, 1999). Also, many recognize that the movement to a location away from a long-familiar house and staff may increase dis- orientation and earlier death (McCallion, 1999).

For many agencies, the pressing concern is rising costs associated with care for peo- ple with dementia. Many are not receiving reimbursements commensurate with chang- ing care conditions and feel forced to discharge the person to more institutional, dementia-capable settings (Chaput, 1998; Cohen, 1999; Udell, 1999a). This is often the result of states' reluctance to revise their daily rates for community care settings once the initial rate is set. Our experience has shown that this generally occurs because of bureaucratic inertia, poor long-term planning for addressing "aging in place," and con- cerns over expanding costs of community care as they affect annual agency budgets. So, it is often more expedient to let care agencies absorb the pressure of changing care conditions than to request appropriate resources (which may run counter to guberna- torial or legislative policies). It is interesting that such restraints often are not observed when initializing services. So, with the growing number of people aging in our com- munities, one may legitimately ask why most state intellectual disabilities agencies will underwrite the expected cost of care for younger people and provide extraordinary supports to maintain them in their community but do not do the same when adults with intellectual disabilities age.

PROGRAMMATIC SUGGESTIONS

Care systems are challenged by trying to provide care for dementia, particularly be- cause the prevailing form of dementia, resulting from Alzheimer's disease, is slow and progressive and results in a profound loss of skills and capabilities. Although early- stage care practices may be less taxing, late-stage care practices often demand sizable resources. General dementia care practices can be accommodated in a range of settings, starting with informal in-home care supports and ending with formal long-term care structured settings. Most home-based care research reveals that dementia care can be a taxing occupation and that caregivers are hard pressed to keep up with the care demands. For example, Gordon, Carter, and Scott (1997) noted that prevalent daily tasks include aiding with mobility, personal care, domestic chores, and management of behavior. Similar demands for personal care and behavior management occupy caregivers during the night. Indeed, predictors of high levels of care include severity of dementia, somatic disorders, and dependency in ADLs (Boersma, Eefsting, van den Brink, & van Tilburg, 1997). The nature of informal caregiving for people with dementia generally mirrors that for adults with intellectual disabilities (i.e., respite, in-home supports, transportation); however, the intensity of care is heightened, and, in most instances, the ages of the caregiver and the dependent adult are more advanced (Alzheimer's Disease and Related Disorders Association, 1999).

Such dementia-related behavior disturbances can pose significant care management concerns but if addressed constructively and purposefully can often be minimized. The behaviors noted next generally are associated with dementia (Warner, 1998) but also may be observed in people with intellectual disabilities who are not affected by dementia (Davidson et al., 1995). Following are some of the common behavior disturbances or abnormalities that often are associated with later-stage dementias, accompanied by some comments on program or home design applications to adults with intellectual disabilities and dementia. These represent both nuisance behaviors (i.e., they are somewhat innocuous but do require special attention from staff) and compromising behaviors (i.e., they can be serious impediments to the equilibrium in the home, can pose danger, and require particular attention and preparatory planning from staff).

Nuisance Behaviors

Rummaging, hiding, and *hoarding* can occur among people who are affected by dementia (Hwang, Tsai, Yang, Liu, & Lirng, 1998). To address these particular behaviors, which can be a nuisance to housemates and family, practices can be instituted to limit access to housemates' rooms and periodically check the person's own space for items that may have been picked up and stored. People with dementia may inadvertently place objects in inappropriate places, such as leaving a bar of soap in the refrigerator. Such behaviors have a logic to them for some individuals (as in storing items to be safe from imaginary adversaries) or are random and seemingly without purpose (Warner, 1998). Rummaging, hiding, and hoarding behaviors can be minimized by careful staff surveillance and interventions (Antonangeli, 1995).

Shadowing also occurs in people with intellectual disabilities who do not have dementia. This behavior is characterized by clinging or remaining in close proximity to others, particularly a favorite staff person or family member (Warner, 1998). For those with dementia, this behavior may be heightened and usually marks a gross insecurity or fear of loss on the part of the person affected. Changes in home configuration, noise, or clutter or installation of assistive devices that help the person gain line of sight or hear the presence of the others in the home all are helpful in minimizing anxieties that result from loss of connection to staff or other caregivers (Antonangeli, 1995). Common spaces in the home that are open rather than closed can help, as can door designs that permit a view to where activities are taking place or others are present.

Repetitive behaviors are found in people with lifelong cognitive impairments as well. These behaviors are characterized by abnormal perseverance at some task or activity.

These behaviors can usually be addressed through thoughtful interventions and therapeutic techniques that anticipate what the person may be doing and why. Although home design features may not affect such behaviors, redirecting activities and assigning productive work tasks that can divert or engage the person can prove helpful (Antonangeli, 1995). Caregivers need to decide whether such behaviors are truly problematic before initiating an intervention.

Pica, or the ingesting of nonfood materials, is seen in some people with severe intellectual disabilities as well as among some adults with dementia (Okuda, Harada, Mizutani, & Hamanaka, 1998). Among people with dementia, it may occur in response to losses for cuing, such that one item may be mistaken for another. Losses for cuing result in generalizations. For example, a colorful, albeit dangerous, cleaning fluid could be mistaken for a favorite beverage of the same color (even if it is clearly marked and in its original container). Obviously, such behavior can be dangerous if the items ingested are harmful. Harmful liquids and household products should be stored in closed cupboards or rooms where they cannot be seen or reached.

Compromising Behaviors

Agitation, combativeness, aggression, and *resistance* are behaviors that can also be found in people with intellectual disabilities with secondary diagnoses other than dementia. However, among the general population, such behaviors generally are associated with dementia and when coupled with dementia in people with intellectual disabilities can be the cause of significant concern among housemates and staff. Design features may need to take into account physical aggression, and items that may become weapons may need to be placed out of sight. More important, staff and housemates need to be told not to personalize the attacks when they are the subject of outbursts or aggression and that these types of occurrences may reflect how the person deals with losses of control or frustrations over continued disorientation caused by the dementing process. Because aggressive acts may be set off by stimuli in the environment, staff may want to log recurring instances, identify the stimuli, and then design ways to mitigate them. Sometimes environmental factors may be the cause of such situations (e.g., the ringing of a loud doorbell or buzzer); thus, alterations in the home are called for. Aggressive or noxious behaviors may also occur when the person is placed in an uncertain situation over which he or she may have no control and may use resistant or aggressive behavior as a response. The person may not have the capacity to internalize reasoning to diminish the behaviors, and care needs to be taken to eliminate or minimize stimuli that set them off.

Catastrophic reactions or extremes in emotional response may occur from a perceived threat or uncertainty. Such behaviors may involve screaming, throwing objects, flailing, and other extremes of emoting or movement. These may also occur in adults with intellectual disabilities who have poor impulse control or who are emotionally immature. When dementia is present, they may become exaggerated and cause great upset to housemates and others in the home because they most likely did not occur in the person's premorbid state. Home design features to minimize damage or injury from the occurrence of such behaviors may include consideration of where typical home objects and furniture are placed and elimination of protruding hard edges and other dangers that could cause injury if struck (Warner, 1998). Clinical responses can include identifying triggers that set off the behavior, calming the situation, and providing reassurance while ensuring the safety of others in the room (Antonangeli, 1995).

Suspiciousness, delusions, and *hallucinations* occur as part of the dementing process as the individual loses familiar physical anchors and memories. Suspiciousness and delusions may have basis in life events or may be a reaction to the home situation. Hallucinations (visual, auditory, or olfactory) may be more problematic and may be reflective of more serious psychopathology. These psychiatric symptoms are not always present but can be difficult to address when they do occur. Given the context of a disease such as Alzheimer's, calming techniques and reassurance of perceptions are the best clinical techniques to use, as well as minimizing events that trigger the person's suspicions. Medications can be productive, particularly if the person is experiencing hallucinations. Physical design features can help, particularly if the person is reacting to environmental features (e.g., poor lighting, reflections, images in wallpaper or other decor).

Sundowning is a particular behavioral phenomenon seen in adults who are affected by dementia (Williams, 1995). It generally occurs later in the day and is manifested by agitation, heightened confusion, or other behaviors that indicate unease and disorientation (Burney-Pucket, 1996; Little, Satlin, Sunderland, & Volicer, 1995). It has been proposed that sundowning may be linked to sleep apnea, deprivation of rapid eye movement sleep, or other factors linked to fatigue or deterioration of the suprachiasmatic nucleus of the hypothalamus (Burney-Pucket, 1996; Vitiello, Bliwise, & Prinz, 1992). Techniques to prevent this behavioral phenomenon are not well defined, although it is useful to be aware of triggering events and attempt to address these. Some have proposed that lighting or access to sunlight might reduce agitation in the late afternoon, although these are not proven applications (Warner, 1998). Others note the positive effects of calm or soothing talking with the person and reduction of sensory inputs (Williams, 1995). There is also some preliminary evidence that massage may improve the quality of sleep of people who are affected by dementia (McCallion & Hegeman, 1998).

Wandering is repetitive, sometimes incessant, roaming, pacing, or attempting to leave the home (Warner, 1998) and generally is associated with greater cognitive dysfunction (Logsdon et al., 1998). It may occur for a variety of reasons: The person may have some specific purpose in mind, may be trying to avoid something, may simply be meandering aimlessly, or may be agitated (Klein et al., 1999). Wandering can be productive behavior as it provides exercise and often is a coping mechanism for reliving stress and tension (Neistein & Siegal, 1996). Home designs for people with dementia often accommodate wandering by building connections among corridors, hallways, and other passage ways; establishing special paths in fenced-in gardens or yards; and constructing dwellings with a central core that provides an interconnection among the main rooms, thus producing a continuous loop for walking and permitting the person to return easily to a starting point (Passini, Rainville, Marchand, & Joanette, 1995; Warner, 1998). Such designs can also provide for needed exercise (Williams, 1995).

Programmatic Adaptations

Many of the general recommendations promoted by Alzheimer's advocacy groups apply to care practices in home settings for people with intellectual disabilities who also have Alzheimer's disease or related dementias (see, e.g., Alzheimer's Disease and Related Disorders Association, 1997). Care and day-to-day supports and services generally do not differ from those provided in specialized housing settings for adults with intellectual disabilities. These include the following general applications (adapted from Sloane, 1997):

- Attention to physical conditioning and exercise
- Attention to personal hygiene
- Involvement in stimulating activities
- Involvement of friends, family, and others
- Maintenance of ADLs
- Management of concomitant medical conditions
- Minimization of discomfort
- Promotion of nutrition and hydration
- Promotion of safety and security
- Support for continence in bladder and bowels
- Support of dignity through respect and attention to appearance
- Support of emotional needs

The dementia care model for adults with intellectual disabilities assumes the following: 1) The condition is progressive, and ever-diminishing abilities are an expectation and 2) even when there is severe cognitive loss, the person remains ambulatory. Thus, the programmatic focus needs to be on compensating for cognitive losses and disorientation, and primary care practices should support safety and mobility and offer protection against injury and disease. Program applications should minimize the presentation of behaviors that can disrupt the equilibrium of the home or pose a danger to the person or others and should help the individual maintain dignity and skills. Even though dementia will eventually lead to debilitation and death, much can be done in the years between recognition of onset and eventual death to make the person feel productive. Within the context of the general applications noted previously, the unique aspects of care for people with intellectual disabilities who are experiencing dementia can fall into three areas: 1) maintaining communication, 2) supporting continued independence, and 3) resolving problem behaviors.

Maintaining Communication   A critical concern is that dementia progressively alters four major components of a person's communication skills: phonology, syntax, semantics, and pragmatics. *Phonology* is the process of forming and producing words, *syntax* involves the processes of sentence comprehension and formulation, and *semantics* is the knowledge of meanings of words. Pragmatics is the learned rules of managing communication, such as maintenance of cohesion and coherence, taking turns, managing topics during a conversation, and reengaging another person when the conversation breaks down (Ripich, 1994; Toseland & McCallion, 1998). Breakdowns in the ability to manage conversations can be dramatic, creating frustrating situations for families, other caregivers, and the person with dementia. For people with intellectual disabilities, the breakdowns may be pronounced because communication skills may have been limited to begin with. Frustrations encourage withdrawal from conversation, even when communication is still possible. Giving up trying to communicate with the person with intellectual disabilities even seems justified, because family members and other caregivers do not want to frustrate the person unnecessarily.

Meaningful communication also requires the processing of words, sounds, and symbols by one's memory to produce and comprehend concepts. There are three levels of memory: sensory, primary, and secondary. Sensory memory is what we hear and see; primary memory is where we interpret, code, and maintain what we see and hear based on coding schemes maintained in secondary memory. Secondary, or long-term, memory also has three subcomponents. Episodic memory contains the conscious recollection of specific events in particular places and times—for example, "I was born on

Independence Day, July 4th, 1941, in Albany." Semantic memory contains vocabulary and general knowledge independent of time and context—for example, "A lot of people barbecue on Independence Day." Procedural memory is about knowing when to do something, what to do, and how to do it—for example, "You need to get the coals nice and gray before you put fish on the barbecue." More and more memories and encoding and interpreting processes are lost with the progression of dementia.

For people with intellectual disabilities, the extent of such memories may be limited and the deterioration may occur at a rapid pace. Long-held procedural memories, however, are usually retained for a long period (Tomoeda & Bayles, 1990). Maintaining communication given these deteriorations is achieved through practicing good communication techniques; using communication aids such as glasses and hearing aids; encouraging the expression of long-held memories using memory photo albums, charts, and audiotapes; and maintaining the effort to communicate even when the person with intellectual disabilities no longer responds (McCallion, 1999; Seman, 1998).

Supporting Continued Independence   Maintenance of people with intellectual disabilities in familiar surroundings, with people they know, and among favored possessions offers the best opportunity to maintain some level of personal independence during the course of the dementia. Regardless of location, however, a series of environmental modifications will assist independence. A four-step process has been found to be helpful: 1) environmental scanning, 2) environmental labeling, 3) environmental flooding, and 4) environmental simplification.

Caregivers need to examine the home or day program site for barriers to independence that will frustrate or confuse the person. This is called environmental scanning. Things to look for include similar looking doors and hallways that make orientation and direction finding more difficult and door mechanisms that are difficult to manage. Helping with orientation or wayfinding (Lawton, 1996) can help compensate for problems with environmental scanning. Some of the frustration and confusion that result can also be reduced through environmental labeling. Putting signs on doors and varying the color of doors, carpeting, and hallways provide visual clues that enable a person with intellectual disabilities to negotiate his or her living or day environment independently. If the person with intellectual disabilities is able to read, then the intervention can be extended to labeling furniture and personal possessions to provide an additional clue to what they are and how they should be used. This is the basis of environmental flooding, a process of giving individuals with dementia multiple clues. For example, a caregiver asks a person with intellectual disabilities who is experiencing dementia to go to the dining room. In many homes, this is a process of choosing between two to three similarly painted closed doors, and many individuals would be unable to find the dining room independently. There is a greater likelihood of success if the caregiver can say that it is the room with the red door and if when the person with intellectual disabilities approaches the door there is a sign that says "dining room," the door is open, the person can hear knives and forks being set on the table, and he or she can smell the food about to be served. Scanning will also identify locations that provide easy access to areas with cleaning supplies, machinery, or tools and egresses that lead to potentially dangerous traffic situations. Restrictions are often placed on independence because the person with intellectual disabilities who is experiencing dementia may wander off, leave a stove on, mistakenly drink cleaning fluids, and so forth. Environmental simplification offers some solutions. Exit from the home can be to a pleasant fenced yard rather than to an open lawn with traffic at its edge; stoves and other appliances can be equipped with shut-off switches; and cleaning fluids and tools can be located in a secure area without totally barring access to kitchens, garages, and basements.

Prior work indicates that a three-step communications-based approach to problem behaviors may be helpful: 1) Find and respond to the need, 2) find the memory, and 3) ensure safety (McCallion, Toseland, Lacey, Freedman, & Banks, 1999). Strategies recommended to discover the nature of the need include 1) asking yes-or-no questions to narrow down what is agitating the person with intellectual disabilities, 2) interpreting the person's gestures and other nonverbal signs, 3) trying to look at the situation through the eyes of the person with intellectual disabilities, and 4) recalling what caused similar incidents in the past. In regard to finding the memory, some experts believe that as people with dementia reminisce more about their past, they also revisit past conflicts and problems. This, in turn, can cause agitation (see, e.g., Feil, 1993). Given preexisting communication limitations, discovering the cause of the agitation may be more difficult with people with intellectual disabilities than with other individuals who are experiencing dementia. Nevertheless, strategies recommended for dealing with this include listening for familiar names and events and asking simple questions that encourage and assist the person with intellectual disabilities to explain what is upsetting him or her. Strategies to ensure safety include 1) staying calm, 2) speaking in soothing tones and keeping all body language nonthreatening, 3) distracting the person with a favorite activity, and 4) getting help if there is a danger of injury to the caregiver or to the person with intellectual disabilities.

CONCLUSIONS

The National Association of State Developmental Disabilities Directors (1997) noted that in the United States, there is a great need for out-of-home housing options. Given that recent estimates put the number of older adults with intellectual disabilities, ages 60 and older, at approximately 500,000, expectations are that the numbers will increase to approximately 1.5 million by 2030 when all of the post–World War II "baby boomers" (those born between 1946 and 1964) are of retirement age. Contributing to these numbers is the issue of longer life span and prolonged survival among adults with intellectual disabilities. It is believed that approximately 80% of adults of all ages live at home and that many, if not most, of these individuals are unknown to state intellectual and developmental disabilities agencies. With life span increasing and greater numbers evident as a result of the baby boom effect, the potential for a significant increase in people of old age with intellectual disabilities is very high. The National Association of State Developmental Disabilities Directors (1997) noted that to accommodate these increases, states will need to be prepared to provide 1) housing options that emphasize small settings with supports, 2) family support programs for adults still living at home, and 3) programs that increase the dignity of the individual and allow older people with disabilities a chance to contribute to and benefit from community life. Given these expectations, the rise of the subpopulation affected by dementia will also present a challenge for providers and public funding resources.

We suggest that agencies consider what the impact of dementia will be not only on people with intellectual disabilities but also on staff and caregivers. Although a detailed examination of staff stress and burden is beyond the scope of this chapter, we can recommend areas of training and support to help staff cope with care management challenges and duties that may take an emotional and physical toll. Everyone should become more aware of the subtle signs of the onset of dementia, such as memory loss and behavior change, and should be trained to become careful observers who keep detailed notes of their observations. Training should also focus on care management techniques and the specific approaches for coping with functional limitations as the disease progresses through the later stages. As the death of affected individuals becomes imminent, end-of-life supports for staff and other caregivers are essential. Such training should be based on beliefs that stress the individuality of the adult with dementia and a perspective that promotes personal dignity, autonomy, and personal welfare. Overall, preparation of staff should include training in the following content areas: normal and pathological aging; Alzheimer's disease; recognition of early signs of dementia; methods for conducting periodic assessments and evaluations; available services; supporting caregivers; general care management; and effective practices for interventions for the early, middle, and late stages of dementia.

In addition to training programs for staff, information should be provided to family caregivers. When the person is still at home, supports and orientation should be provided to family caregivers to enable them to maintain their relative's functioning more effectively and to know from where to seek needed services. Information about program supports, such as day services and respite, as well as in-home services should be made available. Families should be connected to support organizations for Alzheimer's disease or to developmental disabilities and other community resources.

With regard to the impact of dementia on care systems, planning for when and to what extent adults with intellectual disabilities will be affected should provide agencies with a rational basis for the allocation of often scarce resources. Greater emphasis should be given to supporting aging in place by providing more staff training and making modifications to physical environments as well as adaptations to programs to make them dementia capable (Chaput, 1998; Cooper, 1997; Janicki et al., 1996; Janicki & Dalton, 1999; Udell, 1999b). Emerging information on the onset and duration of dementias is telling in that it can help pinpoint at-risk age groups and provide information on when agencies need to begin planning and budgeting for long-term specialized supports for adults with dementia. In addition, given the implications of the increasing number of older adults, managers need to determine whether they want to support individual instances of aging in place or develop specialized community supports for groups of similarly affected individuals. Knowing about the duration and changes related to stages of dementia can help program managers plan proactively for staff deployments and retraining at critical junctures.

Given that progressively more adults may be aging within their own families or in supportive settings, agencies should be more proactive at helping families and other caregivers become trained to raise their "index of suspicion" and to be prepared to provide special services, such as supports for changing behavioral competence and cognitive decline (Pollack, 1998; Walker & Walker, 1998). Care management resources are often allocated on the basis of reasoned estimates of when onset may occur and to what degree dementia may be found in any service population. Agencies that specifically serve older adults with Down syndrome will need to be more vigilant for early-onset signs and provide additional resources earlier in the life course because of the increased occurrence of dementia in this group of people with intellectual disabilities.

In this chapter, we have laid out some of the considerations of confronting dementia as a compounding disability and have presented some thoughts as to what needs to be considered and when. It is hoped that this information will be useful in designing specialized services for older people with intellectual disabilities.

REFERENCES

Alfredson, B.B., & Annerstedt, L. (1994). Staff attitudes and job satisfaction in the care of demented elderly people: Group living compared with long-term care institutions. *Journal of Advances in Nursing, 20,* 964–974.

Alloul, K., Sauriol, L., Kennedy, W., Laurier, C., Tessier, G., Novosel, S., & Contandriopoulos, A. (1998). Alzheimer's disease: A review of the disease, its epidemiology and economic impact. *Archives of Gerontology and Geriatrics, 27,* 189–221.

Alvarez, N. (1996). The natural evolution of Alzheimer's disease in persons with Down syndrome. *British Journal of Developmental Disabilities, 42,* S82.

Alzheimer's Disease and Related Disorders Association. (1992). *Guidelines for dignity: Goals of specialized Alzheimer/dementia care in residential settings.* Chicago: Author.

Alzheimer's Disease and Related Disorders Association. (1997). *Key elements of dementia care.* Chicago: Author.

Alzheimer's Disease and Related Disorders Association. (1998). *Residential care: A guide for choosing a new home.* Chicago: Author.

Alzheimer's Disease and Related Disorders Association. (1999). *Who cares? Families caring for persons with Alzheimer's disease.* Chicago: Author.

American Psychological Association. (1998). Guidelines for the evaluation of dementia and age-related cognitive decline. *American Psychologist, 53,* 1298–1303.

Antonangeli, J.M. (1995). *Of two minds: A guide to the care of people with the dual diagnosis of Alzheimer's disease and mental retardation.* Malden, MA: Cooperative for Human Services.

The Arc of the United States. (1995). *Developmental disabilities and Alzheimer's disease: What you should know.* Silver Spring, MD: Author.

Assisted Living Quality Coalition. (1998). *Assisted living quality initiative: Building a structure that promotes quality.* Chicago: Alzheimer's Disease and Related Disorders Association.

Aylward, E., Burt, D., Thorpe, L., Lai, F., & Dalton, A.J. (1995). *Diagnosis of dementia in individuals with mental retardation: Report of the task force for development of criteria for diagnosis of dementia in individuals with mental retardation.* Washington, DC: American Association on Mental Retardation.

Aylward, E., Burt, D., Thorpe, L., Lai, F., & Dalton, A.J. (1997). Diagnosis of dementia in individuals with intellectual disability: Report of the task force for development of criteria for diagnosis of dementia in individuals with mental retardation. *Journal of Intellectual Disability Research, 41,* 152–164.

Boersma, F., Eefsting, J.A., van den Brink, W., & van Tilburg, W. (1997). Care services for dementia patients: Predictors for service utilization. *International Journal of Geriatric Psychiatry, 12,* 1119–1126.

Brawley, E.C. (1997). *Designing for Alzheimer's disease: Strategies for creating better care environments.* New York: John Wiley & Sons.

Brodtkorp, E. (1994). The diversity of epilepsy in adults with severe developmental disabilities: Age of seizure onset and other prognostic factors. *Seizure, 3,* 277–285.

Burney-Pucket, M. (1996). Sundown effect: Etiology and management. *Journal of Psychosocial Nursing and Mental Health Services, 34*(5), 40–43.

Burt, D.B., & Aylward, E. (1999). Assessment methods of diagnosis of dementia. In M.P. Janicki & A.J. Dalton (Eds.), *Dementia, aging, and intellectual disabilities: A handbook* (pp. 141–156). Philadelphia: Brunner/Mazel.

Chaput, J.L. (1998). *Housing people with Alzheimer disease as a result of Down syndrome: A quality of life comparison between group homes and special care units in long term care facilities.* Unpublished master's thesis, University of Manitoba, Department of City Planning, Winnipeg, Manitoba, Canada.

Cohen, A. (1999, May). *Perspectives on nursing home diversion for individuals with mental retardation who are aging.* Paper presented at the annual meeting of the American Association on Mental Retardation, New Orleans, LA.

Cohen, U., & Weisman, G.D. (1991). *Holding on to home: Designing environments for people with dementia.* Baltimore: Johns Hopkins University Press.

Cooper, S.-A. (1997). High prevalence of dementia among people with learning disabilities not attributable to Down's syndrome. *Psychological Medicine, 27,* 609–616.

Dalton, A.J., & Janicki, M.P. (1999). Aging and dementia. In M.P. Janicki & A.J. Dalton (Eds.), *Dementia, aging, and intellectual disabilities: A handbook* (pp. 5–31). Philadelphia: Brunner/Mazel.

Davidson, P.W., Janicki, M.P., Landrigan, P., Houser, K.D., Henderson, C.M., Cain, N.N., & Brown, C.B. (1995, September). *Age span characteristics of adults with intellectual disability and psychiatric and behavioral symptoms: An exploratory study.* Paper presented at the First European Association for Mental Health in Mental Retardation, Amsterdam, The Netherlands.

Davis, D.R. (1999). A parent's perspective. In M.P. Janicki & A.J. Dalton (Eds.), *Dementia, aging, and intellectual disabilities: A handbook* (pp. 42–50). Philadelphia: Brunner/Mazel.

Duggan, L., Lewis, M., & Morgan, J. (1996). Behavioural changes in people with learning disability and dementia: A descriptive study. *Journal of Intellectual Disability Research, 40,* 311–321.

Evans, D.A., Sherr, P.A., Albert, M.S., Funkenstein, H.H., Hebert, L.E., Wetle, T.T., Branch, L.G., Chown, M., Hennekens, C.H., & Taylor, J.O. (1990). Estimated prevalence of Alzheimer's disease in the United States. *Milbank Quarterly, 68*(2), 267–289.

Evenhuis, H.M. (1997). The natural history of dementia in ageing people with intellectual disability. *Journal of Intellectual Disability Research, 41,* 92–96.

Feil, N. (1993). *The validation breakthrough: Simple techniques for communicating with people with "Alzheimer's-type dementia."* Baltimore: Health Professions Press.

Folstein, M.F., Bassett, S.S., Anthony, J.C., Romanoski, A.J., & Nestadt, G.R. (1991). Dementia: Case ascertainment in a community survey. *Journal of Gerontology, 46,* M132–M138.

Folstein, M.F., Folstein, S.E., & McHugh, P.R. (1975). "Mini-Mental State": A practical method for grading the cognitive state for the clinician. *Journal of Psychiatric Research, 12,* 189–198.

Fray, M.T. (2000). *Caring for Kathleen: A sister's story about Down's syndrome and dementia.* Worcestershire, UK: BILD Publications.

Gordon, D.S., Carter, H., & Scott, S. (1997). Profiling the care needs of the population with dementia: A survey of central Scotland. *International Journal of Geriatric Psychiatry, 12,* 753–759.

Governor's Commission on Mental Retardation. (1996). *Nursing homes as residential placements for persons with mental retardation.* Boston: Author.

Grant, L.A., & Sommers, A.R. (1998). Adapting living environments for persons with Alzheimer's disease. *Geriatrics, 53,* S61–S65.

Grant, L.A., Kane, R.A., Potthoff, S.J., & Ryden, M. (1996). Staff training and turnover in Alzheimer special care units: Comparisons with non-special care units. *Geriatric Nursing, 17,* 278–282.

Hammond, B., & Beneditti, P. (1999). Perspectives of a care provider. In M.P. Janicki & A.J. Dalton (Eds.), *Dementia, aging, and intellectual disabilities: A handbook* (pp. 32–41). Philadelphia: Brunner/Mazel.

Heller, T., Factor, A.R., Hsieh, K., & Hahn, J.E. (1998). Impact of age and transition out of nursing homes for adults with developmental disabilities. *American Journal on Mental Retardation, 103,* 236–248.

Hepburn, K., Petrie, M., Peterson, C., & VanLoy, W. (1995). A moving experience: Reconfiguring a special care unit for Alzheimer's patients. *Gerontologist, 35,* 831–835.

Holland, A.J. (1999). Down's syndrome. In M.P. Janicki & A.J. Dalton (Eds.), *Dementia, aging, and intellectual disabilities: A handbook* (pp. 183–197). Philadelphia: Brunner/Mazel.

Hurley, A.C., & Kennedy, K. (1997). Human resources. In *Key elements of dementia care* (pp. 51–66). Chicago: Alzheimer's Disease and Related Disorders Association.

Hutchings, B.L. (1999, May). *Aging carers and adults with developmental disabilities: Needs and preferences.* Poster presented at the 123rd annual meeting of the American Association on Mental Retardation, New Orleans.

Hwang, J.P., Tsai, S.J., Yang, C.H., Liu, K.M., & Lirng, J.F. (1998). Hoarding behavior in dementia: A preliminary report. *American Journal of Geriatric Psychiatry, 6,* 285–289.

Janicki, M.P. (1998, November). *Community care for older adults with intellectual disabilities with dementia and increasing frailty.* Paper presented at the 51st annual scientific meeting of the Gerontological Society of America, Philadelphia.

Janicki, M.P., & Dalton, A.J. (1997a, April). *Prevalence of dementia and impact on intellectual disability services.* Paper presented at the International Congress III on the Dually Diagnosed-Mental Heath Aspects of Mental Retardation, Montréal, Quebec, Canada.

Janicki, M.P., & Dalton, A.J. (1997b, October). *Planning for the occurrence of dementia among adults with Down syndrome.* Paper presented at the 6th World Congress on Down's Syndrome, Madrid, Spain.

Janicki, M.P., & Dalton, A.J. (1999). Dementia in developmental disabilities. In N. Bouras (Ed.), *Psychiatric and behavioural disorders in developmental disabilities and mental retardation* (pp. 121–153). Cambridge, UK: Cambridge University Press.

Janicki, M.P., & Dalton, A.J. (2000). Prevalence of dementia and impact on intellectual disability services. *Mental Retardation, 38,* 277–289.

Janicki, M.P., Dalton, A.J., Henderson, M., & Davidson, P.W. (1999). Mortality and morbidity among older adults with intellectual disabilities: Health services considerations. *Disability and Rehabilitation, 21,* 284–294.

Janicki, M.P., Heller, T., Seltzer, G., & Hogg, J. (1996). Practice guidelines for the clinical assessment and care management of Alzheimer's disease and other dementias among adults with intellectual disability. *Journal of Intellectual Disability Research, 40,* 374–382.

Klein, D.A., Steinberg, M., Galik, E., Steele, C., Sheppard, J.M., Warren, A., Rosenblatt, A., & Lyketsos, C.G. (1999). Wandering behavior in community-residing persons with dementia. *International Journal of Geriatric Psychiatry, 14,* 272–279.

Koenig, B.R. (1995). *Aged and dementia care issues of people with intellectual disability: Literature review and survey of carers.* Brighton, South Australia, Australia: MINDA.

Lawton, C.A. (1996). Strategies for indoor wayfinding: The role of orientation. *Journal of Environmental Psychology, 16,* 137–145.

Little, J.T., Satlin, A., Sunderland, T., & Volicer, L. (1995). Sundown syndrome in severely demented patients with probable Alzheimer's disease. *Journal of Geriatric Psychiatry and Neurology, 8,* 103–106.

Logsdon, R.G., Teri, L., McCurry, S.M., Gibbons, L.E., Kukull, W.A., & Larson, E.B. (1998). Wandering: A significant problem among community-residing individuals with Alzheimer's disease. *Journal of Gerontology, 53B,* 294–299.

Lovestone, S. (1998). *Early diagnosis and treatment of Alzheimer's disease.* London: Martin Dunitz.

Marler, R., & Cunningham, C. (1994). *Down's syndrome and Alzheimer's disease.* London: Down's Syndrome Association.

May, H.L., Fletcher, C., Alvarez, N., Zuis, J., & Cavallari, S.G. (1996). *Alzheimer's disease and Down syndrome: A manual of care.* Wrentham, MA: Alzheimer's Committee of Wrentham Developmental Center.

McCallion, P. (1999). Maintaining communication. In M.P. Janicki & A.J. Dalton (Eds.), *Dementia, aging, and intellectual disabilities: A handbook* (pp. 261–277). Philadelphia: Brunner/Mazel.

McCallion, P., & Hegeman, C.R. (1998). *Keeping in touch: Attentive touch for nursing home residents with dementia* (Final report). Albany, NY: Foundation for Long-Term Care.

McCallion, P., Toseland, R., Lacey, D., Freedman, K., & Banks, S. (1999). Educating nursing assistants to communicate more effectively with nursing home residents with dementia. *Gerontologist, 39,* 546–558.

McVicker, R.W., Shanks, O.E.P., & McClelland, R.J. (1994). Prevalence and associated features of epilepsy in adults with Down's syndrome. *British Journal of Psychiatry, 164,* 528–532.

McWalter, G., Toner, H., McWalter, A., Eastwood, J., Marshall, M., & Turvey, T. (1998). A community needs assessment: The care needs assessment pack for dementia (CARENAPD). Its development, reliability and validity. *International Journal of Geriatric Psychiatry, 13,* 16–22.

Meyers, B.S. (1999). Depression and dementia: Comorbidities, identification and treatment. *Journal of Geriatric Psychiatry and Neurology, 11,* 201–205.

Mittelman, M.S., Ferris, S.H., Shulman, E., Steinberg, G., & Levin, B. (1996). A family intervention to delay nursing home placement of patients with Alzheimer disease: A randomized controlled trial. *Journal of the American Medical Association, 278,* 1725–1731.

Monmaney, T. (1997, November 28). Thankful for a place called home. *The Los Angeles Times,* pp. A1, A36.

Moss, S., & Patel, P. (1997). Dementia in older people with intellectual disability: Symptoms of physical and mental illness, and levels of adaptive behaviour. *Journal of Intellectual Disability Research, 41,* 60–69.

Moss, S., Lambe, L., & Hogg, J. (1998). *Ageing matters: Pathways for older people with learning disabilities.* Kidderminster, UK: British Institute of Learning Disabilities.

National Association of State Developmental Disabilities Directors. (1997). States confront dilemma in serving aging DD population. *Community Services Reporter, 4*(6), 1, 4–5.

Nearly one-fifth of nursing homes offer Alzheimer's specialized care. (1998, July). *Housing the Elderly Report, 98*(7), 5.

Neistein, S., & Siegal, A.P. (1996). Agitation, wandering, pacing, restlessness, and repetitive mannerisms. *International Psychogeriatrics, 8,* 399–402.

Newroth, S., & Newroth, A. (1981). *Coping with Alzheimer disease: A growing concern.* Downsview, Ontario, Canada: National Institute on Mental Retardation.

Okuda, M., Harada, H., Mizutani, H., & Hamanaka, T. (1998). Pica in demented patients. *Seishin Igaku [Clinical Psychiatry], 40,* 1103–1105.

Olsen, R.V., Ehrenkrantz, E., & Hutchings, B.L. (1993). *Homes that help: Advice from caregivers for creating a supportive home.* Newark: New Jersey Institute of Technology.

One facility's approach: A homey setting for Alzheimer's patients. (1993, February 15). *The Los Angeles Times,* p. B1.

Passini, R., Rainville, C., Marchand, N., & Joanette, Y. (1995). Wayfinding in dementia of the Alzheimer type: Planning abilities. *Journal of Clinical Experimental Neuropsychology, 17,* 820–832.

Pollack, B.G. (1998). Behavioral disturbance of dementia. *Journal of Geriatric Psychiatry and Neurology, 11,* 201–205.

Prasher, V.P. (1999). Adaptive behavior. In M.P. Janicki & A.J. Dalton (Eds.), *Dementia, aging, and intellectual disabilities: A handbook* (pp. 157–178). Philadelphia: Brunner/Mazel.

Prasher, V.P., & Corbett, J.A. (1993). Onset of seizures as a poor indicator of longevity in people with Down syndrome and dementia. *International Journal of Geriatric Psychiatry, 8,* 923–927.

Prasher, V.P., & Filer, A. (1995). Behavioural disturbance in people with Down's syndrome and dementia. *Journal of Intellectual Disability Research, 39,* 432–436.

Reisberg, B., Ferris, S.H., & DeLeon, M.J. (1989). The stage specific temporal course of Alzheimer's disease: Functional and behavioural concomitants based upon cross-sectional and longitudinal observation. In K. Iqbal, H.M. Wisniewski, & B. Winblad (Eds.), *Alzheimer's disease and related disorders: Proceedings of the First International Conference on Alzheimer's Disease and Related Disorders* (pp. 23–41). New York: Wiley-Liss.

Ripich, D.N. (1994). Functional communication with AD patients: A carer training program. *Alzheimer Disease and Associated Disorders, 8,* 95–109.

Seman, D. (1998, November/December). Meaningful pursuits. *Assisted Living Today,* 80–93.

Service, K.P., Lavoie, D., & Herlihy, J.E. (1999). Coping with losses, death and grieving. In M.P. Janicki & A.J. Dalton (Eds.), *Dementia, aging, and intellectual disabilities: A handbook* (pp. 330–351). Philadelphia: Brunner/Mazel.

Sloan, F.A., Shayne, M.W., & Conover, C.J. (1995). Continuing care retirement communities: Prospects for reducing institutional long-term care. *Journal of Health Politics, Policy and Law, 20*(1), 75–98.

Sloane, P.D. (1997). Ongoing resident care. In *Key elements of dementia care* (pp. 25–36). Chicago: Alzheimer's Disease and Related Disorders Association.

Tomoeda, C., & Bayles, K. (1990). The efficacy of speech-language intervention: Dementia. *Seminars in Speech and Language, 11,* 311–320.

Toseland, R.W., & McCallion, P. (1998). *Maintaining communication with persons with dementia: An educational program for nursing home staff and family members.* New York: Springer Publishing Co.

Toward nursing home reform [Editorial]. (1999, May 29). *New York Times,* p. A26.

Udell, L. (1999a, June). *Housing people with Alzheimer disease as a result of Down syndrome.* Paper presented at the Sixth International Conference on Aging and Disability, Rapid City, SD.

Udell, L. (1999b). Supports in small group home settings. In M.P. Janicki & A.J. Dalton (Eds.), *Dementia, aging, and intellectual disabilities: A handbook* (pp. 316–329). Philadelphia: Brunner/Mazel.

Visser, F.E., Aldenkamp, A.P., van Huffelen, A.C., Kuilman, M., Overweg, J., & van Wijk, J. (1997). Prospective study of the prevalence of Alzheimer-type dementia in institutionalized individuals with Down syndrome. *American Journal on Mental Retardation, 101,* 400–412.

Vitiello, M.V., Bliwise, D.L., & Prinz, P.N. (1992). Sleep in Alzheimer's disease and the sundown syndrome. *Neurology, 42*(Suppl. 6), 83–93.

Walker, C.A., & Walker, A. (1998). *Uncertain futures: People with learning difficulties and their ageing family carers.* Brighton, UK: Pavilion Publishing.

Warner, M.L. (1998). *The complete guide to Alzheimer's-proofing your home.* West Lafayette, IN: Purdue University Press.

Weaverdyck, S.E. (1997). Assessment and care/service plans. In *Key elements of dementia care* (pp. 11–24). Chicago: Alzheimer's Disease and Related Disorders Association.

Weaverdyck, S.E., Wittle, A., & Delaski-Smith, D. (1998). In-place progression: Lessons learned from the Huron Woods' staff. *Journal of Gerontological Nursing, 24*(1), 31–39.

Williams, M.E. (1995). *The American Geriatrics Society's complete guide to aging and health.* New York: Harmony Books.

22

Dealing with the End of Life

Anne L. Botsford

A 55-year-old man who was living with his mother at home is admitted to the psychiatric unit of a hospital with severe depression after his mother suddenly dies. A 40-year-old man is brought to a mental health clinic for assessment after police find him wandering and confused. He had lived at home with his parents, unknown to any agencies. After their deaths, he tried to manage the finances and home. He then lost the home and was living on the streets for the past 6 months. The brother of a woman who is living in a group home tells the service coordinator that one of their parents has died, but the family does not want the woman to know because it would upset her. A 76-year-old man in a group home is diagnosed with pancreatic cancer; he wants to remain in the home as long as possible with familiar staff and housemates he has known for 30 years. Three older women from a group residence are killed in a bus accident. Survivors include other residents, family members, and staff.

With increasing frequency, staff of agencies that support people with developmental disabilities are confronting similar scenarios that challenge their knowledge, skills, and values. People die in many ways, in many places, and under many different circumstances. In addition, there are different reasons for death: prolonged illness, sudden death, suicide, accidents, and Alzheimer's disease. Each of these deaths presents distinct issues and elicits different responses. Each individual's experiences, history, and relationship with a terminally ill or dying person are unique. All of these factors come into play when we face the terminal illness or death of an adult with a developmental disability. Some of the questions we may ask include the following: What should I say? What should I do? How can I help? How should I expect the person and family to behave? How do I take care of a person who is dying or grieving? What are my responsibilities? What are my responsibilities when other agencies, such as public health, hospice, or home care, are involved in providing care? How do I know what is typical or atypical in this situation?

Responses to these questions have changed as theories, practices, values, and agency policies and procedures have changed with the times. This is true of our ways of caring for people who have terminal illness and are dying and for people with developmental disabilities. As a society, we have a history of avoiding people with disabilities and of trying to avoid illness, dying, and death. The similarities in how we treat people with developmental disabilities and people with terminal illnesses are linked to fears and lack of understanding of illness, death, and disabilities. Looking back at care practices in the past, we can see how our fears and lack of understanding were expressed in these practices.

HISTORICAL BACKGROUND

For many years, individuals with developmental disabilities or mental illness were stigmatized by society, locked away and out of sight in dehumanizing institutions. During this institutional era, people with terminal illnesses also were stigmatized, segregated, and often isolated in separate areas in hospitals to minimize contact with staff and other patients. Talking about dying and death was considered taboo, and grieving behavior was often perceived as "crazy." Typical responses to ill and dying people with developmental disabilities during the institutional period are illustrated in the following description:

> The dead person was shrouded and wheeled out of hospital ward quietly and covertly. Some resident patients assumed their ward-mate had gone to be admitted to the general hospital. Others sensed that he or she had died. Nocturnal visits of Roman Catholic priests and Protestant chaplains, followed by the absence of a fellow patient at meals, workshop or recreation next day, were observed by verbal and nonverbal residents. Conclusions were reached intuitively, if not cognitively. (Carder, 1987, p. 20)

Just as society devalued the lives of people with disabilities, their dying, death, grief, and bereavement also were devalued and minimized. The opportunity to mourn and grieve loved ones, friends, and other losses was routinely denied. Common professional beliefs about people with disabilities were that they could not comprehend the finality of death, that they did not truly experience grief, and that they just forgot their loved ones once they were gone. Consequently, it was not considered necessary or important to include them in rituals, such as funerals, because they might become upset and act bizarrely, which would upset or embarrass the family.

Fortunately, our theories, practices, and values change with the times. This is true of our practices both with dying and with adults with developmental disabilities. In the 1970s, public policy changes, brought about by legislation and judicial decisions at state and national levels, compelled states to move from an institutional to a community-based system. These public policy changes shifted the focus and organization of services from custodial care in large, congregate environments to an array of individualized supports in the community (Mary, 1998). The contemporary support model of service delivery is still being defined in terms of community integration; supported work; self-advocacy; and client-driven, individual program planning. The goals of the support model are community inclusion, individual and family satisfaction, and individualization. Values include self-determination, individuality, independence, and participation. Services are person centered within a community context.

A similar revolution occurred with the founding in 1967 of the hospice care movement by Dame Cecily Saunders, a London physician, and the introduction of hospice care to the United States by Elisabeth Kübler-Ross, a physician who wrote the seminal text *On Death and Dying* (1969). The hospice movement shattered the silence of the terminal wards in hospitals and introduced death as an issue for public discussion, professional training, and reexamination of care practices. The values of death with dignity; respect for the individuality of the dying person; and empowerment of the dying person to make decisions about her or his care, dying, and funerals emerged from this period. The focus was on the needs, preferences, and wishes of the dying individual and the need to support the survivors through their grief and bereavement. The following scenario illustrates the difference that these changes made (J.S. Evinger, personal communication, August 19, 1998).

> When a man in his 40s, living in a group home, was admitted to a hospital, everyone in his home thought that he would soon recover and return to them. However, his health steadily declined, and, after a month, he died in the hospital. Immediately after his death, several older residents in the home displayed "disruptive" behaviors, both in their work program site and in the group home. This continued for several days. The supervisor of the home told the staff that they would have to tighten controls to eliminate these troublesome outbursts. Staff analyzed the problem differently and contacted a chaplain who was experienced in working with people with developmental disabilities. He organized a house meeting that included a ritual of remembrance for the man who had died. The meeting began with a discussion of the facts of his death and people's feelings about the facts. Art media were used for the expression of feelings, because many of the people who lived in the home were nonverbal. The discussion moved to a sharing of memories prompted by displaying personal objects that the man had kept in his room. After this, scriptures were read, prayers were offered, and a candle was lit. One older woman whose brother had died earlier in the year was encouraged to hold a candle in memory of him. Simple songs were shared, and the gathering concluded with a special meal arranged by the staff. Within one day, all "disruptive" behaviors of the older people in the home had disappeared.

This scenario also illustrates three developments that have influenced care of this population since the shift from the institutional to the support model and the inception of the hospice movement: 1) Case studies and research have expanded our understanding of how people with disabilities and their families experience and deal with terminal illness, dying, death, and the dynamics of the mourning and bereavement processes that follow; 2) program models and interventions have been developed to assist people in dealing with loss and grief and to increase their skills in working with individuals and families; and 3) the community context of care necessitates that agencies and staff work collaboratively on many levels to provide appropriate care. These collaborative arrangements present both opportunities and dilemmas for staff. In the following sections, these developments are explored.

GRIEF PROCESS: HOW PEOPLE DEAL
WITH TERMINAL ILLNESS, DYING, AND DEATH

Kübler-Ross (1969) identified five stages of grief: denial, anger, bargaining, depression, and acceptance. She observed that people's reactions to grief and loss typically could be characterized in terms of these stages. Although there are individual variations for each person, these stages are helpful in understanding and describing the behaviors, feelings, and coping styles of people who are dying or grieving (Wortman & Silver, 1989).

As is the case with people without intellectual disabilities, people with intellectual disabilities have been found to pass through the stages characterized by Kübler-Ross (Corr, 1993). In addition, to cope, they use whichever past experiences they have had (Carder, 1987; McLoughlin, 1986). What is different about the grief of people with a profound disability is their reliance on nonverbal communication, often through increased behavioral disturbance, which is one of the few avenues for communication. Whether having a intellectual disability significantly alters a person's reaction to loss and grief has been explored in terms of the following factors (Harper & Wadsworth, 1993; Kauffman, 1994; Wadsworth & Harper, 1991): learning and experience, intellect, special risks, communication, family perceptions, and staff perceptions. Each of these is explored next.

Learning and Experience

The role that learning and experience play in our reactions has to be considered. If people are shielded from the experience of death; have not seen family members or others grieve; or have been excluded from family, religious, or cultural rituals (such as funerals), then their behavior, feelings, and reactions are unquestionably affected because they lack experience to help themselves cope. The example cited previously from the institutional era (Carder, 1987) illustrated how institutional restrictions excluded people from participating in such social rites. The residents were not incapable of mourning; they were not invited. Having the benefit of experience with participating in family, cultural, and religious rituals, all people are better able to express and deal with grief and mourning.

Intellect

Another factor identified as significant is the intellectual level of the individual and the extent to which understanding of death is impaired when a person has an intellectual disability (Hollins, 1995). Studies of this factor support the conclusion that, except for people with profound retardation, a person's responses and the processing of their grief are the same or similar to those in their age group. Loss and grief are universal experiences. The signs of grief are also universal and recognizable: tears, sorrow, anger, disbelief, fear, and panic. A person's developmental stage—whether child, adolescent, or adult—influences the expression of grief, not whether grief is felt. Similarly, a person's intellectual level influences how he or she expresses loss and grief, but it does not influence whether he or she feels the loss and experiences the ensuing grief.

Special Risks

Other studies have found that individuals with intellectual disabilities are at high risk for special problems in grieving (Doka, 1989; Wadsworth & Harper, 1991). A major risk is the extent to which the individual may be dependent on the person that he or she has lost. If it is a parent with whom he or she has lived all of his or her life, then the loss includes not only the person and the relationship but also his or her "world": home, personal belongings, income, other significant relationships in the community or family, loss of self-esteem, and identity. The person subsequently experiences emergency moves to one or more residences with roommates who may or may not be appropriate for him or her. In these cases, the losses can be sudden, multiple, traumatic, and sometimes catastrophic. These risks reinforce the preventive value of including advance planning and planned separations from parents in working with families (Kauffman, 1994).

Communication

Other special problems are any communication and speech difficulties that individuals may have and the difficulty that caregivers and staff have in recognizing and responding to individuals' efforts at verbal expression of grief or need for more information or support. If these efforts fail, a person is likely to express distress by withdrawing, striking out, or becoming depressed. These behaviors, in turn, may result in the individual's having to move to a more restrictive environment, having a repressive behavior plan, being treated with medications that may inhibit the grief, or being admitted for psychiatric treatment. In addition, Emerson (1977) evaluated crisis intervention approaches, which routinely try to identify a precipitating stress, and found that approximately half of the time, either the death or the loss of an individual close to the person preceded the onset of crisis symptoms among people with a developmental disability. Studies have also noted that individuals experience "anniversary reactions" at the time of the deceased person's death and at birthdays, holidays, and times when the person who died might previously have visited the person (Kauffman, 1994). A person's communication difficulties at these anniversary times, combined with the caregivers' lack of awareness of the significance of the dates, may result in withdrawal, depression, or acting-out behaviors as expressions of distress.

Family Perceptions

Another special difficulty is the quality of the relationships of some families and individuals with intellectual disabilities. In addition to dependency, ambivalence and guilt are common in long-enduring family relationships and can complicate the grief and mourning process for both the family and the individual. Families may withhold information or give incomplete or inappropriate information in an attempt to protect the individual. They may also attempt to limit the person's response or expressions of grief or not allow time to deal with and adjust to the loss. Families may also become angry at an individual who is expressing grief when their anger is related to the death and their own grief (Emerson, 1977).

Staff Perceptions

When staff reactions are concerned, it has been found that staff express a sense of responsibility to care for dying or grieving individuals but often with much stress and much uncertainty about how to help, support, and respond as well as what to expect (J. Arentson, personal communication, August 19, 1998). The needs of individuals who have a terminal illness also are likely to change, which requires that staff reassess the person's needs, learn new procedures, and perhaps obtain additional resources, such as environmental modifications or waivers of code to help with the change in care.

Like families, staff who have long relationships with a person who has a terminal illness or is grieving may feel guilt and ambivalence, especially when dealing with difficult behaviors. Staff may respond inappropriately or not provide adequate time or support to help the person respond and adjust. A special problem identified among staff in supervisory roles is a tendency to focus on the needs of the staff who work directly with individuals to the exclusion of their own feelings about the person. A nurse described her experience with staff who were supporting frail and older adults at a group home:

> In orienting staff, I gave them a brief medical history on each lady with an explanation of what each diagnosis meant and what signs and symptoms they needed to watch for. I also included some guidelines as to what their response should be in different situations, when to call the doctor, an ambulance, or me. To my surprise, their questions and concerns dealt with fear and paranoia surrounding their liability at the time of a death. The health and welfare of the older women became a secondary issue. To describe staff as apprehensive regarding their new assignment was a gross understatement. In the past, if they had any concerns, they could run to the "Med Room" and get a nurse or call the nurse respondent who was always available. Now they were often on their own. They expressed fears of not knowing what to do, missing signs and symptoms, and finding someone dead in bed. (J. Arentson, personal communication, August 19, 1998)

This example illustrates the importance of considering staff needs and questions and concerns about their skills, knowledge, and values when making assignments for care situations involving older adults. It also indicates that staff want and need education, emotional support, and assistance in dealing with end-of-life issues. Frequent exposure to dying and death without proper training and support reduces the ability of staff to respond effectively and sensitively to people for whom they are caring. Some of the interventions and program models that have been developed to assist staff, individuals, and family members who are facing these issues are described in the following section.

INTERVENTIONS AND MODELS TO ASSIST PEOPLE IN COPING WITH LOSS AND GRIEF

The quality of life of older people can be improved by helping them to understand that changes may occur in their environment as a result of the death of friends, loved ones, and caregivers and by assisting them in expressing their losses. Some of the strategies for assisting people in dealing with terminal illness, dying, and death include death education, grief counseling, support groups, bereavement services, crisis teams, certified staff, and end-of-life committees (Rothberg, 1994; Service, Lavoie, & Herlihy, 1999).

Education

Death education is primary prevention—a pragmatic approach to helping individuals and families communicate about dying, death, and bereavement in the process of learning new information and new coping skills (Lavin, 1989). Educating people about death is as essential as educating them about transportation, sexuality, and money management. Analysis of skills and tasks relevant to death education and examples of materials and approaches that can be adapted for use in educational programs are provided by Hedger and Smith (1993) and Yanok and Beifus (1993).

Death education for individuals with an intellectual disability has been incorporated into recreational or other learning activities, for example, through teaching them about the life cycles of plants and animals (Hedger & Smith, 1993; Kloeppel & Hollins, 1989; Lavin, 1989). This approach can also be used with a variety of professional caregivers, therapists, social workers, pastoral counselors, and personal care staff (Hedger & Smith, 1993). Hedger and Smith (1993) found that the life cycle approach effectively modified staff beliefs about the ability of people with intellectual disabilities to express grief and increased staff members' confidence about their ability to support individuals in grief.

An experiential learning approach includes community-based instruction that emphasizes experiential learning within the natural environment. The goal of this approach has been described as "emotional inoculation" of adults to the experience of death (Wadsworth & Harper, 1991; Yanok & Beifus, 1993). An experiential death education curriculum includes field trips to area funeral homes, cemeteries, and houses of worship and can be augmented by guest presentations from morticians, physicians, and clergy. Behavior rehearsal or role playing can allow for the practice of public and private displays of grief, such as prayer or meditation, deportment at funeral services, and offering condolences to the next of kin. Generalization of these bereavement behaviors could be enhanced, if adults are afforded the opportunity to practice in the natural environment of a house of worship, funeral home, and cemetery (Yanok & Beifus, 1993). In an evaluation of the effectiveness of the experiential approach among expressive adults with an average IQ score in the mid-50s and an average age of 35, Yanok and Beifus (1993) found that adults who were randomly assigned to the experimental group significantly increased their knowledge and attitudes about death and grief behavior.

Advance Directives

Discussing advance directives with the family and the individual at planning meetings can provide opportunities not only for advance planning but also for death education (Kauffman, 1994; King, 1996; New York State Office of Mental Retardation and Developmental Disabilities, 1994). Reviewing the individual's and the family's burial preferences, health care proxies and wills can promote participation and communication among the family, individual, and staff in preparing for the inevitable separation. (See King [1996] and Friedman [1998] for discussions of the nuances related to the application of advance directives.)

Grief Counseling

Counseling for individuals, families, and groups is a supportive response to an individual, family, and group's loss and grief. Grief counseling may be an anticipatory approach to help prepare an individual, a family, staff, or other group (residents of a group home) for a long-term illness; to help them cope with the shock and denial that follow a sudden death; or to support them in the bereavement process (Luchterhand & Murphy, 1998). Such counseling may be provided by an agency team, by individuals who are trained and assigned to do grief counseling (e.g., social workers, clergy, volunteers), or by staff at agencies that provide end-of-life care (e.g., hospice workers, hospital staff). For example, in a descriptive report of a support group designed to increase coping skills and expression of grief of adults living in a group home, McDaniel (1989) reported a positive experience for eight older men. The goals of such groups are to help people learn about the bereavement process, to reinforce positive coping skills, to encourage expression of participants' grief, and to assess participants' need for additional support.

Inclusion

Staff, clergy, and families can assist individuals with an intellectual disability to participate fully in the grief and mourning process and in all of the social rituals and supports that society offers when someone dies. An example of sensitive grief work is described in the following vignette:

M.L. was in her late 20s and carried herself with a direct bearing and rough swagger that on any given day fully displayed all of her anger, confusion, or frustration. In between, she also displayed all of her joy, wonder, and gratitude. When a worker at her group home died, a woman to whom she was very attached, it opened a rush of old memories and unhealed wounds regarding the death of her father 18 years prior. M.L. recalled being excluded by her mother from his funeral and burial because her parents were estranged at the time. Now she was preoccupied by her intense desire to visit his grave in order to say "good-bye" in person. A visit was scheduled. She dressed in her nicest clothes and brought a small bouquet paid for with her own money. When M.L. and the staff arrived, they checked with the office and were directed to an older portion of the cemetery. They easily found the gravesite. M.L. refused to believe that was where her father was buried. There was no headstone or grave marker on the plot, in sharp contrast to all of the other graves nearby. To her, no headstone meant no grave and she refused to leave the flowers on the plot.

The key to helping M.L. work through her bereavement was arranging a way for her to buy a simple grave marker with her own funds. M.L. took an active role in the selection process and helped compose the inscription for the gravesite plaque. Once the marker was installed, another visit was scheduled. Again M.L. put on her best clothes and brought flowers. Upon seeing it, she beamed at the plaque with her father's name and was openly proud of her act of caring for him in his death. She laid her flowers on the plot, told him her good-byes, and offered her own prayers. We took a picture of her kneeling with the flowers next to the marker. She went home content, consoled, knowing that she could always visit her father. (J.S. Evinger, August 19, 1998)

In contrast with situations in which expression of grief is denied people with intellectual disabilities, staff in this situation demonstrated sensitive grief work that was essential to this individual's resolving and accepting the death of her father.

There are some processes that staff can follow that will ensure inclusion and support: 1) Actively seek out nonverbal rituals, which are particularly helpful to someone who may not find comfort in verbal rituals; 2) respect both the avoidance and the choice of photos and mementos that can be helpful in dealing with loss; 3) minimize major changes for at least a year; 4) postpone assessment of skills and behaviors; 5) assist appropriate searching behavior to support emotional recovery; 6) support formal observance of anniversaries; and 7) seek consultation with specialists in bereavement if behavior changes occur, such as aggression, depression, regression, mutism, self-injury, wandering, and tearfulness (Hollins, 1995).

Staff Education

If staff are unprepared to deal with terminal illness and death, then they will not permit grieving among the people in their care. Some of the goals of death education for staff are to 1) train staff in the dying and bereavement processes; 2) increase skills and competence in talking with individuals and families about dying and bereavement; 3) increase staff members' knowledge of and sensitivity to cultural and religious preferences; 4) introduce staff to bereavement resources for support of individuals, families, and themselves; and 5) know the value and roles of other community agencies and staff who may be collaborating in the care of the individual and family.

In addition to learning how to help individuals and families deal with these issues, staff often find that as a result of death education, they are better able to deal with their own issues of death, grief, and bereavement. People who have not healed from one loss are hesitant to risk another (Deutsch, 1985). Support groups for staff who work with individuals who have a terminal illness or are grieving for an individual with whom they may have had a long, established relationship are also essential to prevent emotional, psychological, and spiritual numbness that result from being overly stressed by frequent or unresolved losses (Kramer, 1998). One of the ground rules of such a support group must be that staff are supported in grieving openly.

Resources are available for developing staff education, orientation, and support programs (e.g., Barbera, Pitch, & Howell, 1989; Botsford & Force, 2000a; Howell & Pitch, 1989). Community resources for staff in-service training include hospices, mental health departments, houses of worship, funeral homes, local colleges, and employee assistance programs. There are also many educational films on dying, grief, and bereavement, that are available through colleges, state film libraries, and local mental health departments (Botsford & Force, 2000b; Sireling & Hollins, 1985). Some sources of information on dying, death, and bereavement are listed in the chapter appendix.

Program Models
A mobile crisis team (Botsford & Force, 2000a) and a bereavement service (Fauri & Grimes, 1994) are models that agencies have developed and implemented to support individuals, families, and staff at the end of life. Other agencies have established ethics committees or end-of-life committees that review individual cases to assist in decision making and care planning. These committees may also review agency practices that affect individuals, families, and staff and review staff development and education in death and bereavement. These committees may also develop collaborative arrangements with hospitals, hospices, home care agencies, volunteer caregivers, and other community providers to establish a responsive support network. The importance of support networks at individual, agency, and community levels is explored in the following section.

SYSTEMS PERSPECTIVE ON STAFF ROLES AND RESPONSIBILITIES IN DEALING WITH ILLNESS, DYING, AND DEATH
Agencies have diverse programs and work with a range of individuals and families in a variety of environments, such as residences, home, work, education, health care, and mental health. Staff have diverse roles and responsibilities and relate to individuals and their families in several contexts. These are illustrated in Figures 1–3, which provide a systems perspective on the complex roles, relationships, and tasks that agencies and staff encounter in working with individuals who are dealing with end-of-life issues.

Figure 1 illustrates the key roles that staff play within the agency and represents the relationship of staff to the individuals whom they support, families, and other agencies in the community. A systems perspective at this level helps to answer the question, "Where do staff fit into all of this?" Within this system, staff generally have multiple roles and responsibilities. They have responsibilities to individuals and families as well as to their colleagues, managers, administrations, and boards of their agencies. Conflicts and dilemmas sometimes result from these multiple roles. For example, family, staff, administrators, and friends or housemates may disagree in their perceptions of the needs and wishes of the individual and in their preferences about how best to

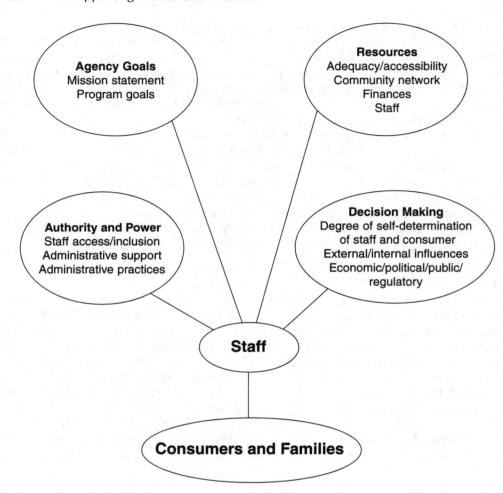

Figure 1. Agency system from a staff perspective. (From McInnis-Dittrich, K. [1994]. *Integrating social welfare policy and social work practice* [1st ed., p. 36]. Pacific Grove, CA: Brooks/Cole; adapted by permission from Wadsworth, a division of Thomson Learning. Copyright © 1994. Fax 800-730-2215.)

honor and remember him or her. One strategy for working out a resolution to this situation is to involve clergy, experienced staff from hospice, or some other person to serve as a mediator.

Staff frequently experience the conflict of caring sensitively for an individual with a terminal illness up to the point of his or her death and then being confronted with the administrative tasks of reporting the death as an "incident" that requires formal investigation and review. Staff may undergo stressful reviews concerned with administrative priorities and processes related to liability and culpability, quite distinct from their role in caring for and supporting the individual. The intimidating nature of the paperwork and process are the reason that staff may express the wish that if a death occurs, even a dignified and peaceful one, it should occur "not on my shift." The following vignette describes the impact of this process on staff (J. Arentson, personal communication, August 19, 1998):

Death is viewed as a major incident. An incident report is generated. An investigation is initiated. Statements are taken from those involved. No stone is left unturned to determine if the death could have been avoided. Not only is there a Mortality Committee, but also a Special Review Committee. Both groups are involved in the investigation. The death of someone you have known for years and grown attached to can be difficult. It is made more difficult when policies and procedures foster feelings of guilt and have one second-guessing his or her actions.

Redefining this process to decrease the adversarial and investigatory quality of the agency's response to the death of a person with a terminal illness would be more supportive and respectful to staff, families, and others. Another practice that adversely affects other individuals and staff is the agency policy of filling the deceased person's place, or their "bed," immediately, as if a group residence were a motel rather than a home. One of the functions of ethics and end-of-life committees is to review such agency policies to enhance the values of dignity and support to individuals, family members, and staff while reducing the depersonalizing and intimidating nature of a one-dimensional administrative response.

Figure 2 illustrates a systems perspective of the relationship between agencies, including the staff and the various systems to which they relate, such as individuals and their families, the community, and the larger society. A systems perspective at this level shows that agencies and staff are "in the middle." They are responsible to the families and individuals whom they support as well as to people in larger external institutions, such as those responsible for the regulations, funding, policies, and procedures. Not only within the agency but also in the community, staff relate to multiple systems and have multiple roles and responsibilities. These roles can be complex, are sometimes conflicting, and can be the source of dilemmas and frustrations, as illustrated in the following vignette:

S.F. was a 64-year-old woman who lived in a group home. She was admitted to a hospital due to gastrointestinal bleeding. She was treated and discharged after a week and then readmitted a month later in a greatly weakened condition with similar symptoms of unknown origin. She was placed on a ventilator to sustain her. Her prognosis was poor and with agency concurrence, a Do Not Resuscitate order was initiated. Within a week, S.F.'s condition unexpectedly improved to the point where she could be discharged and returned to her residence.

The next night, she was discovered dead, having died in her own bed in her sleep. The unattended death prompted a routine call between the county medical examiner's office and the agency physician. Because of the preexisting medical condition and her age, both parties agreed that there would be no need for the medical examiner's office to conduct an autopsy. This was a relief to staff, since the woman was Jewish and an autopsy would have violated her religious practices. With the sign off from the medical examiner's office, one direct care worker proceeded to clean the woman's body as a final act of compassion, since upon her death, her bowels had discharged.

The worker's efforts were interrupted abruptly, however, when an agency representative arrived to investigate this unattended death. He declared the area of the woman's bedroom a crime scene and prohibited any further contact with the woman's body. Soon after, the worker became the object of an investigation since

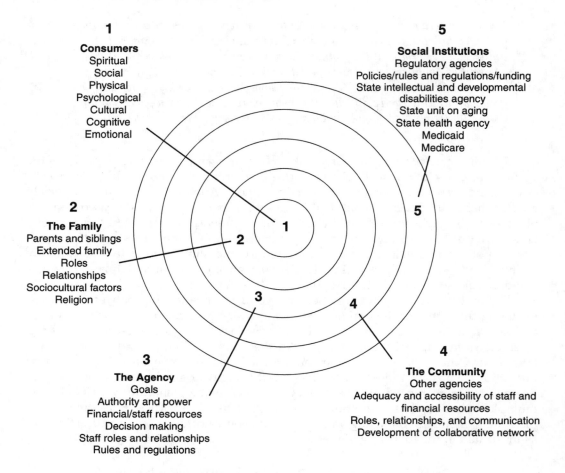

1
Consumers
Spiritual
Social
Physical
Psychological
Cultural
Cognitive
Emotional

5
Social Institutions
Regulatory agencies
Policies/rules and regulations/funding
State intellectual and developmental
  disabilities agency
State unit on aging
State health agency
Medicaid
Medicare

2
The Family
Parents and siblings
Extended family
Roles
Relationships
Sociocultural factors
Religion

3
The Agency
Goals
Authority and power
Financial/staff resources
Decision making
Staff roles and relationships
Rules and regulations

4
The Community
Other agencies
Adequacy and accessibility of staff and
  financial resources
Roles, relationships, and communication
Development of collaborative network

Figure 2.   Systems influencing the care of individuals with intellectual disabilities.

the agency representative regarded the washing of the body as tampering with evidence. The worker was suspended from direct care service, transferred to house-keeping, and only much later allowed to return to direct care. The declaration of the bedroom as a crime scene prevented the dead woman from being completely washed, a fact that, understood out of context, caused the local Jewish burial society, which later prepared her body, to raise questions about her general care at the residence. (J.S. Evinger, August 19, 1998)

In this situation, the staff's sense of responsibility to the individual conflicted with the administrative representative's interpretation of agency procedure. The conflict resulted in a punitive response to the staff and an unfavorable perception of the agency in the community.

Figure 3 illustrates a systems perspective that includes the community and the various agencies with which staff may relate depending on their role, the type of service, and the needs of the individual and family. This perspective shows a complex relationship between the agency and the community system, which is different for each agency,

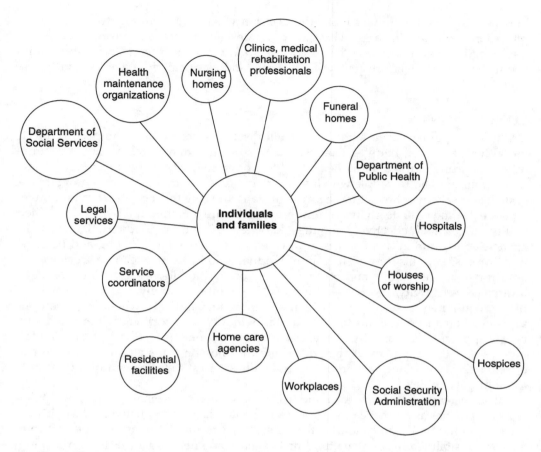

Figure 3.   Community services for people who are dealing with terminal illness, dying, and death.

community, and individual. At this level of the system, the challenges for staff include how to navigate the system successfully while also providing appropriate services according to each individual's needs. Additional challenges include how to interpret one's responsibilities, the regulations, the available finances, and communications while collaborating with other agencies to provide optimal care to individuals and their families and attempting to reduce interagency barriers to efficient and flexible collaboration.

In the case of an adult with a terminal illness in a group home, it is not unusual for a service coordinator to be working with the individual, with other members in the group home, with the area hospice for skilled nursing services, with direct care staff of the group home, with the hospital, and with the family. Issues that typically emerge when the care plan involves multiple providers are who makes decisions and about which areas, who bills and who pays, and who reports to whom about what. Examples of typical questions that arise include the following: Will the individual's Do Not Resuscitate request on record with the agency be honored by the rescue squad and by the hospital? If hospice is involved with a person who has lived in a group home for a long period but hospice has not been involved with his or her family, who will contact the family when the person dies—the agency or hospice staff? If there are no family members involved, who will make the decision whether to continue treatment if the physician at the hospital asks? These are questions about roles, responsibilities, boundaries, regulations, policies and procedures, funding, and ethics. Staff uncertainties about these issues warrant review, evaluation, and clarification at agency and interagency levels.

CONCLUSIONS

Death among older adults with intellectual disabilities has a broad impact. It affects individuals and their families, friends, roommates, staff, and providers in the community. Supporting individuals at the end of life is often complicated by policies, rules, and regulations applied to people who live in group homes or are involved in programs. A systems perspective shows that the roles of staff who care for individuals and families who are dealing with death in a community context are dynamic and demanding. Their ability to respond effectively requires knowledge about individuals, families, the agency, and community resources. It also requires knowledge of dying and bereavement processes; skills for assisting an individual who is dealing with death as well as assisting his or her family and other members of the individual's social network; and awareness, sensitivity, and respect for individual, cultural, family, and social values. If these requirements seem extraordinarily ambitious and overwhelming, then the urgency of a concerted effort to provide staff with death education, training, and support is apparent. The capacity of agencies to provide humanistic, dignified care to individuals and their families at the end of life depends on the staff's competence and effectiveness in working with individuals, families, and systems on end-of-life issues in a community context.

The systems perspective also underscores the need for agencies to review administrative policies and practices to promote 1) greater agency and network flexibility for meeting individual, family, and staff needs; 2) clarification and support of staff roles and responsibilities; 3) adequate funding at agency and network levels for care requirements of individuals who are dealing with death bereavement; and 4) program and staff development to support this expanding population. To deal humanely with end-of-life issues, agencies need to initiate evaluation of administrative practices, rules, regulations, and funding that affect the care of individuals who are dealing with death and bereavement. Such evaluation should serve as a starting point for agencies to institute realistic and respectful policies to fulfill their mission of supporting individuals with developmental disabilities and their families at the end of life.

REFERENCES

Barbera, T., Pitch, R., & Howell, M. (1989). *Death and dying: A guide for staff serving adults with mental retardation.* Boston: Exceptional Parent Press.

Botsford, A., & Force, L. (2000a). *End of life care: Resource manual.* Delmar: New York State Arc.

Botsford, A., & Force, L. (2000b). *Supporting the end of life: A guide for staff supporting individuals with intellectual disabilities.* Delmar: New York State Arc.

Carder, M. (1987). Journey into understanding mentally retarded people's experiences around death. *Journal of Pastoral Care, 41,* 18–31.

Corr, C. (1993). Coping with dying: Lessons we should and should not learn from the work of Elisabeth Kübler-Ross. *Death Studies, 17,* 68–83.

Deutsch, H. (1985). Grief counseling with the mentally retarded client. *Psychiatric Aspects of Mental Retardation Reviews, 4*(5), 17–20.

Doka, K. (1989). *Disenfranchised grief: Recognizing hidden sorrow.* Lanham, MD: Lexington Books.

Emerson, P. (1977). Covert grief reactions in mentally retarded clients. *Mental Retardation, 15*(6), 46–47.

Fauri, D., & Grimes, D. (1994). Bereavement services for families and peers of deceased residents of psychiatric institutions. *Social Work, 39*, 185–190.

Friedman, R.I. (1998). Use of advance directives: Facilitating health care decisions by adults with mental retardation and their families. *Mental Retardation, 36*, 444–456.

Harper, D.C., & Wadsworth, J.S. (1993). Grief in adults with mental retardation: Preliminary findings. *Research in Developmental Disabilities, 14*, 313–330.

Hedger, C., & Smith, M.J.D. (1993). Death education for older adults with developmental disabilities. *Activities, Adaptation and Aging, 18*, 29–36.

Hollins, S. (1995, May/June). Managing grief better: People with developmental disabilities. *Habilitative Mental Healthcare Newsletter, 14*, 3.

Howell, M., & Pitch, R. (1989). *Ethical dilemmas in caregiving: A guide for staff serving adults with mental retardation*. Boston: Exceptional Parent Press.

Kauffman, J. (1994). Mourning and mental retardation. *Death Studies, 18*, 257–271.

King, M.P. (1996). *Making sense of advance directives* (Rev. ed.). Washington, DC: Georgetown University Press.

Kloeppel, D., & Hollins, S. (1989). Double handicap: Mental retardation and death in the family. *Death Studies, 13*, 31–38.

Kramer, B.J. (1998). Preparing social workers for the inevitable: A preliminary investigation of a course on grief, death and loss. *Journal of Social Work Education, 34*, 211–228.

Kübler-Ross, E. (1969). *On death and dying*. New York: Macmillan.

Lavin, C. (1989). Disenfranchised grief and the developmentally disabled. In K. Doka (Ed.), *Disenfranchised grief: Recognizing hidden sorrow* (pp. 229–237). Lanham, MD: Lexington Books.

Luchterhand, C.M., & Murphy, N.E. (1998). *Helping adults with mental retardation grieve a death loss*. Philadelphia: Accelerated Development.

Mary, N.L. (1998). Social work and the support model of services for people with developmental disabilities. *Journal of Social Work Education, 34*, 247–260.

McDaniel, B. (1989). A group work experience with mentally retarded adults on the issues of death and dying. *Journal of Gerontological Social Work, 13*, 187–191.

McInnis-Dittrich, K. (1994). *Integrating social welfare policy and social work practice*. Pacific Grove, CA: Brooks/Cole.

McLoughlin, I.J. (1986). Bereavement in the mentally handicapped. *British Journal of Hospital Medicine, 36*, 256–260.

New York State Office of Mental Retardation and Developmental Disabilities. (1994). *Advance directives*. Albany: Author.

Rothberg, E.D. (1994). Bereavement intervention with vulnerable populations: A case report on groupwork with the developmentally disabled. *Social Work with Groups, 17*, 61–75.

Service, K., Lavoie, D., & Herlihy, J. (1999). Coping with losses, death, and grieving. In M.P. Janicki & A.J. Dalton (Eds.), *Dementia, aging, and intellectual disabilities: A handbook* (pp. 330–351). Philadelphia: Brunner/Mazel.

Sireling, L., & Hollins, S. (1985). *The last taboo: Mental handicap and death* [Film]. London: St. George's Hospital Medical School.

Wadsworth, J., & Harper, D. (1991). Grief and bereavement in mental retardation: A need for a new understanding. *Death Studies, 15*, 281–292.

Wortman, C., & Silver, R. (1989). The myths of coping with loss. Journal of Consulting and Clinical Psychology, 57, 349–537.

Yanok, J., & Beifus, J. (1993). Communicating about loss and mourning: Death education for individuals with mental retardation. *Mental Retardation, 31*, 144–147.

Appendix
Resources on Death Education

The following resource list is intended to introduce staff and families to a variety and range of agencies committed to end-of-life care. Each offers resources and assistance for formal and informal carers. The list is by no means exhaustive of the available resources.

American Association of Retired Persons (AARP)
601 E Street, NW
Washington, D.C. 20049
800-424-3410
Many brochures for widowed persons and a guide, "Customs of Bereavement," for cross-cultural assistance
www.aarp.org

Americans for Better Care of the Dying (ABCD)
2175 K Street, NW, Suite 820
Washington D.C. 20037
202-530-9864
www.abcd-caring.com

The Arc of the United States
1010 Wayne Avenue, Suite 650
Silver Spring, Maryland 20910
301-565-3842
Publications include a list of materials and other resources on people with intellectual disabilities, dying, death and grief support.
www.thearc.org

Beth Israel Medical Center–Phillips Ambulatory Care Center
Department of Pain Medicine and Palliative Care
First Avenue at 16th Street
New York, New York 10003
212-844-8970
Provides the latest innovations in pain care and palliative care as well as information on hospice and end-of-life care
www.stoppain.org

Center to Improve Care of the Dying (CICD)
Institute for Health Policy, Outcomes, and Human Values
George Washington University Medical Center
1001 22nd Street, NW, Suite 820
Washington, D.C. 20037
202-467-2222
E-mail: cicd@gwis2.circ.gwu.edu
An interdisciplinary team engaged in research, advocacy, and educational activities to improve the care of the dying and their families.
www.gwu.edu/~cicd

(continued)

Choice in Dying
1035 30th Street, NW
Washington, D.C. 20007
202-338-9790
800-989-9455
Provides state-specific advance directives,
extensive resources, and links.
www.choices.org

Compassion in Dying
PMB 415, 6312 SW Capitol Highway
Portland, Oregon 97201
503-221-9556
Advocates change in medical care for
terminally ill people and insists that
meaningful reform must include legislation of
assisted dying.
www.compassionindying.org

The Compassionate Friends
Post Office Box 3696
Oak Brook, Illinois 60522-3696
630-990-0010
www.compassionatefriends.org/index.html

DeathNet
Search engine founded by Canadian Right to
Die and the U.S. National Hemlock Society;
offers large collection of "right to die" books,
links, on-line library, and bookstore. The
information is predominately Canadian, but
resources are global.
www.rights.org/deathnet/open.html

**EPEC Project (Education for Physicians on
End-of-Life Care)**
Institute for Ethics
American Medical Association
515 North State Street
Chicago, Illinois 60610
312-464-5619
Supported by a grant from the Robert Wood
Johnson Foundation, the EPEC Project is
designed to educate physicians about end-of-
life care. The web site provides a core
curriculum, an extensive resource guide of
books, and audiovisuals.
www.ama-assn.org/ethic/epec/

Family Caregiver Alliance
690 Market Street, Suite 600
San Francisco, California 94104
415-434-3388
Resource center with an on-line caregiver
group, a clearinghouse, and research and
publications for caregivers and those working
with them.
www.caregiver.org

Growth House Inc.
San Francisco, California
415-255-9045
A search engine with vast resources on key
issues in terminal illness, hospice, dying,
death, grief, and bereavement.
www.growthhouse.org

Hospice Education Institute
190 Westbrook Road
Essex, Connecticut 06426-1510
860-767-1620
800-331-1620
www.hospiceworld.org

Hospice Foundation of America
2001 South Street NW, Suite 300
Washington, D.C. 20009
800-854-3402
www.hospicefoundation.org

Hospice HelpLine
800-338-8619

Hospice Net
401 Bowling Avenue, Suite 51
Nashville, Tennessee 37205
Provides resources for patients, caregivers,
survivors; provides links and information on
rules that govern Medicare coverage of and
payment for hospice care.
www.hospicenet.org

Hospice Web
A search engine with many questions and
answers about hospice, links, and list of
state-by-state hospices.
www.teleport.com/~hospice/

(continued)

Last Acts
A national interdisciplinary coalition
representing many organizations and
providing education and advocacy for
improved care of dying people; extensive
resource directory.
www.lastacts.org

Home Care Online
National Association for Home Care
228 Seventh Street SE
Washington, D.C. 20003
202-547-7424
Comprehensive database of home care and
hospice agencies and information on how to
choose a provider.
www.nahc.org

National Center for Death Education
Mount Ida College
777 Dedham Street
Newton Center, Massachusetts 02459
617-928-4649
Resource directory of books and audiovisual
materials
www.mountida.edu

**National Family Caregivers Association
(NFCA)**
10400 Connecticut Avenue, Suite 500
Kensington, Maryland 20895-3944
Supports caregivers and offers bereavement
programs
www.nfcacares.org

**National Funeral Directors Association
(NFDA)**
13625 Bishop's Drive
Brookfield, Wisconsin 53005
800-228-6332
www.nfda.org

**National Hospice Organization National
Hospice and Palliative Care Organization**
1700 Diagonal Road, Suite 300
Alexandria, Virginia 22314
703-243-5900
www.nho.org

Natural Death Centre
20 Heber Road
London, NW2 6AA
United Kingdom
+44(0)20 8 280 2853
Ideas for supporting dying people at home
and in their careers and helping them to
arrange funerals.
www.globalideasbank.org/
naturaldeath.html

Partnership for Caring, Inc.
1035 30th Street NW
Washington, D.C. 20007-3823
800-989-9455
A national coalition of advocates for dying
people and their families; resources of many
types, including directory, on-line refereed
journal, publications, feature stories, and
state-by-state resources
www.partnershipforcaring.org

Project on Death in America
Open Society Institute
400 West 59th Street
New York, New York 10019
Extensive resource directories of agencies,
services, publications, and facts
www.soros.org/death/index.html

Zen Hospice Project
Links, an extensive reading list, and articles
www.zenhospice.org

IV Essay

What Are You Dying Of?
Natural Causes

Jean B. Zink

A man gradually identifies himself with the form of his fate; a man is, in the long run, his own circumstances.—Borges (1949)

"I am dying, and I would like you to help me live as abundantly as possible while this process takes place." These are the words with which I greeted my new doctor. I am aware that doctors are jealous of the diagnostic initiative and are not given to mere speculations on the part of the patient, so I was not the least surprised when he looked at me a bit quizzically and inquired, "What are you dying of?" "Natural causes," I replied.

Aging with a disability has generated in me an intense desire to have some control over my increasingly complicated medical challenges. With less than 15 minutes budgeted by doctors for each patient, I knew that a long explanation of how aging has altered my health goals would not be heard. So, I decided on the above greeting to move as quickly as I could to the conduct of my medical care. No longer can I expend energy to meet the expectations that quell the fears of society. Conservation of energy must replace relentless striving that is so admired by people who are able as well as disabled.

At age 16, polio took hold of my body and left me what at the time was labeled an "acute paralytic." Those words appeared under my name on my hospital room door. High spirited as teenagers are, I was fond of introducing myself as "a cute paralytic." This cheeky greeting was met with a look of horror rather than mild amusement as it was intended. This was my first inkling that direct confrontation of disability was unac-

433

ceptable. Even though I was less than 6 months away from having been able-bodied, I was now firmly in the disabled community. I had crossed that mystical barrier that separates the able from the disabled. My world would be defined by the perceptions of the able-bodied despite that I would struggle tirelessly to create my own definition of the world in which I had been abruptly thrust.

I absorbed the unspoken but intense lessons of how to live in the able-bodied world and did not question the following 5 years of therapy in which I learned to walk with the assistance of a body brace, long leg braces, and crutches. The goal was that I not use a wheelchair. Abject misery brought on by devastating fatigue was my daily experience. When I told my doctor that at night I had spasms of tremors throughout my body and had to put my hand in my mouth to keep from biting my tongue, he said he felt the same way after a long day—physical therapists, occupational therapists, and social workers concurred. On some level of consciousness, I knew that they were merely encouraging me by identifying with my plight, but it was difficult for me to defy their orders to eschew the wheelchair at all costs. It took me years to decide that I would use every piece of equipment available to me, including the wheelchair, to be in control of my life. I wanted to be able to go through the day without constant reference to how I was going to accomplish the next task. I wanted my mind free of the bondage of my physical limitations. This has been a lifelong struggle.

Balancing the needs of a demanding body with the intellectual, emotional, and social needs of the mind is an intimidating goal. It is a goal that must also allow consideration of the needs of the people who inhabit one's life. I initiated the conversation with my doctor in this unconventional way in the hope of maintaining this balance, as my life draws to a close and aging makes additional demands on my already fragile physical resources.

People with disabilities understand without explanation how difficult it is to discuss any medical problem with a new physician. The disability is seldom discussed, it is merely noted. It is the implicit assumptions that are so disturbing. One is always uncertain as to whether the medical personnel see the life of a person with a disability as a life worth living. We all give lip service to the notion that everyone's life has worth, but more often than not, people view the lives of disabled people as marginal at best, a burden at worst, and certainly not a life that they themselves would want to live.

Most people who have disabilities would not have chosen to be disabled, but somehow the audacity to keep on living implies a choice. The choice is not, of course, to be or not to be disabled but to live or not live. Clearly, people with disabilities who do not choose to live, do not. This is true of the able-bodied as well, but the death sentence is not as immediate. People with disabilities must choose life every day or they will not survive (Hockenberry, 1995). Not only is the will to live for one's self paramount, but the able-bodied community must also will the life of people with disabilities. Dr. Kevorkian has helped depressed disabled people to end their lives while the disabled community watches breathlessly as the able-bodied community voices their consent. Choosing life with the medical service provider community becomes a matter of one's capacity for "activities of daily living." This definition is derived from the burden that people with disabilities put on able-bodied people. I do not deny this burden, but I question the definition of life based on these activities. Instead of being a pure measure of functionality or capability, "activities of daily living" can be so easily compromised. Economic status and class distinctions determine how we think about helping others and about receiving help. For example, wealthy people have everything done for them—from very personal services such as drawing one's bath, doing one's hair and nails, and dressing to cooking, cleaning, and laundry. It is considered beneath their station in life to do these things for themselves. This service frees people of wealth to do other things. In the disability service provider community, doing for oneself takes on a moral dimension. Good people toil. We speak of the indignity of being waited on. Added to the confusion of the quality of life is the attitude of the disabled community itself, insisting that it is insulting to accept help. People must do for themselves no matter the cost. The acceptance of the genteel graces of polite society (e.g., opening doors) is left behind in the zeal to be thought of as competent and independent in every way.

The most recent and clearest example of the assumptions of able-bodied people and the alienation of people with disabilities from themselves is the $20 million Franklin D. Roosevelt Memorial that was dedicated on May 2, 1997. Contemporary people with and without disabilities assume that FDR did not wish to be portrayed as a disabled person (Gallagher, 1994). In other words, they wish to honor his memory and not to remember him with the "dishonor" of his disability. FDR expressed explicitly that he did not want a memorial, but if one were created to honor him, he wanted it no bigger than his desk. Yet this wish is overridden (the memorial covers seven acres) by the assumption of contemporary people that this was not a real wish but an expected humility. He made no explicit wish about people knowing that he had a disability. Throughout his life, he did what he had to do to be accepted by the able-bodied community—he hid his disability. Contrary to public opinion, FDR did not deny that he had polio. He created the March of Dimes, and he opened a rehabilitation center in Warm Springs, Georgia, where he spent a great deal of time and where he died. In his last address to Congress, he apologized for sitting down and noted that carrying 10 pounds of steel on his legs had greatly tired him. I think FDR would have been relieved to have been able to conduct his life with his disability known. It cost him a great deal of his psychic as well as his physical energy to meet the demands of a society that believed disability to be unacceptable. But the perceptions of 65 years ago, which still prevail today, would not release him from the burden of being perceived as able-bodied—no matter what his other strengths may have been.

Unfortunately, as the controversy over the memorial demonstrates, disability remains not an honor but somehow a failing to be swept away. FDR's concern about the disabled community is ignored by those who believe in the "righteousness" of his decision to hide his disability. He did the right thing, and he should not have this veil stripped from him. FDR, I believe, did not have to make the transitions in his life that are expected of the average person of low or middle economic status. He was accustomed to being waited on and having all of the traditional activities of daily living performed for him. He was not demoralized by service. He expected and accepted it. Even as he hid his disability from the general public, he expected those around him to help him create this illusion, and there is nothing to indicate that he thought himself unworthy of this sacrifice on the part of his family and friends. The burden of being a burden is a constant hardship to those of us who try to meet the demands of the able-bodied community, and often the disabled community as well, to be what we are not. So I seek a safe haven with the provider community by trying to be what I am, an aging disabled person, and at the same time living my life in a manner that reflects my humanity and respects the humanity of others.

Was I successful with my diversionary communication tactic with my doctor? Well, yes and no. I am sure he sees me as eccentric and perhaps a relic from the past. Nevertheless, on a recent stay in the hospital, I said to my doctor, "I need physical therapy." "Why?" he asked. "Because I am in bed 24 hours a day and I need to get out of bed!" He replied, "You get up to go to the bathroom. That is enough." I said, "No, I don't. I don't walk when no one is looking." He smiled and left the room. A couple of hours later, a young man appeared at my door and introduced himself as a physical therapist. Surprised, I said, "Who sent you?" He said, "Your doctor." A miracle! I do believe in miracles and especially the small ones that push back our preconceived ideas and let a little light into our lives.

I look forward to the miracle of experiencing joy and sorrow, laughter and tears, and hope and hopelessness and having these things define not my disability but me—a disabled person. Disability makes life richer some days and filled with poverty on others. Willa Cather (1927) said, "Miracles rest not so much upon faces or voices or healing power coming to us from afar, but on our perceptions being made finer, so that for a moment our eyes can see and our ears can hear what there is about us always." I am dying. Help me to live as well as I can during the process that is life itself.

REFERENCES

Borges, J.L. (1949). *El Aleph*. Buenos Aires: Editorial Losada.
Cather, W. (1927). *Death comes for the archbishop*. New York: Alfred A. Knopf.
Gallagher, H.G. (1994). *FDR's splendid deception* (Rev. ed.). Arlington, VA: Vandamere Press.
Hockenberry, J. (1995). *Moving violations: War zones, wheelchairs, and declarations of independence*. New York: Hyperion.

V

NETWORKING SERVICES FOR COMMUNITY SUPPORTS

Focus on Organizational Dynamics

Community supports are strengthened when resources, both human and material, are networked. This last section features specific efforts undertaken to broaden the services that are available for aging adults with lifelong disabilities and their families. Many of these stem from a time, in the 1990s, when the U.S. federal government underwrote or encouraged states to initiate projects that were designed to increase knowledge of system change and services for older adults with lifelong disabilities. Thus, each of these approaches illustrates a "variation on a theme," but the lessons learned from them should help others structure similar initiatives and, it is hoped, find these easier to accomplish. In the broadest sense, the intention to help older families has been at the forefront of each care system's list of goals. However, the means to attain such a goal have not always been explored so fully. We see in Chapter 23, by Hacker, McCallion, and Janicki, how area agencies on aging (AAAs), the cornerstone of local eldercare services, can expand their programs effectively to target people with lifelong disabilities and their aging caregivers. These AAA-oriented endeavors, built on local collaboration between aging and disability agencies, demonstrate the efficacy of a "low-tech," low-cost approach to service capacity building that was undertaken in New York. AAAs can respond meaningfully to the local needs of this constituency. Among the lessons learned is a call for replication of this approach throughout the United States and other parts of the world in which the aging and disability networks exist side by side.

In the same manner, Ansello and Coogle report in Chapter 24 on the results of their Partners III Project to facilitate intersystem cooperation. Their work combined the three components of collaboration, outreach, and capacity-building into the Integrated Model of Service to Older Adults with Developmental Disabilities, which was field-tested in Maryland and Virginia. They describe both statewide and local activities to advance intersystem cooperation, in the belief that these can be used to guide responsive initiatives by human service agencies that find themselves operating at the "intersection" of aging and developmental disabilities. Their integrated model serves as a primary vehicle for helping agencies in the aging network and developmental disabilities system to negotiate collaborative endeavors so that all interested parties benefit. The overriding goal of their collective experiences has been to improve the prospects for continued independence and community living of adults who grow old with lifelong impairments.

Suttie, in Chapter 25, expands on the use of AAAs and aging network resources and demonstrates how a university-initiated project can link the disparate systems in a community, using a collaborative teaming process model. She draws upon her team's experiences with a demonstration project that was carried out in Hawaii. This chapter contributes a number of key concepts that are designed to enhance services. Specifically, it illustrates how the teaming model can work in the context of a multicultural environment through collaboration involving the aging and disability sectors. Central to the success of the project was identifying people who were willing to make a commitment to the goals of program review and improvement. Several small case studies are used to portray the experiences of aging individuals who were involved in the project. Finally, Suttie appraises the effectiveness of the model in a multicultural context and its potential for the implementation elsewhere.

With the largest proportion of older residents in the United States, Florida is home to many older parents and their dependent adult children. Most of these families require assistance of some kind to remain self-reliant community participants. To respond effectively to these new needs, Sherman and Bloom in Chapter 26 describe how Florida's aging and disability systems created a local collaborative service model, using both top-down and bottom-up tactics. Their approach identified existing capacities in community services systems, assessed the needs of aging individuals and their families, and then helped the families plan for the delivery of collaborative services. The strategies used by the authors and their team for developing primary activities, the key role played by mentors, and the successes and problems encountered throughout the experience are detailed in this chapter. To help with replication, the chapter concludes with lessons learned, contributions made, and recommendations for other, similar projects.

In Chapter 27, Stone summarizes an effort undertaken by the Texas Planning Council for Developmental Disabilities to develop and implement supports and services to older adults with lifelong disabilities and their families. The Texas approach involved two major activities. The first was directed at developing an integrated system of service supports to help older adults and their families to have options and choices based on individual needs and preferences reflecting cultural and ethnic life experiences. The second was directed toward developing a service system that could be accessed easily from multiple entry points. Stone describes the model's four steps—coalition building, interagency training, community awareness, and needs assessments—and provides insights on lessons learned.

Last, Sears gives us a bird's-eye perspective of how people who work for local government and who try to change systems manage to persevere. Her essay details how well-intended efforts get enmeshed in the "give and take" of politics and seemingly never-ending funding crises.

23

Outreach and Assistance
Using Area Agencies on Aging

Katharine S. Hacker, Philip McCallion, and Matthew P. Janicki

In the United States, federal legislation, in the form of the Older Americans Act of 1965 (PL 89-73), provides the basis for the structure of social support programs that are designed to accommodate the varied needs of older Americans. This far-reaching legislation supports the existence of a network of local services for older adults and frames the relationships among the various levels of governmental concerns in the areas of policy, planning, and services. In 1987, the act was amended (PL 100-175) to include older adults with disabilities among the specific constituents of concern to both state and area agencies on aging (AAAs). The 1992 amendments (PL 102-375) to the act expanded the province of the nation's AAAs to include initiatives for outreach and service delivery to older individuals with developmental disabilities and their aging caregivers. These amendments also included provisions for a series of demonstration programs in the area of developmental disabilities. One of these demonstration programs was awarded to New York State, which received a grant to find aging caregivers and operate outreach programs from 1994 to 1996 using AAAs as service providers.

This chapter uses the results of that endeavor to explore how AAAs can effectively expand their services to people with developmental disabilities and their aging caregivers in the community. The chapter also discusses how AAAs can have an impact on the structures through which services are delivered to people with developmental disabilities and to their aging caregivers. Lessons learned and recommendations are offered for replications of these efforts throughout the United States and other parts of the world.

BACKGROUND

Until recently, large numbers of people with developmental disabilities did not survive to old age (Janicki, Dalton, Henderson, & Davidson, 1999), and those who did generally were hidden because families, their primary caregivers, were able to provide lifetime care (Roberto, 1993) or they lived out their old age in public institutions. The likelihood that aging people with developmental disabilities will live into retirement years and outlive family caregivers has created an increased awareness of the need for new services and additional resources, a factor for which many aging and developmental disabilities agencies had not planned (Ansello & Rose, 1989; McCallion & Janicki, 1997).

Furthermore, the needs of older caregivers have not received the attention that workers in the field have indicated they should (Jennings, 1987; McCallion & Tobin, 1995; Roberto & Nelson, 1988; Seltzer, 1992), and to a large extent, many of these older caregivers have become the "lost generation" within our services (Breitenbach, 1996). Responses to address the growing needs of these caregivers have been stymied by the following conflicts:

1. Which is the responsible service system—aging or developmental disabilities?
2. Who is the primary client—the aging caregiver or the person with a developmental disability?
3. What are appropriate service models—maintaining the family living situation, planning for transitions to other-than-home living, or promoting the independence of the person with a developmental disability?

It has also been noted by developmental disabilities service workers that there are frequently long-standing conflicted relationships between older caregivers who provide long-term care and formal service providers (McCallion & Tobin, 1995; Smith & Tobin, 1993). These conflicts and an emphasis on responding to the needs of other populations have resulted in little attention being paid by the formal service system to such families. The families themselves also have been reluctant to seek assistance until a crisis occurs. This means that when a caregiving parent dies or becomes too ill to continue care, formal agencies are most likely to be asked to provide out-of-home care on an emergency basis for the individual with a developmental disability. Often, no other plan for continued care exists, or there is no time to develop one. This represents the most expensive level of care within both the aging and the developmental disabilities service systems. Over the past decade, amendments to the Older Americans Act and similar initiatives by the Administration on Developmental Disabilities resulted from a recognition that prior engagement with these families and planning for their needs are likely to result in the use of less costly and less traumatic service options (McCallion & Janicki, 1997). These initiatives also revealed the need to find answers to who the lead agency in these efforts should be and how the two service systems, aging and developmental disabilities, can best cooperate.

Although the indicators are clear that such cooperative endeavors are a sound venture and should be pursued, many barriers still impede successful cooperation between the aging and developmental disabilities service systems (Ansello, 1992; LePore & Janicki, 1997; Wu, 1987):

1. The two systems have differences in language, philosophy, and priorities; indeed, the same words often mean different things.
2. There is uncertainty about who has a "developmental disability" and the numbers of people involved.
3. Not knowing the specific needs of older families who are caring for adult children with developmental disabilities makes it difficult to plan for their inclusion in services.
4. There are major differences in how services are funded and organized within each system.
5. Lack of clear-cut goals in either system for aging people with developmental disabilities and their families makes joint planning more difficult.
6. The meetings, training sessions, and consultations involved in responding to the demands of a unified approach are often perceived by workers in both service systems as an additional hindrance to efforts to meet needs that they poorly understand.
7. There is resistance from aging network constituents to including people with developmental disabilities in aging services planning.
8. In a time of declining resources, there are suspicions that cooperative efforts to serve people with developmental disabilities and their aging families are more likely to draw away resources from populations that are already being served rather than add to service options.
9. It is difficult for those who are brokering cooperative efforts to present themselves as impartial and nonthreatening to both service systems.
10. There is a lack of personnel who are trained in both service systems, although such training seems critical to cooperative efforts.

Four principal strategies have been advocated to address these hurdles: brokering cooperation through an impartial third party, emphasizing cross-training, reformulating public policy, and having aging organizations take a lead role. The first three strategies are discussed elsewhere (see, e.g., Ansello, 1992; Ansello, Coogle, & Wood, 1997; Ansello & Roberto, 1993; Janicki, 1993; Sutton, Sterns, Schwartz & Roberts, 1992; Turner, 1994). While recognizing the merits of these three approaches, this chapter concentrates on the fourth, having aging organizations, the AAAs, take a lead role.

WHY AAAs?

The enactment of the Older Americans Act in 1965 recognized the increasing numbers of older people who needed supports to maintain themselves in the community and who wanted a life free of isolation and poverty. Thus, as crafted, a key objective of the act was to maintain "freedom, independence, and the free exercise of individual initiative in planning and managing their own lives, full participation in the planning and operation of community-based services and programs provided for their benefit, and protection against abuse, neglect, and exploitation" (National Association of State Units on Aging, 1985). To meet this objective, the act defined the elements for what today has become the "aging network." Beginning with the federal agency that is responsible for administering the act, the Administration on Aging, there were to be designated state entities, the state units on aging, and local AAAs. The state units on aging are generally the state offices or departments that are charged with administering each state's system of services for older adults, except those involving long-term care. Locally, the act designated AAAs to be responsible for planning and service delivery. These state units on aging and local AAAs were also mandated to develop and maintain state and area plans for aging services on a 2-, 3-, or 4-year basis.

The Older Americans Act provided for the setting up of a network of programs and advocacy for all older people. It also defined people who are eligible for services as all people age 60 and older, with programs targeted to the "elderly with the greatest economic and social need," including those who are frail, disabled, of low income, and/or from diverse cultures. Attention was to be focused on

> The full restoration services for those who require institutional care, and a comprehensive array of community-based, long-term care services adequate to appropriately sustain older people in their communities and in their homes, including support to family members and other people providing voluntary care to older individuals needing long-term care services. (Act § 321[a])

Practical methods for reaching these objectives were not as clearly prescribed. The act outlined a structure for the operation of programs throughout the United States to provide a range of services to older people, including information and assistance, legal services, nutrition, community-based long-term care, and advocacy and prevention services of various types. These services were to be delivered locally by AAAs, which may operate on a regional or local basis, or by subcontract with community-based agencies. The nation's 655 AAAs, which are governmental or quasi governmental entities, serve to link each locality's services for older citizens with an administrative structure that is responsible for planning; service delivery; and the coordination of the distribution of federal, state, and local funds. In support of these services, major funding for Older Americans Act programs goes to nutrition services, supporting both congregate and home-delivered meals. Although other services receive smaller amounts of financial resources, the delivery of AAA programs generally receives widespread support. In addition, state and local funding significantly supplements federal funds.

Subsequent amendments to the Older Americans Act in 1987 and 1992 included provisions that enable older people with disabilities, including people with developmental disabilities, to be more readily involved and served within programs and services that are regularly provided by AAAs. These amendments also provided specific mandates to state units on aging and AAAs to cooperatively plan, develop, and provide services for older people with disabilities in conjunction with state and local disabilities agencies, target informal aging caregivers for assistance, ensure that congregate meal sites serve adults with disabilities who are dependent and younger than 60 years of age (when accompanied by an eligible parent or caregiver), link the long-term care ombudsman program to advocacy and protection programs, and authorize funding for cross-training and research between service systems (Janicki, 1993).

COMMUNITY AND ORGANIZATIONAL CONTEXT: WHAT AAAs DO

There are many organizational forms to AAAs throughout the United States. A majority of the 655 AAAs serve single counties or metropolitan areas; others include several counties in their catchment area, and, in a few cases, the state agency for aging and the AAA are the same unit (e.g., in Delaware and North Dakota). Across the United States, the AAAs are found in a variety of forms. In New York, for example, the state's 59 AAAs are predominantly county based, with some exceptions: one encompasses the five counties of New York City, two are located on Native American reservations, and one is a two-county joint agency. Nationally, the AAAs are usually public agencies, but in some cases, some or most of their activities are subcontracted to nonprofit entities. Although federally funded, AAAs are usually a part of local government (the exceptions are contract agencies that are not part of the local or state governmental structure).

AAAs have a legislative mandate to plan and to provide assistance to aging people, including people with disabilities. The mandate to plan includes cataloging services and allocating funds, but many AAAs also recognize their responsibility to organize and inform the community about a range of issues. AAAs provide a wide range of advocacy and information materials, usually have newsletters that reach large numbers of people in the community, and have developed extensive cooperative networks in the regions they cover. Agency staff and community-based advisory committees serve as advocates for a range of issues, from transportation to housing. They can, for example, be helpful to developmental disabilities service agencies that need to support individuals in the community, by offering a variety of information about community resources and about financial benefits and related issues. The public activities they carry out make AAAs visible and widely known, making them a frequent first stop for people who are aging and need information on how to find new resources and make adjustments to the changes that come with aging.

Another feature of AAAs is that they employ people from the communities in which they are located. Staff are often hired for their knowledge and understanding of their own community. This makes them less likely to be seen as adversaries and more likely to be accepted as advocates. They help facilitate the inclusion and long-term support of individuals in the community, especially in times of transition. Outreach and interventions by AAAs are, therefore, more likely to be seen as a support. In contrast, developmental disabilities service agencies and social services agencies often are reported to be perceived by families as adversaries (McCallion & Tobin, 1995).

The following illustrates how AAAs may serve older people with a developmental disability as well as their families:

> Mr. Jones and his sister contacted the local AAA. He is a man with an intellectual disability in his late 60s who now lives by himself in an apartment in a small city. He had lived with his brother until 3 years ago, when his brother died. His brother's physician stated that Mr. Jones was not able to take care of himself or live on his own. His two sisters did not want him to live with either of them and had him screened for eligibility for services by the state developmental disabilities agency. He was referred to a group home approximately 60 miles from where he had been living. Mr. Jones was very upset about this and, with the help of a lawyer, sued to be allowed to live on his own. He won the suit and happily moved into his own place, back in the neighborhood where he had previously lived. He knew he needed help, so he and his sister contacted the AAA. A senior companion was assigned to visit him on a regular basis to check on him and help him with bill paying and mail and to provide help with some light shopping and cleaning. He had some medical problems that made it important that he take his medications and receive good nutrition, so AAA staff arranged for him to receive

home-delivered meals 3 days a week. His income made him ineligible for Medicaid, so the worker signed him up for a small amount of needed home care from a state program operated by the AAA. This program also provided some case management services. He also got a ride most mornings in the local senior center van to the center to play cards with a men's club that included several other men with developmental disabilities. No other service needs have been identified; however, AAA staff continued to monitor his situation.

AAAs AS SERVICE PROVIDERS

In its efforts to facilitate successful adherence to the 1987 and 1992 amendments to the Older Americans Act, the Administration on Aging (AoA) recognized a need for technical expertise and information in the following areas: building local coalitions, enabling aging and disability agencies to coordinate and cooperate with regard to services, and facilitating greater access to community support services for families and their adults with disabilities ("Fiscal Year 1993 Program Announcement," 1993). In 1993, the AoA funded a series of demonstration projects to identify, demonstrate, and disseminate best practices in this area. One project funded was a cooperative effort among the New York State Office of Mental Retardation and Developmental Disabilities, the New York State Office for Aging, the New York Developmental Disabilities Planning Council, and several university-based research and service centers (for a full description, see Janicki, McCallion, Force, Bishop, & LePore, 1998). Primary activities of the project were to demonstrate ways that AAAs could locate and help older caregivers who continue to care at home for an adult family member with a developmental disability. McCallion and Grant-Griffin (Chapter 6) report on findings from a separate component of the project that examined how AAAs could reach out and provide assistance to families from diverse cultures.

The AAAs were asked, over the course of an 18-month period, to test the feasibility of incorporating into their daily practice low-cost and low-tech outreach, linkages with developmental disabilities agencies, and supports for households with adults with a developmental disability. All told, 13 of New York state's 59 AAAs participated in the project. The populations in their catchment areas ranged from 55,000 to approximately 1 million inhabitants, with densities ranging from 100 people per square mile for rural AAAs to 1,000–2,000 people per square mile in urban areas. Per capita income in the catchment areas ranged from $20,000 to $45,000, and the percentage of people older than 60 years ranged from 12% to 21%. Annual budgets from all sources for the AAAs ranged from $1.0 million to $8.4 million, with an average of $3.0 million (Janicki et al., 1998).

Approximately 300 families who were interested in receiving services were identified under the project. Of these, approximately 50% had previously been identified by the developmental disabilities service system as including a person with a developmental disability. The outreach methods used included community orientations; sponsorship of workshops; radio and television public service announcements; stories in the local press and AAA-sponsored newsletters; contacts with clergy, police, postal workers, pharmacists, hair stylists, and other community vendors; and posters placed in churches, senior centers, clinics, public offices, and other local meeting places. The effectiveness of these methods varied by community; no one method was superior to another. Yet such outreach methods, in whichever form, can be useful in reaching out to families. We found that approximately 50% of the families that contacted the AAA directly did so as a result of these outreach efforts. Another 30% were referred by other agencies that were now better aware of AAA interest in serving this population. What follows will be drawn from the experiences gleaned from this demonstration.

MAKING CONTACTS

Most contacts to AAAs are made because families need services or because the families are seeking some type of information. In this context, "families" are primarily mothers or sisters, although other relatives, such as fathers and grandparents, also may be present. Caregiving grandparents are proving particularly challenging for AAAs because care recipients in these situations are more likely to be young children. This aspect may require the AAAs to become involved with local school districts, a relationship they had not developed in the past. Grandparents as the object of special initiatives are gaining more attention, and several projects have been developed to assist local agencies with helping this group. People with lifelong disabilities who AAAs encounter are usually adults with mental retardation, but often others with physical and other cognitive disabilities are found as well. Generally, they are evenly split between males and females. In addition, there are now situations in which people with a developmental disability are the primary caregivers for older parents. In addition, frequently there are other people in the household in need of care, including frail older spouses of the caregiver, the caregiver's own parent, and/or other siblings with ongoing illness or mental health concerns.

The services that AAAs provide vary depending on what is readily available or needed. Some AAAs located families and made referrals to local developmental disabilities service agencies. However, when they did not already have a working relationship with such agencies, they were more likely to offer casework and other supports themselves. When AAAs provided direct aid to families, their assistance included some combination of information and referral, securing federal assistance (e.g., Supplemental Security Income, Medicaid), respite, transportation, homemaker services, home weatherization, heating assistance, nutrition programs, legal aid, and other senior services.

An important aspect of the demonstration was its networking and community planning component, which brought together providers from both the aging and developmental disabilities service systems to discuss ways to work more closely for the benefit of families and individuals in the community. Workshops and county-level committees that focused on specific joint programming proved useful for exchanging information and developing working relationships, which improved the quality of services to families in the community. Four areas of changing the interactions between service systems are particularly noteworthy.

First, accompanying the increase in life span of people with developmental disabilities is an increase in the number of these people with common ongoing disabling conditions, such as heart disease, diabetes, arthritis, and Alzheimer's disease. Because staff who work in a local developmental disabilities service agency generally work only with a younger population, they are not familiar with these conditions. The hospitalization of an individual with a developmental disability thus can lead to conflicts over where the person should go after he or she leaves the hospital. Long-term care specialists at the AAA can provide an understanding of the structure and workings of the local long-term care system so that informed decisions can be considered. In another situation, as with someone with severe arthritis, it may be difficult for developmental disabilities services staff who are unfamiliar with the range of limitations caused by this condition to develop a good plan for personal care for the family caregiver to implement. Because such information generally is more readily available through the AAA, a project worker can aid the developmental disabilities agency staff to develop a plan to help the person. One result can be greater recognition from developmental disabilities service agencies of the aging expertise available through AAAs and an increase in requests for assistance with information and planning.

Second, because AAAs are required to serve anyone ages 60 years and older, developmental disabilities service agencies can gain access to these services for older people with developmental disabilities. Thus, either agency has an obligation to provide services to older adults with a developmental disability, depending on what their needs are. Local social services or public welfare departments also have obligations and responsibilities for such adults, particularly if they are covered by Medicaid. A typical situation is when an aging caregiver who is covered by Medicaid and caring for someone with a developmental disability requests home care for herself. Questions can arise as to which service system is responsible (the real question is whose budget will cover the costs). Taking the time to resolve this type of dispute usually delays the delivery of needed services. An approach to resolve this can be to use the AAA project staff person as a consultant for the various organizations that are working with cases that involve family caregivers of the person with a developmental disability. Linking the various workers involved in such a case and explaining the possible use of a range of programs to serve the family can lead to the development of a service package and potential cost sharing among agencies. The AAA worker can act as an advocate, providing one-to-one training and support for agency staff and making frequent telephone contact to answer questions. The staff member also can go to higher-level administrative and policy staff within the region to clarify rules and restrictions when situations prevent a family from receiving needed services.

Third, workers can help families plan for the future. In some instances, workers may encounter situations in which older parents cannot live at the residence they chose because administrators will not permit their dependent son or daughter also to live there. There may also be a lack of willingness or an inability for residential programs for adults with a disability to permit a parent to live with their son or daughter. This may encourage AAA staff to work to maintain families in their existing living situation. Sometimes, this may not be possible. These types of impediments to planning can vex even the most innovative agencies and can continue to represent a major challenge to service systems to explore means of greater cooperation and cost sharing.

Finally, AAAs can often run into difficulties when referring older adults with a disability because the adults have not received a diagnostic evaluation at an earlier point in their lives and thus do not have documentation of a lifelong disability. This can result in their being declared ineligible for services by developmental disabilities service agencies. One way to overcome this problem is to have the state mental retardation and developmental disabilities agency agree to declare individuals eligible for services on the basis of "presumptive disability" and to accept ad hoc case summaries prepared by AAA staff as sufficient rationale for establishing such eligibility. In this manner, AAAs can help eliminate a substantial barrier to the receipt of needed services.

ORGANIZATIONAL DESIGNS

Generally, AAAs can organize an AAA-based initiative to aid older adults with a developmental disability or their caregivers by using any of the following operational approaches: 1) direct operation, 2) contract operation, and 3) multiorganizational operation. In our experience, when AAAs are county based and operated and located in rural and less densely populated regions, they are more likely to use a direct operation design. In this design, they undertake the initiative themselves, either using part of the time of an existing staff or hiring a part-time staff person. However, one concern that can arise for existing staff is ensuring that the time allocated for this project is protected from the infringements of other responsibilities. AAAs using this approach need to ensure that a dedicated staff person is used, irrespective of whether that person works full or part time. Without the internalization of responsibility for such an initiative by a key person, these activities may not receive the attention they require and the initiative may be put in jeopardy.

Independent of location, if an AAA traditionally subcontracts operations to local nonprofit agencies, then such an initiative can also be subcontracted. AAAs are directed by the Older Americans Act to subcontract out, whenever possible, to help support local community-based organizations. With limited funding available, some AAAs may find it easier to contract out at least part of the initiative to an organization with existing funding to serve people with developmental disabilities. The positive aspects of this approach can include the development of formal ties with local agencies and an increased level of interaction and joint training. Also, collaboration with a local developmental disabilities or family services agency can reduce initial training and start-up needs and costs. The negatives of this approach may be that families do not perceive that the services are aging related rather than developmental disabilities related. Also, when AAAs do not develop the internal capacity to serve older people with a developmental disability, there may be uncertainties about how to maintain linkages and services once such an initiative is no longer a focus of AAA activities.

In another approach, several jurisdictions can use the opportunity to expand their current efforts at joint programming and undertake a collective or multiorganizational approach. We observed three AAAs undertake such an initiative and share regional outreach and information and referral activities but handle their own casework and household assistance. In this instance, the regional developmental disabilities service agency aided the three AAAs by assigning a quarter-time administrator to help coordinate the activities, which in turn created an opportunity to have several graduate-level social work interns be assigned to the project. However, although such a coordinated approach attracted additional resources, the network's own processes of coordination, joint program development, and relationship building proved to be time consuming. This type of approach can work best in an environment where cooperative endeavors are already the norm and where the territory, because of its rural nature or clearly defined boundaries, helps facilitate cooperation. Depending on local administrative and fiscal circumstances, all three approaches can prove to be useful. Important is that an AAA choose an approach that is likely to be cost- and service-effective and sustainable over the long term.

When it comes to staffing, AAAs need to ensure that staff can be available for families who are identified and that such caregivers receive appropriate services and information. One successful method is to identify a key staff person to specialize in serving these families and establish linkages with outside agencies and with in-house information and assistance units, home-delivered and congregate meals programs, legal services, home care units, and other programs. Such a staff specialist should provide consultation and information to other staff and sometimes elect to provide services, such as assessment and case management, themselves. A key factor in selecting such an individual is motivation. The task of learning about developmental disabilities and maintaining needed contacts in the community requires an individual with a genuine interest in developing and maintaining the extra skills needed. We observed that staff, particularly those who had a family member with a developmental disability, were usually very effective in working with families. However, such a person would have to dedicate time to make one-to-one contacts and serve as the primary contact person to families. We observed that many families were hesitant to talk to just anyone about their plans (or lack of plans) for the future and about the concerns they had. Time was needed to develop a trusting relationship that could be used to facilitate recognition by families of the need to take action, and it helped to have a staff person with the allocated hours and personal experience to do this. To accomplish this sensitive form of outreach, the time commitment for a staff person to fulfill these responsibilities should be no less than, on the average, 2 days per week.

AAAs can run into barriers as they try to implement such an initiative. No two AAAs will have exactly the same experience. The barriers they may experience include limited funds, having to respond to multiple regulations and funding requirements, burdensome regulations for subcontractors, resistance and resentment from other agencies or from others within one's own agency because they were not involved in developing or running the initiative, little support from local developmental disabilities service agencies, little understanding within the aging and disabilities networks of each other's services, a historical lack of collaboration among agencies within the local community, and the untimely reorganization and restructuring of key agencies during the course of such an endeavor.

Such barriers can be surmountable. However, they require a greater level of collaboration and communication among agencies than some AAAs may have pursued in the past. It is interesting that a number of AAA directors who participated in our project recommended that AAA administrators who are undertaking such an initiative assume that these will be concerns and be forewarned that these issues will consume considerable time during the early stages of any outreach effort. They recommended, to the extent possible, setting up networks and communication arrangements in advance. Most critical, they noted, was ensuring a good relationship with local developmental disabilities service agencies. This applies regardless of whether an AAA subcontracts or operates the outreach and services programs themselves.

When it comes to ensuring that a good relationship will accompany tackling this type of endeavor, the following are suggested:

- Identify a core group of aging and developmental disabilities service agency representatives and family caregivers to advise the project.
- Involve existing networks and coalitions of aging and/or developmental disabilities service agencies.
- Have key service and political decision makers in the community endorse the collaborative efforts.
- Agree to share information about what each group of agencies is doing.
- Agree to exchange referrals.

- Agree to work together on furthering a specific service-related goal for the local community.
- Encourage staff exchanges and cross-training.

One AAA director summed it up this way:

> Be sure to have a direct line of communication by holding regular meetings. Get everyone to agree to participate in cross-training on what each of the members of the network does. Be sure to set up agreements on how to handle casework or follow-up of families who are referred. Agree beforehand who will be the gatekeeper of the system.

In undertaking this type of initiative, AAAs may experience varying levels of cooperation from local developmental disabilities service agencies. If they have not invested a lot of time in networking with these agencies, they may find that they will have to do this as the initiative develops. One method that seemed to work was frequent telephone calls by the AAA worker to the disabilities system intake worker to review new referrals. For each referral, the possible actions that could be taken were reviewed and discussed. The AAA worker helped both the families and the disabilities system worker by undertaking much of the preliminary work needed to get the family declared eligible and enrolled in the disability system and clarifying what services could be provided by each of the systems.

They will also find that funds for developmental disabilities services generally are tied to individuals served rather than to programs. We observed that some local developmental disabilities service agencies were reluctant to participate in more open referral processes, stating that they feared that AAAs would begin to gain access to "their" funds. Our advice: Local services will be enriched when time is taken to develop good communication and cooperation and allay the fears of local disabilities providers who feel threatened by the aging network.

TARGETING

In many instances, the primary targets of AAA outreach efforts are parents and other caregivers. These present special needs that require more than simple delivery of typical AAA services. Often, they may not want to be found for fear of having their son or daughter with a disability "taken away" and may require intensive outreach and counseling to get them to begin to confront the difficult decisions they need to make regarding the future. Sometimes such planning-focused assistance is more effective when done with a specialist from a developmental disabilities agency who is familiar with specialized disability-related legal issues and experienced in providing family counseling around the issue of transition to an out-of-home living setting. Thus, with this target group, the AAA may be more effective in simply finding the family and making the linkage to a developmental disabilities agency. In some instances, older caregivers may seek out aging network services for themselves, such as home-delivered meals; while receiving information from the meals program, they can also be provided with information about other services in which they might have an interest. During the course of these contacts, sometimes just talking about their situation can lead to their seeking out support services that they might never have admitted they needed. For example, an older woman contacted an AAA to request home-delivered meals for her "retarded brother" who lived in his own trailer next to hers. She was going in the hospital and was concerned about whether he would eat well while she was away. She then described the great preparations she was making to cook and freeze large amounts of food for herself for when she would return from the hospital. She saw herself as the survivor who would always be there to protect her brother. After several telephone discussions, she had realized that she needed to involve several other relatives and the local AAA congregate meal site in the care of her brother while she was in the hospital.

AAAs place a priority on community-based long-term care services. These services, although similar to those provided by the developmental disabilities systems, are different in several significant ways. The services provided to most older people are focused on maintaining independence while addressing the need to make major transitions into more intensive services. Thus, there is a need for more frequent assessments and changes in services while maintaining the highest level of independent living. As the numbers of older adults with developmental disabilities increase and more are living in the community, similarities for transitions with other older people will become more evident. AAAs have a great amount of knowledge and experience in helping people through these transitions and can provide help to local developmental disabilities providers who need to adjust their programs to better serve older people. Often, community planning activities can be the vehicle that brings together providers from both systems to discuss ways to work more closely for the benefit of families and individuals in the community. Workshops and local-level committees that focus on specific joint programming are often useful for exchanging information and developing working relationships that improve the quality of services to families and other caregivers in the community.

One outcome of increased life span among people with a developmental disability is an increase in the number of adults with common chronic disabling conditions, such as heart disease, diabetes, arthritis, and Alzheimer's disease. These conditions create problems in all types of community living situations, whether they directly involve families or not. Staff who work in the developmental disabilities system and who have always worked with a younger population often are not familiar with these conditions, and many are unprepared to make accommodations for the changes in lifestyle that may be needed as adults age in place. For example, the hospitalization of a resident of a group home can lead to a nightmare of conflicts over where a person should go after he or she leaves the hospital. Some residence staff may not know anything about changes in diets needed by people as they age or are affected by certain conditions. Developing a good plan for personal care services for someone who has, for example, severe arthritis, may be a completely new job for someone who is not familiar with the range of limitations caused by this condition. In another example, a family who has been caring for an adult who attends an occupational center each day may suddenly be unable to care for their family member, requiring immediate work on getting support services into a home. All of these problems can create a crisis that could overwhelm a worker who is unfamiliar with the aging service system.

There are a number of specific things that can be done in conjunction with AAAs that can be useful in preventing crises and improving planning and provision of services. First, developmental disabilities service providers can use the long-term care specialists at AAAs to gain an understanding of the structure and workings of the local long-term care system. This means getting copies of written materials regarding local assessment and services provision agreements, obtaining directories of services available and rules and regulations regarding their use, and developing one or two good contacts who can explain what to do in a variety of circumstances. Most AAAs are a part of any central intake system for long-term care, where these exist, and know the rules for any joint assessment tools that are used. AAAs should incorporate in their assessments information on the presence of any disabilities among the families that they are serving. The developmental disabilities agencies can set up procedures to link their assessments with the locally used tools to eliminate the duplications and confusion that often exist when two people are assigned to assess the same person. These linkages have been made with consideration of confidentiality and concerns over who is legally responsible for an individual. Decisions have to be made regarding which service system will be the primary system. An individual who is admitted to a nursing facility may lose all connection to the developmental disabilities system. AAA staff, familiar with these types of problems, can be helpful in guiding staff on designing methods to reduce the amount of trauma and confusion that often accompany changes in level of service.

Although AAAs are supposed to serve anyone who is 60 years of age and older, because of inadequate resources, they often are unable to accommodate the needs of people with severe disabilities and will prefer that another organization take full responsibility for someone who is seen as difficult or costly to serve. This may become a big issue when a caregiver needs a service such as home care and the person who needs the home care was caring for someone with a developmental disability. Ideally, services could be paid for by both systems, but in reality, the AAA or its subcontractors may not want to provide any service if it can be paid for by another system. The local department of social services may also become involved if someone in the house is eligible for Medicaid, complicating matters even more. AAAs are not permitted to provide services available from Medicaid to people who are eligible for Medicaid. One way to deal with this type of problem is to use the AAA staff person who is the specialist on aging and disabilities as a consultant. By linking the various workers involved in a case and explaining the possible use of a range of programs to serve families, service and support packages can be developed to meet the needs of such families. The AAA worker can also provide advocacy to make sure contacts are made in a timely fashion and uninformed or resistant workers are supported so that they can provide the services or supports needed. Making this work may involve providing one-to-one training and support to various agency staff and making frequent telephone contact to answer questions. In some cases, it may mean going to higher level administrative and policy staff to clarify rules and restrictions that may prevent individuals from receiving needed services. This is the type of advocacy work often performed by AAAs and is especially helpful for cases in which community-based long-term care is needed.

To provide long-term care–related advocacy to families that are caring for a person with developmental disabilities, strong linkages between information and assistance units, home-delivered congregate meals programs, legal services, and home care services need to exist. Programs cannot be run so separately that no one knows what anyone else is doing. A staff person who is trying to provide advocacy must be able to obtain adequate information about services being provided. Access to records and history of work with families is essential to understanding what needs to be done. In an area with a large population and highly specialized services structure, this may be a very difficult task; however, in this type of environment, it is even more likely that a family's needs might get lost in the system.

The following is an example of how such advocacy might work. This example is drawn from a composite of several situations:

An outreach flier in a senior center led to a call to an AAA. The woman who called was the sister of a 60-year-old man with an intellectual disability who had always been cared for by their mother. The father had died 10 years before, and the sister and her husband had been helping out with paperwork and other support since then. The mother had developed signs of dementia but was not aware that she had any problems. She had never allowed her son to be involved in local services and had not taken him to a physician in more than 25 years because she was afraid someone would make her send her son to an institution. No one else was allowed to do anything for her son except his sister. The sister's husband had decided that when the mother became unable to care for her son, he would not be allowed to move in with him and his wife. The sister and her husband wanted to take some action but were unsure of what to do. They were advised to see a lawyer to straighten out several problems with the mother's financial accounts (for which they had power of attorney) and were told about a number of financial benefits for which the son might be eligible. They were given the names of several people to speak with regarding his possibly living in a local group home and establishing eligibility for developmental disabilities services. They were also given some suggestions on how to cope with the mother's Alzheimer's dementia and some information on how to effect a placement in a nursing facility if her needs led to this.

After this initial contact, the AAA worker, with the permission of the family, contacted several key people among the locality's developmental disabilities agencies and a protective services worker in the social services department to fill them in on the situation. This allowed those workers to be prepared for the eventual arrival of the mother and brother into the service system and helped the sister when she made telephone calls to get more information. A year after the initial contact, the mother fell and broke her hip. The sister's first response was to contact the AAA to get the telephone numbers of the people she had been told about earlier. With the assistance of the people she called, she was able to find a group home quickly for her brother and get her mother admitted to a nursing facility. When there were some problems along the way, the AAA worker placed several key telephone calls to people who could be relied on to help. The adult protection department stepped in quickly to assist with moving the individuals involved and getting needed legal paperwork done. At last report, the son was very happy in his new home, had made several new friends, and had become involved in a variety of new activities.

This type of situation is not atypical and is found with increasing frequency. The type of information and assistance provided in this situation concerned both long-term care and developmental disabilities issues. The major problem that this family faced was addressing the need to move quickly to react to the crisis created by the mother's condition. The AAA staff person's familiarity with the long-term care system and ability to focus on the mother's problems helped the sister to have a significant role in the positive resolution of the case. If the first contact had been to a developmental disabilities agency, the staff person there may or may not have known how to make a referral to the AAA to give the sister the information she needed to help her mother. The important point here is that the established linkages between AAA staff and the various other service systems in an area can be very helpful in addressing complex cases that require advocacy and access to different levels of services.

CONCLUSIONS

AAAs can successfully reach out to older families that are caring for someone with a developmental disability, particularly individuals who were not already connected with services. The strengths that an AAA can bring to this activity include expertise in outreach; a nonthreatening public image; emphasis on low-cost strategies; accessibility to welcomed services such as benefits information, home energy/weatherization grants, and nutrition services; emphasis on service planning; and experience in networking with other agencies. Thus, AAAs are uniquely positioned to provide greater coordination, facilitate policy changes, bridge services networks, and approach families in a nonthreatening way and build trust. Continued commitment to expanding such efforts and resolution of some of the identified problems can help draw AAAs more fully into the support structures for older adults with a developmental disability and their families. Analyzing the capacity of a particular AAA and other organizations in the community to take on the responsibility of aiding older caregivers and older adults with a developmental disability requires a bit of soul searching to determine organizational commitment, understanding, and resources. In closing, we pose the following thoughts, which can be used to assess what needs to be considered before an AAA can assume these responsibilities:

- What level of staff capacity, interest, and motivation exists? Do any staff members know enough to provide quality services to adults with a developmental disability and their families? Are staff members interested in this type of initiative, or do they see it as another burden? Is there a motivated person who will take on the job to learn what needs to be learned and motivate and interest others in joining?
- What level of service intervention can be implemented? Are available staff entry level or experienced? Are they able to do in-depth family-oriented counseling and casework with assessments, or are they information and assistance providers with constraints on what they are allowed to do?
- What is the agency's capacity for change? Are civil service rules, bureaucratic requirements, or political problems going to sabotage efforts for change?
- What types of services can be offered? Are there particular programs that can be targeted as a good starting point? What programs are being used by the locality's adults with developmental disabilities? What motivated the people to seek out these particular services? What additional programs can be offered to the families?
- What are the size and character of local communities in the AAA's service area? Do some communities seem to be better as places to start an outreach effort or other program? Are there organizations in one of the communities that could help? What other types of targeting efforts have been tried that could be linked with a new targeting initiative?
- What are the relationships among aging service providers, the AAA, and developmental disabilities agencies? What agreements and networking arrangements exist? Would a new committee help?
- What is the capacity of the local developmental disabilities system? How much training and experience does it have in working with older people? Do administrators seem receptive to working with organizations outside the developmental disabilities system (do they say things like "our people")? Are there motivated people

who are willing to commit themselves to the extra time and effort to help the AAA implement such an initiative? Are there individuals who seem flexible enough to work with the AAA's looser rules and procedures? Are there people with expertise with developmental disabilities who are willing and able to provide guidance and consultation by telephone?

- Are funding constraints overwhelming? How can a program be developed without having to cut back some other type of service?
- How many staff are available to plan and work with other systems? Are there skilled community organization staff available to develop the community network needed to expand services to a new group of people?

REFERENCES

Ansello, E.F. (1992). Seeking common ground between aging and developmental disabilities. *Generations, 16*, 11–15.

Ansello, E.F., Coogle, C.L., & Wood, J.B. (1997). *Partners: Building inter-system cooperation in aging with developmental disabilities.* Richmond: Virginia Center on Aging, Virginia Commonwealth University.

Ansello, E.F., & Roberto, K.A. (1993). Empowering elderly caregivers: Practice, research and policy directives. In K.A. Roberto (Ed.), *The elderly caregiver: Caring for adults with developmental disabilities* (pp. 173–189). Thousand Oaks, CA: Sage Publications.

Ansello, E.F., & Rose, T. (1989). *Aging and lifelong disabilities: Partnership for the twenty-first century.* Palm Springs, CA: Elvirita Lewis Foundation.

Breitenbach, N. (1996). The lost generation. In M.P. Janicki, *Help for caring for older people caring for an adult with a developmental disability.* Albany: New York State Developmental Disabilities Planning Council.

Fiscal year 1993 program announcement: Availability of funds and request for applications. (1993, May 18). *Federal Register, 58*(95), 29,256–29,294.

Janicki, M.P. (1993). *Building the future: Planning and community development in aging and developmental disabilities.* Albany: New York State Office of Mental Retardation and Developmental Disabilities.

Janicki, M.P., Dalton, A.J., Henderson, C.M., & Davidson, P.W. (1999). Mortality and morbidity among older adults with intellectual disabilities: Health services considerations. *Disability and Rehabilitation, 21*, 284–294

Janicki, M.P., McCallion, P., Force, L., Bishop, K., & LePore, P. (1998). Area agency on aging outreach and assistance for households with older carers of an adult with a developmental disability. *Journal of Aging and Social Policy, 10*, 13–36.

Jennings, J. (1987). Elderly parents as caregivers for their adult dependent children. *Social Work, 32*, 430–433.

LePore, P., & Janicki, M.P. (1997). *The wit to win: How to integrate older persons with developmental disabilities into community aging programs* (3rd rev.). Albany: New York State Office for the Aging.

McCallion, P., & Janicki, M.P. (1997). Area agencies on aging: Meeting the needs of persons with developmental disabilities and their aging families. *Journal of Applied Gerontology, 16*, 270–284.

McCallion, P., & Tobin, S.S. (1995). Social worker orientations to permanency planning by older parents caring at home for sons and daughters with developmental disabilities. *Mental Retardation, 33*, 153–162.

National Association of State Units on Aging. (1985). *An orientation to the Older Americans Act* (Rev. ed.). Washington, DC: Author.

Older Americans Act Amendments of 1987, PL 100-175, 101 Stat. 926, 42 U.S.C. §§ 3001 *et seq.*

Older Americans Act Amendments of 1992, PL 102-375, 106 Stat. 1195, 42 U.S.C. §§ 3001 *et seq.*

Older Americans Act of 1965, PL 89-73, 42 U.S.C. §§ 3001 *et seq.*

Roberto, K.A. (1993). Family caregivers of aging adults with disabilities. In K.A. Roberto (Ed.), *The elderly caregiver: Caring for adults with developmental disabilities* (pp. 3–20). Thousand Oaks, CA: Sage Publications.

Roberto, K.A., & Nelson, R.E. (1988). The developmentally disabled elderly: Concerns of service providers. *Journal of Applied Gerontology, 8,* 175–182.

Seltzer, M.M. (1992). Family caregiving across the full lifespan. In L. Rowitz (Ed.), *Mental retardation in the year 2000* (pp. 85–100). New York: Springer-Verlag.

Smith, G.C., & Tobin, S.S. (1993). Practice with older parents of developmentally disabled adults. *Clinical Gerontologist, 14,* 59–77.

Sutton, E., Sterns, H.L., Schwartz, L., & Roberts, R.S. (1992). The training of a specialist in developmental disabilities and aging. *Generations, 16,* 71–74.

Turner, K.W. (1994). Modeling community inclusion for older adults with developmental disabilities. *Southwest Journal on Aging, 10*(1–2), 13–18.

Wu, I. (1987). *Barriers and strategies: Barriers to and strategies for the integration of older persons with developmental disabilities within aging network services.* Albany: New York State Office for the Aging.

24

Building Intersystem Cooperation

Partners III Integrated Model

Edward F. Ansello and Constance L. Coogle

The two previous Partners Projects funded by the U.S. Administration on Aging, as well as four other related initiatives on disabilities supported in Maryland and Virginia by the respective Developmental Disabilities Councils, the U.S. Department of Education, and others, have demonstrated that cooperation between the aging network and the disabilities system in delivering services is greatly helped when three basic ingredients are present: 1) some formal means of collaboration for ongoing communication between the systems; 2) strategies of two-way outreach to aging adults with lifelong disabilities and informal caregivers (family and friends) who provide community-based assistance; and 3) methods of building the capacities of formal providers of assistance (agency staff), informal providers (family and friends), and aging adults with lifelong disabilities to identify and use appropriate resources that maximize the community functioning of these older adults. The experiences of the original Partners Project in Maryland (1987–1990) and Partners II in Virginia (1990–1992) suggest that the three ingredients are effective both when aging adults with developmental disabilities are already known to the service system(s) and agencies seek better coordination and use of their resources in serving them and when these individuals are unknown and unserved and agencies seek either to initiate direct services or to assist older adults with developmental disabilities (consumers) or their families to use existing resources.

This chapter was supported in part by Grant No. 90AM0680 from the U.S. Administration on Aging, U.S. Department of Health and Human Services.

The Partners III Project combined these three components (collaboration, outreach, and capacity building) into the Integrated Model of Service to Older Adults with Developmental Disabilities (see Table 1) and secured the support of the U.S. Administration of Aging from 1993 to 1996 specifically to field-test the application of the Integrated Model in a variety of contexts, with an eye toward refining it from practical experience and disseminating it broadly. The project's executive committee selected five community-based coalitions of aging and developmental disabilities agencies in Maryland and Virginia, from among 20 applicants, for modest subawards to field-test the model over a 15- to 18-month period.[1] The project staff conducted leadership development workshops to train participant committees from each coalition in the model's three principal components of collaboration, outreach, and capacity building (Coogle, Ansello, & Wood, 1998). Each local coalition selected from among the model's essential and optional elements in applying the model in a variety of geographic and sociodemographic settings. Results have been incorporated into a practical how-to manual (Ansello, Coogle, & Wood, 1997) that objectively reviews strategies for achieving not only intersystem cooperation but also, more important, coordination of resources to serve aging adults with developmental disabilities and their families.

Furthermore, the experiences of the three Partners Projects have shown that there are a number of initiatives that agencies can exercise within each of the three basic components that will serve the purpose of improving services to aging adults with developmental disabilities and their families, given the differences among agencies in their resources, priorities, funding streams, and so forth. In other words, the Integrated Model provides a framework to guide and encourage initiatives. Its simplicity, three working parts, so to speak, belies the years of determining the basics of intersystem cooperation. But its simplicity also increases the prospects of the model's being implemented. A discussion of the rationale for each of the three basic components of the Integrated Model of Service follows, along with examples of initiatives within each, how-to suggestions, and the results of real-world applications of the components. In essence, this chapter is "lessons learned."

COLLABORATION

Rationale

There is only brief history of interaction between the aging and developmental disabilities systems of researchers, policy makers, planners, and providers in organizing and delivering services to meet the needs, maximize the abilities, and alleviate the problems of aging adults with lifelong disabilities (Coogle, Ansello, Wood, & Cotter, 1995; Factor, 1993; Hawkins & Eklund, 1990; Jenkins, Hildreth, & Hildreth, 1993). As Ansello and Rose noted,

> Adults with developmental disabilities are surviving to later life. In this sense, the aging-related and developmental disabilities systems are intersecting; and it is prudent to build bridges between them, bridges that will carry people, ideas, and information and assistance across in both directions. For not only is the developmental disabilities system of providers, programs, and services encountering greater numbers of adults with lifelong disabilities, but also the aging network is experiencing and will continue to experience more and more formerly unimpaired adults who suffer later-life disabilities. Lessons learned in respond-

---

[1]This chapter distills the implementation and results of the field testing. For a further description, see Ansello, Coogle, and Wood (1997).

Table 1.   Essential and optional elements of the integrated model of service delivery for older adults with developmental disabilities

Collaboration
Statewide mechanisms*
   Memoranda of understanding
   Professional/consumer advocacy council
Area planning and service committee*

Outreach
Resource fair*
Home visitor survey
Focus groups
Telephone surveys

Capacity building
Cross-training of staff*
Training in self-care and advocacy for consumers and informal caregivers*
Integration of older people with lifelong disabilities into community services
Internships across systems

*Essential element.

ing to the needs of older adults with lifelong disabilities enrich the capacity to respond to the needs of those with late-onset impairments. (1989, p. 6)

For collaboration to occur between two systems that are relatively unfamiliar with each other and for that collaboration to result ultimately in improved services to aging adults with lifelong disabilities as consumers and to their caregiving families, there should be both top-down and bottom-up mechanisms for collaboration—that is, both statewide and local focuses for collaboration.

Statewide mechanisms for collaboration include a memorandum of understanding between the state unit on aging and the state unit(s) on developmental disabilities (there are sometimes several relevant agencies; see Sutton, Sterns, Schwartz, & Roberts, 1992). This memorandum should pledge cooperation and the sharing of information and policy development relative to older adults with developmental disabilities and should formalize practices of interagency cooperation to promote resource sharing and coordinated services. These agreements are sometimes more valuable for their symbolic than their governing value. They sanction initiative. Another statewide mechanism for collaboration is a Professional/Consumer Advocacy Council (see Chapter 9). This council is composed of older adults with developmental disabilities, family caregivers, and community-based service providers from the aging and developmental disabilities networks, as well as others. They work to ensure the activation of the statewide memorandum of understanding, as well as policy and systems improvements for older adults with developmental disabilities. The Executive Council of the Partners III Project worked to effect both memoranda of understanding and Professional/Consumer Advocacy Councils in Maryland and Virginia.

At the same time, the identification of client needs and the provision of appropriate services will most likely occur on a local level. The overwhelming majority of aging adults with lifelong disabilities live in community settings, often with their families. In the Integrated Model, the local means of intersystem cooperation is called the Area Planning and Service Committee (APSC). With a limited geographical focus, APSCs can operationalize locally the statewide memorandum of understanding, as well as instigate a number of practical examples of its intent, such as to identify appropriate content for staff cross-training and consumer service coordination training, promote interagency collaboration, define the rationale and methods for integrating older adults with developmental disabilities into existing aging services such as senior centers, and provide leadership development of agency staff. Membership on the APSCs should include older adults with developmental disabilities, family caregivers, and agency staff from the aging and disabilities systems and from other community organizations that are concerned about the well-being of these older adults, such as advocacy, religious, recreation, and protective services, and so forth. The APSC becomes its own entity, a blend of the contributions by all of its participants. It is neither "aging" nor "disabilities" but both and more. The APSC acts, essentially, as a nonthreatening "neutral broker" (Ansello, 1992), facilitating the model's processes between the systems. It develops the initiatives listed next, and it issues the invitations.

How to Facilitate Collaboration

As a necessary first step in applying the Integrated Model, each coalition forms an APSC. This committee oversees the implementation of the three basic components of the Integrated Model: collaboration between the systems, strategies for outreach to older adults with developmental disabilities and their caregiving families, and mechanisms to build the capacities of these individuals and of agency staff. The initial tasks of this committee are to host, at a site of their choosing, a leadership development workshop for members of the committee and to participate fully in it. This workshop reviews both the Integrated Model and a range of issues related to successfully implementing the model. These may include 1) techniques for identifying unserved aging adults with developmental disabilities and their families and for identifying older caregivers of these aging adults (Cotter, Ansello, & Wood, 1992), 2) techniques for identifying local resources that might assist older adults with a developmental disability and their families, 3) strategies for interagency collaboration in service planning and delivery (Janicki, 1993; Pederson, 1993; Stroud & Sutton, 1988), 4) integration of older adults with developmental disabilities into the community and, as appropriate, into aging services (Stroud & Sutton, 1988), 5) consumer service coordination (Zirpoli, Wieck, & McBride, 1989) and self-advocacy training for older adults with developmental disabilities and their caregivers (Pederson, Chaikin, Koehler, Campbell, & Arcand, 1993; Zirpoli, Hancox, Wieck, & Skarnulis, 1994), and 6) person-centered planning and service delivery for older adults with developmental disabilities (Heller & Factor, 1991; Smith, Tobin, & Fullmer, 1995; Wood, 1993).

Other tasks relate to taking action on the issues outlined in the leadership workshop. The APSC members plan and implement cross-training sessions for other service providers, such as senior center staff, transportation workers, staff at congregate meal sites, and other community gatekeepers. They also are the prime movers in implementing training in consumer service coordination and self-advocacy for older adults with developmental disabilities (both consumers and potential consumers of services) and their families and advocates. Another function of the APSC is to promote interagency collaboration in planning and service delivery for older adults with developmental disabilities. The APSC, in practice, becomes a forum for people from different agencies, family members, and some consumers to assess the status quo and to develop ways in which aging and developmental disabilities agencies can work together to harmonize their services, to identify unserved older adults with a developmental disability, and to use untapped resources for providing services. Finally, the APSC works to facilitate the integration of older adults with developmental disabilities into the community and, as appropriate, into aging services when this integration is both desired by the older adult and beneficial.

Groups that should be recruited for representation on the committee include providers of aging, health, mental health, mental retardation, physical and sensory rehabilitation, and social services; groups that have responsibility for input into planning services, such as the disability services boards; local chapters of advocacy groups, such as The Arc or United Cerebral Palsy; and older adults with developmental disabilities and their families. The size of the committee will vary from locality to locality, depending in part on the numbers of service providers and advocacy groups that are available. The exact number of people on the committee is less important than is the number of active, regularly attending participants. The projects found that sometimes a relatively neutral third party, such as an institution of higher education, can be a nonthreatening broker in bringing together personnel from the aging and disabilities systems to address their common needs and resources. Essential to the success of the APSC is having a "spark" (Janicki, 1993) to coordinate and to inspire fellow participants, as well as having participants commit, at the outset, to continue for a set number of months and to communicate the APSC's activities to their peers.

Field-Test Experiences

Those who field tested the model considered the APSC to be the most central element in ensuring the successful implementation of the model and, more important, cooperation between the systems so that aging adults with lifelong disabilities benefit. The activity rated by the five field-testing agencies as the most important for a successful APSC is the leadership development workshop. These workshops not only produced statistically significant gains in participants' knowledge of aging and developmental disabilities subject matter (see Coogle et al., 1998) but also gave everyone on the APSC a common language and understanding of the components necessary for intersystem cooperation.

Some observations and recommendations from the subawardees include the following: 1) Organizations, more so than individuals, need to commit to the APSC, 2) good networking occurred between systems because of the APSC, and collaboration was the single best aspect of the project, 3) cross-affiliations improved because of the APSC, 4) concrete meeting agendas, signed letters of commitment, and frequent mailings ensured a successful APSC, and 5) the APSC should be composed of administrative staff.

Issues identified by the subawardees include 1) the need to ensure that members of the APSC do, in fact, keep the rest of their agency alerted to APSC activities, 2) the need to spell out benefits to consumers of employing the Integrated Model, 3) collaboration requires an extensive time frame, more than 1 year, to become effective, 4) coordination of the APSC is central to its success, and the coordinator needs to be neutral and committed to the process, yet participating agencies may not be able to assign a staff member to this role long term, 5) the concept of rotating or fixed-term coordinators may have merit, 6) subawardees had varying success in involving consumers on the APSC, 7) having specific, achievable tasks seemed to help recruit and keep consumers, and 8) the leadership development workshops proved to be essential in understanding and applying the Integrated Model.

OUTREACH

Rationale

A very large percentage of older adults with developmental disabilities are not known to or served by any formal human services system, whether it be aging, developmental disabilities, health, or something else. This observation dates to at least Rose and Ansello (1987) and is likely not limited to Maryland and Virginia. Several researchers have noted that the majority of adults with mental retardation in the United States grow old in their families without use of any developmental disabilities system services (Roberto, 1993; Seltzer, Krauss, & Heller, 1991; Seltzer, Krauss, & Janicki, 1994). Simply, family and friends provide assistance or care that enables the older adult with developmental disabilities to remain at home in the community. However, as these caregivers age and their offspring survive to later life, they constitute "two-generation geriatric families" (Ansello, 1991) in which the older person is becoming increasingly challenged by declining strength or inability to continue to provide assistance. Family caregivers and aging adults with developmental disabilities need to become better aware of existing services and resources within the community so that they might continue to remain in a community environment. The Partners Projects found that often family caregivers were not well informed regarding such resources. Service agencies need to know of the existence and status of such caregiving families so that the agencies can prepare for the eventual request for assistance when the caregiving parent dies or when the parent or the older adult with a developmental disability becomes incapable of continuing without help. The Partners III Project conceptualized outreach as a two-way bridge: sending information out and carrying information in. To inform older adults and their families about existing services that may help them and to aid agencies in planning for future needs, the Integrated Model suggests four different outreach strategies: 1) resource fairs, 2) home visitor surveys, 3) focus groups, and 4) telephone surveys.

Resource Fair   The APSC assembles under one roof a variety of people and materials that can be of assistance to the family caregiver or the consumer. Resource people might include agency personnel who can explain the services of their respective agencies, whether governmental, civic, for-profit, or whatever; representatives of pharmacies, hospitals, home care, insurance, funeral, and other businesses; advocates from associations on aging or disabilities; and representatives from support groups, faith communities, and so forth. Material resources might include self-help audiovisuals, brochures, books, how-to manuals, pamphlets, and so forth. Experience has shown that an effectively publicized resource fair will identify numbers of previously unknown family caregivers and consumers.

Home Visitor Survey   Home visits by agency staff often are purpose specific (e.g., to assess the status of a frail older adult). The Partners II Project discovered that expanding the purpose of the visit revealed relevant information. For example, in Virginia, when aides from aging agencies visited frail older adults and simply asked questions about others who lived in the home and about care that the frail older adult might be giving to another, a substantial number of aging adults with developmental disabilities were "discovered."

Focus Groups   Identifying the unknown can be made easier by convening focus groups in a limited geographical area. Focus groups that are composed of clergy, health care providers, home association or neighborhood leaders, and so forth have proved effective in identifying families that contain older adults with developmental disabilities who are not currently being served by any human services agency.

Telephone Surveys   On occasion, random "cold calls" to local telephone numbers will reveal family caregivers or older adults with developmental disabilities who are not currently known to the direct services agency. Although some potential recipients of services may be identified, large numbers of homes need to be called before one can confidently predict prevalence of such individuals in a catchment area. Nonetheless, agencies may find this outreach strategy to be a good use of volunteers.

How-To: Resource Fair

The resource fair is, in practice, the most effective means of two-way outreach. In fact, it is an essential element of the Integrated Model. Experience has shown that an effectively publicized resource fair will draw and identify numbers of previously unknown family caregivers and consumers. Resource fairs can accomplish at least three things: assistance to or capacity building of older adults with developmental disabilities and their caregivers, identification for service agencies of potential future consumers, and practical cooperation between the systems. An effective resource fair does require extensive cooperative planning, and the very act of planning for a fair tends to foster interagency collaboration, but the subawardees recommended that it be scheduled several months into the collaboration process.

The resource fair is ideally suited to the broad composition of the APSC. It should be jointly planned, marketed, and offered by personnel in both the aging and developmental disabilities systems to serve as a demonstration of resources available throughout the community. Inasmuch as resource fairs offered during Partners II and III each required approximately 100 person-hours of planning and management, the APSC is ideally suited to distribute the work load. The event should be marketed to professionals, as well as to consumers and caregivers. Agency personnel themselves will benefit by becoming aware of the local assistance and resources they can draw upon to help them respond more appropriately to those they serve with both aging-related and developmental disabilities–related needs. Consumers and caregivers will be encouraged to begin thinking about possible needs they may have if they become incapacitated, advancing "permanency planning," and they will become more knowledgeable about help that is available to them through community-based agencies.

In practice, APSCs incorporated the following components into the resource fair: 1) display booths staffed by knowledgeable representatives from organizations offering assistance to the target populations; 2) hands-on demonstrations of equipment, adaptive devices, and so forth; 3) demonstrations of stress-relieving techniques conducted by a psychologist, counselor, social worker, chiropractor, or other professional; 4) expert presenters conducting workshops on relevant topics such as stress management, nutrition, assistive technology, legal issues, financial and estate planning, Social Security, Medicare, and Medicaid; 5) information on services to maintain the home physically, such as home chore services and house weatherization programs; and 6) "brown bag" medications checks conducted by pharmacists (attendees must be told to bring *all* medications, both prescription and over-the-counter). Resource fairs included other enticements that served to encourage attendance, such as free blood sugar checks and blood pressure screening, distribution of donated giveaways, distribution of identification and discount cards, and provision of a light lunch.

Field-Test Experiences

Resource fairs were universally successful. This is not to say that they are effortless. They are an ideal mechanism for interagency cooperation and two-way outreach (sending information out to community members and drawing in information about consumers' and caregivers' situations and needs). Among other things, resource fairs tend to serve the role of reinforcing the capacities of family caregivers to continue doing what they are doing, for the fairs offer information on agencies, services, and fellow caregivers.

Like other forms of outreach discussed later, resource fairs did *not* result in increased caseloads for APSC member agencies. This was an unfounded fear among some agency staff, who were reluctant to initiate any outreach for fear that it would be promising agency services to those who were contacted. Instead, caregiver and consumer participants in the resource fairs pointedly stated that they did not want agency services but, rather, wanted to continue doing what they were doing (e.g., providing care, living relatively independently in the community) for as long as they could.

Additional comments from the field-testing agencies include the following:

1. Outreach is a long-term process that may yield results in years rather than months.
2. Outreach was sometimes affected by strict jurisdictional lines.
3. One APSC found that public forums held in a central library were the best outreach effort.
4. Outreach across large, diverse geography means success must be measured in small numbers.
5. Public awareness campaigns (e.g., radio, brochures) tended to benefit both the resource fair and capacity building simultaneously.
6. The resource fair required the greatest effort of all of the project activities, taking 6 months or more to plan.
7. The resource fair gave rise to a support group and demonstrated that outreach does not necessarily equal added caseloads.
8. One APSC was ambivalent about conducting outreach for fear of stirring up a hornets' nest of consumers' expectations.
9. The resource fair was very successful in serving both outreach and capacity-building (training) roles.
10. The resource fair has the potential to be a regular event that is self-supporting through exhibitor fees.

Issues identified by the subawardees include the following:

1. There is a fundamental difference between how aging and developmental disabilities staff conceptualize "outreach."
2. The purpose of outreach should be clarified for all members of the APSC.
3. The size and homogeneity of catchment areas affect outreach efforts; smaller, more homogenized districts tend to have centralized media and news sources.
4. Agencies may overanticipate need for services.

The outreach strategies other than the resource fair were optional during the implementation by the five subawardees of the Integrated Model. The home visitor survey was the most often tested option. It proved to be a cost-effective means of identifying frail older adults who are responsible for the care of an aging relative with life-long impairments. Knowing that these caregiving scenarios exist is important for human services agencies so that they can anticipate and plan for future needs; staffing projections and fiscal planning documentation can incorporate information about these caregiving families. Other reports from the field-testing include the following:

1. Distribution of refrigerator magnets advertising a shared hotline number was productive.
2. Staffing an information booth at the county fair was another mechanism for outreach.
3. Some success was achieved through use of an eye-catching brochure, a local public affairs program, and a community calendar to publicize events.
4. Several APSC member agencies started screening information and referral request calls from older adults to investigate the existence of unserved adults with developmental disabilities.
5. Large, and mostly rural, service areas presented significant challenges.
6. Outreach involved working with multiple and very localized media resources.
7. A planned telephone survey was not implemented because of funding difficulties of a partnering agency.
8. Seminars on creating neighborhood networks served both capacity-building and outreach purposes.
9. One APSC member agency established a position for a developmental disabilities coordinator within their family and aging department to accomplish outreach.
10. Outreach through neighborhood and faith communities was effective.

CAPACITY BUILDING

Rationale

The Partners Projects sought both to expand the awareness of personnel in the human services systems to the needs, concerns, and contributions of older people with developmental disabilities (Gibson, Park-Choi, & Cook, 1993; Koenig, 1996; Kultgen & Rominger, 1993; Sutton et al., 1992) and to increase for older people and their caregivers the availability of and access to appropriate services. While recognition seems widespread regarding the primacy of families in the care of frail older adults, the research literature on the vital role that family caregiving plays over the dependent adult child's life course is also growing (e.g., Brunn, 1985; Grant, 1986; Heller & Factor, 1993; Pruchno, Patrick, & Burant, 1996; Roberto, 1993; Tobin, 1996). Consequently, the aim of the Integrated Model of Service is to develop the capacities of all those who are involved in the community functioning of older adults with developmental disabilities. Aging individuals with disabilities who live in the community and their primary caregivers have assumed the responsibility of coordinating services and therefore function as "service coordinators." The aging individual with a lifelong disability has learned to communicate needs or concerns to this caregiver, trusting the caregiver to provide or secure the supports needed.

This often happens without the benefit of knowing the service system and without formal training. The service coordination abilities of individuals with disabilities, caregivers, and service providers can be enhanced through cross-training. Family caregivers and people with disabilities who want support from the service system need to be aware of the community resources available to them. Cross-training offers the information needed to be effective service coordinators, defining and pursuing their own service needs. Cross-training can reinforce their ability to choose and control their lives and can play an important part in preventing a crisis intervention and institutionalization. At the same time, service providers in the aging and disabilities networks need to know how to facilitate community-based, person-centered, long-term care. Cross-training can prepare providers to ask the right questions in the right way and to see individuals with disabilities and caregivers as capable service coordinators. This approach maximizes the usefulness of both the informal and formal support systems already in place.

Capacity-building strategies should include, therefore, cross-training of staff in aging and developmental disabilities content and training in self-care and advocacy for older adults with developmental disabilities and their family caregivers. Strategies found effective by the Partners Projects follow. (Capacity-building strategies also include the integration of older adults with lifelong disabilities into aging-related community centers and intersystem internships. The how-to and field experiences of these are discussed later.)

Cross-Training Staff   To be meaningful, cross-training of staff must be in response to identified needs for knowledge and skills. The APSC, with its broad local constituency, is well equipped to identify what aging and developmental disabilities staff do and do not know about aging and developmental disabilities issues. Aging personnel might know little about the various developmental disabilities, for example, or about the priorities and practices of the developmental disabilities system. Developmental disabilities personnel may be unaware of the Older Americans Act of 1965 (PL 89-73) mandates or the composition and purpose of various services provided by the area agencies on aging. The APSC is also well equipped to identify local expertise to conduct such cross-training. The Partners Projects found that the most positively evaluated cross-training sessions were "Inter-Agency Coordination," "The Impact of Aging upon a Developmental Disability," "Client Identification Strategies," "Working with Family Caregivers," and "Focus on Consumer Needs" and that there are substantial variations in identified needs for cross-training from one locality to another.

Training in Self-Advocacy and Service Coordination   Older adults with developmental disabilities and family caregivers can benefit from training that strengthens their capacities to continue community living. Relevant topics include self-advocacy, identification of available community resources, access and overcoming barriers, navigation through bureaucratic "red tape," management of personal assistance services, self-support group networking, permanency planning (provision of care after the caregiver is no longer capable), and means of contributing one's own services to others. The Partners Projects found that the integral involvement of people with developmental disabilities in the operation of the projects helped to provide ready expertise and relevance for such training. As well, the resource fairs proved to be effective not only as outreach mechanisms but also as means of improving the capacities of consumers and their families for self-care and service coordination.

Integration of Older Adults with Developmental Disabilities   Older adults with lifelong disabilities may want to be part of local community centers. Integrating an older adult with developmental disabilities into existing aging-related services is itself likely to be a capacity-building experience for that adult and the organization. It is necessary to prepare the way for such integration into community senior centers by training center staff and by conducting awareness programs for the community's older adults who are already attending the center. Despite initial fears about introducing older adults with developmental disabilities into these senior centers, the experiences have proved to be highly successful and beneficial, with the key being the preparation of all involved and the emphasis being on reciprocal benefits of integration.

Internships Across Systems   Internships have provided a deeper level of understanding of the "complementary system" for a fair number of staff who had previously participated in cross-training sessions. Interns spend 2–3 days at a similar level of responsibility, in an environment that is comparable or parallel to their own, learning about the host agency's philosophies, language, priorities, funding streams, staffing patterns, and daily practices. For example, by interning at a developmental disabilities day center, a staff person from an aging network senior center comes to learn how the other agency works, as well as make personal contacts for future reference.

How-To: Cross-Training Staff

Geographical regions and human services organizations within them have their own personality, their own thumbprint, so to speak. Matters that are problems in one region may not be so in another. The APSC, if it has a broad representation in its membership, is usually an effective means of identifying where there are problems or issues that need attention at the intersection of aging and developmental disabilities. Often, the APSC meetings provide the first substantive opportunity for the local aging and developmental disabilities networks to meet. The APSC can identify local training needs, knowledge gaps among service providers, and local resources for meeting these local needs. The nominal group process can prioritize such matters. Some topics appear consistently on the lists that different APSCs develop for cross-training. These seem to reflect that the aging and developmental disabilities systems have been parallel historically, so they know little about each other. Generally, the topics identified relate to the need to understand better how the aging network works or how the various developmental disabilities are defined and which service systems address them. At the same time, different localities tend to identify their own set of special needs, sometimes reflecting special characteristics of residents in the area, prevailing agency regulations, recent legislation, and so forth.

The following is a rough composite of requested cross-training content, arranged by frequency; it may serve as an orientation for APSCs in attempting to assess knowledge and knowledge gaps among service provider and community members in their area:

1. Definition of developmental disabilities (including criteria and classifications)
2. Understanding functional similarities and differences between older adults with and without a developmental disability
3. Overview of resources in the aging and developmental disabilities systems
4. How to develop and share resources in the community with other organizations and agencies
5. Service coordination (discharge planning, care plan development, crisis intervention, dementias)
6. Integrating older adults with developmental disabilities into aging-related services
7. Which resources and services are available in the developmental disabilities system that could be shared with the aging network
8. Ethical issues (including confidentiality, record keeping, needs assessment, and advocacy)
9. Breaking barriers to service integration and effecting creative policy changes

10. How to deal with behavior challenges in older adults
11. How to enable the older adult with developmental disabilities to "retire" from services (i.e., engage in leisure activities rather than vocational rehabilitation)
12. Caregiver resources and support for families (including respite and permanency planning)
13. Basic processes of aging
14. Adverse drug reactions and geropharmacy (i.e., the mix of medications and aging)
15. Day support services
16. Health and medical issues of later life (including medication management)
17. Criteria for gaining access to services in both the aging and developmental disabilities systems
18. Long-term care planning and advance directives
19. Using older adults as "service providers" for other older adults
20. Accessibility issues and adaptive equipment or assistive devices
21. Legal issues (including guardianship, wills, permanency planning, and client rights)
22. Uniform functional assessment of aging adults and those adults with developmental disabilities
23. Personal assistance (e.g., home health, home chores)
24. Curriculum development in skills training for home visitors and aides

How-To: Training Providers and Consumers in Self-Advocacy and Service Coordination

In the spirit of cross-training, it is most effective to have all of the key players involved in processes to improve self-advocacy and the coordination of services. A partnership approach to planning the training works well. This approach taps the acquired expertise of each. An aging adult with a lifelong disability and an aging caregiver can raise the awareness of the service providers to the expertise they have gained through direct experience that will position them to be partners with the providers. Consumers and their families know the intimacies of aging and disabilities, they know family issues, and they know what they need but may not be able to get it. The same is true for the providers. They know the services, they know the resources in the community, and they know how the system works. The consumer will be able to experience the position and role of the service providers and vice versa, thereby strengthening the networking. An opportunity for informal socializing as part of the self-advocacy planning can reinforce growth in mutual respect.

As members of a team, each learns what expertise the others have to offer, develops interest in what was previously unknown, and begins communication that can be carried throughout the coordination of services. Self-advocacy training sessions set goals to reinforce the capacity of individuals with developmental disabilities and their caregivers to act as self-advocates in coordinating the services they receive and to enhance the ability of service providers from the aging and disabilities networks to act as facilitators in service coordination.

The Partners Projects have found that these goals led to a number of consumer-oriented training topics:

1. What it means to be a self-advocate
2. Self-determination: Problem solving and decision making
3. Disability rights: Laws, resources, and responsibilities

4. Common experiences and coalition building
5. Assertiveness to get needed services
6. Being involved in service planning and coordination
7. The roles of service providers in supporting self-advocacy and informed choice
8. Service resources—what, where, who, why, and when
9. Communication skills
10. Advocacy strategies
11. Letting go (for parents and/or caregivers)
12. Participating in community activities
13. Systems advocacy
14. How public decisions are made

Field-Test Experiences: Cross-Training, Self-Advocacy, and Service Coordination

All five subawardees implemented cross-training of staff and training in self-care and advocacy for consumers and caregivers. These were generally well attended. APSCs that conducted these experiences were gratified to learn that the trainer costs were effectively eliminated because of the composition of the APSC: Its membership produced the trainers, who provided the training at no charge. One subawardee converted all of its budget for trainer fees to other purposes.

Findings from the field-testing include the following:

1. The APSC suggested speakers for cross-training and obtained their participation readily.
2. Training forums were professionally videotaped for repeated usage and inclusion in an agency's resource library.
3. Forums identified more than 80 previously unknown adults with developmental disabilities.
4. The APSC held a self-advocacy workshop series that led to a futures planning program for caregivers.
5. An APSC subcommittee identified the training topics.
6. Cross-training was so beneficial to consumers and family caregivers that one of the partner agencies in the APSC will continue to compile lists of available training, even if it is not being offered by the partnering agency itself.
7. The APSC conducted full-day workshops that included case reviews for practical problem solving.
8. Training incorporated site visits to different aging and developmental disabilities agencies.
9. The APSC conducted separate training needs assessments for consumers and for service providers.
10. One APSC is using a computer link to promote training provided by other agencies.
11. The training introduced aging personnel to Circles of Support.
12. An APSC developed a futures planning guide for consumers.
13. An APSC updated an existing local resource guide by adding developmental disabilities service agencies and services that might assist people with disabilities, and then distributed the guide to various agencies.
14. An APSC found that focus group information sessions (brown bag luncheons and roundtable discussions) helped to accomplish consumer self-advocacy training.

INTEGRATION OF OLDER ADULTS WITH DEVELOPMENTAL DISABILITIES

Rationale

Enabling older adults to participate in senior activities and programs is a worthy goal for any community-oriented organization and a reasonable expectation for an older adult, irrespective of physical characteristics or conditions. An older adult's impairments may disable him or her in physical, sensory, or mental functioning, but these disabilities should not disenfranchise him or her from enjoying aging-related opportunities. Unfortunately, we are all too human in seeking to exclude people who are "different" from our personal experiences. This is where the historical invisibility of adults with lifelong disabilities creates an ironic twist: Because they so often grow older unobtrusively in family environments, most older adults have little experience or contact with them; so when adults with a disability first encounter aging-related services, they represent the "unknown" to the adults who are already using the services.

Integration of older adults with developmental disabilities into senior centers, for example, can be awkward, even a failure, if planners are not sensitive to a certain fear of the unknown that can affect adults without disabilities and human services staff alike. The principles of integration that the Partners III Project found to work follow the basic reality that although older adults with lifelong disabilities have every right according to law to participate in aging-related services and programs, careful preparation is necessary if all parties are to benefit. Integration should be a harmonious, growth-enhancing experience for the various older adults and staff.

How-To

The integration of an individual older adult with a developmental disability into aging-related programs occurs occasionally through the help of a caregiving parent or friend. The parent or friend knows the senior center and visits with the son or daughter, and both are recognized as part of the community. The "unknown" not being present, the son or daughter with developmental disabilities is incorporated readily. At other times, an agency representing older adults with developmental disabilities seeks to develop more aging-related experiences for its participants. For instance, staff at a day program for adults with developmental disabilities recognize that vocational preparation training for clients 60 years old is not so fulfilling as opportunities to garden or play pool. The staff seek to find places that offer social recreational experiences and discover the local senior center. To the extent that integration of these individuals mimics the process that the caregiver takes, staff likely will create a successful experience.

The Partners III Project found five principles to be effective in guiding integration:

1. Introduce small numbers of older adults with developmental disabilities to the desired program, not a whole busload.
2. Prepare the staff of the program, alerting them to the abilities, interests, and potential contributions that the new participants might make.
3. Prepare the leaders among the general older population who are already participating in the program.
4. Monitor the integration, being sensitive to the impact on each party.
5. Explore reciprocity so that the service or program being integrated has tangible opportunities to benefit from further interaction with the developmental disabilities system.

INTERNSHIP ACROSS SYSTEMS

Rationale

It is important to reiterate that education and training are desired because of their capacity-building consequences, not as ends in themselves. Education and training can take multiple forms. Certainly, there is need for aging- and developmental disabilities–related content to be taught (e.g., information about client characteristics, services, funding streams, resources, the other system). At the same time, such training, especially if it is cross-training, leads to exposure to the complementary system; its components are seen as people, and people and expertise are identified for future reference. Finally, exposure may lead to the fullest form of education and training: exchange. In exchange, personnel from the two systems spend mini-internships, perhaps a day or two, at each other's organization. Exchanges occur at similar administrative levels, and participants gain valuable insights into the policies, operations, goals, and characteristics of the complementary system. In this manner, realistic partnerships are made more possible, and interagency cooperation becomes more likely. These forms of capacity building should enable participating organizations to progress in meeting the needs of older citizens with developmental disabilities.

How-To

The Partners Projects' experiences with mini-internships have been gratifying and, in one respect, surprising. The Partners Projects initially set up fairly elaborate mechanisms to reimburse the agencies that released their employees for the internship. The Partners Projects even planned to reimburse mileage for the interns. None of it proved necessary. The mini-internships were mutually rewarding in themselves for all parties. The Partners Projects did learn six strategies to help ensure success: Broker, set eligibility, set goals, set time, sequence, and multiply.

Broker   The APSC is in an ideal position to act as a neutral broker in arranging internship exchanges between agencies. The idea is to enable individuals from an organization in one system to gain firsthand experience in the complementary system and in the process to learn its priorities, funding streams, eligibility criteria, practices, and resources. There is nothing quite like this firsthand experience to build both an understanding and an appreciation of how the "other side" works. To be most meaningful, the internship should be in a similar level of responsibility (e.g., manager to manager, direct service to direct service).

Set Eligibility   The Partners Projects have found that internships are most beneficial to all parties when the would-be intern has achieved some level of knowledge about the system into which the placement occurs. It seems prudent to set a certain number of hours of participation in cross-training as the necessary prerequisite for an internship.

Set Goals   Before spending time at the complementary system at an equivalent position to one's own, the would-be intern should set practical goals for the experience. For example, one may set a modest goal of meeting a certain number of the host agency's clients or participating in the agency's staff meetings, or one may set a more ambitious goal of collaborating with the agency in identifying barriers to joint programming or developing a grant proposal together to be submitted to a foundation, or it can be anything in between. In any event, the APSC can ensure that the intern sets realistic goals to be achieved through the brief placement at the host organization. As important, the intern should prepare a report to the APSC after the internship experience.

Set Time   In brokering approximately 3 dozen internships, those who field-tested the model found that a 2- to 4-day experience usually provides the individual with enough opportunity to reach the goals set. At the same time, the organizations that are releasing the intern generally can accommodate this length of absence. When even this brief period away posed a problem, some interns have allocated their internship time over a period of weeks, say, part of 1 day a week for 1 month. Inevitably, the releasing organizations reported that they are pleased that they allowed the experience.

Sequence   The Partners I Project originally conceived the internship to be an exchange (i.e., staff in the systems simultaneously "swapping" positions). This worked modestly well but in practice meant that there was no peer at the host site to guide the visiting intern. We quickly learned that the APSC must broker sequential mini-internships whereby one intern, then the other, visits the complementary system.

Multiply   Given the broad range of organizations, programs, and agencies that constitute the developmental disabilities system or the aging network, the Partners Projects have encouraged mini-interns to multiply their exposures by crossing segments. That is, those who work in a government-funded direct service agency can profit greatly from a mini-internship in a different segment, say, a citizen-developed advocacy group, and vice versa.

Field-Test Experiences: Integration and Internships

Integration and internships have a lot in common. Each seeks to help make the participant more comfortable in a new environment. The agencies that field tested strategies to integrate older adults with a developmental disability into generic services found that reciprocity was the key to success. An aging-related agency that is receiving or welcoming an older adult with a developmental disability needs to know that the developmental disabilities agencies in the community likewise will provide assistance to it when called upon. The "principles of integration" worked in practice to help ensure some give-and-take between the systems. The same spirit of reciprocity guided internships across systems.

Related findings include the following: 1) An APSC facilitated four internships for its members; 2) another APSC member wanted to have internships, but the employing agency was hesitant to release; 3) APSC members from developmental disabilities agencies spent time at a continuing care community that specialized in dementia care to learn about late-onset disabilities; and 4) an APSC conducted seven or eight extensive site visits exclusively for APSC members in lieu of internships.

Issues identified by the sub-awardees include the following: 1) Integration of older adults with developmental disabilities into senior centers was uneven within the area, being well advanced in one county and in the earlier stages elsewhere, 2) reciprocity between the aging and developmental disabilities systems seems central to success, and 3) both systems must see a benefit to themselves and to those they serve from the senior center integration.

CONCLUSIONS

The information in this chapter has been shared as a guide to aid responsible initiatives by human services agencies that find themselves operating at the "intersection" of aging and developmental disabilities, encountering older adults with lifelong impairments who are experiencing the "gift of time." The Integrated Model, it is hoped, will help aging network and developmental disabilities systems agencies to negotiate this intersection safely and productively so that all interested parties benefit. The overriding goal of this and all of our previous projects has been to enhance the prospects for continued independence and community living of adults who grow old with lifelong impairments. We believe that the Integrated Model's simplicity, just three "working parts," and especially its emphasis on creating a neutral broker (the APSC) should increase the likelihood of sustained interaction and cooperative initiatives between the systems.

At the same time, we acknowledge the enlightening feedback gained from the five subawardees that field tested the model. Some of the Integrated Model's elements, both essential and optional, work better in one context than in another; for example, the less populated areas had more success with some types of media outreach. This is alright. The Integrated Model is, after all, a menu. The field tests also demonstrated in practice some things that we knew from the beginning of Partners III but that had to be learned in local implementation by the participating agencies themselves. These included 1) the inescapability of the need to set shared goals at the outset; 2) the importance of continuity among the membership to meet these goals; 3) the fundamental differences in how the aging and developmental disabilities systems see "outreach," the former more or less as information dissemination, the latter more or less as case identification; 4) the potentially deadly consequences for intersystem cooperation if differences in meaning, such as in "outreach," are not worked out publicly; and 5) the resounding effectiveness of the resource fair as a focus for collaboration among the APSC's members, a vehicle for two-way outreach, and a place to conduct friendly and effective capacity building of consumers and family caregivers. Again, the Integrated Model is drawn from the recommended practices of previous work at the intersection of aging and developmental disabilities; so the Partners III Project staff anticipated some of these developments, but it was reinforcing to see them verified in diverse applications.

Finally, there is the question of money. Some have asked how critical to success was the monetary subaward, or, more pointed, is there a minimal amount necessary to ensure successful intersystem cooperation? Feedback from participating agencies varied. For some, the subaward enabled their hiring a person or expanding the hours of a current employee so that time was dedicated to aging and developmental disabilities; other agencies used their subawards more for the collaboration, outreach, and capacity-building activities themselves, such as expenses related to the resource fair. When the Partners Projects staff asked participants at the project's final plenary questions about how much money they thought was necessary to implement the model, answers were typically "a modest amount," and suggestions tended to be approximately $5,000 a year or less. Much more critical, participants said, was to commit personnel to the APSC over time. There is so much mutuality in the operation of the APSC that many expenses are shared or, at times, obviated.

REFERENCES

Ansello, E.F. (1991). Aging issues for the year 2000. *Caring Magazine, 10*(2), 4–12.

Ansello, E.F. (1992). Seeking common ground between aging and developmental disabilities. In E.F. Ansello & N.N. Eustis (Eds.), *Aging and disabilities: Seeking common ground* (pp. 9–24). Amityville, NY: Baywood Publishing Co.

Ansello, E.F., Coogle, C.L., & Wood, J.B. (1997). *Partners: Building intersystem cooperation in aging with developmental disabilities.* Richmond: Virginia Center on Aging, Virginia Commonwealth University.

Ansello, E.F., & Rose, T. (1989). *Aging and lifelong disabilities: Partnership for the twenty-first century.* Palm Springs, CA: Elvirita Lewis Foundation.

Brunn, L.C. (1985). Elderly parent and dependent adult child. *Social Casework: The Journal of Contemporary Social Work, 66,* 131–138.

474   Networking Services for Community Supports

Coogle, C.L., Ansello, E.F., & Wood, J.B. (1998). Partners III—Bridge-building between the aging and developmental disabilities service networks: An integrated model of collaborative planning and service. *Southwest Journal on Aging, 14*(2), 69–78.

Coogle, C.L., Ansello, E.F., Wood, J.B., & Cotter, J.J. (1995). Partners II—Serving older persons with developmental disabilities: Obstacles and inducements to collaboration among agencies. *Journal of Applied Gerontology, 14*(3), 275–287.

Cotter, J.J., Ansello, E.F., & Wood, J.B. (1992). *Improving services to older persons with developmental disabilities: Policy, training, services* (Grant No. 90AM0484). Washington, DC: Administration on Aging.

Factor, A.R. (1993). Translating policy into practice. In E. Sutton, A.R. Factor, B.A. Hawkins, T. Heller, & G.B. Seltzer (Eds.), *Older adults with developmental disabilities: Optimizing choice and change* (pp. 257–275). Baltimore: Paul H. Brookes Publishing Co.

Gibson, J.W., Park-Choi, Y.R., & Cook, D. (1993). Service providers' knowledge and misconceptions about old age: Comparison of three service networks. *Educational Gerontology, 19,* 727–741.

Grant, G. (1986). Older carers and the care of the mentally handicapped. *Ageing and Society, 6,* 331–335.

Hawkins, B.A., & Eklund, S.J. (1990). Planning processes and outcomes for an aging population with developmental disabilities. *Mental Retardation, 28,* 35–40.

Heller, T., & Factor, A. (1991). Permanency planning for adults with mental retardation living with family caregivers. *American Journal on Mental Retardation, 96,* 163–176.

Heller, T., & Factor, A. (1993). Aging family caregivers: Support resources and changes in burden and placement desire. *American Journal on Mental Retardation, 98,* 417–426.

Janicki, M.P. (1993). *Building the future: Planning and community development in aging and developmental disabilities* (2nd ed.). Albany: New York State Office of Mental Retardation and Developmental Disabilities.

Jenkins, E.L., Hildreth, B.L., & Hildreth, G. (1993). Elderly persons with mental retardation: An exceptional population with special needs. *International Journal of Aging and Human Development, 37*(1), 69–80.

Koenig, B.R. (1996). Survey of practitioners and developmental care workers in supported accommodation facilities for adults with developmental disabilities. *Adult Residential Care Journal, 10*(1), 4–27.

Kultgen, P., & Rominger, R. (1993). Cross training within the aging and developmental disabilities services systems. In E. Sutton, A.R. Factor, B.A. Hawkins, T. Heller, & G.B. Seltzer (Eds.), *Older adults with developmental disabilities: Optimizing choice and change* (pp. 239–256). Baltimore: Paul H. Brookes Publishing Co.

Older Americans Act of 1965, PL 89-73, 42 U.S.C. §§ 3001 *et seq.*

Pederson, E.L. (1993). The research and training consortium process. In E. Sutton, A.R. Factor, B.A. Hawkins, T. Heller, & G.B. Seltzer (Eds.), *Older adults with developmental disabilities: Optimizing choice and change* (pp. 345–369). Baltimore: Paul H. Brookes Publishing Co.

Pederson, E.L., Chaikin, M., Koehler, D., Campbell, A., & Arcand, M. (1993). Strategies that close the gap between research, planning, and self-advocacy. In E. Sutton, A.R. Factor, B.A. Hawkins, T. Heller, & G.B. Seltzer (Eds.), *Older adults with developmental disabilities: Optimizing choice and change* (pp. 277–313). Baltimore: Paul H. Brookes Publishing Co.

Pruchno, R.A., Patrick, J.H., & Burant, C. (1996). Mental health of aging women with children who are chronically disabled: Examination of a two-factor model. *Journals of Gerontology, 51B,* S284–S296.

Roberto, K.A. (Ed.). (1993). *The elderly caregiver: Caring for adults with developmental disabilities.* Thousand Oaks, CA: Sage Publications.

Rose, T., & Ansello, E.F. (1987). *Aging and developmental disabilities: Research and planning. Final report to the Maryland State Planning Council on Developmental Disabilities.* College Park: University of Maryland, Center on Aging.

Seltzer, M.M., Krauss, M.W., & Heller, T. (1991). Family caregiving over the life course. In M.P. Janicki & M.M. Seltzer (Eds.), *Aging and developmental disabilities: Challenges for the 1990s. Proceedings of the Boston Roundtable on Research Issues and Applications in Aging and Developmental Disabilities* (pp. 3–24). Washington, DC: American Association on Mental Retardation, Special Interest Group on Aging.

Seltzer, M.M., Krauss, M.W., & Janicki, M.P. (Eds.). (1994). *Life course perspectives on adulthood and old age.* Washington, DC: American Association on Mental Retardation.

Smith, G.C., Tobin, S.S., & Fullmer, E.M. (1995). Elderly mothers caring at home for offspring with mental retardation: A model of permanency planning. *American Journal on Mental Retardation, 99*, 487–499.

Stroud, M., & Sutton, E. (1988). Appendix B. Consortium: A planning model. In M. Stroud & E. Sutton (Eds.), *Expanding options for older adults with developmental disabilities: A practical guide to achieving community access* (pp. 227–235). Baltimore: Paul H. Brookes Publishing Co.

Sutton, E., Sterns, H.L., Schwartz, L., & Roberts, R. (1992). The training of a specialist in developmental disabilities and aging. *Generations, 16*(1), 71–74.

Tobin, S.S. (1996). Non-normative old-age contrast: Elderly parents caring for offspring with mental retardation. In V.L. Bengston (Ed.), *Adulthood and aging: Research on continuities and discontinuities* (pp. 124–145). New York: Springer Publishing Co.

Wood, J.B. (1993). Planning for the transfer of care: Social and psychological issues. In K.A. Roberto (Ed.), *The elderly caregiver: Caring for adults with developmental disabilities* (pp. 95–107). Thousand Oaks, CA: Sage Publications.

Zirpoli, T.J., Hancox, D.H., Wieck, C., & Skarnulis, E. (1994). Partners in policymaking: The first five years. *Mental Retardation, 32*, 422–425.

Zirpoli, T.J., Wieck, C., & McBride, M. (1989). Case management: A new challenge for families. In M.H. Linz, P. McAnally, & C. Wieck (Eds.), *Case management: Historical, current, and future perspectives* (pp. 125–136). Cambridge, MA: Brookline Books.

25

Collaboration in Multicultural Environments

Janene N. Suttie

People with developmental disabilities are living longer and posing new challenges to caregivers and service providers. In many ways, this is not surprising, as the aging of this population is a relatively new phenomenon, made possible by advances in medical technology and the positive effects of deinstitutionalization policies (Factor, 1993; Lubin & Kiely, 1985; Rice & Feldman, 1985). An understanding of later-life development and the characteristics and needs of aging individuals is essential in providing quality services for appropriate aging experiences for older adults with developmental disabilities. In the continuing quest for normative experiences and as a rationalization of services in the current economic climate, principles of full inclusion (equity, access, participation, equality, and rights) are particularly relevant.

Collaboration between aging and developmental disabilities agencies can combine resources to facilitate recommended practices for all aging individuals, thus benefiting participants with a range of choices in service options and inclusive programs. Typically, service providers express concerns regarding the needs of a particular population—aging or those with developmental disabilities. With an enhanced understanding of the characteristics and commonalities of both populations, the needs of all aging people and their caregivers can be met. This chapter considers a number of key concepts in the enhancement of services through a teaming model that considers

This chapter was supported in part by Grant No. 90-AM-0677 from the Administration on Aging, U.S. Department of Health and Human Services.

collaboration between generic aging and disability sectors in the context of a multi-cultural environment.

CONTEXT FOR COLLABORATION

As the number of older adults with developmental disabilities increases, so too does the need for appropriate policies, programs, and services to meet the needs of this aging population. In the early 1980s, an increased interest in the characteristics and needs of older adults with developmental disabilities resulted in projects to test models of integration of this population into generic programs, including senior centers, nutrition sites, and adult day services (Janicki, 1991). Although some initial reluctance was noted, collaboration resulted in innovative programs and substantial cost benefits. Recommendations that arose from these early initiatives stressed that programs should reflect social adult day service models, be cost-efficient, include people with and without developmental disabilities, use community-based resources and facilities, and preferably be located away from traditional environments for developmental disabilities services (Janicki, 1991).

Perhaps the most important messages to emerge were the need to stress the commonalities of the characteristics and needs of all older adults, develop opportunities for cross-training personnel from both aging and developmental disabilities agencies (Ansello & Zink, 1990; Kultgen & Rominger, 1993), and inform and maintain close communication with networks and provider groups. As Janicki reminded us, "Networks composed of persons with like interests committed to a particular issue . . . address issues, develop training, provide technical assistance, and help educate the public at large" (1991, p. 10).

The extent to which interagency collaboration has been effective has been investigated in a number of studies (Cotten & Spirrison, 1988; Factor, 1993; Janicki, Knox, & Jacobson, 1985; Pederson, 1993; Seltzer, 1988; Seltzer, Krauss, Litchfield, & Modlish, 1989). In particular, concerns were expressed regarding the duplication of services and the low numbers of aging adults with developmental disabilities who were actually benefiting from inclusion in programs of integrated activities. Janicki et al. (1985) identified a four-step planning process model to guide initiatives in aging and developmental disabilities: 1) identifying the population; 2) assessing needs and services; 3) defining the service system, including gaps and barriers, particularly in relation to needs; and 4) determining solutions to service system gaps. Since then, many have used this process in policy development and innovative programming, using task forces or working groups to initiate change (e.g., Cotten, Britt, & Moreland, 1986; Hawkins, Eklund, Garza, Garza, & DiOrio, 1987; Janicki, 1992; Wanninger & Pederson, 1986).

A central concern related to including older adults with disabilities in generic programs is the need for broad-based training at all levels. Without an understanding of the characteristics, needs, and issues related to both aging and developmental disabilities, interagency cooperation and coordination are less effective (Hawkins & Eklund, 1990). Cross-training is important for agencies that are striving toward the full inclusion of aging individuals with developmental disabilities. Members of both services networks—aging and disabilities—benefit from training across the broader spectrum of both domains. Those in the disabilities area gain from an enhanced understanding of later-life development as many more people with developmental disabilities survive into older age, while those experienced in generic aging gain insights into the nature of developmental disabilities and the particular characteristics and needs of these aging people. As Kultgen and Rominger (1993) pointed out, cross-training facilitates success-ful inclusion in community participation and access.

Kultgen and Rominger also suggested differences in the perceptions of service systems. Those surveyed in the developmental disabilities system expressed a strong need for training in the general areas of later-life development, including age-related changes and age-appropriate programming. Personnel from the aging services network, however, were less familiar with the numbers of aging people with a developmental disability and were therefore in need of information related to incidence figures, characteristics of developmental disabilities, and the types of service provision most likely to be used. These professionals were less likely to be familiar with the developmental services network and the range of services already in place.

A further consideration in service provision is the increase in diverse ethnic groups in multicultural environments (see Chapter 6). Significant population changes are occurring in many Western countries, leading to a number of specific services issues. Kuehn and Imm-Thomas (1993) identified issues of availability, access, affordability, accommodation, and cultural appropriateness as critical factors that have an impact on the ways in which services are used. They highlighted the need for cultural appropriateness above all else while pointing out that it is impossible for any one individual to be able to accommodate all needs in a diverse population.

Problems related to access to services (e.g., medical, day programs, nutrition programs, senior centers) include language barriers, differences in traditional practices, and cultural enclaves that tend to preclude the inclusion of individuals from other ethnic groups. For instance, programs may be offered by individuals who speak one language, with practices that alienate others who are attempting to participate in the programs or activities offered. Cultural perceptions of caregiving differ between ethnic groups. Although services may be accepted and used by some, others believe that the caregiving role should be maintained within the family or the community. Service providers therefore need an awareness of diversity within a community and need not only to attend to predominant minority groups but also to be aware of minority groups in areas where very few individuals are represented but whose needs may be great.

A CASE MODEL OF MULTICULTURAL
COLLABORATION: THE HAWAII EXPERIENCE

Hawaii is an excellent example of an area with rich cultural diversity. The state has no single ethnic group that is in the majority—in fact, none comprises more than a quarter of the overall population. According to estimates (State of Hawaii, 1998), the four largest groups are people of European (22%), Japanese (20%), Hawaiian (21%, virtually all being part Hawaiians with only 0.8% considered "pure" Hawaiians), and Pilipino (10.0%) ancestry. There are also significant numbers of people of Chinese, Korean, Indochinese, African, and Pacific Islander (e.g., Samoan) heritage. Although scant attention has been paid to the breakdown of ethnicity of older adults with developmental disabilities in Hawaii, one study (Hawaii University Affiliated Program, 1989) suggested high numbers of people of Japanese (32.4%) and Hawaiian or part Hawaiian (26.9%) ancestry. Also included are substantial numbers of adults of Portuguese (12.0%) and Pilipino (10.6%) heritage. These figures stress the need for services and programs that are culturally sensitive and that address the issues of availability, access, affordability, accommodation, and cultural appropriateness for racial and ethnic minority populations (Kuehn & Imm-Thomas, 1993).

Hawaii consists of seven main islands, making culturally appropriate access to many services difficult, particularly for those on islands other than Oahu, the main center of government and business. For instance, the makeup of particular ethnic groups is unevenly distributed across islands. On Oahu, people of European and Japanese descent predominate in the Honolulu area, whereas many Pilipino families reside in the central rural district of Oahu. There are considerably more Pilipinos than Japanese or Europeans on the island of Kauai. However, the numbers of Chinese, native Hawaiians, Koreans, and African Americans are particularly low on Kauai, putting these groups at a further disadvantage in the provision of services. The majority of native Hawaiians live on the islands of Hawaii and Molokai. Services to people who are aging (e.g., health care, nutrition, senior centers) are aimed at the "majority" groups of particular geographical areas, tending to provide for English- or Japanese-speaking groups.

Thus, Hawaii's unique ethnic mix adds an element that must be taken into account when developing and implementing programs for aging adults, particularly in view of current recommended practices that stress individualized planning and family participation. When dealing with the family, for example, it is important to know the culturally patterned roles of its members, especially with regard to decision making (Hanson, Lynch, & Wayman, 1990; McDermott, Tseng, & Maretzki, 1980). Efforts to promote the participation of families are enhanced if made culturally appropriate (Hanson et al., 1990; Harwood, 1981). Further concern is raised by differing ethnic longevity rates. Japanese American and Chinese American women, for instance, typically survive into their eighth decade, whereas adults with native-Hawaiian backgrounds have shorter life spans and experience more health problems and functional impairments in older age (Takamura, 1991). This creates the need for a diversity of services to meet individual needs.

Within the state, older adults with developmental disabilities had, until recently, received little attention to their increasing aging needs. In particular, the areas of policy planning and program development had been slow to respond to this group of people who were progressing from adulthood into later years. The response to increased demands for services for aging adults had been reactive rather than proactive, with a tendency to extend existing adult services rather than to develop age-appropriate programs for older adults with developmental disabilities.

A report by the University of Hawaii found that there were differences in the types of services available to older adults in general and to those aging with developmental disabilities (Hawaii UAP, 1989). The general older adult population has available socially oriented services and meal and homemaker assistance, whereas aging adults with disabilities have available specialized medically oriented services, residential care, training, and habilitation. Both service sectors offer recreation, day care, and respite programs, but these are limited and particularly difficult for aging adults with developmental disabilities and their families to gain access to. This is generally attributed to 1) negative community attitudes toward adults with disabilities, 2) lack of support services within the community, 3) lack of staff training and development in relation to the aging needs of this consumer group, and 4) difficulties in distinguishing the particular needs and services of aging adults with developmental disabilities as distinct from those of older adults in general. Furthermore, local agencies identify the unmet needs of older adults with disabilities as social/recreational programs, residential services, and social supports including respite, outreach, and service coordination. These unmet needs generally were similar to those identified as of concern to older adults in general. The findings of the report, while identifying many of the characteristics and needs of aging adults with developmental disabilities, highlighted that many programs and services for older adults were indeed duplicated across the two systems.

To address these system problems, the report recommended, among other things, the development of integrated generic services to serve people with developmental disabilities with their peers without disabilities, cross-training opportunities for generic and disabilities services personnel, and interagency collaboration between the service systems to promote joint planning and program development. These recommendations were consistent with findings from other states, which noted that the major barriers to improving services included entrenched policies, low levels of consciousness among administrators and legislators about the aging needs of people with developmental disabilities, a lack of adequate personnel and programs, poor channels of communication between agencies, negative attitudes toward people with developmental disabilities in the general community, and limited access to training and information (Wu, 1987).

Therefore, it was considered that the collaboration of developmental disabilities and aging agencies in Hawaii might further enhance the understanding of the characteristics and needs of aging adults and provide diverse options to older adults both with and without developmental disabilities. By augmenting or restructuring existing programs and services, implementing recommended practices, and cross-training to increase expertise, quality service provision and support could become a reality for the state's aging adults and their caregivers.

A MODEL FOR COLLABORATION IN A MULTICULTURAL ENVIRONMENT

In response to the needs identified in the previous section, a project, "Teaming to Promote Inclusive and Appropriate Aging Experiences for Persons with Developmental Disabilities," was proposed and eventually funded by the United States Administration on Aging in Washington, D.C. The project aimed to combine two pertinent areas—identifying current issues in the care and development of aging adults with developmental disabilities in Hawaii (including inclusion in day care programs and services, generic seniors programs, and support for family caregivers) and cross-training personnel who are involved in integrated programs for aging adults. Central to the success of the project was the cooperation of aging services personnel in a teaming process involving the collaboration of the whole range of relevant agencies and individuals. The teaming process model was developed by the University of Hawaii's University Affiliated Program for Developmental Disabilities (HUAP). Although initially designed for systems change in schools, the teaming model (Stodden, 1991) adapted well for use with agencies and services involved in systems change and collaboration across agencies.

The project was undertaken cooperatively with the State Council for Developmental Disabilities, the State Executive Office on Aging (Hawaii's state unit on aging), and the University of Hawaii and involved personnel from a broad range of community-based services and programs. A collaborative teaming process model (see Figure 1) was used to restructure programs and services across both aging and developmental disabilities agencies and networks to facilitate a breadth of options and inclusive experiences to meet the aging needs of people with developmental disabilities living in the community. The model comprised three phases: interdisciplinary team building, action planning for desired program improvements, and program restructuring.

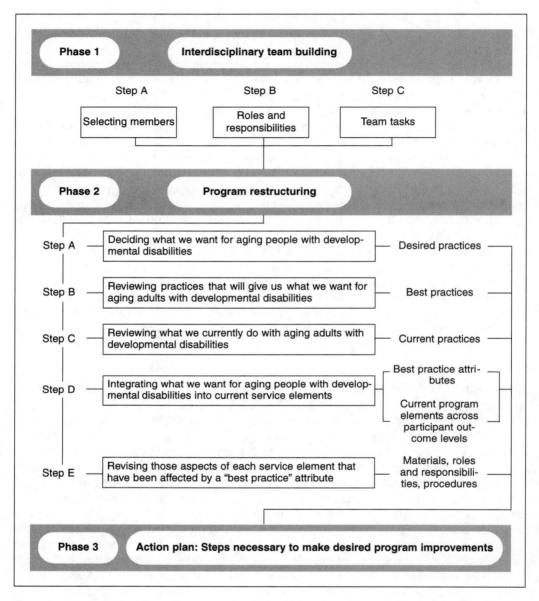

Figure 1.   Team-building process for restructuring programs for aging adults with developmental disabilities.

Phase 1: Team Building

The first step in implementing such a project is to identify and recruit potential team members. Careful planning is essential in the overall success of such a project. In our case, the project time line was a 2-year period—a relatively short time to achieve the stated goals—but this was dictated by the funding span of the grant received to underwrite the project. Therefore the team model structure was implemented with a view to initiate the local networking and team building in the shortest time possible, yet permit intrinsic support for the teams to be self-directed after the project period expired. To begin, an all-day workshop was designed to present key considerations in the development of cooperation and collaboration between service agencies that were providing supports to aging or disability populations.

Invitations to the workshop were disseminated widely to attract as many interested people as possible. After the workshop, attendees expressed interest in participation in an extended project. Furthermore, visits were made to government and nongovernment agencies and service providers to identify those interested in making a strong commitment to the objectives of the project and enlist their cooperation to support the project teams and efforts.

Acknowledging the diversity of groups across the spread of islands, we endeavored to enlist commitment from people across the various islands in the state. To encourage participation, we provided assistance with paying for airfares to attend team meetings and scheduled meeting times to accommodate airline and work schedules. Initial concerns by members suggested that they felt restrained by a lack of services in rural areas, in comparison with the perceived range and variety of services in urban areas. In reality, these members became an inspiration for others on the teams, as they had developed skills in adapting scant existing resources to meet individual needs of aging adults.

Phase 2: Action Planning

The second step is to compose a working network. In our case, working teams were established around three focus areas: day care programs and services, inclusion in generic seniors programs, and support for family caregivers. The teams were charged with undertaking program improvement activities, which began with creating a mission statement that specified desired outcomes for successful aging experiences and led to revisions in procedures, practices, and policies. Each team was made up of eight members who had indicated an interest in one of the three content areas (day care programs, seniors programs, or support for family caregivers) and included a mix of older adults with and without developmental disabilities; family members of aging individuals; representatives from state, regional, and local government and private agencies; direct care personnel; and community members. A mix of people from diverse cultural backgrounds was also apparent in the makeup of teams, although this was perhaps more a function of the widespread acceptance of diversity within the community rather than a result of any selection criteria.

After an initial combined team session, individual teams met on a regular monthly basis. From time to time, the three teams met at combined meetings to discuss common progress and issues and to work on action plans. We found that these teams worked well together; in particular, the rapport developed between team members was excellent. Team members visited each other's sites and shared and discussed many issues related to the barriers of including older adults with developmental disabilities in general aging programs. Each team developed a unique profile with its own set of working rules and procedures, meeting times, and venues. Decisions were made by consensus and served to promote optimal commitment by each member to the team's objectives. Meeting venues varied—teams either rotated around several members' work locations or chose to meet regularly at one convenient site. At the end of each meeting, teams would agree on the best date and meeting time for all involved. Consideration was given to such factors as wheelchair access, transportation, and times to facilitate best involvement of both workers and family members.

We found that it is crucial to offer guidance and support to the teams through a process of needs assessment, planning, and implementation. This was the role of the university personnel, who were acting as facilitators and managing the project. An initial activity of each team was to create a vision of the ideal world for people who are aging and from this to develop a mission statement. Thus, the team members developed mission statements that described desired outcomes for all older adults rather than specifically those with developmental disabilities.

Each of the three teams (day care, seniors programs, family caregivers) decided on a number of focus areas for consideration at team meetings (see Table 1). Subsequent team meetings included the consideration of recommended practice initiatives in these areas by way of journal articles, conference papers, video presentations, guest presenters, and general discussion. To facilitate a knowledge and understanding of the circumstances of aging adults with and without developmental disabilities, interviews were videotaped with a number of older adults with and without developmental disabilities living in urban and rural areas of the state, including the islands of Kauai, Oahu, and Hawaii. These tapes illustrated the life status and needs of a variety of aging individuals and enhanced discussion of the identified focus areas.

Phase 3: Program Restructuring

The third step is to involve the participants of each team in a process of identifying ways to solve identified problems and to affect change in the local system. In our case, team members were particularly aware of the need to restructure or further develop certain aspects of current programs. In particular, general aging program personnel were proactive in considering ways to include older adults with developmental disabilities in existing programs. Critical discussion of programs centered around the ability to achieve desired outcomes as measured by each team's vision and mission statement. From these discussions, members of each of the three teams developed a series of action plans designed to restructure or enhance current programs (see Table 2) on the basis of their discussions of recommended practice and measured by the teams' visions and mission statements.

An important component of such action plans is the consideration of time lines and identification of specific personnel who should see each task through to its completion. Generally, the preparation for the implementation of such action plans is supported by staff discussions, in-service training, and workshops. In our case, our primary goal was to replicate and institutionalize processes and products found to be effective in promoting inclusive and appropriate aging experiences of adults with developmental disabilities. However, we found that this goal was, perhaps, the most difficult to accomplish because of the state's changing fiscal situation. Approximately 1 year after the project was funded, the state—as did many other states in the United States—found itself with a severe tax revenue shortfall as a result of a depressed economy and began a period of cutbacks in social and human services. Unfortunately, we were trying at the same time to enhance needed services, and this became an area of conflict. What should have been a fairly dispassionate process proved to be one vested with competition for scarce resources and significant interagency difficulties.

Notwithstanding the fiscal problems of the state, we proceeded to develop plans and activities that would take advantage of the momentum we had built and that did not rely solely on the allocation or reallocation of state funds. Thus, although some action plans developed by team members required major changes or advance planning and needed the support and commitment of higher level personnel—planners, policy makers, administrators—most of the action plans required few, if any, fiscal resources

Table 1.   Focus areas for consideration at team meetings

Focus areas for consideration at seniors programs team meetings

Friendships/social contact

Recreation activities: Range, access, choice

Transportation

Information and support for individuals and families with regard to services and access

Health care: Services, access; complementary health practices

Attitudes toward aging/ageism, role models, intergenerational issues, and disability

Physical accessibility

Education/knowledge, public's attitudes

Advocacy: Role, legal issues

Employment, volunteers, foster grandparents, opportunities

Communication/mobility/assistive technology

Safety: At home, on the streets, on public transportation (bus, van)

Nutrition

Housing

English: Communication, facilitation, bilingual communication

Cultural diversity

Focus areas for consideration at day care team meetings

Consumer input, opportunities for choice and flexibility

Differing levels of functional abilities

Funding for discrete groups

Innovative staffing/scheduling/time flexibility, and staff training

Activities: Breadth and scope

Behavior issues

Quality assurance

Cultural issues

Education: Consumers, service providers

Medical issues

Nutrition and meal environment

Physical accessibility

Regulations: Constant review

Focus areas for consideration at support for caregivers' team meetings

Education and training, including community attitudes toward the caregiving role

Respite

Futures planning

Legal issues

Finances

Formal and informal individual support

Mourning, death, and dying

Interpersonal relationships

Spiritual

"Gap groups": Those that fall through the cracks

Table 2.   Ways to support team visions

Transition to a retirement-oriented lifestyle (seniors programs team):

Preretirement training and/or programs to aid transition of people with developmental disabilities

Cross-training of staff in general areas of developmental disabilities, aging-related changes and needs

Access to age-appropriate, community-integrated, generic aging services and programs (seniors programs team)

Locate "willing" programs: Identify types, locations, and diversity of programs and sites

Identify and offer incentives for generic programs to include people with developmental disabilities

Recruit companions to accompany older adults to programs

Cross-train staff

Offer specific training (e.g., management of challenging behaviors)

Transportation:

Representation on Mayor's transportation committee

Encourage breadth of options (e.g., carpooling, share-a-van, informal networks with families and friends)

Waive transportation fee for volunteer escorts

Coordinate group pickup points

Use city bus with companion (i.e., practicum students)

Driver's liability coverage

Train and support volunteers and drivers in an understanding of aging individuals with developmental disabilities

Access to health and rehabilitative services that are sensitive to aging-related change (adult day care team):

Provide for special medical needs in adult day care programs

Train and hire appropriate staff

Reimburse for special services

Bring specialized services to centers (e.g., physician visits, physical therapist, occupational therapist, speech-language therapist)

Provide ongoing medical monitoring and service coordination

Link levels of care to cost determination

Actively encourage care homes to participate in funding the day care needs of individuals

Empowerment for personal decision making, including access to information needed for conducting life in a self-determined manner (all teams):

Provide aging individuals with developmental disabilities with personal training for choice making

Identify a range of choices and possible options in an individual's daily life

Provide choices and options in available programs:

Inventory existing programs: Availability, appropriateness, day, location, cost

Train staff to increase opportunities for individual choice

Survey individuals with developmental disabilities for interests, abilities, needs

Develop additional activities based on survey information

Provide choice in the degree of participation

---

and were based on attitude or procedural changes. Subsequently, a number of these were included in the teams' action plans.

In addition, to deal with the broader state-level issues, a meeting of key state planners and policy makers was held to generate long-term support. This meeting proved successful, and we obtained a commitment from the meeting's participants to build further on the work of the teams and to try to accomplish many of the recommendations that would lead to the greater inclusion of aging adults with developmental disabilities in generic aging programs and services. The state-level meeting led to a commitment by program directors to support collaboration among agencies in the area of training; an agreement for the flexibility of funding for client-based, rather than agency-based, programs (a representative of the state council for developmental disabilities participates on the home community-based services waiver task force and continues to advocate for and monitor client-based funding); and an agreement to clarify liability issues, particularly in regard to agencies' serving unfunded people, and issues related to the use of volunteers. In addition, these agreements produced a commitment to develop a directory of available services, agencies, sources of information, and training contacts to support aging adults with and without developmental disabilities. We were also able to obtain a verbal commitment from key state personnel (representing the State Council for Developmental Disabilities and the State Health Department) and agency directors to convene future meetings to consider ongoing progress in the identified actions and to keep faith with an existing memorandum of agreement between the Health Department and the State Council for Developmental Disabilities.

At a final plenary meeting of the teams, participants agreed to continue to meet at regular intervals and continue planning and coordination. At the close of the university-sponsored phase of the project, a subcommittee of six team members met with the university's coordinator to discuss the facilitation, purpose, and structure of future meetings. From this, it was agreed that existing members would recruit interested others, in particular, people or services identified as filling the gaps in representation; that a resource list of services and providers of programs for aging adults with and without developmental disabilities would be compiled using the group's knowledge and the networking of team members; and that the action plans would be continually reviewed. Members agreed to continue to account for actions to be undertaken, discuss progress and barriers to implementation, and review what supports would be needed to achieve the outcomes.

PEOPLE AFFECTED BY THE COLLABORATIVE MODEL

To help put the use of the collaborative teaming process model in perspective, several case studies—presentations of how select aging individuals with developmental disabilities were affected by the project—are proffered.

P.M. is a 62-year-old woman of Japanese-Hawaiian background with a developmental disability. She lives in a care home on the island of Kauai with four other women, also with developmental disabilities; two caregivers; and the caregivers' families. Until 2 years ago, she attended a day program offered by the local intellectual disabilities agency and enjoyed participating in the program's activities with her friends. As she grew older and began to experience some aging-related problems, staff considered alternatives that were more appropriate to her changing health and mobility needs. In consultation with one of the island's day services program team members, an arrangement was made to have her attend the local adult day services center, a service provided for older individuals from the general community. In P.M.'s words: "When I retired from Arc ... I never liked it ... I cried and cried, and they missed me." Staff responded to her sadness and arranged for her friends to visit with her at the day services center. With this new arrangement, she began to feel better about attending. She enjoyed showing her friends around, and they often participated in the center's activities, including exercise class and lunch. Occasional visits still occur, and P.M. also takes new friends from the day services center to visit at The Arc [the intellectual disabilities agency day program]. These reciprocal visits have greatly assisted her integration into the day services program. Now she feels more comfortable and accepted and participates in a greater number of activities. Her friends from The Arc also have a sense of what to expect when they retire, and staff from the general program have an enhanced understanding of the needs of people with disabilities.

K.K., a 55-year-old woman of part-Hawaiian ancestry, lives in Honolulu with her sister. She is blind and has an intellectual disability. She attends a local senior center several days per week with a companion. Although she is the youngest participant at the center, she is a warm, friendly person and is a welcome member of the group. K.K. has a special gift for music, and the center has organized a special program, "Music with K.," once a week. Staff acknowledged that they had some concerns when initially approached about including K.K. in their program; however, they now have only positive comments of her involvement and would welcome other adults with developmental disabilities who wish to participate. Connections made between staff from a neighboring program for people with developmental disabilities and staff of the center have further enabled proactive programming and inclusion in this neighborhood of Honolulu.

D.P., a lively woman in her 60s, has cerebral palsy and gets about by using a wheelchair. She was an early joiner of one of the project teams and never missed a meeting. She always had much to contribute by way of personal experiences and words of wisdom. Her creative thinking brought many issues down to earth and assisted in keeping simple many solutions to "difficult problems." She tested the new wheelchair-accessible versions of "The Bus"—Hawaii's main form of public transportation—on a daily basis, ensuring that the city of Honolulu was kept on its toes throughout the early phase of identifying problems. She was instrumental in testing the accessibility of most major tourist hotels on the Waikiki strip [the beachfront area of Honolulu], much to the chagrin of many embarrassed managers. Throughout the project, D.P. served as an inspiration to the team members and continued to be an advocate for the well-being of all seniors, with or without a disability.

CONCLUSIONS

Because of the balanced multicultural nature of Hawaii, issues of divisiveness or territoriality did not become significant in the introduction of the collaborative teaming process model in trying to bring these two disparate networks together. Each recognized its strengths and weaknesses and brought to the team structure the cultural influences of the main cultures of the state. Because of a history of closely working within a multicultural domain, key individuals, such as planners, policy makers, and agency administrators, were committed to building on the work of the teams and facilitating the recommendations and actions that would lead to the greater inclusion of aging adults with developmental disabilities in generic programs and services. At the final plenary team meeting, participants overwhelmingly elected to continue to meet as a network of interested people and agencies for aging adults with and without developmental disabilities. To ensure that this would happen, a subcommittee was formed to facilitate planning and communication among team members. The original group also suggested increasing numbers of participants by inviting interested others to become involved in future meetings. Notwithstanding the diverse cultures represented by the state's population, the collaborative efforts of participants from disability and generic groups concerned with aging individuals heightened a general awareness of the needs of people with developmental disabilities and encouraged participation in a broad range of programs within the community. In a state where life expectancy far exceeds the national average, aging finally came of age.

Although the project described in this chapter addressed the needs of a particular state, the collaborative teaming process model could be applied in any community. The model offers the framework for community development teams that are formed for purposes of program review and restructuring through a step-by-step process across three phases of development—team building, program review and restructuring, and the development of action plans to bring about desired program improvements. Central to the success of any similar project is the identification and recruitment of people who are willing to make a commitment to the goals of program review and improvement. A team or teams may have a specific focus at the time of initial development or may develop a focus after a period of discussion of the specific needs of an identified group or community. Programs need not be restructured in their entirety; rather, features that are working well can be enhanced further with program modifications or additions that reflect current recommended practices. Teams may be formed for a specific time period to address a specific task or for an indefinite period to review continually programs and components for effectiveness or need for adjustment. Above all, service providers must be aware of the diversity of cultural backgrounds in populations and strive to provide culturally sensitive access and opportunities for all citizens, young or old, with or without disabilities.

For those who are interested in implementing a similar effort, in particular where the society is represented by many diverse cultures, the following thoughts about application are offered:

- Time spent up front in team building considerations is a key to the success or failure of such a project. It is essential to take time to identify key people from the diverse cultures represented in your area; to visit with and talk about specific programs and services and to understand how that culture views aging, caregiving, and disability; and to discover the breadth of program or service areas or cultural groups from which team members may be recruited.
- To promote equal power bases across diverse cultures, ensure appropriate representation from groups to be served. The Hawaii experience was, in many ways, unique as no one group makes up a majority; thus, minority groups have become accustomed to working together in a multicultural context. When other cultures play a predominant role, the balance of power in teamwork will need to be addressed.

- People who nominated themselves for team membership tended to be more committed than those who had been directed to participate by an employer or other high-level person. Thus, it is imperative to spend time with key individuals whom you want involved to help them accept the initiative as their own and commit to making an impact.
- Build in considerations for supporting participation from people in outlying communities (e.g., provision for transportation to meetings) or for those who need special provisions (e.g., access, mobility, speech facilitation) to participate fully.
- "Dropping out" of a team (e.g., as a result of agency staff turnover or realignments within a cultural society or association) poses a problem to ongoing team membership as it leads to less cohesiveness among team members. New members need to develop some sense of the history of the group before being fully accepted as part of the team, and the team leaders must take the time to draw new members into the existing group process and network.
- Team-building skills and role identification or task sharing (e.g., as facilitators, record takers, time keepers) underpin and support a team's ability to continue after the formal period of such a project expires. Be sure responsibilities are shared equally among the predominant cultural groups and that communications are in the language of the cultural groups represented.
- Recruiting support from heads of departments, key providers, and agencies enables program restructuring or development to be more readily accepted and institutionalized. Furthermore, a mix of key individuals from various cultures brings a more balanced focus on the needs of specific cultural groups and the ways in which provisions are implemented.

REFERENCES

Ansello, E.F., & Zink, M.B. (1990). Targeting community-based research and education on aging and developmental disabilities. In W.M. Rivera & N.W. Clarke (Eds.), *1990 Lifelong Learning Research Conference proceedings* (pp. 118–124). Fairfax, VA: George Mason University, School of Continuing and Alternative Learning.

Cotten, P.D., Britt, C.R., & Moreland, C. (Eds.). (1986). *Services for elderly mentally handicapped Mississippians: A coordinated plan.* Sanatorium: Mississippi Department of Mental Health.

Cotten, P.D., & Spirrison, C.L. (1988). Development of services for elderly persons with mental retardation in a rural state. *Mental Retardation, 26,* 187–190.

Factor, A.R. (1993). Translating policy into practice. In E. Sutton, A.R. Factor, B.A. Hawkins, T. Heller, & G.B. Seltzer (Eds.), *Older adults with developmental disabilities: Optimizing choice and change* (pp. 257–275). Baltimore: Paul H. Brookes Publishing Co.

Hanson, M.J., Lynch, E.W., & Wayman, K.I. (1990). Honoring the cultural diversity of families when gathering data. *Topics in Early Childhood Special Education, 10,* 112–131.

Harwood, A. (1981). *Ethnicity and medical care.* Cambridge, MA: Harvard University Press.

Hawaii University Affiliated Program. (1989). *Aging persons with developmental disabilities in Hawaii: Preliminary observations.* Honolulu: University of Hawaii at Manoa University Affiliated Program.

Hawkins, B.A., & Eklund, S.J. (1990). Planning processes and outcomes for an aging population with developmental disabilities. *Mental Retardation, 28,* 35–40.

Hawkins, B.A., Eklund, S.J., Garza, J.M., Garza, T., & DiOrio, R. (1987). *Aging/aged persons with developmental disabilities in Indiana: An interagency planning task force report.* Bloomington: Indiana University, Institute for the Study of Developmental Disability and Center on Aging and Aged.

Janicki, M.P. (1991). *Building the future: Planning and community development in aging and developmental disabilities.* Albany: New York State Office of Mental Retardation and Developmental Disabilities, Community Integration Project in Aging and Developmental Disabilities.

Janicki, M.P. (1992). *Integration experiences casebook: Program ideas in aging and developmental disabilities.* Albany: New York State Office of Mental Retardation and Developmental Disabilities, Community Integration Project.

Janicki, M.P., Knox, L.A., & Jacobson, J.W. (1985). Planning for an older developmentally disabled population. In M.P. Janicki & H.M. Wisniewski (Eds.), *Aging and developmental disabilities: Issues and approaches* (pp. 143–159). Baltimore: Paul H. Brookes Publishing Co.

Kuehn, M.L., & Imm-Thomas, P. (1993). A multicultural context. In E. Sutton, A.R. Factor, B.A. Hawkins, T. Heller, & G.B. Seltzer (Eds.), *Older adults with developmental disabilities: Optimizing choice and change* (pp. 327–343). Baltimore: Paul H. Brookes Publishing Co.

Kultgen, P., & Rominger, R. (1993). Cross training within the aging and developmental disabilities services systems. In E. Sutton, A.R. Factor, B.A. Hawkins, T. Heller, & G.B. Seltzer (Eds.), *Older adults with developmental disabilities: Optimizing choice and change* (pp. 239–256). Baltimore: Paul H. Brookes Publishing Co.

Lubin, R.A., & Kiely, M. (1985). Epidemiology of aging in developmental disabilities. In M.P. Janicki & H.M. Wisniewski (Eds.), *Aging and developmental disabilities: Issues and approaches* (pp. 95–113). Baltimore: Paul H. Brookes Publishing Co.

McDermott, J.F., Tseng, W.S., & Maretzki, T.W. (Eds.). (1980). *People and cultures of Hawaii: A psychocultural profile.* Honolulu: University of Hawaii Press.

Pederson, E.L. (1993). Appendix: The research and training consortium process. In E. Sutton, A.R. Factor, B.A. Hawkins, T. Heller, & G.B. Seltzer (Eds.), *Older adults with developmental disabilities: Optimizing choice and change* (pp. 345–369). Baltimore: Paul H. Brookes Publishing Co.

Rice, D.P., & Feldman, J.J. (1985). Living longer in the United States: Demographic changes and health needs of the elderly. In M.P. Janicki and H.M. Wisniewski (Eds.), *Aging and developmental disabilities: Issues and approaches* (pp. 9–26). Baltimore: Paul H. Brookes Publishing Co.

Seltzer, M.M. (1988). Structure and patterns of service utilization by elderly persons with mental retardation. *Mental Retardation, 26,* 181–186.

Seltzer, M.M., Krauss, M.W., Litchfield, L.C., & Modlish, N.J. (1989). Utilization of aging network services by elderly persons with mental retardation. *Gerontologist, 29,* 234–238.

State of Hawaii. (1998). *State of Hawaii Data Book 1998: A statistical analysis* (Available http://www.hawaii.gov/dbedt/index.html). Honolulu: State of Hawaii, Department of Business, Economic Development and Tourism.

Stodden, R.A. (1991). *Career/vocational preparation for students with disabilities: A program improvement guide.* Tallahassee: Florida State Department of Education.

Takamura, J.C. (1991). Asian and Pacific Islander elderly. In N. Mokuau (Ed.), *Handbook of social services for Asian and Pacific Islanders* (pp. 185–201). Westport, CT: Greenwood Publishing Group.

Wanninger, B., & Pederson, E.L. (1986). *Older adults with mental retardation and developmental disabilities.* Cincinnati, OH: Cincinnati Center for Developmental Disorders.

Wu, H.-I. (1987). *Barriers and strategies: Barriers to and strategies for the integration of older persons with developmental disabilities within aging network services.* Albany: New York State Office for the Aging.

26

Statewide
Organizational Development

Jean M. Sherman and Patricia A. Bloom

The emergence of a substantial yet previously hidden population of older people—those who have developmental disabilities—caught some observers in Florida by surprise. Where have these seniors been? When did they arrive? What services do they need? What is the best way to help them? This chapter suggests some answers to these questions and describes a model used to respond to these issues. Furthermore, to encourage replication in other areas of the United States, the specific application of this model in Florida is explored, along with an explication of the barriers and benefits that were encountered.

BACKGROUND

In terms of its elderly residents, Florida is often viewed as a bellwether state, because it presages by 10 years the demographic trends of the rest of the country. Florida is home to the largest proportion of elders in the United States. More than 19% of its residents are older than 60 years; within 25 years, that number is expected to climb to almost 30% (Campbell, 1996). As they migrated to Florida, some older citizens brought along their dependent adult children. Frequently, these families were unprepared for what they found: an adopted state that consistently ranks close to last in the amount

---

Editors' note: The system term *developmental disabilities* is not used in Florida; instead, the system is called *developmental services.* To maintain consistency with other chapters in this book, however, the term *developmental disabilities services* is used when the term is used generally.

of funds it expends for the care of people who have developmental disabilities. This is exacerbated by the realization that the number of older adults with developmental disabilities is unprecedented and growing. The majority of people with intellectual disabilities (the largest single diagnostic category of developmental disabilities) live in the community with their families, often with elderly parent caregivers (Seltzer, Krauss, & Heller, 1990). With offspring approaching age 60 or older, these parents are in their late 70s, 80s, and older.

As they move toward the end of their family life cycles, both the adults with disabilities and their parents are likely to be experiencing age-related difficulties and are, therefore, potential candidates for traditional kinds of health and social services. Although many of these individuals will achieve a good "fit" within the aging system, there are some who will require service modifications; still others will need completely new services or supports. In any case, many of these families will require some kind of assistance from the formal services system if their family stability is to be maintained. Ansello (1996) pointed out that any interventions for aging adults with lifelong disabilities must also respond to the realities of their family circumstances and the need for continued self-reliance. Should such families fail to gain access to necessary community resources or become less self-reliant, then, ultimately, both the elderly parent caregivers and their adult children will suffer.

If service systems are to assume a proactive stance to aid these families, two things must occur: First, models of service collaboration between the aging and developmental disabilities services networks must be constructed. Second, to forestall caregiving crises, elderly parent caregivers of adults with developmental disabilities must be identified, their needs assessed, participation in service planning invited, and supportive assistance offered. However, before embarking on any activity, it is useful to study similar efforts already made by others. We examined the services models used in Ohio, New York, Illinois, Maryland, and Virginia and found that each includes some degree of grass roots control and that all incorporate some form of collaboration, outreach, and capacity building. In New York, for instance, the area agency on aging feasibility model allowed each of four demonstration sites to develop its own outreach methodology (LePore & Janicki, 1997). The Florida model also had four sites that developed their own outreach strategies and supplemented their own capacities through the use of volunteers, paid companions, or shared staff.

In Maryland and Virginia, the integrated model built on earlier inclusion efforts. Five sets of service partners field tested an integrated and collaborative services model (see Chapter 24). Some commonalities existed across the five sites: each one used community resource fairs as an outreach strategy, conducted cross-training with local aging and developmental disabilities staff, and offered consumers training in self-care or advocacy. The Florida model borrowed from the foregoing models' attributes, adding its own strategies for forming community-based coalitions as it evolved. In general, Florida's approach was to identify existing capacities of the local service systems, as well as the needs of the individuals, and to plan collaboratively for services. The implementation of the model marked the first time in Florida that the aging and developmental service systems worked in concert to serve their mutual clientele.

In this chapter, we describe the statewide and local organizational activities undertaken in Florida to include older adults with developmental disabilities within aging network programs. To obtain the desired result, the following questions were asked:

1. What sort of overarching structure should be in place at the highest state level to encourage widespread local collaborative efforts?
2. Which grass-roots model would lead to successful inclusion of older adults with developmental disabilities at the community level?
3. Would the same local model and activities prove equally effective in four distinctly different areas of this state?

Before such specific questions are addressed, it is necessary to understand Florida's social service system for older adults with developmental disabilities.

STATUS OF THE SYSTEM

Since the late 1960s, the community aging network in the United States has evolved from a system of congregate or center-based services and programs to one that emphasizes the supports necessary to maintain frail elders in their own homes. This change in focus came from the gradual realization that, over time, people "age in place," requiring more individualized supports as they reach their later years. During approximately this same time frame, the developmental services network began shifting from institutional care to total community inclusion with individually tailored supports. In past years, the emphasis from early childhood on was to help individuals acquire and maintain job skills. Only recently have activities at the far end of the life spectrum been acknowledged.

Florida's System

Florida uses a decentralized social services structure with parallel networks for each category of service. Within this system, part of the administration and the funding for each network is at the state level; part is at the local or district level. Each local service network is actually a sublayer of the decentralized state system, claiming a certain degree of autonomy within that geographic locale. Specifically, the Florida aging network is composed of the Department of Elder Affairs (DOEA) and the 11 area agencies on aging (AAAs) and their 400 subcontracted provider agencies. The developmental service network is composed of the state office and 15 district program offices—all part of Florida's Department of Children and Families (DCF)—along with their various subcontracted provider agencies. Another network component is Aging and Adult Services (now called Adult Services), which is also part of DCF.

Both formal networks face the same fiscal reality: The generous annual flow of public funds for social services has slowed to a trickle. Approaching the new millennium, many service programs funded by federal or state governments have experienced significant reductions in their annual budgets or have barely been subsisting with maintenance-level funding. Add to this the fact that although most experts cite the age group of people older than 85 years as the fastest growing group in the United States, the fastest growing segment of this population, in fact, is centenarians—people age 100 years and older (Campbell, 1996; Manton, 1996). More people living to older ages translates into more requests for services; more people are requesting more services from programs that have fewer dollars.

Although hardly new, the need to maximize existing funds has resulted in the creation of a number of service collaborations around the country. An obvious benefit of this strategy is more appropriate use of existing services. An important bonus is the recognition of informal services as part of the shared delivery system. A third benefit—

which may be less obvious to professionals—is the active participation of consumers and family members in the service planning process. This last element is based on a growing recognition of the need to include consumer rights and choices. Such consumer participation can result in truly responsive services, enabling families and consumers to enjoy the fruits of practical empowerment firsthand.

State and Local Initiatives

As recently as 1992, the unique needs of older people with developmental disabilities and their aging parent caregivers in Florida had yet to be formally addressed. In October of that year, a state-level interagency agreement became the catalyst for an organizational development sequence to occur on both the statewide and the local levels. In many ways, Florida's attempt to serve older people with developmental disabilities and their families resembled models from other states, such as New York and Virginia. However, in one very distinct way, Florida's endeavor was unusual. In Florida, the seeds of service collaboration were sown and came to fruition via an incremental series of top-down and bottom-up strategies. The seeds came from the top down, with the formation of a statewide coordinating entity, the Aging and Developmental Disabilities Interagency Effort (ADDIE). A cross-network training project (Dare to Dream) was a bottom-up approach, as were the grass-roots action groups of Project FLAGs (Florida's Local Action Groups).

Aging and Developmental Disabilities Interagency Effort

Background   Historically, individuals with developmental disabilities typically did not survive to old age. Therefore, professionals in the disabilities field had little experience serving older people. Similarly, those who worked in aging programs had few encounters and little experience with providing services for people with lifelong disabilities. On the network level, there was scant interaction between the aging and developmental disabilities systems. It takes little imagination to realize that members of an aging population, who share lifelong disabilities and are outliving their parents, could easily fall through gaps in the service system. No one had organized the delivery of services to this group of older people and their elderly caregivers. So, in 1992, at the instigation of the Center on Aging and Developmental Disabilities (CADD) at the University of Miami, the Florida Developmental Disabilities Council brokered the signing of a joint statement of cooperation between the Florida DOEA and the Department of Health and Rehabilitative Services (now the DCF) Adult Services and Developmental Services programs. The signing of this joint statement was the first top-down step taken.

Data from the state's Developmental Services office showed that the system was serving only approximately 10% of the probable number of elderly individuals with developmental disabilities in Florida (State of Florida DOEA, 1996b). As a result of the joint statement, aging and disability agencies and other involved entities were to 1) join to educate the public about the plight of individuals with developmental disabilities who are aging, 2) inform the community about family-caregiver concerns, 3) identify the service needs of these older consumers and their families, and 4) create new, coordinated service options to meet the unique needs of this population. The ADDIE was established to oversee these mandates. Florida's governor, an advocate for the state's elders, was most supportive and demonstrated his endorsement with a statewide proclamation of ADDIE. The joint statement of cooperation and ADDIE (the second top-down initiative) were part of Florida's response to the Older Americans Act

Amendments of 1987 (PL 100-175) mandate to make aging services available to elders with developmental disabilities.

Objectives of the Aging and Developmental Disabilities Interagency Effort   ADDIE membership included older adults and families of older adults with developmental disabilities, along with representatives of related state agencies, advocacy groups, university affiliates, AAAs, and private service providers. The committee's stated mission was to "secure a collaborative network of services for Florida's elders with developmental disabilities and their caregivers that will maximize opportunities for self-sufficiency and personal independence" (Aging and Developmental Disabilities Interagency Effort, 1994). ADDIE members held meetings on a regular, quarterly basis, and their role was to recommend strategies and to review the results of current collaborative efforts. The overarching role of ADDIE was to serve as a catalyst and a visible partnership among professionals, caregivers, and consumers while overseeing all joint activities of the aging and developmental disabilities services networks. ADDIE embraced the premise that older adults with developmental disabilities can live successfully in the community, in places of their own choosing, while making positive contributions to the lives of their families and communities and having access to services and supports that promote choice and full citizenship.

Methods and Activities   For collaborative efforts to occur between Aging and Developmental Services, both networks had to acknowledge their shared clientele and become familiar with each other's system and professionals. Consequently, in 1993 the CADD embarked on the sponsorship of a series of regional cross-training workshops, called Dare to Dream. These workshops gathered together local aging and disabilities providers, often for the first time. Held at various locations across the state, these sessions also introduced the district administrators of the state's Developmental Services and Adult Services to the local AAA directors while providing cross-network training to them, their staffs, and provider agency personnel. These workshops were the impetus for systems collaboration and constituted the initial bottom-up initiative.

Outcomes   Building on the success of the Dare to Dream workshops, several aging and developmental disabilities efforts were initiated by ADDIE. These included the 1994 gubernatorial proclamation of ADDIE, presentations by members at several state and national conferences, oversight of Project FLAGs, and a statewide FLAGs summit meeting with three subsequent regional minisummits.

In 1994, ADDIE sponsored a statewide invitational summit, which featured three state-level department heads from the DOEA, Developmental Services, and Adult Services. The 15 district or local office administrators from the state's Developmental Services and Adult Services offices and the executive directors of the 11 AAAs in Florida also attended. This summit communicated clearly to local decision makers that this aging–developmental disabilities collaboration was endorsed at the highest levels. Bringing together the top echelon of social services administrators allowed for the onsite creation of cooperative agreements and collaborative action plans in all 15 districts. Between late 1995 and early 1996, ADDIE scheduled three regional mini-summit meetings. These occurred in the northern, central, and southern parts of the state and focused on learning about best collaborative service practices around the United States; sharing FLAG experiences and problems; and answering questions from parents, advocates, and consumers.

The early success of ADDIE attracted other projects to it, but some of these ancillary programs drew ADDIE's attention away from FLAGs. As a result of this distraction, oversight for some of the collaborative activities reverted to the individual group leaders. Fortunately, when this occurred, the FLAG members demonstrated that their groups were mature enough to carry on. A second problem concerned the lack of consistent meeting attendance by some ADDIE representatives. When last-minute substitutions were made, the well-meaning proxies often were not well informed about their regional FLAG activities. Consequently, much valuable meeting time was spent bringing the substitutes up to date. Also, important issues would be left in abeyance and unresolved. A third problem dealt with the continuation of ADDIE. Given its overarching role, it seemed that statewide oversight of FLAGs should continue through ADDIE. However, funding for the support of this coordinating body was curtailed as of mid-1997. Cross-state travel costs were its primary expenses, so efforts were begun to create "regional ADDIEs," without the need for distance travel.

Project FLAGs

To promote regional collaboration, Project FLAGs was undertaken to develop formal mechanisms for building local bridges of understanding and collaborative service delivery between the aging and developmental disabilities service networks. The intent was to involve older adults with developmental disabilities and their families with administrators and service providers in planning and gaining access to local services that would meet their needs. Though initiated on the state level as a joint project of the state's DOEA and Developmental Disabilities Council, Project FLAGs was the second bottom-up activity in Florida (Dare to Dream was the first). After a 1994 request for proposals from the DOEA, four community sponsors accepted the challenge of developing local service collaborations. The following describes these FLAG sites, each of which served a different demographic population.

The Tri-County FLAG was located in northwest Florida, a sparsely populated, rural area of more than 1,700 square miles. Here, services for elders and those for people with developmental disabilities were delivered by a limited number of local agencies. A multiservice aging provider was the original sponsor for this FLAG. Delivering services to people who were living in scattered rural communities inherently required cooperation and coordination. The small-town flavor of the area lent itself naturally to the idea of coalition building, because nearly all of the service providers were already known to one another. However, the idea of increasing services was approached with caution because placing increased demands on this delivery system could easily strain already-stretched resources.

The Gold Coast FLAG, sponsored by a local developmental service agency, served a county on the state's west coast that consisted of both suburban and rural areas and a population of more than 250,000 people. Fully one-third of that total was older than age 60 years. Composed largely of clustered retirement villages, the area is known for its large transient snowbird population. The presence of so many seasonal residents presented a challenge for outreach and identification of families.

The Urban FLAG, located in the ever-expanding city of Orlando, served all of Orange County. Initially sponsored by a multifaceted aging services provider, this FLAG later was led by a developmental disabilities service provider. The area covered by this FLAG site was both urban and suburban, near the east-central coast. In 1996, it was estimated that this area had more than 110,000 people older than 60 years of age (State of Florida DOEA, 1996c). Both the aging and disabilities networks had well-established provider systems in this area, along with the obligatory waiting lists and consequent funding limitations.

The Central Florida FLAG was located in the middle of the state and sponsored by the sole provider of aging services. This FLAG covered a rural area with an estimated 24,000 people who were older than 60 years of age (State of Florida DOEA, 1996c). Here, too, the aging and developmental disabilities service networks were well established. This county had two senior centers, one congregate senior nutrition site, and two vocational training workshops for people with disabilities.

Objectives of the FLAGs   The first major objective was to provide cross-training in each FLAG to foster mutual knowledge, understanding, and relationships among representatives from the aging system, the developmental service system, older consumers, and family members. A second objective was to coordinate strategies for bringing older adults with disabilities into aging network programs while still retaining any needed developmental services. A third and more crucial objective was to create procedures to identify older adults with developmental disabilities, whether affiliated with the service system or not, who could benefit from aging services. The final objective was to recruit mentors who would be matched with and facilitate the transition of older adults with developmental disabilities into senior programs.

The first two objectives, cross-training and coordination of inclusion strategies, were met primarily through a series of training programs that were conducted by the University of Miami's CADD. In addition, regional mini-summit meetings hosted out-of-state experts and afforded members the opportunity to learn from the efforts of others. These educational activities were key to changing the perceptions of some professionals in the aging system who were hesitant to welcome seniors with developmental disabilities. Training also gave assurance to disabilities representatives that they would not lose control of their consumers or their funding. Both networks came to understand that the inclusion of adults with disabilities into aging network activities was by no means a relinquishing of care under the auspice of the state's developmental services agency. In the process, group members became familiar with the procedures, possibilities, and limitations of each respective system. Professional friendships formed, and real efforts were made to cooperate and learn from each other. The rigid restrictions of each system's structure gave way to more creative yet statutorily compliant responses.

The third objective addressed the need to identify older adults with developmental disabilities who could benefit from aging services. To do so, FLAGs used a number of strategies that included reviewing the client databases of member agencies to determine the presence of eligible older individuals, analyzing outreach data, and placing recruitment advertisements in local newspapers and newsletters encouraging individuals who were caring for an elder with a disability to call. To support these outreach efforts, an informational guide for families—a packet of salient fact sheets and a list of community aging resources—was prepared by the CADD (Alfassa-White & Bloom, 1995). These materials were given to identified adults with disabilities and their caregivers, to FLAG members, and to community residents.

As their first identification activity, staff from the state's developmental services office reviewed their current client rosters. There were few adults who were older than age 60 years, but there were large numbers of individuals between the ages of 45 and 59. One FLAG even made the serendipitous discovery that the aging and developmental service programs shared some of the same clients. Finding families that were not connected to the service system proved to be more difficult, yet this endeavor produced the most creative efforts undertaken by each FLAG; grass-roots activities used informal information outlets that were unique to the characteristics of each site. Ultimately, the most successful identification strategies were those that were tailored to the social dynamics of the specific community. For example, the rural multicounty site in northern Florida opted to use naturally occurring community "meeting places," such as a grocery store or gas station, as an information dissemination base. The following vignette considers how that worked.

> *A local resident noticed that one of the FLAG members had the habit of stopping at a certain gas station as she made the long drive home from work. After filling her tank one afternoon, the professional was hailed by "Alice," a waiting local. (Alice could have called the FLAG member at her office during the day but chose to approach her in this more personal way.) Explaining that she had been waiting and watching for nearly a week, Alice shared her concerns about a certain older gentleman. The man, in his mid-50s, had been living comfortably with his mother in a distant town until her death several months ago. Now he has moved to their locale to live with his older sister and her husband, who own the hardware store across the street. After taking some time off to help her brother settle in, the sister had to return to work, leaving her brother alone at home each day. When the brother became depressed because of his social isolation, his sister began taking him to work with her. To her neighbor, the sister confided her desire to find a program that her brother could attend during the day. For this reason, Alice had been waiting at the gas station to talk with the FLAG member and obtain information about such activity programs. After subsequent contact with the sister, the FLAG member arranged a meeting with her and her brother. It was clear during the meeting that the brother had no intention of going to any program. He was content to pursue his new job in the hardware store, meeting and greeting patrons as they came in and watching the day's passersby. Though there is no immediate service need in this situation, the sister is now aware of the programs available in the community. She promised to contact the services agency in the future, if assistance became necessary.*

This sort of "referral" is characteristic of the interpersonal dynamics that are regularly at work in small, rural communities. A second example is the public park that hosted the monthly surplus foods distribution—another good information dissemination location. Large posters describing developmental disabilities and offering assistance to families of adults with such conditions were displayed at the registration tables. As a result of this one strategy, nearly 60 families eventually made contact with this FLAG. Because the urban and suburban FLAGs generally boasted a more developed network of services, their identification efforts targeted existing service entities such as senior centers and nutrition programs. For outreach purposes, churches, neighborhood stores, and the local media were chosen. Another strategy—leaving materials in doctors' offices and clinics—met with little success. Dissemination via more naturally frequented venues, such as pharmacies, and public service spots on local radio and television stations accomplished more. Two FLAGs requested that their AAA modify its intake system, adding a query about anyone with a developmental disability living in the household. Responses there led to the discovery of unknown older clients with developmental disabilities. Unfortunately, not all were 60 years old and so did not meet the age criteria for Older Americans Act of 1965 (PL 89-73) programs. By far, the largest age group uncovered in the four FLAG areas were those in the 45- to 59-year age range.

Identifying seniors with disabilities is one thing, but enabling their inclusion into community aging programs is quite another. Because the aging programs are funded primarily by the Older Americans Act, the fourth objective matched eligible individuals who were 60 years or older with a senior volunteer mentor. Later, individuals who were younger than 60 years were brought in on a case-by-case basis. The role of the mentor was to ease entry into the local senior program or assist the person to participate in generic community activities. The CADD provided a "train-the-trainers" program for staff who were responsible for volunteer recruitment and conducted this training for the initial volunteer mentors. The matching of mentors and consumers with disabilities typically occurred in the following way. The FLAG coordinator met with the older individual and his or her caregiver to explain the program, determine the individual's interest in participating, and identify the types of leisure activities the individual would enjoy. Later, the consumer's profile was reviewed, and a plan was developed for a companion. When a consumer was matched with a mentor, the volunteer was given information on safety, transportation, and any services being provided. The companions met initially at either the consumer's home or the senior center, and a mutually convenient meeting schedule was established.

Outcomes   If locating older adults with disabilities in the communities posed unique challenges, recruiting sufficient numbers of volunteer mentors was even more problematic. The most successful outcomes were reached in the two FLAG areas where aging network volunteer agencies (RSVP and Senior Companions) did the actual recruiting. Taking a different tack, one FLAG appointed a part-time volunteer coordinator, who was assigned exclusively to recruiting, training, and matching volunteers. The fourth FLAG simply added volunteer coordination duties to an existing staff position and then focused on recruiting seniors who were already involved in local aging programs. Though there was some early discomfort and even reluctance on the part of potential mentors, as time passed and consumers and volunteers interacted with one another, their growing relationships evolved to the point that they resembled naturally occurring friendships. However, as the FLAGs program continued, there was a greater number of individuals with disabilities than there were volunteer mentors.

To address this shortfall, a new component, the Companion-Link program, was added. The companions who participated were subsidized volunteers drawn from the Senior Companions program, sponsored by the Corporation for National Service. The goal of this augmentation was to develop (and expand) a more consistent volunteer mentor system that would enable entry of older adults with developmental disabilities into community senior activities statewide. The concept of using a peer companion to achieve community inclusion is not new. It has been used in different areas of the United States for a number of years, as regular participants at senior centers became mentors for older adults with disabilities. But the use of Senior Companions broadened the mentorship. This program could mentor individuals with disabilities who were as young as age 55 years into generic community activity programs. (Senior Companions receive specific training for their assignments, regular in-service training sessions, modest tax-free stipends, reimbursement for transportation and meals, annual physical examinations, and accident and liability insurance while on duty.)

The first phase of integrating older individuals with disabilities into senior programs occurred at a moderate but steady rate, with one or two at a time taken to their local community senior centers each week. Center staff and volunteer mentors were mindful of the need for flexibility and patience in their responses; there were considerable variations in the physical and emotional capabilities of their new participants. For example, two older women initially required home visits from their mentors. Similarly, two other adults were uneasy about leaving their homes; their attendance at the program was sporadic at first. Undaunted, FLAG members knew that each of these small successes would eventually lead to the larger goal of inclusion. Conversely, there were several newly mentored adults who began to attend the senior center regularly, delightedly making the most of this opportunity for inclusion. Striking successes include an elderly woman who had been socially isolated. When she first attended the senior center, her volunteer companion spent considerable time talking with and listening to her. As a result, this woman became more comfortable in her new social setting and became sociable and outgoing. Another older woman who had been attending a congregate meal site was easily confused and needed a guide. A volunteer mentor served as a sounding board, providing a "willing ear" and much needed personal attention. The woman improved so much that eventually she met a gentleman who also attended the meal site and they married.

Nevertheless, success at matching consumers and mentors varied across and even within the FLAGs. Although the training received by each volunteer emphasized sensitivity awareness and communication skills, the ultimate match-up was necessarily determined by the personalities and chemistry between the two people. None of the successful pairings were—nor should they have been—forced. They resulted naturally from social opportunities to learn more about one another, as mentors facilitated their companions' entry into the aging network program. The positive acceptance of the new member with a disability by other participants was definitely aided by the presence and the cuing of the mentor. Such ease of assimilation should be encouraging to others who may be considering using the FLAG model. Several of the senior volunteers were family caregivers of adults with developmental disabilities, but they generously agreed to serve as mentors for others. In doing so, these volunteers also became service recipients. By chance, during training, some of these volunteers spoke of needing certain information for their own families. As a result, these older caregivers were given the information that provided them with assistance in making future-care plans for their own loved ones. This proved to be a win–win situation for all concerned.

Successful attempts at inclusion were significant in another way, because of their impact on several staff members from the aging network. Evincing beliefs reminiscent of historical stigmas, they openly confessed their misgivings about integrating individuals with developmental disabilities into their senior programs. To counter this, FLAG members selected the highest functioning candidates with the best potential for successful inclusion. When those successes came and the program continued, the functional criteria were gradually relaxed and people with more severe limitations were chosen. It is notable that the more rural areas achieved particular success in developing their mentor programs, possibly because of small-town familiarity and the ease of making one-to-one approaches. Indeed, several of the mentors in those areas decided to exceed their schedules and arranged extra visits and special outings with their companions.

Meetings of the rural FLAG often discussed implementation problems and drafted individualized solutions to overcome identified barriers. However, in the absence of administrative support, some of those solutions proved difficult to effect. In addition, when one FLAG encountered stereotypical attitudes and superstitions among community residents, the group developed the objective of educating the local community. Because it was recognized that this could be a lengthy process, members agreed to take every opportunity to educate individual area residents on the topic of developmental disabilities. Another problem, more urgent in rural areas, consistently surfaced—the scarcity of transportation. Because the area did not have a local hospital, medical transportation for elders in these areas always took priority over social purposes. Consequently, volunteers with cars became prized assets. Having cars, these mentors solved the transportation riddle, opening up a new world for those who had been waiting.

In the arena of volunteer coordination, one FLAG designated staff to assume the additional responsibilities. Its poor recruitment rates contrasted sharply with the group in which a new position was created specifically to recruit, train, and supervise the volunteers. Overall, the difficulty encountered in the recruitment of volunteers emphasized the importance of a dedicated, coordinated effort for this task. It also suggested the value of using an experienced, recognized volunteer agency to obtain sufficient senior mentors. Another obstacle to volunteer recruitment for one FLAG was the transience of many area residents, making it difficult to recruit seniors who could commit to long-term relationships. This FLAGs' members recognized that the inability of a volunteer to provide consistent, ongoing contact would be detrimental to the development of a trusting relationship. Though it significantly reduced the potential pool, only volunteers who could commit to year-round assignments were accepted.

Most FLAG members were service professionals who were enthusiastic about the prospect of shared service delivery. Yet in their efforts to achieve collaboration, they needed administrative support from all participating agencies. Authorizing necessary spending, assigning appropriate staff, and acknowledging the importance of FLAG activities took administrative time but proved to be essential. Family caregivers who were isolated from the service system posed a unique problem. With these parents, professionals first had to prove their worth. Only when they demonstrated their intent to maintain the high quality of care that these families had so diligently provided over the years did caregivers accept their assistance. The following illustrates this:

> One elderly mother was unwilling to let go of her older son and allow him to participate at the community senior center. To increase the caregivers' confidence and familiarity, both parents and their son were invited to attend the senior center. In time, all of the family members came, and they enjoyed the program. The son was able to spend time with his companion while his parents were active in other areas of the center. Later, the mother fell ill. However, by that time, the companion was warmly welcomed as he made visits to the son at home.

Finally, another problem involved the lack of discretionary funds available to older adults with disabilities, which they needed to participate in certain senior activities. To resolve this situation, one FLAG used some of its allocated administrative funds to subsidize the attendance of a number of older adults with developmental disabilities at several of the area's nutrition sites and on outings.

GENERALIZABLE FINDINGS

It is clear that the existence of a top-down commitment to collaboration between the aging and developmental services networks was essential to the long-term success of the bottom-up or grass roots efforts of FLAGs. The endorsement by the governor of Florida, as well as by the DOEA and the DCF Offices of Developmental Disabilities and Adult Services, communicated to administrators on the district level that collaboration among the various aspects of Florida's social services networks was both encouraged and expected. The creation of a statewide internetwork advisory body (ADDIE) successfully provided oversight from the perspective of multiple stakeholders and ensured that priority issues for aging and developmental disabilities collaboration were addressed and followed.

Several generalizable findings emanated from the local FLAGs. Among the most important were 1) the effectiveness of grass roots systems collaboration, 2) mentoring as an inclusion methodology, 3) the value of training mentors, 4) having an exclusive volunteer coordinator, and 5) earning the trust of unaffiliated families. The desire to serve an emerging population of elders with developmental disabilities in a new way was the *raison d'être* of Project FLAGs. This rationale for a change in the social services system was clearly observed by the outside evaluator of FLAGs. The most significant systems change—responsive local, collaborative programming—was the result of both the successful mentoring and the creative networking activities of this project. As the evaluator concluded, "It is highly unlikely that this type of innovative conceptualization would have occurred outside of the impetus provided by FLAGs" (State of Florida DOEA, 1996a).

Beyond an orientation to developmental disabilities and the specific responsibilities of a mentor, supplemental volunteer training also proved to be valuable. This additional training consisted of the mentor's spending a day with an older adult at home or at a developmental service program site, observing how the adult and caregiver interacted. The purpose was not for the volunteer to become a substitute caregiver; rather, it was intended to acquaint the mentor with some of the skills and abilities that the older person used in his or her daily life. The FLAG's experience also shows the necessity of a long-term commitment by a volunteer companion. Equally important is the volunteer's ability to see each individual as a person first. The durability of several companion matches underscores the importance of mentors' being sensitive to the unique needs of each older person with a lifelong disability. Project FLAGs showed these characteristics to be essential in mentors, if their efforts are to result in the successful transition of older individuals with lifelong disabilities into generic aging programs. A final note on mentoring: Staff were unanimous in their belief that one person must be assigned to coordinate the volunteer mentor program in each area and be given the resources to do this.

One interesting finding from FLAGs seems particular to rural communities, where some rural residents frown on any form of outside dependence, espousing instead a philosophy of "taking care of our own." This view takes on added meaning when it is held by a family caregiver of a person with a developmental disability. With such an attitude, the needs and worries of an aging caregiver might sometimes be hidden from public view. Yet this attitude could also result in the formation of important neighborhood support networks. However, for families that are not in supportive environments or when the need for assistance becomes too complex for informal caregivers, this isolationist attitude is a detriment to meeting a family's needs.

Despite the fact that some neighbors might become involved in care, other rural residents had a limited understanding of developmental disabilities. Like many in the general population, when seeing no relevance to themselves, they did not take advantage of educational opportunities. Furthermore, social isolation and high rates of illiteracy, particularly in the poorer rural areas, probably helped to sustain the belief that developmental disabilities are due to demonic possession or the results of witchcraft. Whether such beliefs are part of the local folklore or spring from some more primitive fears is open to speculation. When unaffiliated families choose not to become involved in the social service system, it is difficult for service professionals to convince them otherwise. This is true, regardless of the need or the potential benefits that might accrue from their participation in a community senior program. Nevertheless, even reluctant families sometimes will accept information when it is conveyed by a caring professional who has earned their trust. In this regard, the value of outreach that serves to inform families rather than specifically involve them should not be underestimated. Information delivered through outreach may be just as important to one family as a particular service is to another.

CONCLUSIONS

In Florida, as in many other states, the aging and developmental disabilities systems are like two trains running side by side. Oblivious of one another, they move along on parallel tracks, never intersecting. Project FLAGs produced intersections. For instance, in one FLAG, the local aging and developmental service administrators first met at a cross-network training workshop (Dare to Dream) 2 years earlier. Project FLAGs was the first opportunity for both administrators to work together. At the end of 2 years, they and members of this group unanimously agreed that the collaborative FLAG experience was most rewarding. As Project FLAGs successfully demonstrated, with collaboration the services of the aging and developmental services networks can be combined and made available to their mutual clients. Collaboration can be a welcome strategy for providers in both service networks as the means by which agencies become more responsive to their communities' needs. The FLAGs collaborative process marked the first time that some consumers in Florida had any real involvement in services planning or implementation.

In itself, participation in a collaborative process is a means of empowering consumers and families. Though empowerment can be more professional rhetoric than reality, collaboration offers a true opportunity to embody this concept. Rather than just discuss empowerment, collaboration presents an occasion to cultivate it. As collaborative services proliferate and invite consumer participation, subsequent consumer satisfaction will become the hallmark of service quality and agency accountability.

The most consistent problem encountered in Project FLAGs was the need for continued strong commitments from the local leadership in the aging and developmental disabilities systems to assist in working out the inevitable glitches and conflicts that arose. At times, exceptions from normal operating procedures were needed. Handled case by case, these exceptions were negotiated by the providers involved but required the formal approval of one or both district system administrators before they could be executed. The authors note that when timely administrative responses are not forthcoming in these situations, progress can be impeded indefinitely. When obstacles that blocked local cooperation arose, they were—more often than not—the sorts of issues that required the attention of district- or state-level administrators. Thus, future collaborations should include regular opportunities for district aging and developmental disabilities administrators to come together with their local service providers, perhaps in problem-solving workshop settings. There, administrators could receive ongoing input and give ongoing feedback to facilitate and strengthen their regional group efforts. This approach would go a long way toward ensuring administrators' understanding of the everyday obstacles involved in carrying out service collaborations.

The diversity of participants in each FLAG was a contributing factor to the strengths and challenges of each group. In addition, a lasting contribution of Project FLAGs has been the creation and enhancement of channels of communication between each group's aging and developmental disabilities members and between service providers and community residents. This seems to be particularly salient at the provider level, where care managers and direct care staff are now more aware of a wider range of services and support options that are available to their older consumers. In the United States, there is one issue that inevitably confronts the aging and developmental disabilities networks whenever their services intersect: chronological aging versus functional decline. Some individuals with developmental disabilities age 10–20 years before what might be expected chronologically. Thus, we see people in their 40s who have multiple, severely disabling conditions or individuals with Down syndrome, whose bodies display the hallmark signs of physical aging. Other individuals, who have spent 30–40 years in a workshop environment, are now ready to retire from a life of total vocational emphasis to one that has more leisure time and meaningful social interactions. These two groups of people with developmental disabilities—who are within the first wave of aging baby boomers—generally fall into the 45- to 59-year-old range. However, the specific age criterion of the Older Americans Act precludes their eligibility for those programs. As has been the case with other collaborative services efforts around the United States, Project FLAGs has had to address this age versus frailty statutory dilemma.

Several approaches were used by the various local FLAG groups to allow older adults who were not yet 60 to participate in community leisure programs. First, the federally mandated exceptions of dependent adults who live with parents age 60 and older were honored. Next, potential participants of a senior program who agreed to volunteer at the senior center were also accepted on that basis. Third, the use of a volunteer mentor to escort an aging person with a disability, one-to-one, to community events and outings was not constrained by any age eligibility. Thus, movie and luncheon dates and shopping excursions were very popular and successful community activities. Of course, these successes also necessitated careful preparation and the setting of realistic expectations on the part of both mentors and mentees. While not addressing the age obstacle to participation in formal senior programs, escorted community excursions did seem to provide an enjoyable, acceptable alternative for those involved.

In any group, a few usually make most of the effort. This was no different in FLAGs. Intended as a collaboration model, the whole was certainly expected to be greater than the sum of its parts. When the lack of unanimous member participation lessened the sum total, it meant the difference between a successful inclusion effort or failure, and an older person in need left waiting. We have learned from our work with the FLAGs model that in areas with differing demographics, no one size fits all. On balance, however, Florida's experience in creating collaborative service vehicles—on both the state and local levels—has definitely been positive. The developmental strategies that have been effective here merit replication (for a replication handbook, see Sherman & Bloom, 1996). The service demands and fiscal environments of our current times truly challenge us. They invite all social services professionals to reach for new heights of creativity and to construct new ways of meeting the needs of the people we are committed to serving.

Achieving inclusion within aging programs for older adults who have yet to attain the age of 60 remains somewhat of a knotty issue. Though individual situations can be circumvented and remedied locally, the issue of age eligibility must be addressed directly. From the results of Project FLAGs, we suggest that criteria for participation in Older Americans Act programs be broadened to include all adults who are functionally appropriate for a particular environment. This should be true whether the disabilities occur in old age or are lifelong. Supports that are more community inclusive must also be created to serve better this new population of people who are growing older. As Project FLAGs illustrated, community inclusion can become a reality when true collaborative services efforts are made.

REFERENCES

Aging and Developmental Disabilities Interagency Effort. (1994). *Mission statement* [Brochure]. Tallahassee, FL: Author.

Alfassa-White, R., & Bloom, P. (1995). *Aging with developmental disabilities: A guide for families.* Miami, FL: University of Miami.

Ansello, E.F. (1996). *Partners III: Testing a model for aging and disabilities inter-system cooperation.* Richmond: Virginia Commonwealth University.

Campbell, P. (1996). *Population projections for States by age, sex, race, and Hispanic origin: 1995 to 2015.* (U.S. Bureau of the Census, Population Division, Report PPL-47). Washington, DC: U.S. Department of Commerce.

LePore, P., & Janicki, M.P. (1997). *The wit to win: How to integrate older persons with developmental disabilities into community aging programs* (3rd rev.). Albany: New York State Office for the Aging.

Manton, K. (1996, August 8). Report on aging: Duke University Center for Demographic Studies. *Charlotte News and Observer*, A17–A18.

Older Americans Act Amendments of 1987, PL 100-175, 42 U.S.C. §§ 3001 *et seq.*

Older Americans Act of 1965, PL 89-73, 42 U.S.C. §§ 3001 *et seq.*

Seltzer, M.M., Krauss, M.W., & Heller, T. (1990, November). Family caregiving over the life course. In M.P. Janicki & M.M. Seltzer (Eds.), *Boston roundtable on research issues and applications in aging and developmental disabilities.* Washington, DC: American Association on Mental Retardation.

Sherman, J., & Bloom, P. (1996). *FLAGs: Project outcomes and recommendations for building community coalitions to serve older adults with developmental disabilities.* Miami, FL: University of Miami.

State of Florida Department of Elder Affairs (DOEA). (1996a). *FLAGs expansion: Project evaluation report.* Tallahassee: Author.

State of Florida Department of Elder Affairs (DOEA). (1996b). *1996–2001 master plan on aging.* Tallahassee: Author.

State of Florida Department of Elder Affairs (DOEA). (1996c, August). *Population projections for Florida.* Paper presented at the meeting of the Florida Consensus Estimating Conference, Tallahassee, FL.

27

Promoting Integrated Services

The Texas Experience

James A. Stone

States have used a variety of methods in striving to provide access to services that specifically support aging and older people with lifelong disabilities and their caregivers (e.g., Bigby, 1994; Janicki, 1993; Turner, 1994). One is the top-down systems change approach, which begins with intersystem efforts at the state level and then transfers efforts to the local level; another is a grass roots intersystems approach that focuses on education and creation of awareness of how each local system provides services and supports. A combination of top-down and bottom-up initiatives seems most logical and effective and has been tried in a number of states (see Ansello & Rose, 1989; Janicki & LePore, 1997; Chapter 26). For example, with the encouragement of the state's unit on aging and developmental disabilities agency, New York tested the feasibility of integrating agency network services on the county level and found general acceptance among those involved (Janicki & LePore, 1997); and Maryland and Virginia tested statewide efforts with top-level memoranda of understanding and advocacy councils, as well as local initiatives to interrelate staff of aging and developmental disabilities services and to develop broad-based coalitions (Ansello, Coogle, & Wood, 1997; Ansello, Wells, & Zink, 1989). These approaches, along with variations used by other states, have led to significant progress since the 1980s in addressing the needs of older adults who are simultaneously confronting aging and disability issues in their lives.

Growing concerns about its increasing population of people who are aging with disabilities or caring for others with disabilities prompted Texas to develop an initiative that would help expand the services options for older Texans with developmental disabilities. In the mid-1990s, the Texas Planning Council for Developmental Disabilities (TPCDD) initiated a 5-year project to develop and implement supports and services to aging and older Texans with developmental disabilities and their families. The Texas Department on Aging (TDoA) became the vehicle for this development. Under an interagency agreement, the TDoA pledged to develop local collaborative systems and supports that would directly benefit people with developmental disabilities who are aging and whose caregivers are aging. The TDoA committed staff and other resources to changing the existing aging and disabilities supports systems so that older adults with disabilities could easily find and obtain needed aging and disabilities services.

THE TEXAS PROJECT

The philosophy of the Texas project reflects a recognition of the ideal support system for the aging adult with developmental disabilities and builds on a foundation of individualized preferences and choices that reflect the person's cultural, environmental, and life experiences. The ideal support system enables the individual to remain active in the neighborhood and the local community for as long as possible without experiencing isolation, abuse, neglect, or loss of control of later-life choices. This allows the ability to communicate, "I want," "I like," and, "I need," or, "I don't want," "I don't like," and, "I don't need!" The community has, in fact, varied resources that may open worlds of opportunity to involve the aging adult with lifelong disabilities, including social, recreational, and leisure activities. Older people with developmental disabilities have demonstrated the ability to grow and learn when provided the chance to participate in self-selecting programs and services that include both formal and informal supports. Their needs are what most people need: homes; medical services; social, recreational, and leisure activities; opportunities for work if desired; friends and family; on-request transportation; and involvement in decisions that affect their futures. Older family caregivers have a different set of needs for supports and services. They need assistance in learning what services are available for both themselves and their family member with developmental disabilities. Older and aging caregivers need to understand a variety of aging-related matters, including wills and trusts, networking, and their child's aging processes, as well as how to gain access to available and appropriate support services and programs.

The approach used in Texas to implement this philosophy involved two major activities. The first was developing an integrated system of services supports to help older Texans with developmental disabilities and their families to have options and choices based on individual needs and preferences reflecting cultural and ethnic life experiences. The second was developing a service system to which these community members could gain access easily from multiple entry points and be assured of receiving assistance from agency staff who were knowledgeable about and responsive to their needs. The model involved four strategies: coalition building, community awareness, interagency training, and needs assessments (Stone, 1998) and set as its goal the development of an integrated services system to which older people with developmental disabilities and older people who are caring for people with developmental disabilities can gain access from single or multiple entry points.

Texas is a state of substantial proportions, with a population age 60 years and older of approximately 2.3 million people, or 14% of the total state population. It has 28 area agencies on aging (AAAs), representing planning and service oversight for older adults all over the state. The AAAs were to be the means of implementing the strategies and attaining the goal in the Texas Project. All of the AAAs have in place core services and staff that can affect the lives of older Texans with developmental disabilities and their older parents, as well as family caregivers who may be responsible for children or grandchildren with developmental disabilities. Support coordination generally is available through their core services. This core includes service coordination, intake and assistance, benefits counseling, and a network of volunteer ombudsmen. These community providers are the first line for coordinating supports and services to what one may consider an "invisible population" of older adults with disabilities. However, to ensure that all of these AAA supports and services were accessible, the Texas Project created and maintained a working partnership with other vital community services and programs. These included the local mental health and mental retardation agencies, human or social services, private providers, and any and all other generic support systems that may be needed on an individual basis at any time. The current service system of the local community, therefore, determined which agencies were available to be involved as members in a coalition or partnership. The Texas model built on this to ensure that working together and sharing information, experiences, and expertise as well as referrals and resources, these agencies developed a working community partnership.

The Texas model built on the available community resources and supports or sought to develop new supports, as necessary, by reaching out to other agencies and initiating interagency activities over several phases. During the initial phase, the model concentrated on four basic foundation activities:

1. Developing ongoing cooperative and collaborative relationships between the aging and the developmental disabilities service agencies and other support services at the local level
2. Identifying community resources and gaps in the supports system and interagency training requirements in the local project areas and developing local plans of collaboration
3. Cross-training key local coalition members to understand and react to the supports needs of older people with developmental disabilities and of older people who are caring for a person with a developmental disability
4. Conducting a local needs assessment for the older adults with developmental disabilities and their families in the local community, which will also identify supports needs and gaps in services delivery

It was not expected that the agencies would begin to provide supports and services to the older population of people with developmental disabilities during the initial phase. Rather, it was assumed that this would result from the natural progression of coalition development. During the second phase, the model focused on continuing to build on the four activities and was expanded to include these functions:

1. Continue ongoing cooperative and collaborative relationships of the work group at the local level.
2. Invite additional public and private advocacy groups to participate in and support the coalition activities and service systems' integration goals.
3. Create an awareness for the key local aging and developmental disabilities providers to learn about individualized permanency plans or person-centered plan-

ning to ensure that the target population has the opportunity to make choices in later life.
4. Develop outreach and intake initiatives to create individual supports plans for older people with developmental disabilities and their family members on an as-needed basis.
5. Provide older adults with developmental disabilities or older family members who are caring for people with developmental disabilities access to existing aging programs (e.g., senior centers, meal sites) and other age-appropriate support services in the local community.
6. Develop volunteer and other generic community resources to assist families to achieve the goals of social supports and financial security for their aging adult children with developmental disabilities. These services may include *pro bono* legal, estate planning, and person-centered planning for the time the caregiving responsibility is no longer provided by the parent or family members.

Expected Outcomes of the Texas Project
Under ideal and well-planned strategic conditions, implementing such an aging and developmental disabilities model should produce the following outcomes:

1. Opportunities will develop for aging and older individuals with developmental disabilities and their families to participate to their full ability in later-life activities and supports to gain access to their community's resources and activities. Retirement, volunteer work, or participation in age-appropriate activities of their choosing are just a few of the options that could be available to this target group.
2. Coalition efforts will improve access to the quality of care for people with developmental disabilities by training care professionals in the needs of both individuals and families.
3. Coalition members, policy makers, and program administrators will be made aware of the unique needs of the aging and older population with developmental disabilities in the state through training, information sharing, and public meetings in which program staff, advocates, aging individuals, and family members express their needs and concerns.
4. Outreach and supports to older families will improve, including underserved minority and rural families who are caring for a relative with developmental disabilities, by focusing on the local aging services systems, disabilities agencies, social services, and the generic resource agencies.
5. Families will receive training, information, and assistance for continued support after death or the inability of the parents to continue day-to-day formal and informal supports. (For example, real estate and family homes are major resources for aging and older people; however, older homeowners nationwide have rarely used the reverse mortgage option to convert their dwelling into income for a fixed time period or life and to stay there, and very few families have made necessary arrangements for futures planning, wills, estate plans, trusts, or advance directives for health care.)
6. Interagency service coordination and service delivery will be supported by establishing working relationships to flow across service systems and enhance access to aging network services and programs for older adults with developmental disabilities.

7. Cross-training should focus on professionals who are working in the fields of aging, developmental disabilities, and other generic services. The training will assist staff to understand the aging processes, needs of aging and older people with developmental disabilities and family caregivers, and how to collaborate to gain access to community programs and resources in a timely way.

It was assumed that at the conclusion of the second phase, implementation of the Texas model would have resulted in a good working relationship among all of the coalition agencies. In practice, when a call was made to one of the participating agencies for assistance or for information by or for an aging Texan with a developmental disability, information would be collected and an intake or referral would be made to begin access to individualized supports and services. It is at this point that additional training of front-line staff may be necessary to keep the effort moving forward, because the model stresses a proactive rather than reactive approach to crisis situations and emergencies. However, knowing that not all events will ever be planned for completely and that the "invisible population" will eventually become visible and need to be provided with new options and choices in later life, a constant renewal and training process is part of the model's functions.

Life Course of the Texas Project
The Texas model was funded by a 5-year, $1 million grant from the TPCDD that was supplemented by $600,000 contributed by the TDoA. To begin this initiative, several preliminary activities were undertaken. First, a statewide steering committee was assembled, made up of key players from the participating agencies (developmental disabilities planning council, state unit on aging, and the state intellectual disabilities authority). Second, a national search was conducted for a statewide project coordinator. Third, a statewide consulting committee was assembled. The members of this committee were given two charges: to contribute their expertise and experience not only in the areas of aging and developmental disabilities but also in other areas that are critical to a well-balanced approach for the project, including self-advocacy skills, insurance matters, financial and estate planning, life planning, and legal issues; and to connect the project with people and entities with influence, such as advocacy agencies, academia, local model programs, and any others interested in serving and supporting this population.

During the initial phase of the project, the steering committee met quarterly, providing input into the goals and objectives of the project. The committee's main activity during this phase was to design and disseminate a request for proposal to the network of the state's 28 AAAs. Each was invited to indicate its interest in participating. To participate, the AAAs had to agree to accomplish the four primary objectives for community development during the early phase of the project, each with a local focus. During the first year, TDoA publicized the aging and developmental disabilities project throughout Texas and nationally and organized a series of orientation and training sessions on aging and disabilities across the state. The statewide project coordinator hired by the TDoA began to provide technical assistance and helped to identify priorities, plans, and activities for each successive year of the project.

After this organizational phase, the TDoA encouraged intersystem exposure by sponsoring a 1-day seminar on aging and disabilities and inviting AAA directors and leaders from the local disabilities communities. A secondary purpose for this meeting was to provide an overview of the application process and to permit the coordinator to provide technical assistance with application development. To encourage attendance at the event, TDoA paid travel expenses of the AAA directors and invited guests from the local disabilities community. The seminar was held in the state capital and included several national experts who are well versed in the development of community-oriented aging and developmental disabilities systems liaisons and cooperative services. The content of the meeting included how other states managed liaisons, the challenges of providing care for individuals with Down syndrome and Alzheimer's dementia, and developing community supports and other program development issues. Time was also set aside for TDoA staff to review the proposals with the AAAs and their guests. Staff reiterated the major components of the proposal and the criteria that would be used in the scoring. The AAAs were then provided with technical assistance with their application efforts. As a result of this meeting, 12 proposals were submitted by the AAAs, 7 of which were funded as demonstration sites during the first year. Five additional AAAs were funded and joined the demonstration project in the second year.

Expectations at the Local Level

The initial seven AAAs functioned as demonstration sites and were given the greatest level of technical assistance and provided with substantial information sharing. To facilitate such a critical foundation, the first year's focus was kept simple and to the point: Each AAA was to raise community awareness, conduct interagency training, and build a local coalition. It was expected that these collaborative efforts would include orientation and training of staff and professionals on aging and developmental disabilities and that they would draw upon state and national experts for assistance. These collaborative meetings were attended by employees of local aging and disabilities agencies and private partners and local stakeholders who were members of the collaborative work group. Other community service provider involved included local disabilities services agencies, independent mental health and intellectual disabilities centers, state schools and hospitals, Texas Rehabilitation Commission regional offices, Independent Living Councils, nursing homes, and individuals from local self-advocacy groups.

TDoA expected that each of these seven awardees would accomplish the four basic objectives in the first year. The AAAs were to develop ongoing cooperative and collaborative relationships between the aging and developmental disabilities service agencies at the local level, identify gaps in the supports system and interagency training requirements in the local project areas and develop local plans of collaboration, orient and cross-train key local aging and developmental disabilities personnel to understand and react to the support needs of aging people with developmental disabilities, and conduct local needs assessment to identify supports needs and gaps in service delivery.

The participating AAAs served as the lead local agency responsible for developing collaborative and cooperative interagency efforts among established community agencies and programs. Together, this local interagency workgroup set out the necessary steps and activities to develop individualized plans that could be used by multiple agencies to assist aging people with disabilities or aging caregivers residing in their areas. These individualized plans offered options and guidance for people in either group (aging with disabilities or aging caregivers) in making appropriate choices in later life. Such options and choices included questions such as, "How can I continue to receive care I need when my parents die?" "Where will I live?" "Who will make decisions about my medical care if I become incapacitated?" These were choices and options that were based on individual needs and preferences and by necessity reflected cultural and ethnic life experiences.

A major product of this individualized planning was the clear identification of gaps, absences, or overlaps in local services and the mechanisms that had to be put in place to address them. Each of the seven projects required some flexibility in developing activities and tasks to ensure successful program operations and outcomes. The ultimate goal for each project was for any person who was aging with a disability or caring for such a person to be able to have easy access to all appropriate aging and disabilities services.

The objectives for the AAAs in subsequent years moved to more complexity. They were to provide supports and open access to services for the target populations, continue ongoing cooperative and collaborative relationships within their local work groups, work with private advocacy groups to support the public agencies and service integration goals, and continue to develop and refine steps to create individual supports plans for aging adults with disabilities and older caregivers that would help them to achieve the highest possible level of independence and social autonomy. It was envisioned that each awardee would also undertake supplementary activities, including 1) mainstreaming older adults with disabilities and older caregivers into the available aging programs (e.g., senior centers, meal sites) and other age-appropriate services in the local community, including the existing disabilities programs, and 2) recruiting volunteers and finding available community resources to assist families in obtaining social supports and a plan for financial security for their aging relatives who have disabilities. This varying of activities specific to each AAA would become a feature of the Texas model.

As the years progressed, the expectations for deliverables were raised. These included functions designed to provide broader supports and access to services, such as continuing the ongoing cooperation and collaboration of the local work group, encouraging private advocacy groups to support the public agencies' service integration goals, and developing more extensive outreach and intake initiatives to create individual supports plans for older people with developmental disabilities and their family members. The agencies also developed volunteer and other generic community resources that assisted families in achieving the goals of social supports and financial security for their aging adult children with developmental disabilities.

During the first 2 years of the project, a total of 12 AAA-oriented subprojects were funded as part of the statewide initiative. Each participating AAA received $25,000 during the first year and $12,500 during the second year. This funding was subsequently changed to 2 years of level funding of $18,750 annually. Funding during the third, fourth, and fifth years was to be the responsibility of the AAAs, and no state project monies were provided. Participating AAAs were told that local funds would have to be used for successive years. However, the experiences of the local projects showed that continued funding into the third and fourth years was necessary.

The AAAs approached the project in different ways. Six AAAs chose to use a staff person or hire a person to coordinate the project from within the AAA. The other six subcontracted the project activities and coordination to other local agencies that had experience in developmental disabilities services. The latter included one "triad leadership" with administrative responsibilities shared by three agencies (the AAA, a rehabilitation agency, and an established community disabilities services agency).

After the first 2 years, seven of the projects were in position to begin "opening the doors of supports and services" in the community. Two years of working on the project objectives provided the foundation for continuing the working relationships when requests for access and assistance were received. The second wave of five projects achieved similar results subsequently.

What the Area Agencies on Aging Accomplished

Twelve of Texas's 28 AAAs participated in the initial phase of the project. The 12 were the Alamo AAA and Bexar County AAA in San Antonio; Central Texas Council of Governments AAA in Belton; Coastal Bend AAA in Corpus Christi; Dallas AAA in Dallas; East Texas AAA in Kilgore; AAA of the Panhandle in Amarillo; North Central Texas AAA in Arlington; AAA of South East Texas in Port Arthur; South Plains Association of Governments AAA in Lubbock; AAA of Tarrant County in Fort Worth; and the Texoma AAA in Sherman. These AAAs represented a wide geographical area with broad cultural diversity and a rural-urban mix. What follows is a brief summary of accomplishments by the 12 projects during the first 24 months.

The 12 projects worked to develop and maintain coalition work groups in each AAA. Consequently, in each AAA region was established a formal structure of interagency members who participated in three subcommittees to build local experience and expertise in supporting aging Texans with developmental disabilities and their caregivers. The projects leveraged public and private monies to assist in their efforts. More than $250,000 was generated as matching funds, including local grants and cash contributions. For example, the Central Texas AAA received $10,000 in community block grant funding and $8,000 from local county governments, the Bexar County AAA received a $10,000 start-up initiative from the local United Way, and the Texoma AAA worked with Austin College to become a research site and a participant in an international study on the effect of vitamin E on aging people with Down syndrome.

Generally, the AAAs interacted purposefully with other community organizations, as illustrated by the growing number of agencies that participated in the local coalitions. Approximately 1,500 community agencies received information about the local projects and were invited to the coalition start-up meetings, and overall the 12 projects included more than 400 agencies as working partners. These partnerships included private and public direct services agencies, local government, staff of elected officials, colleges and universities, individuals with disabilities and advocacy groups, and parents and other family caregivers. Data from the Texas Department of Mental Health and Mental Retardation estimated that approximately 10,000 people with developmental disabilities older than 50 years may have been and most probably will be affected by these projects.

The AAAs reported a new willingness to work together and share agency information and expertise. Staff at the agencies involved began to understand how other agencies operated and what services they provided. As examples, the Central Texas AAA reported that the local mental health and intellectual disabilities agency, which had previously taken up to 90 days to conduct referral evaluations, now completed these in less than a week after this was described at a coalition meeting as a barrier to having services coordinated. In this AAA region, members of the coalition participated in developing local transportation plans that included the needs of people with disabilities. The Texoma AAA supported the creation of a new chapter of The Arc (a parent-based voluntary membership organization) when its local coalition project identified a lack of advocacy groups in their community.

Working products developed by the 12 projects included community resource directories specific to the needs of the aging and developmental disabilities population and training manuals for interagency cross-training and for family financial planning. Other products included a marketing plan for services by one AAA and numerous seminars and training activities within the others. Some of the agencies developed a separate identity for their projects, using special letterhead stationery and logos as recommended by Ansello et al. (1997).

Whereas urban projects were able to take advantage of diverse and concentrated media outlets in their outreach activities, rural projects needed to be more creative to deal with their absence. Rural efforts by the Panhandle and South Plains AAAs focused on using the Rural Electric Cooperative. Information about these two projects was inserted in a monthly magazine circulated to more than 42,000 customers living in rural homes. Twelve families responded by mailing back a postcard requesting specific information about the projects. This illustrated that for dissemination in rural areas, an innovative type of outreach informed large numbers and stimulated some readership to respond, but the return was very small and other methods should be considered. What was accomplished by the Dallas AAA is a good example of how urban-oriented AAAs handled information dissemination. This metropolitan AAA managed to publish two news articles in the local paper, and its staff participated in a local radio talk show with a large listenership. Corpus Christi, a more moderate-size city on Texas's Gulf Coast, also succeeded in having two articles about its project appear in the local paper, resulting in community response. Other AAAs used the press with success.

To help with statewide dissemination, the TDoA generated a number of products, including an informational brochure, a project guideline for new projects referencing materials and efforts from previous projects, and a training module on aging and developmental disabilities for the TDoA ombudsman volunteers.

LESSONS LEARNED

At the midpoint of the project, the sites were asked what was working in their projects. The following are their responses: acceptance and recognition of issues, people and agencies have been brought together, education and training on developmental disabilities, opportunity to expand the information and referral components to include developmental disabilities, increased participation validated integration of senior centers, developmental disabilities issues included in advocacy services, allowing individual projects to develop differently according to local needs allows players to "own" the project and enables the overall project to develop many more products, funneling project through AAAs brought in the caregivers and stimulated future planning for both caregivers and providers, hiring a consultant to facilitate projects, training, shared products, overall structure was helpful to play against, raising agency and community awareness, building a coalition, designating as coordinator a person with a disability, involving consumers at the front end, educating and involving elected officials, leveraging local funding, cross-training and educating coalition members about AAA resources, understanding other agencies' procedures, educating the medical community on medication issues, including graduate students in the coalition, and building awareness and utilization of Council of Governments resources.

At the same time, these projects were asked what they still needed to do to become successful models. Of the 2 dozen issues they identified, they judged the following six as most important: long-term funding, automatic referral to AAA for eligible clients, interagency sharing of client information, postplanning implementation funds, effective outreach to rural areas, and state-level data by county.

The Texas experience produced a number of key lessons, which are described in the following subsections.

Focused Leadership

The key element in the success of these projects was the involvement of the executive directors of the AAAs and their collective willingness to take on the challenges of coalition building and systems change to serve aging Texans with developmental disabilities and their older family caregivers. The executive directors' understanding of the problems and the need to assist this invisible population was central to the success of the coalitions and accomplishing the goals and objectives of their project. Furthermore, under the directors, each of the projects had a coordinator; just as the statewide project coordinator hired by TDoA served the role that Janicki (1993) called the "spark," assisting and stimulating groups across the state, the local project coordinators worked hard in meeting the objectives and developing local expertise in the community and sparked the community to participate.

Access to an Experienced Consultant

Having the statewide project coordinator serve as a readily available consultant provided the project sites with a view from outside their community and the state as to what had previously been developed in other parts of the United States. This enabled the project to adapt materials and resources to the local environment and model their project from their community's resources. These projects were able to obtain technical assistance via fax, telephone, and e-mail. The statewide project coordinator visited the local projects at least twice a year and more often when requested. The regular contact and on-site assistance he maintained with each site proved invaluable.

Flexibility

Having the flexibility to develop the local model of access on the basis of available resources and supports services provided each site with choices and helped to ensure that their future consumers' options were individualized. Sites did not have to seek components directed by a specific model and were encouraged to have the coalition agencies and the people with disabilities determine what their model would be. Each AAA had the basic aging services components of intake and assistance, service coordination, and benefits counseling and of possible outreach through the volunteer ombudsman programs. The other supports services that may be used were determined by which agencies were operating within the service region.

Simple Budgets

Keeping the annual budget simple allowed flexibility at the local levels. From among the nonapplicants, only one AAA considered the amount of funds available to be insufficient, giving this as its reason for not applying for the project. After the project began, it was noted that the funding for the first 2 years needed to be restructured; this was due to the lengthy start-up time that each site experienced before being able to gain access to funds. It was also observed that having a third year of funding that focused on start-up costs to gain access to the community's supports and services could benefit the projects and be a catalyst for leveraging other funding sources that are available. In the third year, the TDoA awarded each site $11,600 to continue the project efforts of community services and supports access. Originally, it was planned that each site would be self-supporting by this point.

Sufficient Funding

Funding available to provide the projects the initiative to pay for key people's time and effort, to subcontract a portion of the funding with other agencies or acquire or develop materials and provide information, or to have outside experts give technical assistance when needed was key to successful coalition building and community agency participation. The $1,550 made available monthly for the first 2 years was found to be the minimum level of funding necessary to provide the projects the foundation and tools to become successful.

BARRIERS DISCOVERED

State Politics

During the period that the Texas Project was being implemented, the Texas Sunset Commission recommended eliminating a number of state departments and consolidating them into one Department of Long-Term Care. Time and effort to respond to these recommendations affected the continued cooperation within local work groups, because many of the agencies were projected to have changes and different responsibilities. Coalition members were less ready to commit resources when the future of their agencies and their jobs were unclear. These activities held up the community team building because of the uncertainty over who would be working for whom and where and how these agencies might be restructured. Certainly, this is a variable that rarely is under the control of a project; however, such occurrences should be taken into account with planning the length and activities of a project.

Deadlines

Fifteen of the state's AAAs did not submit proposals to participate in this project because the request for proposal cycle coincided with the end of the fiscal year for AAAs and the workload requirements associated with submitting their annual reports. The proposals were due at the same time that the AAAs had to resubmit their annual plans and proposals for the next fiscal year and close out the current year. Despite the concerns raised by the AAAs, the administrators at the state unit on aging declined to change the due date, thus eliminating several viable AAAs from the competition. Flexibility and understanding of local agency workload requirements should also be a consideration.

No Common Tool

Efforts were made, but with little success, to develop a standardized client intake form that could be used by all providers that were participating in the project. Two of the projects did work-up and began to use a standard referral form that is now being used by their agencies. Often, such an effort is time-consuming and fraught with political considerations. Experience has shown that the adoption of a universally applicable instrument usually is most palatable when instituted from the top down with consultation from local users. This was attempted in this case, but because of other vagaries it was not possible within the scope of this project.

Unknown Number of Potential Consumers

It proved difficult to provide local projects with accurate and concise data on the number of people who may be aging and who may have a developmental disability, because the state's data systems did not capture such data by disability and age (see Chapter 1). The Texas Department on Mental Health and Mental Retardation was able to produce data on the number of older adults (age 50 and older) in residential programs and receiving services from day services agencies. However, these data were not universal and reflected only an active service population. Furthermore, data from the state's Medicare/Medicaid agency were not collected in a way that could determine the number and type of services being provided on the basis of age and disabilities. Such data deficiency issues are always a problem in any such undertaking and may present a challenge in situations in which local planners need viable estimates for projecting workload and resource allocation. Alternative estimate methods are in place (see Janicki, 1993, and Chapter 1 for varying means for arriving at such estimates).

Grandparents as Caregivers

A number of the projects discovered an unanticipated population of caregivers, namely, grandparents who were responsible for grandchildren with developmental disabilities. Other projects elsewhere have reported similar findings (see, e.g., Janicki, McCallion, Force, Bishop, & LePore, 1998). Although the projects had not prepared special outreach or training activities for these grandparents, the presence of grandparents as caregivers offers an added source of help for community living. The issue of grandparents as caregivers is one that deserves more attention and thoughtful investigation.

Leadership Turnover

Staff changing jobs and leaving positions of importance within the project's domain affected the project at both the local and state levels. In the first year, two AAA executive directors resigned and another was reassigned to other duties. In the second year, another two executive directors chose to retire. All of the projects continued moving forward because these sites had subcontracted with outside agencies to manage the day-to-day operations of the local effort. However, long delays in implementation were observed in two sites where the project coordinators resigned; it took 6 months before new administrators were assigned or hired. These long delays affected the continuation of the local coalitions and required some rededication and re-education on the project's goals and objectives and on how access to community supports and service delivery was being shaped locally. At the state level, there was a nearly 50% turnover in staff members who oversaw the Texas Project. Turnover in top management and in local project coordinators hampered the development of the Texas Project. In the most dramatic example, one AAA had four coordinators over the course of the project's life. Such turnover obviously affects continuity and commitment but also reflects the reality under which any effort, such as this one, must operate.

Oversight Complications

Over the course of this project, there was a complete turnover among the individuals at TPCDD and TDoA who were responsible for overseeing the Texas Project. A key person who was overseeing this project within the state unit on aging was promoted and took on new responsibilities within her agency; there was also a change in staff at the developmental disabilities council. In addition, there was a change in the statewide project coordinator who was hired to implement and oversee the project. A decision within the main administrative agency to replace the statewide project coordinator with someone from within "the system" was made at the end of the third year and caused a significant disruption in the administrative scope and structure of the project.

CONCLUSIONS

The Texas Project, using a statewide approach for local networking and allocating community responsibility for a target population, proved to be a productive exercise in community development. Under the model, the state unit on aging and the state's developmental disabilities planning council collaborated on a project designed to change a system of existing services. This aging and developmental disabilities project was unusual in that funding and responsibility were given directly to the AAAs. These entities had to initiate the leadership and invite other community agencies to participate in enhancing the later-life years for older adults with developmental disabilities and their older caregivers. There was a commitment to reasonable funding over multiple years to develop access or "one stop entry." The interest to make the necessary changes was demonstrated by a significant number of the state's AAAs. Although expectations were for a complete statewide involvement in the aging and developmental disabilities project, it was found that this required more than a 4-year time frame to get all of the AAAs involved and working at the same level. However, the main objective—to make a difference in the lives of people who have developmental disabilities and who are aging—was achieved. None of the areas will ever be the same. New opportunities have been opened for aging adults with lifelong disabilities and for family caregivers to exercise options and make choices on the basis of personal preferences, experiences, and needs and to be involved in doing what they want to do in their homes and local communities.

REFERENCES

Ansello, E.F., Coogle, C.L., & Wood, J.B. (1977). *Partners: Building inter-system cooperation in aging and developmental disabilities.* Richmond: Virginia Commonwealth University, Virginia Center on Aging.

Ansello, E.F., & Rose, T. (1989). *Aging and lifelong disabilities: Partnership for the twenty-first century.* Palm Springs, CA: Elvirita Lewis Foundation.

Ansello, E.F., Wells, A.I., & Zink, M.J. (1989, November). *The Partners Project: Research and training on aging and developmental disabilities.* Paper presented at the Annual Scientific Meeting of the Gerontological Society of America, Minneapolis, MN.

Bigby, C. (1994). A demographic analysis of older people with intellectual disability registered with Community Services Victoria. *Australia and New Zealand Journal of Developmental Disabilities, 19,* 1–10.

Janicki, M.P. (1993). *Building the future: Planning and community development in aging and developmental disabilities* (2nd ed.). Albany: New York State Office of Mental Retardation and Developmental Disabilities.

Janicki, M.P., McCallion, P., Force, L., Bishop, K., & LePore, P. (1998). Area agency on aging outreach and assistance for households with older caregivers of an adult with a developmental disability. *Journal of Aging and Social Policy, 10,* 13–36.

LePore, P., & Janicki, M.P. (1997). *The wit to win: How to integrate older persons with developmental disabilities into community aging programs* (3rd ed.). Albany: New York State Office for the Aging.

Stone, J.A. (1998, November). *Developing supports and services for aging and older Texans with developmental disabilities and the aging family/caregivers.* Paper presented at the annual scientific meeting of the Gerontological Society of America, Philadelphia.

Turner, K.W. (1994). Modeling community inclusion for older adults with developmental disabilities. *Southwest Journal on Aging, 10*(1–2), 13–18.

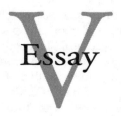

Essay

Bridging Madison County

Christine N. Sears

A few years ago, I was involved in several efforts to bridge or link the aging and disability networks in my county. At the time, I was working for the local area agency on aging. I have since gone to work for the local Arc chapter. My story speaks to two particular efforts we undertook to help older adults with intellectual disabilities and their families. Madison County, where I work, can be characterized as a fairly rural county with a population of approximately 70,000 people. In the late 1980s and early 1990s, when I was working for the county aging office, we became aware of a number of older county residents with an intellectual disability. We were also aware that there were virtually no, or only limited, programs that could accommodate older people with a life-long disability. For example, no formal retirement programs were in place and we did not have any special initiatives to target this population whose disability was compounded by the effects of aging.

To begin to deal with this deficit, we developed a local team that consisted of various human services agencies, including the local area agency on aging, the local Arc, the state's developmental disabilities services office, the Retired and Senior Volunteer Program, the county health department, and a number of other service provider and volunteer organizations. Together, we worked out a plan that would help integrate older adults with a developmental disability into the available generic aging services, which included adult day programs, senior nutrition programs, and some other services already available to older people in our rural county. With limited funding options, we undertook a creative approach that focused mostly on shared services, the use of volunteers and organized training on aging and developmental disabilities for the team's organizations. We soon realized that the needs of the aging population and the needs of adults with developmental disabilities were similar. Many of the older adults served by the area agency on aging were experiencing an increase in late-life disabilities—we saw a number who had a stroke or who were affected by debilitating conditions such as dementia or arthritis. The same was true for those older people with developmental disabilities whom we knew. Because their needs were so similar, it made sense to blend the two networks' (aging and developmental disabilities) older populations.

The blending, or integration, of senior citizens with disabilities into community programs for older adults was successful. To begin, we used a gradual approach to allow for an acceptance period between the two groups. Volunteers of similar age were asked to be companions for their age-peers with a lifelong disabilities and to help introduce them to these new programs and new friends. Soon, seniors with a developmental disability were participating in many community-based programs that were typical of the aging population. They went on day trips, played bingo, attended adult day programs and senior nutrition programs—and they loved it. Most important, they were participating in retirement programs. We were able to get the two networks, aging and developmental disability, to work together and help create a retirement program where there once was none. Other needs were identified. The one major need in a rural county is accessible transportation. The Arc had a fleet of vehicles that were fully accessible. Thus, we were able to get the two networks again to work together to meet an unmet need. The importance of this effort was magnified when the Arc was asked to transport an older couple to a doctor's office. The husband had sustained a severe stroke, and the wife could not drive and she desperately wanted to help her husband who could no longer communicate. She called a private ambulance but found that the service could transport only her husband, not her. Upset by this, she called us at the area agency on aging and asked for help. We, in turn, called the Arc, which was more than willing to transport the couple to the doctor's office.

On a local level, the two networks generally worked together as a team. There were some minor problems along the way, but nothing we could not settle. However, one major problem that vexed us was triggered by the issue of funding. The state Office for the Aging questioned which agency (aging or developmental disability) was funding people with developmental disabilities at the county's nutrition programs. They also wanted to know who was attending the senior nutrition program and who had a developmental disability and resided in state-supported homes. Federal regulations for the nutrition program require only that an individual be age 60 or older. Under the program's guidelines, a confidential "suggested" donation is asked from all program participants. No one is refused a meal because he or she cannot pay for the meal. For some reason, the Office for the Aging wanted us to charge back the actual cost of the meal to the developmental disability agencies whose adults were coming to the meal sites. Not only did this charge-back exceed the daily allotment for meals for those agencies, but it would have been cheaper for the participants to go out to lunch at a local diner. It would have been prohibitively expensive for adults with a developmental disability to attend the program and even perhaps have been a violation of the Older Americans Act, which governs the program. Tensions developed between the two networks that had been working so well together. It resulted in the Arc's considering to charge the actual cost of transporting someone for the area agency on aging, which would have been prohibitively expensive. Everything that we had worked for was in jeopardy.

Both the sharing of services on a local level and meeting genuine needs were being threatened. It was extremely important that the team not let this challenge go unattended. Letters were written, telephone calls were made, and visits to the state's Office for the Aging took place—all advocating for our program and the people whose needs we were trying to meet. Our efforts were successful, for soon the questions from the state Office for the Aging dissipated and we were able to resume our program. However, our team always remained attentive and prepared in case this issue were ever raised again. Such issues of funding are a constant challenge, as our other effort illustrates.

As I mentioned, obtaining services in a rural county can be a challenge. A year or two later, we undertook another project involving adults with disabilities. The state's Office of Mental Retardation and Developmental Disabilities had identified an initiative that it wanted to undertake in a select number of counties. It was linked to a significant unmet need—that of older parents who had adult children with a developmental disability living with them and not receiving services. Under this initiative, we received a small grant to assist in locating and helping these older caregivers and to help them obtain services for their adult children.

Historically, many parents from the "Depression Era" generation or even older had little or no services to aid them as they raised their children with a disability at home. More recently, the state system has improved and is now providing services for people with disabilities and their families. Institutions are closed or closing, and services are community based and consumer driven. However, many of these older caregivers still fear the "old way" and reject help from the developmental disability network. It was thought that the area agency on aging could help attract these older parents and assist them with obtaining available services for their adult child. This approach would reduce their fears and at the same time educate them about the community-based services that were available. Our county office for the aging was asked to identify these parents, develop a trusting relationship with them, and then bring in the developmental disability agency to provide services. It all sounded so simple. We identified a number of such families by getting the word out in creative ways—we used churches, hairdressers, nutrition programs, doctor's offices, and neighbors, all of whom were asked whether they knew of anyone who was caring for an adult with a developmental disability.

One of the concerns of the area agency on aging was the terminology we used or the need to be "politically correct." It was decided that it was more important to be understood than to be politically incorrect. Older caregivers had trouble understanding the term "developmentally disabled," when many years ago the term "retarded" was acceptable. Therefore, announcements that included the words "retarded" or "mentally retarded" were used to help these parents know what we were talking about. The next step after identifying the family was to develop a trusting relationship. This was crucial to the success of this program. It could take up to a year or more to develop this trust. It was also very important that once trust was established and the disabilities provider was brought in that the parents see results in an expeditious manner.

Once the county aging office identified the families, contact was made with the local developmental disability provider. However, the problem of determining eligibility for state-funded services soon became an issue. We believed that it was important that the area agency on aging not make the determination as to whether someone has a developmental disability. We had expertise on the aging process, but not with disabilities. Yet we were placed in the role of gatekeeper in terms of the eligibility issue. To make a referral, we have to indicate that the adult has a developmental disability. But in many cases, a previously made determination of a developmental disability could not be found or had not been made. Local records, particularly in rural areas, may not show whether a developmental disability existed before the age of 22. In some cases, the individual with a developmental disability was old and had outlived his or her parents. In one case, a man with a developmental disability lived on his own and the community took care of him, buying his groceries, helping him manage money, and fixing meals for him. He had no records that were easily accessible and would document a lifelong disability. Determining whether a developmental disability existed seemed to be a tedious process; it required much research and for the parents or family members was intrusive because it forced them to reveal personal information. This was frustrating to us at the area agency on aging because the sole requirement to receive our services was that a person be age 60 or older.

Funding for the project came from the state. The program required a full-time staff person to find and work with the families. To help the families, we needed to maintain continuity, which meant continued funding and support for this program. It was believed that these older parents, who believed the system let them down so many years ago, should not be let down again. But our worst fears came true. About a year into the project, the state cut the funding completely. The staff person who was hired to run this program was moved to another department, and the families were at risk of being left alone. The county aging office did everything it could to advocate for funds to keep the program running. Eventually, we thought we found a solution: use of the Medicaid waiver. However, this created another set of problems. The paperwork for waiver funding was so time consuming that an evaluation was done to determine whether it was cost-effective to continue the program. Although formally the program ended, the awareness that was created from this project continued.

Certainly, one lesson learned from these experiences is that the reality of funding often interferes with the good intentions of providing a needed service at the local level. State regulations can often impinge on common sense and make the bridging of services between two different networks a difficult challenge. Moreover, the most frustrating part of providing a service to people in need is the "politics" that seem to intervene everywhere. Everything can change with the wave of the electorate to either "pro" or "con" or through the whims of a bureaucrat. There are years when funding seems plentiful, and there are times when funding is cut back or eliminated. We found that sharing services was cost-effective and met an unmet need. What worked in our county was demonstrating a unified front and having two different networks working together and meeting a need. But trying to maintain a needed service at the local level is difficult when funding is controlled elsewhere. It is a fickle process, but when one is willing to deal with the frustration, it is well worth it when the goal is to improve the lives of people in need.

VI

ASSESSING THE PRESENT, DESIGNING THE FUTURE

28

Supports for Community Living

Evolution of an Aging with Lifelong Disabilities Movement

Matthew P. Janicki and Edward F. Ansello

> Ageing is about life, not just the continuation of life statistically, but life as an ongoing endeavor, engaging change, solving new problems, growing, learning, creating and sharing. (Alvarez, 1999, p. 21)

Movements have a life history and a trajectory. Aging with lifelong disabilities is a movement in that it has a body of opinion that is shared by a number of people and that is expressed in words and actions. A movement is an impetus toward new development. This final chapter presents an opportunity to step back from the detail-rich chapters that have preceded it, to reflect on both the significant developments that have encouraged this movement and the prospects for the maturing field of aging and lifelong disabilities. Like all histories, the history of this movement is one of events and individuals. Like all projections, prospects may or may not be realized. We acknowledge the limitations of this reflection, especially the inability to be both concise and exhaustive in our commentary. It is important, however, to recognize the movement's history and the big picture or *Zeitgeist* that influenced and will likely further shape its stages. The following sections represent our assessments of 1) the history of the aging with lifelong disabilities movement, 2) the continuing evolution of aging with lifelong disabilities, 3) some policy implications of increasing numbers of older adults with lifelong disabilities, and 4) the three stages of contemporary society, a conceptual analysis of large, mostly demographic changes in society since approximately 1960 and loosely correlated changes in the field of aging and lifelong disabilities.

A HISTORY

Approximately 40 years ago, what was probably the first article on aging and intellectual disabilities appeared. Gunnar Dybwad, a respected authority and advocate for people with intellectual disabilities, described the emergence of adults and their aging as a "new social phenomenon," noting both an increase in their life spans and their greater visibility in the community (Dybwad, 1962). He proposed a continuous program of public education and a systematic expansion of services as the best strategies for improved and continued acceptance. He referenced Tarjan, who asked in his 1959 presidential address to the precursor of the American Association on Mental Retardation whether the adult with an intellectual disability is not

> Entitled to the same benefits as any other unemployed adult or aged individual? Recreational, church, and other community programs make no special provisions for him and he is forgotten as soon as he is unable to participate in the usual activities. While at home, health resources are also often denied him. Should we not make every effort to support him or render him special services at home, in his own community, among his family members and friends? (Tarjan, 1959, p. 10)

Dybwad raised a number of public policy issues that were relevant to this emerging group of work-age adults, including their opportunities for work, community participation, and socialization, while recognizing their fragility, for they faced risks posed by the illness or death of older parents and by the dangers of losing the supports of family and friends. However, even in Dybwad's enlightened report, his focus was on work-age adults (perhaps extending to those in their 50s) and their needs, and not on the aging as this term is interpreted today. When Dybwad revisited this topic in the foreword to Herr and Weber's (1999) text on aging and rights, he noted that the definition of aging now represents a different perspective over the life course and commented that "today, the picture is far brighter. With improvements in health care, human services, and legally based supports and public attitudes, more and more individuals with lifelong disabilities are not just surviving, but thriving in their later years" (Herr & Weber, 1999, p. xv). He recognized what many in the field now see, namely, that, like all who grow old, aging adults with lifelong disabilities face a myriad of opportunities and risks and that their lengthening life expectancy poses questions for each individual and "brings new puzzles to a group once falsely thought of as 'eternal children'" (Dybwad, 1999, p. xvii). The line from Dybwad's earlier comments to his recent appraisals was drawn by the aging with lifelong disabilities movement.

The late 1970s and the 1980s brought to light the challenges of aging for people with intellectual and other developmental disabilities. Several major reports in the United States (Schalock, 1987; Segal, 1978; Sweeney & Wilson, 1979) foreshadowed much of what we do and are concerned with today. Segal (1978) identified a number of now-familiar aging-related needs, including transportation, counseling, diagnostic assessments, adult activities (including vocational training and employment), financial assistance, residential placement, and information and referral services, and noted that there were clear gaps in service provision in both health and social services. He voiced other concerns, such as needs for sexual and spiritual expression, personal stability, and coping with feelings resulting from death and dying experiences. Segal (1978) posed several questions that were presented to the field as challenges for further inquiry:

1. Do people with developmental disabilities tend to age more quickly than do other people in the general population?
2. Does residing in the community rather than in an institution prolong life?
3. Does group home living encourage infantilization and dependency?
4. Is coordination of community services possible given the need for organizational territoriality and boundary maintenance?
5. How can the right to privacy and human decency be guaranteed to older people with developmental disabilities who are living in institutional environments?
6. How can people with developmental disabilities best be prepared for the aging process?

In the often-cited report *Double Jeopardy: The Plight of Aging and Aged Developmentally Disabled Persons in Mid-America,* Sweeney and Wilson (1979) compiled chapters by workers who were experienced in the aging-related issues of that time. Sweeney (1979) cited the dearth of available information about aging or aged people with developmental disabilities; he recognized the problems of extrapolating prevalence estimates on the old from those available on children and of not having useful information about differential longevity. Part of his contribution to addressing these deficits was undertaking a study that examined the questions of estimating numbers of services recipients who were older, defining services being provided, identifying needed services, and identifying barriers to service provision. His study's results were disappointing; many agencies reported having little or no contact with older adults or, if services were being provided, little age-specific attention. Sweeney characterized older adults as "invisible clientele," being virtually unserved by mainstream disability agencies, attributing this to what we now term "ageism" and "handicappism" (i.e., pervasive discrimination against older adults and people with disabilities). He reported a lack of consensus on what was considered "aging" and interpreted this to be a boundless barrier to agencies in focusing on this group; he found the lack of specificity in federal statutes, especially the precursor versions of the Developmental Disabilities Bill of Rights Act of 1987 (PL 100-146) and the Older Americans Act of 1965 (PL 89-73), to be particularly troublesome obstacles to agencies in assuming responsibility for the development and provision of aging-related services.

As the number of known older adults with disabilities in a variety of care systems grew, the 1980s brought forth several state efforts to investigate this phenomenon, both as planning and service development exercises (Janicki, 1993). Examples include dedicated studies in Indiana (Hawkins, Eklund, Garza, Garza, & DiOrio, 1987), Maryland (Rose & Ansello, 1987), Mississippi (Cotten, 1987), and New York (Puccio, Janicki, Otis, & Rettig, 1983). Each produced a report and recommended a plan of action to address their state's population of adults with disabilities and their particular aging-related issues. Consistency of identified needs and actions characterized these four plans, and they were emulated by other states and jurisdictions around the world. These first investigations generally involved state-level task forces that were charged to examine definition issues, identify needed services, explore services being provided, determine what services needed to be organized, and identify barriers to services provision, be they structural, programmatic, financial, or attitudinal. Overall, the plans began with attempts to address definition issues (e.g., age criteria, disabilities involved, degree of impairment), because no federal guidance was apparent. Although there were variations in age criteria, there was general consensus that "middle age" was the starting

point for aging-related concerns and services. Although there was considerable variation on when middle age occurs, most adopted 55 or 60 as the starting point of old age.
However, interstate consistency was absent, because services under the Older
Americans Act, the only relevant federal legislation in effect at the time that included
an age criterion for eligibility, were not commonly being used by people with disabilities. At that time, the states had not adopted uniform definitions of their service populations; some used the federal developmental disabilities definition, others limited
eligibility to people with intellectual disabilities, whereas still others used some combination. States also had not made community-dwelling adults targets for service provision because of a preoccupation with deinstitutionalization.

Once definition issues were identified, generally necessary to determine the scope
and structure of the population being considered (i.e., age criterion, definition of disability, extent of inclusion for numerical assessment), the states were able to undertake
some form of demographic analysis. If they had registry or data systems in place, they
came up with numbers of some certainty as to who was receiving services and where
they were. Others, lacking such data systems, relied on approximations or best estimates often derived from general surveys of service providers. The absence of clear
delineations of the service population vexed these early investigations. Mississippi's
plan noted that "it is impossible to determine the exact number of individuals who fall
in the category of 'elderly mentally handicapped'" (Cotten, 1987, p. 15). The Indiana,
Maryland, and New York projects derived numbers from their state databases or reg-
istries and extrapolated reasoned projections for the potential service population. The
phenomenon of earlier aging among some adults with intellectual disabilities, especially with Down syndrome, aggravated age criterion consensus. As Indiana's report
observed, there was a need to reexamine eligibility criteria "to allow individuals who
are under 60 to receive needed services related to the aging process" (Hawkins et al.,
1987, p. 23).

With regard to the identification of service needs, service agency capabilities, and
potential for overcoming barriers to meeting the needs, the early state plans were more
on target, almost prescient. They stated that the needs of older people with lifelong disabilities were the same as the basic needs of older people, such as a place to live, financial resources, a range of in-home supports, health and medical services, transportation,
and a day service or place to go for continued activities and involvement. They identified deficits in state financing, availability of general services, and provision of cross-
services between the disabilities and aging systems. They also recognized the critical
importance of educating support staff—that is, cross-training personnel in the aging
network for work with people with disabilities and cross-training personnel in the disabilities system for work with people who are aging. Issues that seemed unresolved
were housing and the use of nursing facilities for long-term care. They acknowledged
the inadequacies of nursing facilities for people with lifelong disabilities but saw few
solutions other than continued new development of costly alternative housing options.
Furthermore, they recognized deficits in existing health care provision; difficulties in
obtaining appropriate geriatric care assessments and medical interventions in light of
these deficits; the need for a more coordinated system of services, appropriately linking
the disabilities and aging networks around the needs of older adults with lifelong disabilities; and the needs of their families and caregivers.

The difficulties of older adults with lifelong disabilities in gaining access to services
within the aging network generally were perceived as impediments to their full use of

the community. The Mississippi plan captured the dilemma that older people with life-long disabilities face when it noted that

> It is true that all individuals 60 years or age and above are entitled to services provided by the aging network. It is also true that there is hesitation on the part of many providers within that network to provide services to individuals who are diagnosed as mentally retarded or developmentally disabled due partly to their lack of training and experience with this population, as well as the myths held by other recipients of their services toward persons so diagnosed. (Cotten, 1987, p. 6)

It was partly this challenge of bridging these two networks that led in 1987 to the organization of the Wingspread Conference on Aging and Lifelong Disabilities, where senior administrators from the state units on aging and the state intellectual and developmental disabilities authorities from across the United States were brought together to discuss issues of common concern and to "assist states in planning their responses to the current and emerging needs of older citizens with lifelong disabilities" (Ansello & Rose, 1989, p. 1). Ansello, in the report that resulted from this conference, encouraged an aging and disabilities partnership, noting that to "develop policy, to plan and to manage programs and opportunities, professionals in the two systems of developmental disabilities and aging must work together" (1989, p. 13). He noted that the two systems were continually being drawn together by the evolving status of their clienteles and that states must seize the chance to read the differences between the two systems not as barriers but as opportunities to broaden their collective expertise and respond to the needs of older adults, both with and without disabilities.

The 1987 Wingspread Conference served as the springboard for many new state and federal efforts and changes in attitudes at both the local and national levels. In 1987, the first of several relevant amendments to the Older Americans Act (PL 100-175) was passed by Congress, enabling older adults with lifelong disabilities to be full recipients of the services provided by states and localities under the Act. The Developmental Disabilities Bill of Rights Act was also amended at this time and included new and far-reaching provisions that significantly expanded the roles of the state developmental disabilities councils, protection and advocacy agencies, and the university affiliated programs (UAPs) with regard to aging. Noteworthy was the provision that expanded the charge of the UAPs to develop aging-related programs and initiatives and to train new personnel, conduct research and service demonstrations, and generally expand the base of knowledge in this area.

These new legislative provisions and the expanding attention being given by states to aging led to a period of progressive development of specialty services. These provisions also stimulated interest in the research community and the development of networks of workers, advocates, and others who wanted to broaden what was known about this topic. In 1990, the first of a growing number of research-based meetings on aging with intellectual and developmental disabilities was held in Boston, Massachusetts. The Boston Roundtable helped provide an international forum for the synthesis of existing knowledge and produced an agenda for research that was to help guide service design and international research activities for many years (Janicki & Seltzer, 1991). Seltzer and Janicki (1991) noted the conceptual and practical changes in the field since the late 1970s and early 1980s. For example, older age as a distinct life stage was by 1990 accepted as a norm for people with intellectual and developmental disabilities, the infrastructure of programs and services had begun to emerge to accommodate the needs of older adults with lifelong disabilities and their families, and national and local organizations recognized and implemented professional training initiatives on aging and developmental disabilities. A critical mass of expertise on aging with lifelong disabilities had arisen, both within the United States and internationally (cf. Breitenbach, 1990; Hogg, Moss, & Cooke, 1988; Maaskant & Haveman, 1989).

The primary topics of discussion at the Boston Roundtable reflected both the consistency and the evolution of the movement: family caregiving, social and community integration, physical and mental health changes associated with aging, and life-span development and trends. Participants noted that additional research needed not only to further consider these topics but also to be tempered by select methodological issues. For example, there was growing evidence that although it might make sense to think of older people with developmental disabilities as a group from a services perspective, from a research perspective, the assumption that aging affects all people with developmental disabilities similarly was problematic. They noted, furthermore, that there was a need to attend to the phenomenon of the aging process and that the family remained as the primary caregiving unit for this population, despite the great strides made by the public services sector during the preceding decade. These more mature directions for research, coupled with consumers' growing sophistication for older adult services and community involvement practices, led in the 1990s to research and practice agendas that were more equivalent to those of mainstream gerontology. Earlier activity in the aging with lifelong disabilities movement related to the scope and nature of the population, diversions of traditional clinical services, and everyday community supports, such as housing, work and transportation, and help for people in caregiving roles. These primary concerns remain today, but to these the 1990s added an extended band of concerns, an acknowledgment of aging as a distinct yet interwoven dimension of the life course, and research and practice regimens that are more mature and self-sustaining.

Developments in aging and lifelong disability grew exponentially worldwide during the 1990s. In the United States alone, these included the following: 1) Major steps were taken on the federal level to ally two major bureaucracies—the Administration on Aging and the Administration on Developmental Disabilities—for common goals related to the aging of people with disabilities (there is now an interagency agreement and shared responsibility for funding and overseeing demonstration projects), 2) national professional and advocacy organizations recognized aging as a distinct public policy issue (e.g., the national Arc promulgated an aging policy statement; the American Association on Mental Retardation developed a policy and legislative agenda on aging), 3) national organizations incorporated special-interest sections on aging and intellectual disabilities within their membership frameworks (e.g., the American Association on Mental Retardation now has a division on gerontology; the Gerontological Society of America has a formal interest section on developmental disabilities), and 4) national research organizations began to sustain research and program development in this area (e.g., the National Institute for Disability and Rehabilitation Research continues to fund a rehabilitation research and training center on aging with intellectual disabilities at the University of Illinois at Chicago; the Administration on Developmental Disabilities has supported a number of university affiliated programs [UAPs] whose focus is aging). Internationally, several universities and civic organizations have expanded their work on the aging of adults with lifelong disabilities. The two main international organizations—the International Association for the Scientific Study of Intellectual Disabilities (IASSID), a nongovernmental organization attached to the

World Health Organization (WHO), and Inclusion International—both have special concentration areas on aging and have taken leadership roles within their respective constituencies, the research and advocacy communities, respectively.

Concerns related to the aging of people with lifelong disabilities reached the level of international organizations by the close of the decade. In 1998, the WHO asked the IASSID to examine a range of health and social issues and to prepare a report on the health-related status of aging people with intellectual disabilities throughout the world. The goal of this effort was to identify key features of health and social policies and practices around the world that would improve the longevity and well-being of people with intellectual disabilities. In response, an international working group of the IASSID and Inclusion International developed a series of reports on health issues, including physical health, women's health, and biobehavioral issues, as well as on social and aging policy (Evenhuis et al., 2000; Hogg, Lucchino, Wang, Janicki, & Working Group, 2000; Thorpe, Davidson, Janicki, & Working Group, 2000; Walsh, Heller, Schupf, van Schrojenstein Lantman-de Valk, & Working Group, 2000). Their work transcended national boundaries and examined aging as a concern in both developed and developing countries.

The main product of the WHO and IASSID collaboration, *Aging and Intellectual Disabilities: Improving Longevity and Promoting Healthy Aging* (Janicki & Breitenbach, 2000), is a significant document for several reasons, not the least of which is its recurring themes of valuing all human life and promoting healthy aging for all of a nation's citizens. Its impact is likely to endure, and the document deserves some discussion here. Most fundamental, it emphasizes that over their life spans, adults with intellectual disabilities have the same basic needs as other members of a nation's population and that to promote healthy aging, nations must maintain policies that support quality of life and well-being throughout the course of life. Furthermore, the WHO/IASSID document recognizes aging as a process that has both a normal and a pathological course; so, to promote their healthy aging, adults with intellectual disabilities need to receive the same protective and ameliorative health services as those offered to the general population. Social services and health care providers throughout the world should include people with intellectual disabilities of all ages in their services, adopt a life-span approach to life care and supports, and understand that under select circumstances, because of the progression or consequences of specific diseases, there is need for therapeutic interventions. However, even within this framework, health services alone will not lead to healthy aging. A lifetime of social inclusion, of engagement with one's community, is central to promoting healthy aging. In this document, the practice of health promotion transcends the arena of basic clinical and programmatic needs and rises to the plane of total societal involvement and inclusion, indeed, to what Ansello (Chapter 1) terms *assisted autonomy* (see Table 1).

The WHO/IASSID document reinforces, conceptually and in specific recommendations, our own practices and beliefs. One need only broaden the focus that WHO/IASSID employed, namely, aging adults with intellectual disabilities, to read "aging adults with lifelong disabilities" to find concordance. To ensure further their general well-being, adults with intellectual disabilities and/or lifelong disabilities and their caregivers should receive appropriate and ongoing education and training on nutrition, exercise, oral hygiene, safety practices, and the avoidance of risky behaviors such as tobacco use and substance abuse. Because of the frequency of late-onset disabilities and the fact that their detection may require a high index of suspicion for clin-

Table 1.   Key recommendations from the World Health Organization summative document on healthy aging and intellectual disabilities

A life-span approach that recognizes the progression or consequences of specific diseases and therapeutic interventions should be adopted by health care providers around the world.

Adults with intellectual disabilities and their caregivers should receive appropriate and ongoing education regarding healthy living practices (e.g., nutrition, exercise, oral hygiene, safety practices, and the avoidance of risky behaviors such as tobacco use and substance abuse).

There should be sufficiently educated and trained medical and health personnel to provide appropriate preventive and treatment-oriented health and social services, and the special health care needs of women with intellectual disabilities should be addressed.

Preventative health strategies should include ways to promote mental health and minimize negative outcomes of mental health problems and to improve the quality of life of older people with intellectual disabilities.

Public policies should promote inclusive societies by recognizing the contributions of adults with intellectual disabilities, ensuring equitable access to generic services, and, when appropriate, providing specialized services and assistance.

Research efforts should be undertaken that include:

Studies of practices in developing nations that successfully promote longevity and healthy aging of people with intellectual disabilities, and practices that promote successful and productive aging of people with intellectual disabilities in developed and developing nations; and studies of the educational and training needs of those providing services to older people with intellectual disabilities to ensure a high quality of life.

Studies of morbidity and mortality of older people with intellectual disabilities in developing nations; and studies of the conditions under which the health and social needs of older people with intellectual disabilities can be met within generic and/or specialized services.

Evaluations of programs aimed at maintaining functional abilities, extending competence in later life, and enhancing quality of life; and studies of factors that increase inclusiveness in society with respect to both age and intergenerational unity.

Studies of a cross-cultural nature that identify common aspects of quality provision; and studies of significant cultural and economic factors that support family caring.

Adapted from Janicki and Breitenbach (2000).

ical diagnosis, nations need to ensure that there are sufficiently educated and trained health care practitioners to provide appropriate preventive and treatment-oriented health services.

The aging with lifelong disabilities movement has matured considerably. It promises to continue to develop. The WHO/IASSID document may represent a high-water mark in this ongoing evolution, for it not only incorporates accumulated wisdom on aging with a particular lifelong disability but also highlights underappreciated issues. These include matters related to women and to mental health: The deficiencies evident in services to women need to be remedied, and women's health across the life span needs to be promoted as part of a global strategy; compelling research priorities remain in reproductive and sexual health; women with disabilities must be directly involved as full partners in the formation of health strategies and interventions to be contributors to their own well-being as they age. The document's position on issues of mental health transcends the usual notions of associating psychopathology with mental health. Adults with intellectual and developmental disabilities can be challenged in the same manner as other adults when coping with the stresses of daily life. Promoting sound mental health involves improving the detection and assessment of life stressors and mental disorders, such as depression, anxiety, and dementia, in these aging adults. The WHO proposed that national preventive health strategies must include ways to promote mental health and minimize negative outcomes of mental health problems in older people with intellectual disabilities. This is true across the spectrum of lifelong disabilities. We expect that the WHO's contribution will be to heighten awareness of aging among people with intellectual disabilities and to stimulate promotion of social and health policies across nations that improve the longevity of people with intellectual disabilities. Like the earlier efforts in the United States in the late 1970s and the 1980s, the WHO's entering this movement will drive innovations and service design well into the early 21st century. It should serve as a model orientation for the range of lifelong developmental disabilities.

CONTINUING EVOLUTION OF AGING WITH LIFELONG DISABILITIES

The next 15–20 years should see a number of developments that will affect the provision of community supports for aging adults with lifelong disabilities. These developments include patterns of aging in the general population and characteristics of those with lifelong disabilities who are at middle age but who soon will be the "aging," those who will attain 50 or 60 years of age or more.

Aging in the General Population

The populations of the developed nations will be considerably older in the next decades as infant mortality declines, life expectancy increases, and the median age at death works inexorably upward. As we noted in Chapter 1, improvements directed toward the early years of life have produced longevity unwitnessed in history. On every continent, the more developed nations are projected to manifest this "graying." Even among nations that are currently developing, infant mortality rates are expected to fall significantly, producing relatively older general populations. The critical issue remains that the aging of the world is occurring largely without commensurate growth or development in the various social institutions needed to deal meaningfully with this aging. To different degrees among the nations, aging of the general population has so far produced little in the way of the enlightened health care, workplace, personal development, or public policy expertise needed to ensure that added years are beneficial years for both the individual and the nation. To be sure, achievements in public health have, at times, been spectacular. In the United States, the Centers for Disease Control and Prevention (1999) reported that deaths from diseases of the heart and from stroke, which together accounted for more than 40% of all deaths for most of the 20th century, declined 56% and 70%, respectively, between 1950 and 1996. The Centers for Disease Control and Prevention attribute the decline to prevention efforts and improvements in early detection that lowered risk factors (smoking, high blood pressure, cholesterol levels) for the overall adult population and to improved cardiovascular diagnoses and treatment. Notwithstanding such remarkable accomplishments, gerontological and geriatric developments have remained modest. Research on the processes of aging, not on specific disease states that may or may not be more prevalent among older adults, is still minimal in contrast. The numbers of programs that educate geriatric practitioners have remained small. Shortfalls exist in geriatric medicine, nursing, and social work, for example. Furthermore, employers have just begun to awaken to the shortsightedness of practices that encourage older workers to leave the workplace, taking expertise, loyalty, and productivity with them. Older adults themselves wrestle, at times, with the ambiguities of early retirement and lengthened life expectancy as they satisfy their socially sanctioned roles and leave for the unknown. Spasms of concern interspersed with years of neglect have characterized how governments tend to develop public policy related to older adults, as in their never-thorough analyses of pension schemes such as Social Security. As counterintuitive as it seems, aging of the general population is still being discovered and its myriad implications are yet to be addressed systematically.

It may be characteristic of social institutions such as those just mentioned to respond primarily to crises. Without a near-term calamity, it may be that they change exceedingly slowly. Certainly, the decreases in mortality and morbidity and the extension of life expectancy carry none of the urgency of crises such as economic depression or virulent epidemics. If this is so, what are the implications for aging with lifelong disabilities when this phenomenon is occurring amidst a demographic evolution that is colored, if at all, with positive and noncrisis tones? For instance, will the general population's improving health status add to or detract from a focus on older adults with lifelong disabilities? Will decreasing rates of morbidity and disabilities highlight the needs of these older adults by contrast, or will their needs become further marginalized as exceptions to overall population well-being? In short, is the aging of the general population good for older adults with lifelong disabilities?

Aging of Midlife Adults with Lifelong Disabilities

A greater percentage of those who will be older adults with lifelong disabilities 15–20 years from now will have experience in self-care and managing personal assistance than do today's older adults. Although the latter have often grown older invisibly in natural family contexts in their communities, those who are at midlife today have grown up the beneficiaries of increasingly enlightened public policies that have encouraged more education, more consumer control of services, and more engagement in the mainstream of life. There is often a gulf between the ideal and the practice, but, overall, adults with lifelong disabilities who are currently at midlife should reach 60 or more years of age healthier and more experienced with managing their own support than today's older adults are. They also will likely be far more numerous than today's older adults. A tripling by 2015 of the number of known older adults with lifelong disabilities is a reasonable estimate for the United States, with increases in the millions worldwide ("Year of 6 Billion," 1999). It is important to note, nonetheless, that during the next 15–20 years, the needs of newly "discovered" older adults—that is, older adults whose family caregivers have become incapacitated or have died—likely will capture more of the time and resources of both the aging and the developmental disabilities services systems. Those who will have grown old invisibly in the care of their families—that is, those whose prolonged family caregiving will have been made possible by the aging evolution—will appear like numerous blips on a previously blank radar screen. Unless managed judiciously, services at that time may be conflicted; demand for agency services for the formerly invisible older adults may contend with demand for continued personal assistance services for those who are currently at midlife and who will have grown older. As Coogle, Ansello, Wood, and Cotter (1995) found, developmental disabilities–related service agencies tend to demonstrate passive attitudes toward outreach to and identification of older consumers and toward the appropriation of human and material resources; they also found that those whose needs were made known to the agencies by others or by the consumers themselves received attention. During the next 15–20 years, advocates for the formerly invisible older adults and consumers who will have managed their own personal assistance as they grew old may find themselves contending with each other for services in a "squeaky wheel gets the oil" scenario.

POLICY IMPLICATIONS

There are a number of policy implications of the increasing numbers of older adults with disabilities, either lifelong or late onset, among the citizens of the world's nations. Clearly, the status quo should not be continued. It ranges from fragmented, uncoordinated services and reactive rather than proactive practices to isolated examples of intersystem cooperation and empowerment of individuals in managing their own lives. Although the rates of morbidity and disabilities are declining among developed nations, the absolute numbers of older adults with disabilities are increasing; each number is a human life that deserves better choices, services, and supports. The increasing numbers of older adults with lifelong disabilities have often been ignored by the aging and developmental disabilities service systems, as Coogle, Ansello, Wood, and Cotter (1997) found in a national survey of state units on aging and developmental disabilities. The growing numbers of these individuals should make acknowledgment of their presence, their abilities, and their needs inescapable. The form that the acknowledgment takes, moreover, can be shaped positively by emulation of the recommended practices so thoughtfully articulated by the contributors to this book and by public policy initiatives that help set the direction for this field. A public policy "wish list" might include more effectively trained staff, greater interagency cooperation, recognition of natural support environments, increases in geriatric specialists, innovative cross-system partnerships, and education and training curricula. Next, we expand on what we see in each of these areas.

Effectively Trained Staff

Having more aging adults with lifelong disabilities requires more mandates and associated funding for the cross-training of staff members in agencies that serve older adults and people with lifelong disabilities. Such cross-training would not only introduce aging-related personnel to the terminology, philosophies, funding streams, and practices of the lifelong disabilities world and vice versa but also would address the fragmentation that often exists within the lifelong disabilities field itself; therefore, those who work in intellectual disabilities would learn of the worlds of cerebral palsy, polio, autism, spinal cord injury, and other subsets of lifelong, developmental disabilities and, again, vice versa. Becoming conversant in another's sphere of operation is the key to resource sharing and other innovations to serve consumers more effectively.

Greater Interagency Cooperation

There need to be public policy initiatives to strengthen cooperation between the aging and lifelong disabilities fields. These might include directives for memoranda of agreement or memoranda of understanding between the highest levels in aging and in lifelong disabilities. Such memoranda have been shown to be a prerequisite for intersystem cooperation, which ultimately occurs in a more local arena. Sanctioning intersystem cooperation enables local agencies to develop area planning committees that make full use of the fragmented and sometimes overtaxed resources of the agencies that would constitute the local cooperative. Pointedly, combining numbers of small and even overtaxed resources tends to produce the critical mass for less taxed, more efficient resource allocation (Ansello, Coogle, & Wood, 1997).

Recognition of Natural Support Environments

There needs to be a progressive evolution of long-term health care policies toward the family or noninstitutional contexts. Nations differ in their use of institution-based care of individuals with lifelong disabilities. Even the individual states or provinces within nations often differ from one another in this matter. The so-called "deinstitutionalization" wave has affected some jurisdictions more than others. It seems that philosophies of self-determination, self-care, and person-centered planning, as well as the costly economics of institutional care, would argue for a shift in focus away from large, institutional, long-term care and toward aging in a manner preferred by the overwhelming majority of the general population, namely, aging among one's family and friends within neighborhoods and communities. Individuals who grow old with lifelong disabilities and those who acquire impairments upon growing old tend to receive most of their chronic care from their families, yet these family caregivers receive little, if any, recognition or training. Funding flows to institutional care and to licensed professionals who, in the aggregate, provide far fewer hours of long-term care than do families. At the same time, one recognizes that individuals with lifelong disabilities who are now at midlife often reach that point in the life span through the exercise of their own decision making and their own management of personal assistance services that enable them to live a more normal life. Continuing to recognize only institutions and professionals as the agents of the long-term care system will not fit with the histories of these midlife individuals as they grow older in the next 15–20 years.

The core apparatus of the long-term care systems (location, funding, and training) needs to shift to include the caregiving family of parents, spouses, siblings, and relatives and the person with lifelong or late-onset disabilities. They deserve more financial support in the form of tax credits, grants, stipends, and allowances, for they are the locus of ongoing care. Their cessation of or inability to continue this ongoing care could have disastrous consequences for the more formalized sector. They deserve training from established health care providers, because family caregivers and individuals with lifelong disabilities regularly face issues of medication management, nutrition, health care coordination, transportation, social engagement, mental health, assistive technology, and so forth without the preparation or training that their formal counterparts receive. It is likely that the illogic of this policy will become increasingly obvious as the decade progresses. Already, Virginia and several other states have begun to legislate some cash assistance to family caregivers, and members of the United States Congress introduce more bills to enlarge the purview and increase the funding of the Medicaid-financed home- and community-based care programs.

Increases in Geriatric Specialists

National legislation should encourage increases in the numbers of professionals who are trained in geriatrics, in disabilities, and in the combination of aging and disabilities. Although shortages of physicians and nurses who are trained in geriatrics are not universal among the developed nations, they are disturbing in the United States. The Alliance for Aging Research reported that approximately 6,800 physicians in internal medicine, family practice, and psychiatry have become "certified geriatricians . . . out of a total U.S. physician population of 684,414" (1996, p. 5). This shortage of practitioners who are trained in geriatrics is being maintained, in part, by managed care practices that limit the amount of time that practitioners may spend with patients. Older adults with disabilities often "present with" multiple complaints and, in effect, frustrate the time allotment process. Their ongoing conditions do not lend themselves to reversals by physicians' interventions. Moreover, the processes of human aging produce "individuation," or increased heterogeneity, within a group as its membership ages. This requires fine-tuning the health care interview to the one individual being seen, a practice that is inconsistent with medicine-by-the-numbers. The infusion of greater numbers of women into health care may benefit geriatric care in the next 15–20 years, for women may prove more efficient in listening to patients and communicating within limited time frames. Increasing the numbers of physicians, nurses, social workers, psychologists, physical therapists, and others who are trained in geriatrics and gerontology is itself a daunting challenge. It may be accomplished through fellowships and stipends to students in training and through changes in funding formulas to teaching hospitals and schools that graduate these practitioners. More challenging still is the need to redress the shortage of these professionals who are trained in their primary disciplines, plus gerontology or geriatrics, plus disabilities. The life experiences of the chair of a state-level advocacy council demonstrate the problem. A midlife attorney with cerebral palsy, the chair developed urological problems in his early 40s and sought medical help. Trying to find a triangulation of medical expertise in urology, aging, and cerebral palsy has proved frustrating for the past several years. Practitioners with training in cerebral palsy have been pediatricians; urologists with geriatrics training have no experience with the special conditions that cerebral palsy presents.

Innovative Cross-System Partnerships

There should be recognition of the differences and commonalities between lifelong and late-onset disabilities and actions to put into place partnerships among the fields of aging, lifelong disabilities, and late-onset disabilities. The aging, lifelong disabilities, and late-onset disabilities triangle represents a concept whose activation offers opportunities for meaningful collaborations between pairs—that is, between aging and lifelong disabilities, lifelong disabilities and late-onset disabilities, and late-onset disabilities and aging. Those who work in each of the currently separate fields have different histories and constituents, but they and their fields share with the other fields in the triangle notable similarities. These include perennial shortages of personnel, unending need for greater public awareness of their issues and correlated greater public support of their efforts, critical reliance on family caregivers for ongoing care, unsteady funding streams, threats of competition from other worthy causes when appropriations are reduced, and consumers who themselves have complex, concurrent disabling conditions, to name a few similarities.

Aging adults who acquire late-onset disabilities such as dementia personify opportunities for partnership between aging-related and Alzheimer's disease assistance agencies and advocacy groups, just as aging adults with lifelong disabilities who acquire late-onset disabilities such as stroke or heart disease personify opportunities for partnerships among all three sectors of aging, lifelong disabilities, and late-onset disabilities. The benefits to be derived from cooperation could be substantial for the individuals, the families, and the organizations.

At the same time, the aging and disabilities triangle as a concept can be made three-dimensional by adding risk factor prevention groups as another base (e.g., anti-violence, antismoking, anti–drunk driving). For instance, medical technology enables many of the usually young victims of criminal violence or drunk driving to survive the trauma. Many will live the rest of their lives with impairments until they eventually become aging adults with disabilities. It seems judicious to partner to prevent the trauma and to apply the existing resources to the needs of those who already have disabilities.

Education and Training Curricula

Too often, curricula developments proceed without a life-span orientation. No wish list would be complete without recognition that reaching old age is becoming so commonplace in the developed nations that educational curricula need to reflect this reality, from elementary education, to the special education of individuals with lifelong disabilities, to the preparation of professionals. In the first instance, grade school–age children need to be exposed to aging issues and to older adults, because they will inherit a world in which aging will drive much of the economic and political activity. Some educators advocate exposing children at the earliest ages to positive images of aging, before ageist attitudes might set in, maintaining that children need to see older heroes and "the elder within" (McGuire, 1999). The University of Texas's Health Science Center at San Antonio has developed for the middle grades an extensive curriculum that borrows content from gerontology and geriatrics to introduce aging-related subject matter without replacing existing curricula (Pruski, 1999). For example, in studying bone density over the life course, students in history class learn the historical and cultural significance of skeletons and bones; in English class, the origins of the names of bones; in natural science, the changes in bone or skeletal structure that are sequential; in mathematics, how to compute the density of selected bone specimens; and in science, the influence of genetic and environmental factors on bone health. Students learn age-related changes naturally and in different disciplinary contexts. With similar motivation, the Association for Gerontology in Higher Education, an international organization headquartered in Washington, D.C., has adopted the concept of aging education in kindergarten through secondary school. If students learn that aging is a normal part of the life span, they can plan for its occurrence and work to maintain their own well-being over the life course. This advantage affects children with lifelong disabilities as well.

The core of aging education is sympathetic to the heart of person-centered planning and the ethic of assisted autonomy. More of us are likely to be privileged to experience the gift of time. Aging and old age are normal parts of the life course and do not necessarily signify an end to our own exercise of choice and self-development.

THREE STAGES OF CONTEMPORARY SOCIETY

Reflections and appraisals sometimes stimulate deeper reflections and appraisals. We cannot help but observe the larger evolutions within which the aging and lifelong disabilities movement has occurred. In this section, we note that contemporary society seems to have evolved through three fairly well-defined stages and that the development of the aging with lifelong disabilities movement has correlated with this evolution. We consider that grand societal evolutions over the past 40 or more years have not only shaped orientations to old age but also influenced the progress of the aging with lifelong disabilities movement. The evolution of society since 1960 has been inextricably woven with its demography. This is not to say that demographics solely have dictated direction. Science and technology have reshaped everyday life fundamentally over this period. But demographics have signified stages of development, as it were, in society across the developed nations. These stages can be named according to the fundamental influence of the time period. First came the Stage of the Child. The early 1960s saw completion of the demographic aberration known as the post-war baby boom, a historical jump in birth rates after World War II. This boom reversed a trend toward older average populations that had typified the developed nations for a century. Unprecedented numbers of children focused the attention of nations on school construction, elementary and secondary education, and commerce related to the young, such as clothing, entertainment, and the media. The Stage of the Child also enabled the emergence of advocacy, service systems, and research related to children with disabilities, as sheer numbers of these children compelled action.

The Stage of the Adult followed as the boom's children reached maturity. This stage was stimulated by economics that were driven by huge numbers of adult workers and were sometimes affected by a surplus of such labor. Large supplies of young adult and middle-age workers fueled economies and influenced the direction of economies, both up and down. The plight of unfortunate older adults, many living below the poverty level in some nations, captured public attention as exceptions to the prevailing value and impelled action. The economic well-being and the larger numbers of non–older adult workers enabled bold action, as when President Nixon and the Congress in the United States so forcefully amended federal programs in 1974 to eliminate age-based disparities in poverty. For the next 20–25 years, the explosion in the numbers of Americans who were older than 60 years took place paradoxically in a society that was focused on things other than older adults. It seems that older adults received attention only as long as was necessary to resolve pension scheme–related crises. The economics of developed nations were wrenched by booms and busts during this time, but the inattention to issues related to later life was remarkable. The aging of individuals with lifelong disabilities and the acquisition of disabilities by individuals who had grown old received some attention. The recommended practices and initiatives reported in this book testify to this. Conversely, the relatively small numbers of such exemplars may be a reflection of a society that is still very much oriented to relatively younger adults.

Now we see the Stage of Diversity dawning across the developed nations. Nations are growing more complex internally; worldwide, they are experiencing great influxes of immigrants who increase the mix of their populations. At the same time, the absolute numbers of older citizens are beginning to compel public attention. By 2016, 18% or more of the populations of France, Germany, Italy, Japan, and the United Kingdom will be 65 years of age or older (Peterson, 1999). The AARP (1999), using U.S. Bureau of the Census data, projects that by 2025, whole continents will have aged: 55% of Europe's population will be older than 60, 15% of Africa's, 20% of Asia's, 14% of Latin America's, 25% of North America's, and 43% of the former Soviet Union's. Aging individuals bring individuation. With large numbers of citizens who grow less like their age-mates every year, one-size-fits-all policies and practices simply will fail. If ever there were a rationale for person-centered planning, it will be evident when increasing numbers of older adults with disabilities grow more heterogeneous. The Stage of Diversity may introduce greater recognition of "consumers" as individuals. It may foster more careful coordination of services and the husbanding of resources, because more older adults with disabilities will be using services and their abilities and needs will be more diverse.

As the Stage of Diversity progresses over the next 15–20 years, it may also stimulate creation of yet another life stage for the human life course. Just as the life stage of adolescence was created by realities of the late 19th century that dictated more educational preparation for work and postponement of entry into the labor force, and just as the life stage of young adulthood emerged in the past 30 years during the Stage of the Adult for the same reasons, so, too, may the existence of greater diversity within nations' older populations prompt creation of new or redefinition of existing life stages. As later life grows to encompass 2 or 3 decades or more of the life span, recognition will grow inevitably that such terms as "young old" and "old old" are virtually meaningless.

In a more broad sense, the human life span may come to be conceptualized as having four "ages" rather than the current three favored in popular culture. Added to stages of childhood, work, and retirement may come a fourth stage that is synonymous with disabilities. As mortality rates remain flat and the demographic curve of survival becomes rectangular, the abrupt slope toward finality may come to be associated with disabilities and disabilities with the end of the life course. A problem with this concept is that it still ties disability to chronological age; entitlements for services and resources are often tied to chronological age. Far better for an ethic to emerge that dismisses aging as a criterion for services and introduces need as the justification. This may, after all, prove to be the greatest challenge that those who work at the intersection of aging and lifelong disabilities will face in the next 15–20 years; that is, as populations grow older and as public policy ties services to mere attainment of chronological age through entitlements, coming older adults may demand continuation of extant services whether they need them or not. An aging lobby that is self-serving rather than one that advocates for those with greatest needs within its numbers could hamper the maturation of the aging and disabilities field. Partnerships between aging and disabilities networks offer the greatest promise for resources being used by members of the community in greatest need of the assistance.

THIRD AGE OF THE AGING WITH LIFELONG DISABILITIES MOVEMENT

Finally, reflection suggests that the aging with lifelong disabilities movement itself has progressed through stages or periods that roughly correlate with the evolution of contemporary society since 1960 that was just reviewed. In the beginning, there was indifference to aging with lifelong disabilities. This was certainly consistent with the prevailing values during the societal Stage of the Child. The fields of aging and lifelong disabilities operated as parallel, nonintersecting systems. The disabilities system focused its attention and resources on children in the belief that early intervention would improve the course of life, however long that might be. Aging was not its concern, nor was disability the aging network's concern. From the perspective of the aging with lifelong disabilities movement, this was the "prehistoric period." Drawn by the aging of its consumers on the one hand and the late-onset impairments of some of its older adults on the other, a few in the two systems began to explore intersections between the systems. Questions arose in the lifelong disabilities network about the onset and meaning of aging, the possibility of retiring from sheltered work, the value of active treatment requirements, and, in both systems, use of the complementary network and the development of specialized services. The movement progressed through this "period of exploration," with its demonstrations and exploratory studies. It seems now to be entering a "period of crystallization." Systemically, the networks have tested strategies and models for intersystem collaboration to benefit aging adults with lifelong disabilities, family caregivers, and agency staff who provide services. Combined efforts, if not combined bureaucracies, are beginning to be undertaken to determine what can be accomplished together for and with people, rather than for "older adults" or for "people with disabilities." This period is also introducing transition points in the life course as critical areas for study and facilitation. This shift may represent a maturing of the movement. For example, during the transition from middle age to older age, the individual needs stable supports to prepare for older age, to ensure health care and promotion of wellness, to maintain housing and work, and to assist aging family caregivers to plan for the continuation of care beyond their own capabilities. How might these be developed, evaluated, and implemented practically to benefit the individual? Another critical transition is retirement. Embedded in this transition are its meaning for the aging adult, families, and caregivers, its impact on regulatory and licensing structures, its modification by preparation (learning or adapting to be a retiree), what it triggers regarding the equitable use of resources within general services and the aging network, and a general lifestyle refocus and consideration of its impact on families and agencies (e.g., budgets, staffing, program). These embedded values need to be determined for the individual and incorporated into an overall plan. Furthermore, the transition to older age may precipitate changes for older adults, families, and caregivers regarding health considerations, pathological aging, access to support services, housing issues, aging in place, and end-of-life issues. Transitions and their impacts must be considered in appraising the lives of aging adults with lifelong disabilities. Ultimately, the next steps of the movement relate to normalizing later life for people with lifelong disabilities. This means ensuring equitable access to health and social supports and enjoying the gift of time with respect, dignity, and autonomy.

We honor the work of colleagues who have advanced our understanding of growing older with lifelong disabilities. Their insights, experiments, pilot programs, and refinements of practices have contributed to a fuller appreciation of the supports required to sustain meaningful aging for adults with lifelong disabilities. We look forward to the further maturing of this movement, and in closing, we offer this thought on timing from Alvarez, a force behind global activities on aging within the United Nations: "If we are not to fall by the wayside, 2020 must be the measure of our foresight, not the year in which we will finally wake up" (1999, p. 3).

REFERENCES

Alliance for Aging Research. (1996). *Will you still treat me when I'm 65?* Washington, DC: Author.

Alvarez, J.T. (1999). *Reflections on an agequake* [Selected quotations from the speeches of Julia Tavares Alvarez, Alternate Permanent Representative of the Dominican Republic Mission to the United Nations]. New York: United Nations Nongovernmental Organization Committee on Aging.

American Association of Retired Persons (AARP). (1999). *Global aging report: Aging everywhere.* Washington, DC: Author.

Ansello, E.F., Coogle, C.L., & Wood, J.B. (1997). *Partners: Building inter-system cooperation in aging with developmental disabilities.* Richmond: Virginia Commonwealth University, Virginia Center on Aging.

Ansello, E.F., & Rose, R. (1989). *Aging and lifelong disabilities: Partnership for the twenty-first century.* Palm Springs, CA: Elder Press (Elvirita Lewis Foundation).

Breitenbach, N. (1990, July). Comments to panel on ageing and mental handicap at the Congress of International League of Societies for the Mentally Handicapped, Paris.

Centers for Disease Control and Prevention (CDC). (1999, August 6). Achievements in public health, 1900–1999: Decline in deaths from heart disease and stroke—United States, 1900–1999. *Morbidity and Mortality Weekly Report, 48*(30), 649–656.

Coogle, C.L., Ansello, E.F., Wood, J.B., & Cotter, J.J. (1997, April). *"Hot button" issues for 1997: State agencies tell us their concerns.* Paper presented at the 18th Annual Meeting of the Southern Gerontological Society, Norfolk, VA.

Cotten, P.D. (1987). *The Mississippi program for elderly developmentally disabled persons.* Sanatorium, MS: Boswell Retardation Center.

Developmental Disabilities Bill of Rights Act of 1987, PL 100-146, 42 U.S.C. §§ 6000 *et seq.*

Dybwad, G. (1962). Administrative and legislative problems in the care of the adult and aged mental retardate. *American Journal of Mental Deficiency, 66,* 716–722.

Dybwad, G. (1999). Foreword. In S.S. Herr & G. Weber (Eds.), *Aging, rights, and quality of life: Prospects for older people with developmental disabilities* (pp. xv–xvii). Baltimore: Paul H. Brookes Publishing Co.

Evenhuis, H., Henderson, C.M., Beange, H., Lennox, N., Chicoine, B., & Working Group. (2000). *Healthy aging—Adults with intellectual disabilities: Physical health issues.* Geneva: World Health Organization.

Hawkins, B.A., Eklund, S.J., Garza, J.N., Garza, T., & DiOrio, R. (1987). *Aging/aged persons with developmental disabilities in Indiana: An interagency planning task force report.* Bloomington: Indiana University, Institute for the Study of Developmental Disabilities.

Herr, S.S., & Weber, G. (Eds.). (1999). *Aging, rights and quality of life: Prospects for older people with developmental disabilities.* Baltimore: Paul H. Brookes Publishing Co.

Hogg, J., Lucchino, R., Wang, K., Janicki, M.P., & Working Group. (2000). *Healthy aging—Adults with intellectual disabilities: Aging and social policy.* Geneva: World Health Organization.

Hogg, J., Moss, S., & Cooke, D. (1988). *Ageing and mental handicap.* London: Croom-Helm.

Janicki, M.P. (1993). *Building the future: Planning and community development in aging and developmental disabilities.* Albany: New York State Office of Mental Retardation and Developmental Disabilities.

Janicki, M.P., & Breitenbach, N. (2000). *Aging and intellectual disabilities: Improving longevity and promoting healthy aging.* Geneva: World Health Organization.

Janicki, M.P., & Seltzer, M.M. (Eds.). (1991). *Aging and developmental disabilities—Challenges for the 1990s: Proceedings of the Boston Roundtable on Research Issues and Applications in Aging and Developmental Disabilities.* Washington, DC: American Association on Mental Retardation.

Maaskant, M., & Haveman, M. (1989). Aging residents in sheltered homes for persons with mental handicaps in the Netherlands. *Australia & New Zealand Journal of Developmental Disabilities, 15,* 219–230.

McGuire, S.L. (1999, November). *Aging education for elementary school children.* Paper presented at the 52nd Annual Scientific Meeting of the Gerontological Society of America, San Francisco.

Older Americans Act Amendments of 1987, PL 100-175, 42 U.S.C. §§ 3001 *et seq.*

Older Americans Act of 1965, PL 89-73, 42 U.S.C. §§ 3001 *et seq.*

Peterson, P.G. (1999). Gray dawn: The global aging crisis. *Foreign Affairs, 78*(1), 42–55.

Pruski, L. (1999, November). *Creating teaching materials for middle school students.* Paper presented at the 52nd Annual Scientific Meeting of the Gerontological Society of America, San Francisco.

Puccio, P.S., Janicki, M.P., Otis, J.P., & Rettig, J. (1983). *Report of the committee on aging and developmental disabilities.* Albany: New York State Office of Mental Retardation and Development Disabilities.

Rose, T., & Ansello, E.F. (1987). *Aging and developmental disabilities: Research and planning. Final report to the Maryland State Planning Council on Developmental Disabilities.* College Park: University of Maryland, Center on Aging.

Schalock, R.L. (1987). Program issues for elderly developmental disabled persons. In S.F. Gilson, T.L. Goldsbury, & E.H. Faulkner (Eds.), *Three populations of primary focus: Persons with mental retardation who are elderly* (pp. 85–94). Omaha: University of Nebraska Medical Center.

Segal, R.M. (Ed.). (1978). *Developmental disabilities and gerontology: Proceedings of a conference.* Ann Arbor: University of Michigan, Institute for the Study of Mental Retardation and Related Disabilities.

Seltzer, M.M., & Janicki, M.P. (1991). Commentary and recommendations. In M.P. Janicki & M.M. Seltzer (Eds.), *Aging and developmental disabilities—Challenges for the 1990s: Proceedings of the Boston Roundtable on Research Issues and Applications in Aging and Developmental Disabilities* (pp. 101–104). Washington, DC: American Association on Mental Retardation.

Sweeney, D.P. (1979). Denied, ignored, or forgotten? An assessment of community services for older/aged developmentally disabled persons within HEW Region V. In D.P. Sweeney & T.Y. Wilson (Eds.), *Double jeopardy: The plight of aging and aged developmentally disabled persons in mid-America* (pp. 54–88). Ann Arbor: University of Michigan, Institute for the Study of Mental Retardation and Related Disabilities.

Sweeney, D.P., & Wilson, T.Y. (Eds.). (1979). *Double jeopardy: The plight of aging and aged developmentally disabled persons in mid-America.* Ann Arbor: University of Michigan. Institute for the Study of Mental Retardation and Related Disabilities.

Tarjan, G. (1959). Prevention, a program goal in mental deficiency. *American Journal of Mental Deficiency, 64,* 4–11.

Thorpe, L., Davidson, P., Janicki, M.P., & Working Group. (2000). *Healthy aging—Adults with intellectual disabilities: Biobehavioral issues.* Geneva: World Health Organization.

Walsh, P.N., Heller, T., Schupf, N., van Schrojenstein Lantman-de Valk, H., & Working Group. (2000). *Healthy aging—Adults with intellectual disabilities: Women's health issues.* Geneva: World Health Organization.

Year of 6 billion people, living dangerously. (1999, October 7). *The New York Times,* p. D3.

Author Index

Page number followed by "t" and "f" indicate tables and figures, respectively.

Subject Index

Page numbers followed by "t" and "f" indicate tables and figures, respectively.